S0-BFD-024

Genome Plasticity and Infectious Diseases

Genome Plasticity and Infectious Diseases

EDITED BY

Jörg Hacker
German National Academy of Sciences Leopoldina
Halle (Saale), Germany

Ulrich Dobrindt
University of Münster
Münster, Germany

Reinhard Kurth
President Emeritus
Robert Koch Institute
Berlin, Germany

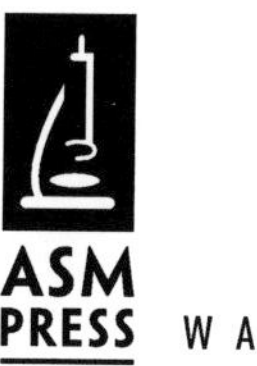

ASM PRESS WASHINGTON, DC

Library of Congress Cataloging-in-Publication Data

Genome plasticity and infectious diseases / edited by Jorg Hacker, Ulrich Dobrindt, and Reinhard Kurth.
p. cm.
Includes bibliographical references and index.
ISBN 978-1-55581-708-4 (hardcover)
1. Communicable diseases—Genetic aspects. 2. Microbial genomes. 3. Pathogenic microorganisms—Genetics. I. Hacker, Jörg (Jörg Hinrich). II. Dobrindt, Ulrich. III. Kurth, Reinhard, 1942–
RC112.G395 2011
362.196′9—dc23
2011032862

eISBN 978-1-55581-721-3

10 9 8 7 6 5 4 3 2 1

Printed in the United States of America

Address editorial correspondence to ASM Press, 1752 N St. NW, Washington, DC 20036-2904, USA
E-mail: books@asmusa.org

Send orders to ASM Press, P.O. Box 605, Herndon, VA 20172, USA
Phone: (800) 546-2416 or (703) 661-1593
Fax: (703) 661-1501
Online: estore.asm.org

Cover photo: Electron micrograph of an *Aspergillus fumigatus* conidiophore. The conidiophore shows the typical columnar, uniseriate conidial head. Phialides are the conidiogenous cells which produce long chains of conidia in basipetal succession. See chapter 19. Photo kindly provided by Jeannette Schmaler-Ripcke (HKI Jena and the Center for Electron Microscopy, Friedrich Schiller University, Jena, Germany).

CONTENTS

CONTRIBUTORS

Niyaz Ahmed
Pathogen Biology Laboratory, School of Life Sciences, University of Hyderabad, and Institute of Life Sciences, University of Hyderabad Campus, Hyderabad, India

J. David Barry
Wellcome Trust Centre for Molecular Parasitology, Institute of Infection, Immunity and Inflammation, University of Glasgow, Glasgow G12 8TA, United Kingdom

Hans-Ulrich Bernard
Department of Molecular Biology and Biochemistry and Program of Public Health, University of California Irvine, Irvine, CA 92697

Martina Bielaszewska
Institute of Hygiene, University of Münster, Robert-Koch-Str. 41, D-48149 Münster, Germany

Axel Brakhage
Department of Molecular and Applied Microbiology, Leibniz Institute for Natural Product Research and Infection Biology—Hans Knöll Institute, and Department of Microbiology and Molecular Biology, Friedrich Schiller University Jena, Beutenbergstraße 11a, D-07745 Jena, Germany

C. Buchrieser
Institut Pasteur, Unité de Biologie des Bactéries Intracellulaires and CNRS URA 2171, 28, rue du Dr. Roux, 75724 Paris Cedex 15, France

Michelle M. Buckner
Michael Smith Laboratories and Department of Microbiology and Immunology, The University of British Columbia, Vancouver, British Columbia, Canada

Ulrich Desselberger
Department of Medicine, University of Cambridge and Addenbrooke's Hospital, Cambridge, United Kingdom

Singamaneni Haritha Devi
Pathogen Biology Laboratory, School of Life Sciences, University of Hyderabad, Hyderabad, India

Ulrich Dobrindt
Institute for Molecular Biology of Infectious Diseases, Julius Maximilians University Würzburg, Josef-Schneider-Str. 2/Bau D15, D-97080 Würzburg, and Institute for Hygiene, University of Münster, Robert-Koch-Str. 41, D-48149 Münster, Germany

Hermann Einsele
Medizinische Klinik and Poliklinik II, Josef-Schneider-Str. 2, D-97070 Würzburg, Germany

Rosana B. Ferreira
Michael Smith Laboratories, The University of British Columbia, Vancouver, British Columbia, Canada

B. Brett Finlay
Michael Smith Laboratories and Department of Microbiology and Immunology, The University of British Columbia, Vancouver, British Columbia, Canada

Matthias Frosch
Institute for Hygiene and Microbiology, University of Würzburg, D-97080 Würzburg, Germany

Michael S. Gilmore
Schepens Eye Research Institute, 20 Staniford St., Boston, MA 02144

L. Gomez Valero
Institut Pasteur, Unité de Biologie des Bactéries Intracellulaires and CNRS URA 2171, 28, rue du Dr. Roux, 75724 Paris Cedex 15, France

Jörg Hacker
Institute for Molecular Biology of Infectious Diseases, Julius Maximilians University Würzburg, Josef-Schneider-Str. 2/Bau D15, D-97080 Würzburg, and German Academy of Sciences Leopoldina, Emil-Abderhalden-Str. 37, D-06108 Halle/Saale, Germany

Seyed E. Hasnain
Institute of Life Sciences, University of Hyderabad Campus, Hyderabad, and School of Biological Sciences, Indian Institute of Technology Delhi, New Delhi, India

Thorsten Heinekamp
Department of Molecular and Applied Microbiology, Leibniz Institute for Natural Product Research and Infection Biology—Hans Knöll Institute, and Department of Microbiology and Molecular Biology, Friedrich Schiller University Jena, Beutenbergstraße 11a, D-07745 Jena, Germany

Hartmut Hengel
Institute for Virology, Heinrich Heine University, Düsseldorf, Germany

Biju Joseph
Institute for Hygiene and Microbiology, University of Würzburg, D-97080 Würzburg, Germany

Deirdre A. Joy
Parasitology and International Programs Branch, National Institute of Allergy and Infectious Diseases, National Institutes of Health, Bethesda, MD 20892

Helge Karch
Institute of Hygiene, University of Münster, Robert-Koch-Str. 41, D-48149 Münster, Germany

Reinhard Kurth
Chairman of the Foundation Council, Ernst Schering Foundation, and President Emeritus, Robert Koch Institute, Berlin, Germany

Vu Thuy Khanh Le
Institute for Virology, Heinrich Heine University, Düsseldorf, Germany

Juergen Loeffler
Medizinische Klinik and Poliklinik II, Josef-Schneider-Str. 2, D-97070 Würzburg, Germany

Mohammad Majid
Pathogen Biology Laboratory, School of Life Sciences, University of Hyderabad, Hyderabad, India

Jelle Matthijnssens
Laboratory of Clinical and Epidemiological Virology, Department of Microbiology and Immunology, Rega Institute for Medical Research, University of Leuven, Leuven, Belgium

Alexander Mellmann
Institute of Hygiene, University of Münster, Robert-Koch-Str. 41, D-48149 Münster, Germany

Markus Mezger
Kinderklinik, Hoppe-Seyler-Str. 1, D-72026 Tübingen, Germany

Stephen Norley
Robert Koch Institute, Berlin, Germany

Peter Palese
Department of Microbiology, Mount Sinai School of Medicine, 1 Gustave Levy Pl., New York, NY 10029-6574

Kelli L. Palmer
Schepens Eye Research Institute, 20 Staniford St., Boston, MA 02144

Claude Pujol
Department of Biology, The University of Iowa, Iowa City, IA 52242

Bryndís Ragnarsdóttir
Department of Microbiology, Immunology and Glycobiology, Institute of Laboratory Medicine, Lund University, Sölvegatan 23, S-223 62 Lund, Sweden

Syed Asad Rahman
EMBL-European Bioinformatics Institute, Wellcome Trust Genome Campus, Hinxton, Cambridge, United Kingdom

Michael Roggendorf
Institute of Virology, University of Duisburg-Essen, Virchowstrasse 179, D-45147 Essen, Germany

C. Rusniok
Institut Pasteur, Unité de Biologie des Bactéries Intracellulaires and CNRS URA 2171, 28, rue du Dr. Roux, 75724 Paris Cedex 15, France

Christoph Schoen
Institute for Hygiene and Microbiology, University of Würzburg, D-97080 Würzburg, Germany

Eckart Schreier
Department of Infectious Diseases, Robert Koch Institute, Nordufer 20, D-13353 Berlin, Germany

Roland Schwarz
Cancer Research UK, Cambridge Research Institute, Li Ka Shing Centre, Cambridge, CB2 0RE, United Kingdom

David R. Soll
Department of Biology, The University of Iowa, Iowa City, IA 52242

Silke Stertz
Department of Microbiology, Mount Sinai School of Medicine, 1 Gustave Levy Pl., New York, NY 10029-6574

Xin-zhuan Su
Laboratory of Malaria and Vector Research, National Institute of Allergy and Infectious Diseases, National Institutes of Health, Bethesda, MD 20892

Catharina Svanborg
Department of Microbiology, Immunology and Glycobiology, Institute of Laboratory Medicine, Lund University, Sölvegatan 23, S-223 62 Lund, Sweden, and Singapore Immunology Network (SIgN), Biomedical Sciences Institutes, Agency for Science, Technology, and Research (A*STAR), 8A Biomedical Grove, Immunos, Biopolis, Singapore 138648

Shivendra Tenguria
Pathogen Biology Laboratory, School of Life Sciences, University of Hyderabad, Hyderabad, India

Joerg Timm
Institute of Virology, University of Duisburg-Essen, Virchowstrasse 179, D-45147 Essen, Germany

Mirko Trilling
Institute for Virology, Heinrich Heine University, Düsseldorf, Germany

Jaroslaw Zdziarski
Institute for Molecular Biology of Infectious Diseases, Julius-Maximilians-University Würzburg, Josef-Schneider-Str. 2/Bau D15, D-97080 Würzburg, Germany

Wilma Ziebuhr
Institut für Molekulare Infektionsbiologie, Universität Würzburg, Josef-Schneider Str. 2, D-97080 Würzburg, Germany

PREFACE

Genetic information determines the characteristics of all living organisms. On the basis of the key principles of Darwinian evolution, differences in genetic composition result in biodiversity. Genetic variation in microorganisms exists at the level of individual genes as well as at the level of genome size and organization. The acquisition or loss of genetic information via recombination or point mutations has been shown to contribute to genetic variation. These processes represent well-known mechanisms for diversification of microorganisms, including microbial pathogens, and the shaping of their genomes. However, genetic variation may affect not only the general genome content or the intrinsic properties of gene products, but also gene expression patterns. Therefore, genome plasticity can contribute to microbial adaptation in response to changing environmental conditions.

Several mechanisms of infectious disease and microbial adaptation have come to be understood through a variety of physiological, biochemical, and genomic studies, and this research has led to the development of vaccines, anti-infectives, and a range of biological control methods. Modern molecular genetic techniques have facilitated the study of genetic variation. The amount of genomic information about microbes as well as their hosts is constantly increasing. Access to complete genome sequences of multiple isolates of a genus or species and comparative genomics enable us to analyze the impact of genetic variation on (macro)evolution and diversification of pathogenic microorganisms. Furthermore, genetic variation as a means of microbial adaptation can be assessed. Valid genetic markers associated with important microbial (virulence) traits or with host susceptibility to different infections can also be identified and used for improved diagnostics and risk assessment. The analysis of microevolutionary processes due to genome plasticity will reveal additional modes of pathogen-host interactions. Although genomic differences between pathogenic and nonpathogenic variants have been described, the processes responsible for the constantly ongoing genome plasticity involved in adaptation or pathogenicity at the molecular level are still insufficiently understood, especially those that occur in vivo.

The impact of genome plasticity on the adaptation of microbial pathogens has been studied with several model organisms. The ability of many pathogens to acquire genetic information from related organisms and, due to close interactions, sometimes even from their hosts has meanwhile been well documented, as has the occurrence of mutations and genomic recombination events. Recombination events play an important role in diversification and adaptation of bacteria, viruses, and eukaryotic pathogens, as they may lead to genomic reassortments and gene rearrangements. Furthermore, genome instability of pathogenic microbes might influence clinical outcomes and has an impact on diagnosis, epidemiology, and evolution. It has become clear that the host response promotes genome plasticity in microbial pathogens and thus represents a driving force for the above-mentioned mechanisms by which pathogens can evade the immune system.

Our knowledge of determinants of host susceptibility to infections and genetic variation that influences host defenses is still limited. Only in recent years, defined clinical risk factors which increase the possibility of infection, as well as single-nucleotide polymorphisms (SNPs) in various genes relevant to immunity, have been shown to genetically determine susceptibility to microbial infection.

In conclusion, the genome plasticity of microbial pathogens represents a significant hurdle for the development of both effective vaccines and novel therapeutic interventions. In addition, there is a great clinical need to identify genetic variants on the host side that improve resistance or increase the susceptibility to infectious pathogens. This book provides an overview of and introduction to the field of genome plasticity of microbial pathogens and genetic variation of the host and its relevance for infection.

JÖRG HACKER
ULRICH DOBRINDT
REINHARD KURTH

BACTERIAL INFECTIONS

I

IMPACT OF GENOME PLASTICITY ON ADAPTATION OF *Escherichia coli* DURING URINARY BLADDER COLONIZATION

Ulrich Dobrindt, Jaroslaw Zdziarski, and Jörg Hacker

1

Bacteria can rapidly adapt to changing environmental conditions. Adaptation can result from active regulation of gene expression on the transcriptional and (post)translational levels in response to diverse internal and environmental stimuli. In addition, the bacterial genome is a flexible entity and responsive to environmental changes. The bacterial genome usually consists of a conserved core gene pool which codes for essential cellular functions, and genetic regions which are required only under certain environmental conditions, the so-called flexible gene pool. The latter represents variable genomic regions and often encompasses mobile genetic elements such as genomic islands, transposons, integrons, plasmids, or phages (Ahmed et al., 2008; Dobrindt et al., 2004; Hacker et al., 2003). These mobile elements can be laterally transferred. Consequently, horizontal gene transfer is one of the driving forces of bacterial evolution (Ochman et al., 2000). Environmental stimuli can induce alterations in the flexible gene pool, e.g., the excision and mobilization of genomic islands or integrative and conjugative elements, entry of the lytic cycle of prophages inserted into the bacterial chromosome, or transfer of plasmids (Frost and Koraimann, 2010; Juhas et al., 2009; Wozniak and Waldor, 2010). In addition, DNA rearrangements, smaller deletions and point mutations can occur which may also affect the expression or functionality of genes. Bacterial genomes also evolve during the course of infection in humans. During infection, a variety of stress conditions and strong selective pressures are exerted on the pathogen. In particular, genomic regions involved in host-pathogen interaction seem to exhibit increased mutation rates (Plotkin and Dushoff, 2003). Furthermore, mutation rates appear to be higher in pathogens in vivo than in vitro (Björkman et al., 2000), suggesting that the interaction of pathogen and host facilitates the generation of variation. Genome plasticity thus leads to the generation and selection of fitter mutants via the key processes of Darwinian evolution (Shapiro et al., 2009). The generation

Ulrich Dobrindt, Institute for Molecular Biology of Infectious Diseases, Julius Maximilians University Würzburg, Josef-Schneider-Str. 2/Bau D15, D-97080 Würzburg, and Institute for Hygiene, University of Münster, Robert-Koch-Str. 41, D-48149 Münster, Germany. *Jaroslaw Zdziarski*, Institute for Molecular Biology of Infectious Diseases, Julius Maximilians University Würzburg, Josef-Schneider-Str. 2/Bau D15, D-97080 Würzburg, Germany. *Jörg Hacker*, Institute for Molecular Biology of Infectious Diseases, Julius Maximilians University Würzburg, Josef-Schneider-Str. 2/Bau D15, D-97080 Würzburg, and German Academy of Sciences Leopoldina, Emil-Abderhalden-Str. 37, D-06108 Halle/Saale, Germany.

Genome Plasticity and Infectious Diseases,
Edited by J. Hacker, U. Dobrindt, and R. Kurth,

of genetic variability together with phenotypic expression of new variants and selection result in microevolution and the ongoing adaptation and modification of bacteria. The resulting genetic changes that occur in extraintestinal as well as in intestinal pathogens might influence clinical outcome and have an impact on diagnosis and epidemiology.

REDUCTIVE EVOLUTION OF *E. COLI:* ASYMPTOMATIC BACTERIURIA AS AN EXAMPLE OF BACTERIAL ADAPTATION TO PROLONGED IN VIVO GROWTH IN THE URINARY TRACT

Urinary tract infections (UTIs) are considered to be the most common bacterial infection in industrialized countries. Seventy to ninety percent of acute community-acquired, uncomplicated infections are caused by *E. coli* (Foxman, 2002). Urinary tract colonization and significant numbers of bacteria in the urine, however, may not always be associated with symptoms: asymptomatic bacteriuria (ABU) is characterized by long-term carriage of bacteria in the bladder with often more than 10^5 bacteria/ml of urine without symptoms, and ABU is estimated to be the most common form of bladder colonization (Lindberg et al., 1978). *E. coli* is the most common organism isolated from patients with ABU (Colgan et al., 2006).

For many years, uropathogenic *E. coli* (UPEC) isolates have been used to characterize virulence traits of bacteria causing symptomatic urinary tract infections (Brzuszkiewicz et al., 2006; Chen et al., 2006; Lloyd et al., 2009; Welch et al., 2002; Wiles et al., 2008). Expression of virulence factors in UPEC is spatially and temporally regulated. Among the first virulence factors required during host-pathogen interaction and the establishment of an UTI are cell surface-associated proteins which function as adhesins or invasins, promote biofilm formation, and are involved in signaling between the microorganisms and epithelial cells. Flagella not only allow ascension from the urethra to the bladder and even further to the kidneys, but can also function as adhesins and invasins. In later stages of an infection, toxins may further support infection by destruction of epithelial cells, the release of nutrients, protection against the host response, and signaling between the pathogens and the host. Capsules, O antigens, and other extracellular polysaccharides protect UPEC against the host immune system. Additional biochemical and metabolic traits are associated with improved fitness, growth, and survival of UPEC in the urinary tract (Fig. 1) (Nielubowicz and Mobley, 2010; Wiles et al., 2008). The ability of UPEC to trigger mucosal and systemic host responses determines the clinical outcome of the infection and correlates with urovirulence (Bergsten et al., 2004; Svanborg et al., 2001). Host response to the important UPEC type 1 adhesins and P fimbriae is mediated via the Toll-like receptor 4 (TLR4)-dependent pathway, but different adaptor proteins are involved in the downstream signaling (Svanborg et al., 2006). As a result, neutrophils are attracted to the bladder (Godaly et al., 1997; Hang et al., 1999), where they internalize and kill UPEC by phagosome formation and secretion of reactive oxygen species and hydrolytic enzymes.

The molecular characterization of *E. coli* ABU isolates was started relatively recently and has demonstrated that many *E. coli* ABU isolates resemble UPEC that cause symptomatic infection, but with reduced virulence traits (Edén et al., 1979; Mabbett et al., 2009; Raz, 2003; Zdziarski et al., 2008). ABU model isolate 83972 is phylogenetically closely related to several archetypal UPEC isolates from patients with symptomatic UTI but does not express classical UPEC virulence factors. Nevertheless, genomic analysis detected a large number of UPEC virulence-associated genes (Dobrindt et al., 2003). Recent analyses of selected pathogenicity factors of strain 83972 suggested that the loss of functional UPEC virulence factors was due to deletions or multiple point mutations (Klemm et al., 2006; Roos et al., 2006a, b) indicative of genome reduction as an adaptation to prolonged colonization of the bladder (Fig. 1) (Zdziarski et al., 2008).

Reductive evolution and gene loss are well-known observations made in (uro)patho-

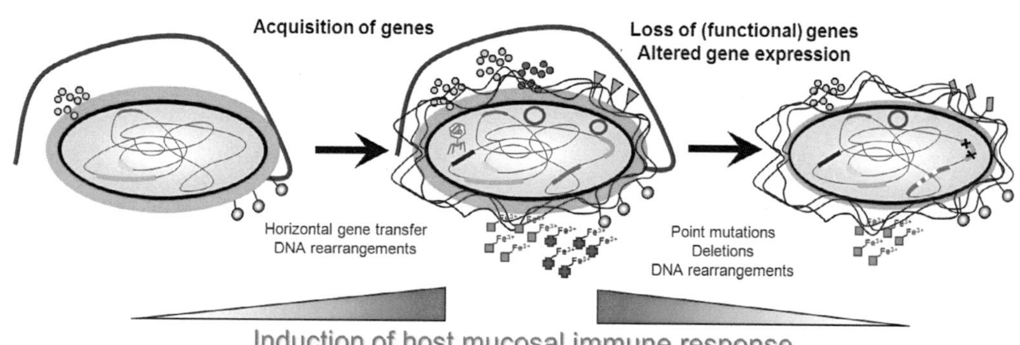

FIGURE 1 Impact of genome plasticity on adaptation and evolution of (pathogenic) bacteria. Plasmids, bacteriophages, and genomic islands may encode virulence-associated traits, such as adhesins, toxins, siderophore systems, and capsules. Acquisition of such mobile and accessory DNA elements contributes to the evolution of pathogenic variants by horizontal gene transfer. Genome plasticity can also result in alterations of gene expression or inactivation of virulence factors due to DNA rearrangements, deletions, or point mutations. Altered expression of virulence factors either as a result of active bacterial gene regulation or selection of corresponding mutants arising from genome plasticity can be advantageous for pathogenic bacteria with the ability to cause persistent infection in order to avoid or reduce activation of the host immune response.

genic *E. coli* strains isolated from patients with persistent infection (Table 1). Deletion of chromosomal regions comprising virulence determinants led to the discovery of pathogenicity islands in the early 1990s (Hacker et al., 1990) and may mirror general bacterial genome plasticity. On the other hand, such deletions may represent a specific UPEC response to the urinary tract-specific growth environment. Deletion of virulence genes may convert highly virulent strains present in the initial phase of an infection to attenuated pathogens during chronic stages of infection. UPEC isolates from patients with chronic UTI carried fewer virulence determinants than did strains isolated from patients suffering from acute UTI (Fünfstück et al., 1986). Similarly, antigenic variation by an altered expression, variation, or even loss of the O antigen, altered capsule or flagellum expression, and changes in the ability to utilize different sugars have been observed during the course of chronic UTI or recurrent extraintestinal *E. coli* infection (Bettelheim and Taylor, 1969; Olesen et al., 1998). Other adaptation strategies to establish persistent infection include the transformation into small-colony variants and the formation of intracellular biofilms (Borderon and Horodniceanu, 1978; Mysorekar and Hultgren, 2006). Both are potent strategies against host defenses and antibiotic therapy.

Genotypic and phenotypic comparison of virulence-associated traits of a collection of UPEC, ABU, and fecal *E. coli* isolates, in combination with molecular epidemiological analyses, demonstrated that about two-thirds of the ABU strains resembled UPEC isolates with regard to genome content and phylogeny but exhibited fewer virulence-associated phenotypes than did UPEC. Interestingly, one-third of the ABU isolates were similar to commensal *E. coli* isolates. These findings suggest that ABU can occur in different ways, e.g., due to reductive evolution of UPEC or colonization by commensals. The occurrence of ABU isolates was not restricted to particular clonal groups. Geno- and phenotypic comparisons of closely related *E. coli* isolates which demonstrated the impact of genome plasticity, i.e., gene acquisition and gene loss, on bacterial evolution as different members

TABLE 1 Examples of in vivo adaptation strategies of uropathogenic *E. coli* during infection

Phenotype	Type of infection	Reference(s)
Loss of virulence genes, pathogenicity islands	Chronic or recurrent UTI	Fünfstück et al., 1986
Antigenic variation, loss of O antigen, altered expression of capsule, flagella, altered metabolic versatility	Chronic or recurrent UTI, bacteremia	Bettelheim and Taylor, 1969; Olesen et al., 1989
Loss of functional adhesion expression, loss of O antigen, altered motility, phenotypic attenuation	Asymptomatic bacteriuria	Bergsten et al., 2005; Klemm et al., 2006; Zdziarski et al., 2008, 2010
Intracellular biofilm formation	Chronic UTI	Mysorekar and Hultgren, 2006; Rosen et al., 2007

of sequence type (ST) 73 represent highly uropathogenic as well as commensal or ABU *E. coli* isolates. Although these strains belong to the same clone, they differed markedly in their genome size and their virulence and fitness-related phenotypes (Zdziarski et al., 2008).

IMPACT OF GENOMIC CHANGES ON BACTERIUM-HOST INTERACTION AND FITNESS

The natural reservoir of UPEC is the large intestine. Successful colonization of the urinary tract requires bacterial adaptation to the different growth conditions encountered in this niche, including the host response during infection. Consequently, successful colonization results in adaptation of UPEC (to, e.g., different nutrient availability, osmolarity, or host response) which appears as (i) reversible and (ii) stable genomic changes (point mutations, deletions, genomic rearrangements) resulting from genome plasticity and selection. Short-term adaptation of *E. coli* to growth in urine relative to Luria broth has been analyzed on the transcriptional and protein level (Alteri and Mobley, 2007; Roos and Klemm, 2006; Snyder et al., 2004) and has led to the identification of many bacterial determinants which were deregulated upon growth in urine and/or in vivo. These studies confirmed that iron uptake systems, certain metabolic pathways, as well as fimbrial adhesion determinants and determinants involved in protection against nitrosative stress belong to the most responsive genes upon growth under these conditions (Hagan et al., 2010; Roos and Klemm, 2006; Snyder et al., 2004).

To investigate microevolutionary and adaptational changes during long-term growth, bacterial populations can be established from a single colony and cultivated under defined conditions for many generations. "Experimental evolution" experiments provide information on the evolutionary dynamics within the population (Lenski, 1991). Experimental evolution experiments with *E. coli* K-12 demonstrated that fitness gains are initially rapidly acquired but the speed of acquisition declines over time. Adaptation results from random mutations and selection (Cooper et al., 2001; de Visser and Lenski, 2002; Lenski and Travisano, 1994; Lenski et al., 2003). This suggests that, in a new growth environment, the fitness of a population will evolve from a generally lower fitness toward an adaptive peak or plateau. Microevolution during experimental evolution is typically driven by the occurrence of relatively few mutations that confer large benefits and a large number of mutations with small benefits (Rozen et al., 2002). Data on genome-wide changes and adaptation during long-term growth of *E. coli* in vitro have started to accumulate only recently (Barrick et al., 2009).

Bacterial adaptation to prolonged in vivo growth in different host backgrounds has been analyzed by comparing the genome structure and virulence- and fitness-related phenotypes of *E. coli* 83972 and three selected reisolates from deliberate human therapeutic urinary bladder colonization. As a control, strain 83972 was cultivated in vitro in a continuous culture in pooled human urine for more than 2,000 generations (Zdziarski et al., 2010). Altogether, the relatively small number of 37 single-nucleotide polymorphisms (SNPs), four small deletions (1, 5, 12, and 165 bp), one 1,731-bp DNA inversion, and one 27-kb DNA deletion have been detected in the four isolates upon prolonged growth in pooled human urine in vivo or in vitro. These genomic alterations occurred only in the *E. coli* 83972 chromosome, whereas the small cryptic plasmid remained unaffected. Regions of the core and flexible gene pool were both affected by mutations which were, with four exceptions, observed in coding regions. Among the mutated loci were many genes encoding pleiotropic regulators or two-component systems, such as *barA*, *fecI*, *gyrA*, *marRA*, and *oxyR*. The occurrence of 5 synonymous versus 32 nonsynonymous or missense nucleotide substitutions among the 37 SNPs detected indicates strong positive selection for the corresponding phenotypes in vivo. Interestingly, the number of genomic alterations in *E. coli* 83972 in vivo reisolates was generally larger than that of the *E. coli* 83972 isolate from the in vitro experimental evolution experiment, where strain 83972 was propagated in pooled human urine without host contact. The number of mutations could also be correlated with the duration of bladder colonization. Interestingly, several genes turned out to be affected by bacterial genome plasticity upon independent deliberate colonizations of different hosts. The existence of these mutation hot spots in the urinary tract which affect the bacterial response to osmotic and nitrosative stress as well as in iron acquisition indicates important selective pressures during bacterial growth in the bladder (Zdziarski et al., 2010).

INTRAVESICLE GROWTH AFFECTS THE MOTILITY OF *E. COLI*

Both murine and human in vivo transcriptome analyses indicated that motility is downregulated during *E. coli* bladder colonization (Roos and Klemm, 2006; Snyder et al., 2004). Although flagellum-mediated motility/chemotaxis was not required, it would be beneficial during colonization of the urinary tract by contributing to bacterial fitness (Lane et al., 2005, 2007). It has been suggested that loss of surface antigens occurs during long-term exposure of *E. coli* to host factors of the urinary tract (Hansson et al., 1989). Furthermore, motility is downregulated in *E. coli* upon bladder colonization (Roos and Klemm, 2006; Snyder et al., 2004). ABU strain 83972 is only barely motile. Several in vivo reisolates, however, displayed different degrees of motility, suggesting that the flagellar determinant was functional and its expression was actively regulated (Zdziarski et al. 2010). Flagella as an important pathogen-associated molecular pattern are immunogenic and stimulate interleukin-8 (IL-8) production (Zhou et al., 2003). Nevertheless, bistable flagellar expression and a heterogenous population with a low percentage of motile individuals (thus causing only minimal host response activation) could play an important role in bladder colonization. Bistable flagellar expression has also been reported for *Salmonella enterica* serovar Typhimurium as phenotypic noise involved in self-destructive cooperation and thus survival of certain parts of the infecting bacterial population (Ackermann et al., 2008; Freed et al., 2008).

INTRAVESICLE GROWTH AFFECTS BACTERIAL GROWTH CHARACTERISTICS AND METABOLISM OF *E. COLI*

Fast growth and efficient utilization of resources available in urine are among the most important factors enabling ABU isolates to colonize the urinary tract. In healthy adults, normal urine production ranges from 1 to 2 liters per day and a single micturition results in the release of 200 to 400 ml of urine. After micturition, about 1 ml of urine remains in the bladder and might function as an inoculum for ongoing bladder colonization. If the growth rate is high enough to guarantee that the number of growing bacteria exceeds the number of those which are lost upon micturition, colonization of the mucosal surface is not required for persistence in the bladder (Gordon and Riley, 1992). The early phase of colonization is critical for the successful establishment of bacteriuria, because in this phase the innate immune system may be able to clear the infection. Therefore, fast growth in the early exponential phase in combination with weak induction of host defense may be a successful strategy to successfully establish ABU. ABU isolates exhibit high growth rates in vitro in human urine and are able to outcompete UPEC strains when grown together in pooled human urine (Roos et al., 2006a, 2006c). Thus, prolonged growth in the urinary tract may select for variants with increased growth rates in urine. The analysis of multiple reisolates of strain 83972 from the deliberate therapeutic colonization indicated that stable bladder colonization for longer periods did not always result in selection of variants with increased growth rates or increased fitness. Only a few reisolates grew faster than their parent strain 83972, whereas in many cases a significantly increased growth could not be observed. In addition, some reisolates exhibited a decreased fitness relative to the parent strain in growth competition experiments with pooled human urine (Fig. 2). This further underlines the importance of the individual host background and in vivo growth conditions for adapatation of these *E. coli* strains.

Upon entry to a new niche, bacteria have to multiply and colonize. This depends on successful adaptation to the growth conditions in the bladder and requires efficient sensing of environmental parameters and the processing of such signals. Bacterial metabolic networks have to be adapted to grow fast and optimally utilize nutrients present in the urine. Transcriptome analysis of selected *E. coli* 83972 reisolates uncovered significant differences not only between in vivo and in vitro reisolates but also among different in vivo reisolates. In individual hosts, *E. coli* 83972 used different strategies to optimize proliferation. Sugar acids such as galacturonate, gluconate, glucuronate, *N*-acetylglucosoamine, and *N*-acetylgalactosamine, as well as sialic acid, are available in urine and often derive from food such as galacturonate (from pectin) or gluconate and ketogluconate (from muscle tissue) (Peekhaus and Conway, 1998). Furthermore, the bladder urothelium is covered by a thick layer of protective glycoproteins and is rich in *N*-acetylglucosoamine, *N*-acetylgalactosamine, and sialic acid and contains lesser amounts of glucuronate and galacturonate. In line with this, in certain in vivo reisolate uptake and metabolic pathways for many of these sugars were up-regulated (Zdziarski et al., 2010). It has also been reported that *E. coli* induces the expression of genes involved in uptake and utilization of sugar acids such as galacturonate, glucuronate, and galactonate during growth in urine (Roos and Klemm, 2006). Another example of an alternative nutritional strategy of strain 83972 during growth in the bladder is the degradation of ribo- and deoxyribonucleosides which may be used as carbon sources via the pentose phosphate pathway (Zdziarski et al., 2010). Nucleic acids can be found in urine since many epithelial cells undergo apoptosis and their DNA is degraded. In addition, bacterial lysis results in freely available nucleic acids in urine.

The *E. coli* BarA/UvrY two-component regulatory system is involved in regulation of gluconeogenesis and glycolysis as well as of many virulence- and fitness-associated traits via the carbon storage regulation system CsrA/B (Babitzke and Romeo, 2007). This two-component system is crucial for efficient adaptation between different metabolic pathways, an essential function for adaptation to a new environment. Based on transcriptome analysis of UPEC isolated from urine of female patients suffering from UTI, it has been recently proposed that UPEC strains grow rapidly in the bladder, exhibiting "overflow metabolism," i.e., rapid growth on excess carbon sources by mixed-acid fermentation (Alteri et al., 2009; Anfora et al., 2008; Hagan et al., 2010). In UPEC, BarA/UvrY affects survival in long-term competition cultures and is a determinant for virulence in a monkey cystitis model (Pernestig et al., 2003; Tomenius et al., 2006). The urine in the bladder contains several different carbon sources, and its composition changes over time. It has been suggested that the inability to efficiently switch between different carbon sources may explain the role of BarA/

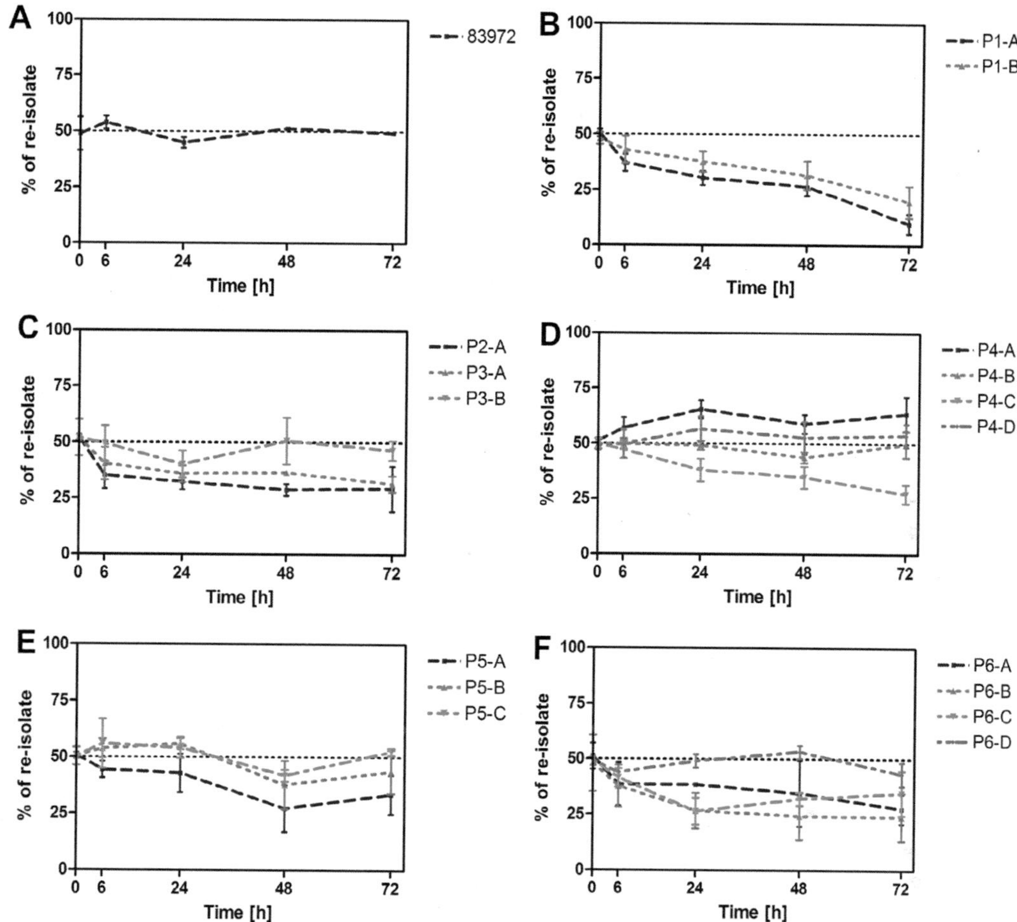

FIGURE 2 Competitiveness of in vivo reisolates of *E. coli* 83972 relative to their parent strain in pooled human urine. For growth competition experiments, the chloramphenicol-resistant derivative of parent strain 83972, *E. coli* 83972*cat*, and one in vivo reisolate were mixed in the same ratio and cultivated at 37°C for 72 h in pooled human urine. At different time points (6, 24, 48, and 72 h), the ratio of the parent strain 83972*cat* to the in vivo reisolate was determined by colony counting on LB agar plates supplemented with chloramphenicol and LB plates, respectively. (A) Results of the control experiment, where the parent strain and its chloramphenicol-resistant variant 83972*cat* were cocultured to demonstrate their identical competitiveness. Competitiveness of consecutive reisolates (as indicated by the order of letters) from individual patients P1 to P6 differed between the patients as well as between reisolates from the same patient (B to F). All experiments were performed in triplicate, and the corresponding mean values of the ratio between parent strain and reisolate and standard deviations were plotted.

UvrY in urovirulence. Interestingly, the functionality of the BarA/UvrY system in *E. coli* 83972 was altered due to point mutations upon long-term bladder colonization, thus supporting the importance of this regulatory system for intravesical growth of *E. coli* (Zdziarski et al., 2010).

ANALYSIS OF HOST FACTORS AND THEIR IMPACT ON ADAPTATION OF *E. COLI*

Asymptomatic bacteriuria is established when the innate immune response, controlled by TLR4, is impaired. Mutations which disturb TLR4 signaling result in an asymptomatic carrier state (Frendeus et al., 2001). Bacterial colonization of the urinary tract activates the innate host response, e.g., the expression of the chemokines IL-6 and IL-8. This activation is much stronger when functional fimbriae are expressed; however, nonfimbriated isolates cause a weaker and delayed response (Samuelsson et al., 2004). On the other hand, the level of immune response may vary due to the patients' susceptibility to UTI (Svanborg et al., 2006). Children with ABU were shown to express lower levels of TLR4 than controls without a history of UTI. Furthermore, functional chemokines and their receptors are crucial for neutrophil recruitment, and for the neutrophil-dependent bacterial clearance (Lundstedt et al., 2007; Ragnarsdóttir et al., 2007, 2008). Neutrophils play a pivotal role in host defense against microbial infection and produce reactive oxygen species as well as nitric oxide (NO) (Wheeler et al., 1997). Furthermore, urine contains significant amounts of nitrate (Tsikas et al., 1994) and anaerobic NO_3 metabolism results in the generation of additional nitric oxide. Nitrosating agents cause mutagenic lesions (Weiss, 2006). Therefore, regarding the frequent occurrence of mutations in the genomes of ABU reisolates, it is tempting to speculate that prolonged growth in urine and exposure to different factors of the immune response, e.g., reactive oxygen or nitrogen species, increases the mutation rate and thus is a driving force for the development of the ABU lifestyle and evolution within the urinary tract. One particularly important effect of NO in this context is its ability to cause mutagenic DNA lesions (Sakai et al., 2006; Weiss, 2006). When DNA is exposed in vitro to HNO_2 or to NO, the exocyclic amines of the nucleobases form unstable *N*-nitroso derivatives that lead to deamination. Thus, adenine is deaminated to hypoxanthine, guanine is deaminated to xanthine, and cytosine is deaminated to uracil (Shapiro and Pohl, 1968). The deaminated products pair with different bases than their aminated counterparts, thereby frequently resulting in mutations upon subsequent replication.

E. coli employs two mechanisms to detoxify NO, i.e., by the use of flavohemoglobin or flavorubredoxin (Poole et al., 1996; Poole, 2005a, 2005b). The periplasmic cytochrome *c* nitrate reductase NrfA, which reduces NO_2^- to NH_3, may also be able to directly reduce NO (Poock et al., 2002). Genes involved in protection against nitrosative stress are induced in ABU strain 83972 upon in vivo growth (Roos and Klemm, 2006; Snyder et al., 2004). Additionally, the transcriptome analysis of *E. coli* 83972 in vivo reisolates also revealed that determinants required for protection against oxidative and nitrosative stress were strongly induced relative to those in the parent strain (Zdziarski et al., 2010). Growth under nutritional stress conditions may cause oxidative stress (Gordon and Riley, 1992; Hull and Hull, 1997; Russo et al., 1999; Seaver and Imlay, 2001a, 2001b; Snyder et al., 2004). Bacterial defenses against oxidative stress include enzymatic components, e.g., superoxide dismutases, catalases, or alcohol dehydrogenases, as well as nonenzymatic components, such as glutathione-dependent reduction systems (Carmel-Harel and Storz, 2000). According to the analysis of reisolates of *E. coli* 83972, the determinants coding for several of these protection systems were mutated or exhibited altered expression patterns upon prolonged bladder colonization (Zdziarski et al., 2010). This suggests that bacterial colonization of the urinary bladder is accompanied by stress due to, e.g., nutrient limitation, as well as oxidative and nitrosative stress. *E. coli* variants which induce a weaker host response and/or are more resistant to stress conditions are selected. High stress resistance in *E. coli* goes hand in hand with an elevated mutation rate and an increased generation of deleterious mutations (Saint-Ruf and Matic, 2006). The observed increased genome plasticity of in vivo-grown reisolates of *E. coli* 83972 relative to control isolates from the in vitro experimental evolution study (Zdziarski et al., 2010) may in part result from stress-induced increased genome plasticity.

CONCLUSIONS

Genome plasticity of *E. coli* and the interaction between UPEC strains and their host play important roles in bacterial adaptation and microevolution in the urinary tract. Altogether, the results indicate that prolonged growth in urine under stress conditions, as well as direct contact with the host tissues and selective pressure in the host, promotes bacterial variability. The acquired mutations which may reduce the sensitivity to stress (Bjedov et al., 2003; Rosenberg, 2001) or changing metabolic requirements point to specific bacterial responses to prolonged growth in the urinary tract. Alteration of other genes may result from the fact that these loci became redundant in the urinary tract and were thus lost in the new environment (Giraud et al., 2008; Novak et al., 2006). Similar evolutionary mechanisms have been observed in genomic analyses of, e.g., sequential *Pseudomonas aeruginosa* or *Helicobacter pylori* isolates obtained from persistently infected hosts. These sequential isolates also showed a loss of virulence as well as altered phenotypes due to changes in genome content and gene expression (Hogardt and Heesemann, 2010; Jelsbak et al., 2007; Oh et al., 2006; Smith et al., 2006). Host factors play an important role in the adaptation of UPEC isolates and other bacterial pathogens which are able to persistently infect their hosts. In *E. coli*, point mutations and genomic alterations, unless they are deleterious, contribute to adaptation and survival in the urinary bladder. Positive selection of clones which do not activate a strong immune response or which exhibit increased stress resistance promotes efficient asymptomatic bladder colonization or chronic urinary tract infection by these bacterial variants. The identification of genomic regions subjected to host-driven mutagenesis might help to discover new potential drug targets.

ACKNOWLEDGMENTS

We thank Catharina Svanborg and Björn Wullt (Lund, Sweden) for generous support, very fruitful collaboration, and helpful discussion.

Our work was supported by the Deutsche Forschungsgemeinschaft (SFB479, TP A1). These studies were carried out within the European Virtual Institute for Functional Genomics of Bacterial Pathogens (CEE LSHB-CT-2005-512061) and the ERA-NET PathoGenoMics (grants 0313937A and 0315436A).

REFERENCES

Ackermann, M., B. Stecher, N. E. Freed, P. Songhet, W. D. Hardt, and M. Doebeli. 2008. Self-destructive cooperation mediated by phenotypic noise. *Nature* **454:**987–990.

Ahmed, N., U. Dobrindt, J. Hacker, and S. E. Hasnain. 2008. Genomic fluidity and pathogenic bacteria: applications in diagnostics, epidemiology and intervention. *Nat. Rev. Microbiol.* **6:**387–394.

Alteri, C. J., and H. L. Mobley. 2007. Quantitative profile of the uropathogenic *Escherichia coli* outer membrane proteome during growth in human urine. *Infect. Immun.* **75:**2679–2688.

Alteri, C. J., S. N. Smith, and H. L. Mobley. 2009. Fitness of *Escherichia coli* during urinary tract infection requires gluconeogenesis and the TCA cycle. *PLoS Pathog.* **5:**e1000448.

Anfora, A. T., D. K. Halladin, B. J. Haugen, and R. A. Welch. 2008. Uropathogenic *Escherichia coli* CFT073 is adapted to acetatogenic growth but does not require acetate during murine urinary tract infection. *Infect. Immun.* **76:**5760–5767.

Babitzke, P., and T. Romeo. 2007. CsrB sRNA family: sequestration of RNA-binding regulatory proteins. *Curr. Opin. Microbiol.* **10:**156–163.

Barrick, J. E., D. S. Yu, S. H. Yoon, H. Jeong, T. K. Oh, D. Schneider, R. E. Lenski, and J. F. Kim. 2009. Genome evolution and adaptation in a long-term experiment with *Escherichia coli*. *Nature* **461:**1243–1247.

Bergsten, G., M. Samuelsson, B. Wullt, I. Leijonhufvud, H. Fischer, and C. Svanborg. 2004. PapG-dependent adherence breaks mucosal inertia and triggers the innate host response. *J. Infect. Dis.* **189:**1734–1742.

Bergsten, G., B. Wullt, and C. Svanborg. 2005. *Escherichia coli*, fimbriae, bacterial persistence and host response induction in the human urinary tract. *Int. J. Med. Microbiol.* **295:**487–502.

Bettelheim, K. A., and J. Taylor. 1969. A study of *Escherichia coli* isolated from chronic urinary infection. *J. Med. Microbiol.* **2:**225–236.

Bjedov, I., O. Tenaillon, B. Gerard, V. Souza, E. Denamur, M. Radman, F. Taddei, and I. Matic. 2003. Stress-induced mutagenesis in bacteria. *Science* **300:**1404–1409.

Björkman, J., and D. I. Andersson. 2000. The cost of antibiotic resistance from a bacterial perspective. *Drug Resist. Updat.* **3:**237–245.

Borderon, E., and T. Horodniceanu. 1978. Metabolically deficient dwarf-colony mutants of *Escherichia coli*: deficiency and resistance to antibiotics of strains isolated from urine culture. *J. Clin. Microbiol.* **8:**629–634.

Brzuszkiewicz, E., H. Brüggemann, H. Liesegang, M. Emmerth, T. Oelschlaeger, G. Nagy, K. Albermann, C. Wagner, C. Buchrieser, L. Emödy, G. Gottschalk, J. Hacker, and U. Dobrindt. 2006. How to become a uropathogen: comparative genomic analysis of extraintestinal pathogenic *Escherichia coli* strains. *Proc. Natl. Acad. Sci. USA* **103:**12879–12884.

Carmel-Harel, O., and G. Storz. 2000. Roles of the glutathione- and thioredoxin-dependent reduction systems in the *Escherichia coli* and *Saccharomyces cerevisiae* responses to oxidative stress. *Annu. Rev. Microbiol.* **54:**439–461.

Chen, S. L., C. S. Hung, J. Xu, C. S. Reigstad, V. Magrini, A. Sabo, D. Blasiar, T. Bieri, R. R. Meyer, P. Ozersky, J. R. Armstrong, R. S. Fulton, J. P. Latreille, J. Spieth, T. M. Hooton, E. R. Mardis, S. J. Hultgren, and J. I. Gordon. 2006. Identification of genes subject to positive selection in uropathogenic strains of *Escherichia coli*: a comparative genomics approach. *Proc. Natl. Acad. Sci. USA* **103:**5977–5982.

Colgan, R., L. E. Nicolle, A. McGlone, and T. M. Hooton. 2006. Asymptomatic bacteriuria in adults. *Am. Fam. Physician* **74:**985–990.

Cooper, V. S., A. F. Bennett, and R. E. Lenski. 2001. Evolution of thermal dependence of growth rate of *Escherichia coli* populations during 20,000 generations in a constant environment. *Evolution* **55:**889–896.

de Visser, J. A., and R. E. Lenski. 2002. Long-term experimental evolution in *Escherichia coli*. XI. Rejection of non-transitive interactions as cause of declining rate of adaptation. *BMC Evol. Biol.* **2:**19.

Dobrindt, U., F. Agerer, K. Michaelis, A. Janka, C. Buchrieser, M. Samuelson, C. Svanborg, G. Gottschalk, H. Karch, and J. Hacker. 2003. Analysis of genome plasticity in pathogenic and commensal *Escherichia coli* isolates by use of DNA arrays. *J. Bacteriol.* **185:**1831–1840.

Dobrindt, U., B. Hochhut, U. Hentschel, and J. Hacker. 2004. Genomic islands in pathogenic and environmental microorganisms. *Nat. Rev. Microbiol.* **2:**414–424.

Edén, C. S., G. L. Janson, and U. Lindberg. 1979. Adhesiveness to urinary tract epithelial cells of fecal and urinary *Escherichia coli* isolates from patients with symptomatic urinary tract infections or asymptomatic bacteriuria of varying duration. *J. Urol.* **122:**185–188.

Foxman, B. 2002. Epidemiology of urinary tract infections: incidence, morbidity, and economic costs. *Am. J. Med.* **113**(Suppl. 1A)**:**5S–13S.

Freed, N. E., O. K. Silander, B. Stecher, A. Bohm, W. D. Hardt, and M. Ackermann. 2008. A simple screen to identify promoters conferring high levels of phenotypic noise. *PLoS Genet.* **4:**e1000307.

Frendeus, B., C. Wachtler, M. Hedlund, H. Fischer, P. Samuelsson, M. Svensson, and C. Svanborg. 2001. *Escherichia coli* P fimbriae utilize the Toll-like receptor 4 pathway for cell activation. *Mol. Microbiol.* **40:**37–51.

Frost, L. S., and G. Koraimann. 2010. Regulation of bacterial conjugation: balancing opportunity with adversity. *Future Microbiol.* **5:**1057–1071.

Fünfstück, R., H. Tschäpe, G. Stein, H. Kunath, M. Bergner, and G. Wessel. 1986. Virulence properties of *Escherichia* coli strains in patients with chronic pyelonephritis. *Infection* **14:**145–150.

Giraud, A., S. Arous, M. De Paepe, V. Gaboriau-Routhiau, J. C. Bambou, S. Rakotobe, A. B. Lindner, F. Taddei, and N. Cerf-Bensussan. 2008. Dissecting the genetic components of adaptation of *Escherichia coli* to the mouse gut. *PLoS Genet.* **4:**e2.

Godaly, G., A. E. Proudfoot, R. E. Offord, C. Svanborg, and W. W. Agace. 1997. Role of epithelial interleukin-8 (IL-8) and neutrophil IL-8 receptor A in *Escherichia coli*-induced transuroepithelial neutrophil migration. *Infect. Immun.* **65:**3451–3456.

Gordon, D. M., and M. A. Riley. 1992. A theoretical and experimental analysis of bacterial growth in the bladder. *Mol. Microbiol.* **6:**555–562.

Hacker, J., L. Bender, M. Ott, J. Wingender, B. Lund, R. Marre, and W. Goebel. 1990. Deletions of chromosomal regions coding for fimbriae and hemolysins occur *in vitro* and *in vivo* in various extraintestinal *Escherichia coli* isolates. *Microb. Pathog.* **8:**213–225.

Hacker, J., U. Hentschel, and U. Dobrindt. 2003. Prokaryotic chromosomes and disease. *Science* **301:**790–793.

Hagan, E. C., A. L. Lloyd, D. A. Rasko, G. J. Faerber, and H. L. Mobley. 2010. *Escherichia coli* global gene expression in urine from women with urinary tract infection. *PLoS Pathog.* **6:**e1001187.

Hang, L., M. Haraoka, W. W. Agace, H. Leffler, M. Burdick, R. Strieter, and C. Svanborg. 1999. Macrophage inflammatory protein-2 is required for neutrophil passage across the epithelial barrier of the infected urinary tract. *J. Immunol.* **162:**3037–3044.

Hansson, S., U. Jodal, L. Noren, and J. Bjure. 1989. Untreated bacteriuria in asymptomatic girls with renal scarring. *Pediatrics* **84:**964–968.

Hogardt, M., and J. Heesemann. 2010. Adaptation of *Pseudomonas aeruginosa* during persistence in the cystic fibrosis lung. *Int. J. Med. Microbiol.* **300:**557–562.

Hull, R. A., and S. I. Hull. 1997. Nutritional requirements for growth of uropathogenic *Escherichia coli* in human urine. *Infect. Immun.* **65:**1960–1961.

Jelsbak, L., H. K. Johansen, A. L. Frost, R. Thogersen, L. E. Thomsen, O. Ciofu, L. Yang, J. A. Haagensen, N. Hoiby, and S. Molin. 2007. Molecular epidemiology and dynamics of *Pseudomonas aeruginosa* populations in lungs of cystic fibrosis patients. *Infect. Immun.* **75:**2214–2224.

Juhas, M., J. R. van der Meer, M. Gaillard, R. M. Harding, D. W. Hood, and D. W. Crook. 2009. Genomic islands: tools of bacterial horizontal gene transfer and evolution. *FEMS Microbiol. Rev.* **33:**376–393.

Klemm, P., V. Roos, G. C. Ulett, C. Svanborg, and M. A. Schembri. 2006. Molecular characterization of the *Escherichia coli* asymptomatic bacteriuria strain 83972: the taming of a pathogen. *Infect. Immun.* **74:**781–785.

Lane, M. C., C. J. Alteri, S. N. Smith, and H. L. Mobley. 2007. Expression of flagella is coincident with uropathogenic *Escherichia coli* ascension to the upper urinary tract. *Proc. Natl. Acad. Sci. USA* **104:**16669–16674.

Lane, M. C., V. Lockatell, G. Monterosso, D. Lamphier, J. Weinert, J. R. Hebel, D. E. Johnson, and H. L. Mobley. 2005. Role of motility in the colonization of uropathogenic *Escherichia coli* in the urinary tract. *Infect. Immun.* **73:**7644–7656.

Lenski, R. E. 1991. Quantifying fitness and gene stability in microorganisms. *Biotechnology* **15:**173–192.

Lenski, R. E., and M. Travisano. 1994. Dynamics of adaptation and diversification: a 10,000-generation experiment with bacterial populations. *Proc. Natl. Acad. Sci. USA* **91:**6808–6814.

Lenski, R. E., C. L. Winkworth, and M. A. Riley. 2003. Rates of DNA sequence evolution in experimental populations of *Escherichia coli* during 20,000 generations. *J. Mol. Evol.* **56:**498–508.

Lindberg, U., I. Claesson, L. A. Hanson, and U. Jodal. 1978. Asymptomatic bacteriuria in schoolgirls. VIII. Clinical course during a 3-year follow-up. *J. Pediatr.* **92:**194–199.

Lloyd, A. L., T. A. Henderson, P. D. Vigil, and H. L. Mobley. 2009. Genomic islands of uropathogenic *Escherichia coli* contribute to virulence. *J. Bacteriol.* **191:**3469–3481.

Lundstedt, A. C., S. McCarthy, M. C. Gustafsson, G. Godaly, U. Jodal, D. Karpman, I. Leijonhufvud, C. Linden, J. Martinell, B. Ragnarsdottir, M. Samuelsson, L. Truedsson, B. Andersson, and C. Svanborg. 2007. A genetic basis of susceptibility to acute pyelonephritis. *PLoS One* **2:**e825.

Mabbett, A. N., G. C. Ulett, R. E. Watts, J. J. Tree, M. Totsika, C. L. Ong, J. M. Wood, W. Monaghan, D. F. Looke, G. R. Nimmo, C. Svanborg, and M. A. Schembri. 2009. Virulence properties of asymptomatic bacteriuria *Escherichia coli*. *Int. J. Med. Microbiol.* **299:**53–63.

Mysorekar, I. U., and S. J. Hultgren. 2006. Mechanisms of uropathogenic *Escherichia coli* persistence and eradication from the urinary tract. *Proc. Natl. Acad. Sci. USA* **103:**14170–14175.

Nielubowicz, G. R., and H. L. Mobley. 2010. Host-pathogen interactions in urinary tract infection. *Nat. Rev. Urol.* **7:**430–441.

Novak, M., T. Pfeiffer, R. E. Lenski, U. Sauer, and S. Bonhoeffer. 2006. Experimental tests for an evolutionary trade-off between growth rate and yield in *E. coli*. *Am. Nat.* **168:**242–251.

Ochman, H., J. G. Lawrence, and E. A. Groisman. 2000. Lateral gene transfer and the nature of bacterial innovation. *Nature* **405:**299–304.

Oh, J. D., H. Kling-Backhed, M. Giannakis, J. Xu, R. S. Fulton, L. A. Fulton, H. S. Cordum, C. Wang, G. Elliott, J. Edwards, E. R. Mardis, L. G. Engstrand, and J. I. Gordon. 2006. The complete genome sequence of a chronic atrophic gastritis *Helicobacter pylori* strain: evolution during disease progression. *Proc. Natl. Acad. Sci. USA* **103:**9999–10004.

Olesen, B., H. J. Kolmos, F. Ørskov, and I. Ørskov. 1998. *Escherichia coli* bacteraemia in patients with and without haematological malignancies: a study of strain characters and recurrent episodes. *J. Infect.* **36:**93–100.

Peekhaus, N., and T. Conway. 1998. What's for dinner? Entner-Doudoroff metabolism in *Escherichia coli*. *J. Bacteriol.* **180:**3495–3502.

Pernestig, A. K., D. Georgellis, T. Romeo, K. Suzuki, H. Tomenius, S. Normark, and O. Melefors. 2003. The *Escherichia coli* BarA-UvrY two-component system is needed for efficient switching between glycolytic and gluconeogenic carbon sources. *J. Bacteriol.* **185:**843–853.

Plotkin, J. B., and J. Dushoff. 2003. Codon bias and frequency-dependent selection on the hemagglutinin epitopes of influenza A virus. *Proc. Natl. Acad. Sci. USA* **100:**7152–7157.

Poock, S. R., E. R. Leach, J. W. Moir, J. A. Cole, and D. J. Richardson. 2002. Respiratory detoxification of nitric oxide by the cytochrome c nitrite reductase of *Escherichia coli*. *J. Biol. Chem.* **277:**23664–23669.

Poole, L. B. 2005a. Bacterial defenses against oxidants: mechanistic features of cysteine-based peroxidases and their flavoprotein reductases. *Arch. Biochem. Biophys.* **433:**240–254.

Poole, R. K. 2005b. Nitric oxide and nitrosative stress tolerance in bacteria. *Biochem. Soc. Trans.* **33:**176–180.

Poole, R. K., M. F. Anjum, J. Membrillo-Hernandez, S. O. Kim, M. N. Hughes, and V. Stewart. 1996. Nitric oxide, nitrite, and Fnr regulation of *hmp* (flavohemoglobin) gene expression in *Escherichia coli* K-12. *J. Bacteriol.* **178:**5487–5492.

Ragnarsdóttir, B., H. Fischer, G. Godaly, J. Gronberg-Hernandez, M. Gustafsson, D. Karpman, A. C. Lundstedt, N. Lutay, S. Ramisch, M. L. Svensson, B. Wullt, M. Yadav, and C. Svanborg. 2008. TLR- and CXCR1-dependent innate immunity: insights into the genetics of urinary tract infections. *Eur. J. Clin. Investig.* **38**(Suppl. 2)**:**12–20.

Ragnarsdóttir, B., M. Samuelsson, M. C. Gustafsson, I. Leijonhufvud, D. Karpman, and C. Svanborg. 2007. Reduced toll-like receptor 4 expression in children with asymptomatic bacteriuria. *J. Infect. Dis.* **196:**475–484.

Raz, R. 2003. Asymptomatic bacteriuria. Clinical significance and management. *Int. J. Antimicrob. Agents* **22**(Suppl. 2)**:**45–47.

Roos, V., and P. Klemm. 2006. Global gene expression profiling of the asymptomatic bacteriuria *Escherichia coli* strain 83972 in the human urinary tract. *Infect. Immun.* **74:**3565–3575.

Roos, V., E. M. Nielsen, and P. Klemm. 2006a. Asymptomatic bacteriuria *Escherichia coli* strains: adhesins, growth and competition. *FEMS Microbiol. Lett.* **262:**22–30.

Roos, V., M. A. Schembri, G. C. Ulett, and P. Klemm. 2006b. Asymptomatic bacteriuria *Escherichia coli* strain 83972 carries mutations in the *foc* locus and is unable to express F1C fimbriae. *Microbiology* **152:**1799–1806.

Roos, V., G. C. Ulett, M. A. Schembri, and P. Klemm. 2006c. The asymptomatic bacteriuria *Escherichia coli* strain 83972 outcompetes uropathogenic *E. coli* strains in human urine. *Infect. Immun.* **74:**615–624.

Rosen, D. A., T. M. Hooton, W. E. Stamm, P. A. Humphrey, and S. J. Hultgren. 2007. Detection of intracellular bacterial communities in human urinary tract infection. *PLoS Med.* **4:**e329.

Rosenberg, S. M. 2001. Evolving responsively: adaptive mutation. *Nat. Rev. Genet.* **2:**504–515.

Rozen, D. E., J. A. de Visser, and P. J. Gerrish. 2002. Fitness effects of fixed beneficial mutations in microbial populations. *Curr. Biol.* **12:**1040–1045.

Russo, T. A., U. B. Carlino, A. Mong, and S. T. Jodush. 1999. Identification of genes in an extraintestinal isolate of *Escherichia coli* with increased expression after exposure to human urine. *Infect. Immun.* **67:**5306–5314.

Saint-Ruf, C., and I. Matic. 2006. Environmental tuning of mutation rates. *Environ. Microbiol.* **8:**193–199.

Sakai, A., M. Nakanishi, K. Yoshiyama, and H. Maki. 2006. Impact of reactive oxygen species on spontaneous mutagenesis in *Escherichia coli*. *Genes Cells* **11:**767–778.

Samuelsson, P., L. Hang, B. Wullt, H. Irjala, and C. Svanborg. 2004. Toll-like receptor 4 expression and cytokine responses in the human urinary tract mucosa. *Infect. Immun.* **72:**3179–3186.

Seaver, L. C., and J. A. Imlay. 2001a. Alkyl hydroperoxide reductase is the primary scavenger of endogenous hydrogen peroxide in *Escherichia coli*. *J. Bacteriol.* **183:**7173–7181.

Seaver, L. C., and J. A. Imlay. 2001b. Hydrogen peroxide fluxes and compartmentalization inside growing *Escherichia coli*. *J. Bacteriol.* **183:**7182–7189.

Shapiro, B. J., L. A. David, J. Friedman, and E. J. Alm. 2009. Looking for Darwin's footprints in the microbial world. *Trends Microbiol.* **17:**196–204.

Shapiro, R., and S. H. Pohl. 1968. The reaction of ribonucleosides with nitrous acid. Side products and kinetics. *Biochemistry* **7:**448–455.

Smith, E. E., D. G. Buckley, Z. Wu, C. Saenphimmachak, L. R. Hoffman, D. A. D'Argenio, S. I. Miller, B. W. Ramsey, D. P. Speert, S. M. Moskowitz, J. L. Burns, R. Kaul, and M. V. Olson. 2006. Genetic adaptation by *Pseudomonas aeruginosa* to the airways of cystic fibrosis patients. *Proc. Natl. Acad. Sci. USA* **103:**8487–8492.

Snyder, J. A., B. J. Haugen, E. L. Buckles, C. V. Lockatell, D. E. Johnson, M. S. Donnenberg, R. A. Welch, and H. L. Mobley. 2004. Transcriptome of uropathogenic *Escherichia coli* during urinary tract infection. *Infect. Immun.* **72:**6373–6381.

Svanborg, C., G. Bergsten, H. Fischer, G. Godaly, M. Gustafsson, D. Karpman, A. C. Lundstedt, B. Ragnarsdottir, M. Svensson, and B. Wullt. 2006. Uropathogenic *Escherichia coli* as a model of host-parasite interaction. *Curr. Opin. Microbiol.* **9:**33–39.

Svanborg, C., B. Frendeus, G. Godaly, L. Hang, M. Hedlund, and C. Wachtler. 2001. Toll-like receptor signaling and chemokine receptor expression influence the severity of urinary tract infection. *J. Infect. Dis.* **183**(Suppl. 1)**:**S61–S65.

Tappe, D., H. Claus, J. Kern, A. Marzinzig, M. Frosch, and M. Abele-Horn. 2006. First case of febrile bacteremia due to a wild type and small-colony variant of *Escherichia coli*. *Eur. J. Clin. Microbiol. Infect. Dis.* **25:**31–34.

Tomenius, H., A. K. Pernestig, K. Jonas, D. Georgellis, R. Mollby, S. Normark, and O. Melefors. 2006. The *Escherichia coli* BarA-UvrY two-component system is a virulence determinant in the urinary tract. *BMC Microbiol.* **6:**27.

Tsikas, D., R. H. Boger, S. M. Bode-Boger, F. M. Gutzki, and J. C. Frolich. 1994. Quantification of nitrite and nitrate in human urine and plasma as pentafluorobenzyl derivatives by gas chromatography-mass spectrometry using their 15N-labelled analogs. *J. Chromatogr. B* **661:**185–191.

Weiss, B. 2006. Evidence for mutagenesis by nitric oxide during nitrate metabolism in *Escherichia coli*. *J. Bacteriol.* **188:**829–833.

Welch, R. A., V. Burland, G. Plunkett III, P. Redford, P. Roesch, D. Rasko, E. L. Buckles, S. R. Liou, A. Boutin, J. Hackett, D. Stroud, G. F.

Mayhew, D. J. Rose, S. Zhou, D. C. Schwartz, N. T. Perna, H. L. Mobley, M. S. Donnenberg, and F. R. Blattner. 2002. Extensive mosaic structure revealed by the complete genome sequence of uropathogenic *Escherichia coli*. *Proc. Natl. Acad. Sci. USA* **99:**17020–17024.

Wheeler, M. A., S. D. Smith, G. Garcia-Cardena, C. F. Nathan, R. M. Weiss, and W. C. Sessa. 1997. Bacterial infection induces nitric oxide synthase in human neutrophils. *J. Clin. Investig.* **99:**110–116.

Wiles, T. J., R. R. Kulesus, and M. A. Mulvey. 2008. Origins and virulence mechanisms of uropathogenic *Escherichia coli*. *Exp. Mol. Pathol.* **85:**11–19.

Wozniak, R. A., and M. K. Waldor. 2010. Integrative and conjugative elements: mosaic mobile genetic elements enabling dynamic lateral gene flow. *Nat. Rev. Microbiol.* **8:**552–563.

Zdziarski, J., E. Brzuszkiewicz, B. Wullt, H. Liesegang, D. Biran, B. Voigt, J. Grönberg-Hernandez, B. Ragnarsdóttir, M. Hecker, E. Z. Ron, R. Daniel, G. Gottschalk, J. Hacker, C. Svanborg, and U. Dobrindt. 2010. Host imprints on bacterial genomes—rapid, divergent evolution in individual patients. *PLoS Pathog.* **6:**e1001078.

Zdziarski, J., C. Svanborg, B. Wullt, J. Hacker, and U. Dobrindt. 2008. Molecular basis of commensalism in the urinary tract: low virulence or virulence attenuation? *Infect. Immun.* **76:**695–703.

Zhou, X., J. A. Giron, A. G. Torres, J. A. Crawford, E. Negrete, S. N. Vogel, and J. B. Kaper. 2003. Flagellin of enteropathogenic *Escherichia coli* stimulates interleukin-8 production in T84 cells. *Infect. Immun.* **71:**2120–2129.

GENOTYPIC CHANGES IN ENTEROHEMORRHAGIC *Escherichia coli* DURING HUMAN INFECTION

Alexander Mellmann, Martina Bielaszewska, and Helge Karch

2

EHEC: OVERVIEW OF EPIDEMIOLOGY AND CLINICAL PATHOGENESIS

Enterohemorrhagic *Escherichia coli* (EHEC) is a pathogenic subgroup of Shiga toxin-producing *E. coli*. EHEC causes diarrhea, bloody diarrhea, and hemolytic-uremic syndrome (HUS) (Levine et al., 1987). *E. coli* O157:H7, the first EHEC serotype identified during two large outbreaks of bloody diarrhea in the United States in the early 1980s (Riley et al., 1983), is the most frequent EHEC serotype implicated in bloody diarrhea and HUS worldwide (Karch et al., 2005; Tarr et al., 2005). Moreover, EHEC belonging to several non-O157:H7 serotypes, most notably O26:H11/H$^-$ (nonmotile), O91:H21, O103:H2/H$^-$, O111:H8/H10/H$^-$, O113:H21, O121:H19, O145:H28/H25/H$^-$, and O157:H$^-$ (sorbitol-fermenting strains), has been recovered from patients with severe human diseases in Europe, North America, and Australia (Karch et al., 2005; Johnson et al., 2006; Brooks et al., 2005; Elliott et al., 2001; Jelacic et al., 2003). In Germany, such non-O157:H7 EHEC accounts for ca. 50% of EHEC strains isolated from patients with HUS (Bielaszewska et al., 2007a) and bloody diarrhea (Bielaszewska et al., 2008). Similarly, *E. coli* O157:H7 is not so predominant in Australian children with HUS (Elliott et al., 2001). However, in the United States EHEC O157:H7 is isolated from the majority (>95%) of patients with HUS (Banatvala et al., 2001).

Cattle and other animal species are colonized with EHEC (Caprioli et al., 2005), shed the pathogen in the environment, and are not ill. Undercooked meat (specifically hamburgers) contaminated by EHEC during production was the most important source of infection in the initial outbreaks caused by *E. coli* O157:H7 (Riley et al., 1983; Bell et al., 1994). The changing epidemiology of EHEC infections during the past decade is reflected by the association of more recent outbreaks with consumption of contaminated raw vegetables such as sprouts (Michino et al., 1999), lettuce (Hilborn et al., 1999), and spinach (CDC, 2006), as well as cookie dough (http://www.washingtonpost.com/wp-dyn/content/article/2009/08/31/AR2009083103922.html; accessed 16 November 2009). Additional sources of EHEC transmission are contaminated water (Holme, 2003), direct contact with animals (Crump

Alexander Mellmann, Martina Bielaszewska, and Helge Karch, Institute of Hygiene, University of Münster, Robert Koch Str. 41, 48149 Münster, Germany.

Genome Plasticity and Infectious Diseases,
Edited by J. Hacker, U. Dobrindt, and R. Kurth,

et al., 2002), and contact with infected humans (Werber et al., 2008). To survive in the different milieus where it occurs, EHEC must quickly adapt its genome for the specific conditions it encounters.

The most severe clinical outcome of an EHEC infection is HUS, which is clinically characterized by a triad of microangiopathic hemolytic anemia, thrombocytopenia, and renal insufficiency (Gerber et al., 2002; Tarr et al., 2005). HUS develops approximately one week (range, 3 to 13 days) after the onset of diarrhea in 10% to 15% of patients under 10 years of age infected with *E. coli* O157:H$^-$ (Tarr et al., 2005). The frequency of HUS after infection with non-O157:H7 EHEC serotypes is unknown. HUS is the most common cause of acute renal failure in children. Although the fatality rate of HUS is nowadays less than 5% (Gerber et al., 2002), morbidity is still ca. 30% and often involves chronic renal and cerebral impairment with hypertension (Garg et al., 2003; Gerber et al., 2002; Tarr et al., 2005). Renal failure can cause chronic morbidity and premature death.

Microvascular endothelial injury, in particular in the renal glomeruli and the brain, is the primary histopathological change underlying HUS (Richardson et al., 1988). The major virulence factor of EHEC responsible for the microvascular endothelial injury is Shiga toxin (Stx). Stx is produced by EHEC which colonizes, after ingestion and passage through an acidic stomach, the large intestine; it is then translocated to the bloodstream and transported to the target organs. Here, Stx binds to microvascular endothelial cells by interaction with its specific receptor, globotriaosylceramide (Waddell et al., 1988; Müthing and Distler, 2010). Binding of Stx to its target cells presumably initiates a complex chain of events, including coagulation and proinflammatory processes, resulting in HUS (Bielaszewska and Karch, 2005). In additon to Stx, several other potential virulence determinants have been identified in EHEC. These include toxins such as the cytolethal distending toxin (CDT)-V (Janka et al., 2003), a new member of the CDT family, and EHEC hemolysin (Schmidt et al., 1995). CDT-V is a genotoxin and cyclomodulin which causes DNA damage in human microvascular endothelial cells, resulting in G_2 cell cycle arrest, inhibition of proliferation, and finally cell death (Bielaszewska et al., 2005a). EHEC hemolysin, a member of the RTX (repeat-in-toxin) family, is a pore-forming toxin which rapidly lyses human microvascular endothelial cells (Aldick et al., 2007). Other putative virulence determinants of EHEC include serine proteases (EspP) (Brockmeyer et al., 2007; Brunder et al., 1997), subtilase cytotoxin (Paton et al., 2004), and fimbrial and nonfimbrial adhesins, the best studied of which is the intimin encoded by *eae*, a part of the pathogenicity island locus of enterocyte effacement (Yu and Kaper, 1992). Some non-Stx virulence factors (e.g., intimin, EHEC hemolysin, and EspP) are widely distributed among EHEC strains, whereas others (e.g., CDT-V and Sfp fimbriae) are restricted to EHEC isolates of particular serotypes (Müsken et al., 2008; Bielaszewska et al., 2004; Janka et al., 2003; Friedrich et al., 2006).

The interaction of EHEC virulence factors with human cells has been analyzed using various cultured cells derived from intestinal epithelial and micro- and macrovascular endothelial cells (Aldick et al., 2007; Bielaszewska et al., 2005a; Friedrich et al., 2006; Müsken et al., 2008). Data from these experiments prompt a reassessment of EHEC pathogenesis, indicating the effects of cocktails of virulence determinants rather than of Stx alone. The rapidly changing conditions which the pathogen encounters during the human infection, in particular during passage through the gastrointestinal tract, require a rapid adaptation to the particular conditions which may be associated with chromosomal changes, specifically with the loss of virulence determinants.

GENOMES OF EHEC

The ca. 5.5-Mb large chromosomes of EHEC O157:H7 strains consist of a core genome of 4.1 Mb, which is similar to the size of the chromosome of *E. coli* K-12 (Leopold et al., 2009; Hayashi et al., 2001; Perna et al., 2001; Ogura et al., 2009). Genes located on the core chromosome exhibit a relatively homogenous G+C content and a specific codon usage. These segments are separated by ca. 1.4 Mb of O-islands, also termed S-loops, that are absent from *E. coli* K-12 (Hayashi et al., 2001; Perna et al., 2001). These DNA stretches harbor genes with a G+C content and a codon usage which differ from those of the "core" genome. This "flexible" gene pool encodes additional traits that contribute to the pathogenesis, fitness, and adaptation of EHEC. The flexible gene pool consists of variable chromosomal regions and includes mobile and accessory genetic elements such as bacteriophages, plasmids, genomic/pathogenicity islands, insertion sequences, and transposons. The genomes of EHEC O26, O111, and O103 have a similar mosaic structure, but they differ markedly with respect to virulence genes from EHEC O157 (Ogura et al., 2009). The lability of horizontally acquired genomic elements, such as pathogenicity islands, and especially of bacteriophages, increases the possibility of genomic alterations during human infections. Most EHEC strains possess one or more large plasmids.

The large EHEC plasmid as a whole is relatively stable but also contains a variety of insertion elements that can lead to mobilization of plasmid-encoded putative virulence factors (Brunder et al., 1999, 2006). Genes or gene clusters identified on the large plasmid pO157 in *E. coli* O157:H7 which have been linked to the virulence and some ecological factors of EHEC include the EHEC-hemolysin operon (EHEC-*hly*); genes encoding a periplasmic catalase-peroxidase (KatP), a type II secretion system, and the secreted serine-protease EspP; and the *toxB* gene, which is involved in adherence. *stcE* is reported to encode a metalloprotease, and the large plasmid of SF EHEC O157:H$^-$ (pSFO157) is approximately 30% larger than pSFO157 but lacks the *esp*, *katP*, and *toxB* genes and possesses a more complete transfer region and a *sfp* fimbrial operon (Brunder et al., 2006).

Differences between EHEC O157:H7 strains have been considered to usually result from *stx* genotypes (Jelacic et al., 2003; Friedrich et al., 2002), from possession of particular virulence factors such as CDT-V (Friedrich et al., 2007), and from discrete chromosomal insertions or deletions rather than from single-nucleotide polymorphisms (SNPs) (Kudva et al., 2002). However, recently more than 500 EHEC O157:H7 clinical isolates have been genotyped on the basis of 96 SNPs to analyze changes in the genome content in general and specific differences of individual O157 lineages with regard to clinical presentation and disease severity. One O157:H7 clade was significantly more strongly associated with HUS than were other O157:H7 lineages (Manning et al., 2008). Leopold et al. (2009) recently demonstrated that SNP profiling, if applied to sufficient loci, could better differentiate strains of *E. coli* O157:H7 because unlike other mutations, SNPs are quite stable. Moreover, the backbone open reading frame sequence is precise and prone to minimal errors of interpretation. They further suggest that an emergent subpopulation of cluster 1 diverged into new clusters and probably was transmitted from the Old World to the New World. Another study aimed to identify SNPs in *tir*, encoding the translocated intimin receptor in *E. coli* O157:H7. *tir* polymorphisms could be correlated with the ability of *E. coli* O157:H7 strains to cause human disease (Bono et al., 2007).

IDENTIFICATION OF GENETIC CHANGES DURING EHEC INFECTIONS

Genome plasticity of *E. coli* is accelerated under in vivo conditions. To investigate genetic changes of EHEC in patients with HUS, we analyzed consecutive stool samples from such patients by detecting *stx* and *eae* genes and by using a cytotoxicity assay to detect free Stx (Mellmann et al., 2005). In initial stool samples from 137 patients, we identified *stx*-positive/*eae*-positive strains of serotypes O157:H7/H$^-$ (nonmotile), O145:H28/H$^-$, O111:H8/H$^-$, O103:H2, and O26:H11/H$^-$, while five patients shed *stx*-negative/*eae*-positive strains of serotypes O26:H11/H$^-$, O145:H$^-$, and O157:H$^-$. When follow-up (approximately 1 week later) stool samples from these patients were analyzed by the same procedures, the proportion of those who shed *stx*-positive/*eae*-positive strains had dramatically decreased whereas the proportion of those who shed *stx*-negative/*eae*-positive strains had increased. In seven additional patients who initially shed *stx*-positive/*eae*-positive strains of serotypes O26:H11/H$^-$(six patients) or O157:H$^-$ (one patient), the initial shed strains were completely replaced by *stx*-negative/*eae*-positive derivatives of the same serotypes. Moreover, free fecal Stx was present in the initial stool samples but absent from the follow-up stool samples of these seven patients.

To determine the origin of the *stx*-negative/*eae*-positive *E. coli* strains in stools of HUS patients, we compared them with the EHEC isolated from the same patients. *stx*-negative/*eae*-positive strains share with the corresponding EHEC isolates serotypes, virulence patterns, and the phylogenetic background as determined by multilocus sequence typing (MLST) (Fig. 1). Thus, a plausible explanation for their presence in stools of patients with HUS, which is typically caused by EHEC, is that the *stx*-negative/*eae*-positive strains derived from the original infecting EHEC strains by the loss of the *stx* gene during infection. Therefore, we designated these strains EHEC-LST (EHEC that lost Stx) (Bielaszewska et al., 2007a). *stx* genes are encoded in the genomes of temperate bacteriophages which can be deleted from their genomic integration sites by different in vitro and in vivo stimuli, and these

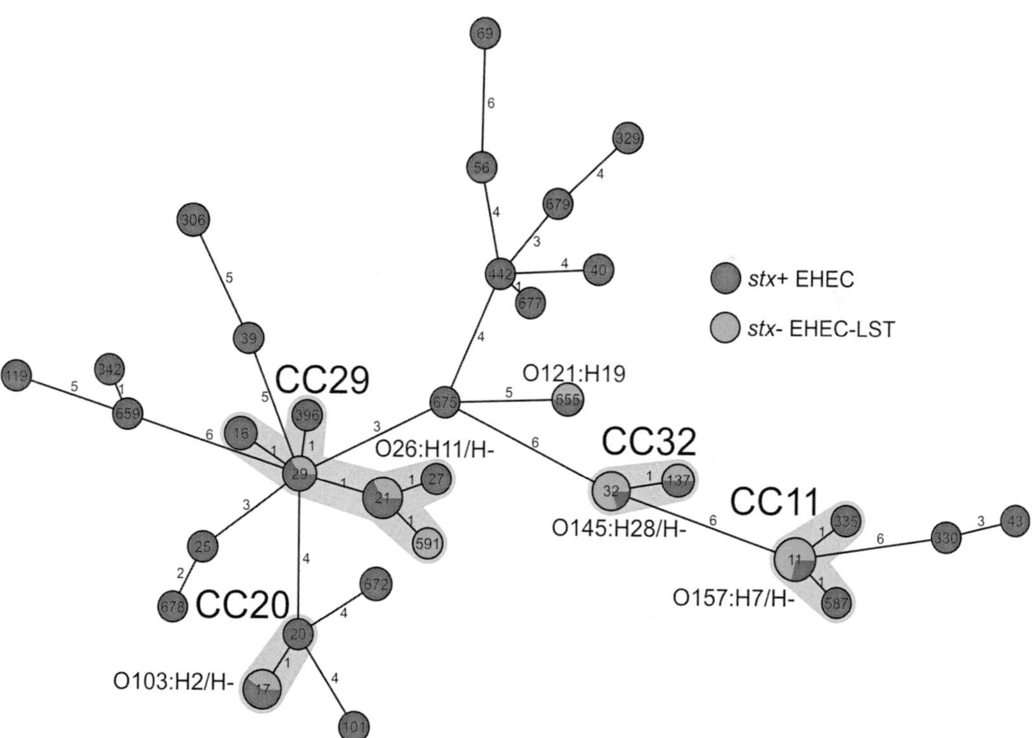

FIGURE 1 Minimum spanning tree based on the allelic profiles of an MLST analysis of 42 *stx*$^+$/*eae*$^+$ EHEC strains (red), representing all currently known serotypes and MLST sequence types (ST) of HUS-associated EHEC, and 17 *stx*$^-$/*eae*$^+$ *E. coli* strains (EHEC-LST; green) from corresponding serogroups O26, O103, O121, O145, and O157. Each ST is represented by a circle labeled with its ST. The numbers on the connecting lines represent the number of differing alleles from the seven housekeeping genes of the MLST scheme. Clonal complexes (CC) are, if applicable, shaded in grey and named in accordance with the *E. coli* MLST website (http://mlst.ucc.ie/mlst/dbs/Ecoli).

data suggest that such conditions might also be present in the human body (Wagner and Waldor, 2002). It is, however, unknown if the complete phages are lost in all strains.

INTERSEROTYPE DIFFERENCES IN CONVERSION OF EHEC TO EHEC-LST

EHEC of different serotypes differ in the frequency of *stx* gene loss. A replacement of the original infecting EHEC strain by a *stx*-negative/*eae*-positive strain of the same serotype during infection was observed in 28.6% of patients infected with EHEC O26:H11/H^- and 3.3% of patients infected with SF EHEC O157:H^- but did not occur in any of 61 patients infected with typical non-sorbitol-fermenting (NSF) EHEC O157:H7 (Mellmann et al., 2005). In another study, the ratio between SF O157:H^- and NSF O157:H7 strains among EHEC-LST isolated from patients with HUS was ca. 7:1, which contrasts with the ratio of these serotypes among EHEC isolated from HUS patients in Germany (1:3) (Bielaszewska et al., 2007a). Furthermore, a significant difference in the frequency of *stx* loss between EHEC O157:H7 and SF EHEC O157:H^- was indicated by our study, where *stx*-negative/*eae*-positive SF *E. coli* O157:H^- were found in stools of 12.7% of patients with bloody or nonbloody diarrhea but *E. coli* O157:H7 strains were found in stools of only 0.8% of such patients (Friedrich et al., 2007). The reason(s) for these apparent differences in the stability of *stx* genes among EHEC of different serotypes, which plausibly reflect differences in stability of *stx* phages in such strains, is unknown. We noted that although EHEC O111:H8/H^- is relatively frequently associated with HUS and bloody diarrhea (Bielaszewska et al., 2007a, 2008; Mellmann, 2005), no *stx*-negative/*eae*-positive strains of this serotype were found in such patients (Bielaszewska, 2007a, 2008; Mellmann et al., 2005). One explanation may be that stx_1, which is the most prevalent *stx* in EHEC O111 (Zhang et al., 2007), is located within a defective prophage which has been immobilized in the EHEC genome (Creuzburg et al., 2005), preventing the *stx* loss by phage excision.

CONSEQUENCES OF IN VIVO GENETIC CHANGES IN EHEC

Epidemiological Implications of *stx* Loss

Loss of *stx* by outbreak EHEC strains has been demonstrated or suspected in several studies (Alpers et al., 2009; Friedrich et al., 2007; Bielaszewska et al., 2007b; Mellmann et al., 2008; Muniesa et al., 2003; Schimmer et al., 2008). However, based on currently used criteria, *stx*-negative strains, even though of the same serotype, would not be considered epidemiologically related to *stx*-positive strains. Therefore, cognizance of the possibility of *stx* loss during infection and subsequent spread of the *stx*-negative derivative, and systematic searching for EHEC-LST in addition to EHEC, in outbreak investigations, can assist epidemiologists in correctly linking epidemiologically related cases, identifying the source of the infection, and tracing modes of its spread and transmission to humans. Notably, in such investigations it should be considered that multiple losses and gains of *stx* phages, which plausibly occur in the strain during the course of the outbreak, might diversify the *E. coli* genomic architecture, as demonstrated by more or less pronounced alterations in pulsed-field gel electrophoresis (PFGE) patterns. Such phage-driven alterations of PFGE patterns have been reproduced in vitro (Bielaszewska et al., 2007b; Feng et al., 2001; Murase et al., 1999). These changes can affect strains which possess a single *stx* gene (Bielaszewska et al., 2007b) but also strains harboring two copies of a stx_2 gene where one copy has been lost. Therefore, the possibility of an altered PFGE pattern resulting from loss of a *stx* phage should be always taken into account when interpreting PFGE patterns of potentially epidemiologically related *E. coli* isolates (Fig. 2).

Diagnostic Consequences of *stx* Loss

The reason why most patients with bloody diarrhea or HUS who shed EHEC-LST at the time of stool analysis are missed by currently used diagnostic protocols is that stool samples from such patients are analyzed solely for EHEC by methods that rely mostly on the detection of the

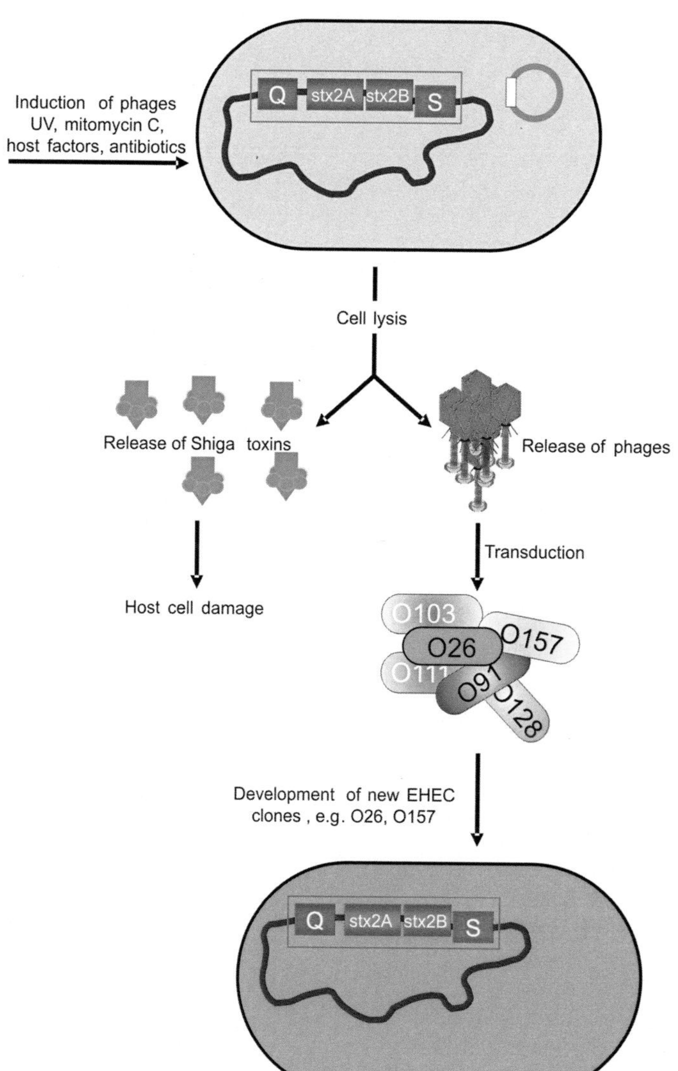

FIGURE 2 Schematic presentation of *stx2* loss and gain during the development of new EHEC clones by phage induction, release, and transduction of *stx* phages. Q, transcription activator, S, cell lysis protein.

stx gene (PCR) or produced Stx (various immunoassays). Such procedures miss *stx*/Stx-negative EHEC-LST. Therefore, to identify both EHEC and EHEC-LST in stool samples, detection of *stx*/Stx must be complemented by detection of *stx*-independent target(s) which are common to both pathotypes. The *eae* gene, which is present in the majority of EHEC strains isolated from patients with HUS and bloody diarrhea in Europe (Karch et al., 2005; Beutin et al., 2004) and the United States (Brooks et al., 2005; Banatvala et al., 2001), and *escV*, another component of the locus of enterocyte effacement, appear to be appropriate additional diagnostic targets (Mellmann et al., 2005; Bielaszewska et al., 2007a, 2008; Müller et al., 2007). The *sfpA* gene, which is a component of the plasmid-borne *sfp* cluster found until now only in SF EHEC and EHEC-LST O157:H$^-$ (Friedrich et al., 2004; Bielaszewska et al., 2007a, 2008) and EHEC O165:H25/H$^-$ (Bielaszewska et al., 2009), would be a suitable non-*stx* target to screen for such strains. However, optimal detection algorithms, and non-*stx* loci, depend on geographically and temporally specific epidemiologic trends and baseline data. Considering the current epidemiology

(Karch et al., 2005; Tarr et al., 2005), the optimal diagnostic strategy for both EHEC and EHEC-LST should consist of culture on sorbitol MacConkey (SMAC) agar (which detects classical *E. coli* O157:H7/H$^-$ based on lack of sorbitol fermentation) and enterohemolysin agar (which detects the most common non-O157:H$^-$ EHEC based on enterohemolytic phenotype) (Bielaszewska et al., 2005b; Sonntag et al., 2004; Zhang et al., 2007; Mellmann et al., 2005), Stx and/or *stx* testing, and targeting of *eae* (or *escV*) and *sfpA* (Friedrich et al., 2004; Bielaszewska et al., 2007a, 2008; Klein et al., 2002). Thus, genetic changes of the pathogen during infection must be considered when developing appropriate diagnostic strategies.

DOES *stx* LOSS MITIGATE CLINICAL OUTCOME?

It is not known whether *stx* loss during infection influences the clinical outcome. We observed that in a subset of patients with bloody diarrhea, the infection progressed to HUS even though they excreted only EHEC-LST and had no Stx in stools at the time of analysis (Bielaszewska et al., 2008). Also, EHEC-LST strains were isolated as the only pathogens from 5.5% of patients who had overt HUS (Bielaszewska et al., 2007a). These studies indicate that *stx* loss during infection does not prevent the development of systemic complications caused by Stx. On the other hand, observations from a cluster of SF *E. coli* O157:H$^-$ infections suggest that loss of *stx* by the outbreak strain might result in a milder disease (Friedrich et al., 2007). The controversial results of these studies suggest that the time point in the infection when *stx* is lost might determine whether systemic complications such as HUS develop. Specifically, *stx* loss very early in infection, before Stx is produced and injures the host microvascular cells, might prevent progression to HUS, but such a scenario is highly speculative at this point. Therefore, all patients with bloody diarrhea who shed EHEC-LST should be considered potentially infected with EHEC and therefore at risk of HUS development.

EVOLUTIONARY ASPECTS AND ADAPTATION

EHEC persists in its natural animal habitats, infects humans (where it only rarely persists for a long time), and is shed into the environment. Therefore, the ability of particular EHEC strains to lose *stx* genes and, in most cases, the *stx*-harboring phages might be related to their capability to adapt to these changing environmental conditions. The lysogenic state is potentially suicidal because it makes the bacterium prone to lysis. Thus, by generating *stx*-negative mutants, a strain can survive without automatically lysing and carrying the burden of toxin production. In this way, the loss of *stx*-encoding phage can offer a selective advantage in the gastrointestinal tract. This hypothesis is supported by findings that EHEC of particular serotypes, such as SF EHEC O157:H$^-$ and O26:H11, has been isolated from cattle as *stx*-negative variants (Lee and Choi, 2006; Anjum et al., 2003). Also, it is noteworthy that cattle surveys generally identify a larger proportion of *stx*$^-$ *E. coli* O157:H7 (Paros et al., 1993). In the human gut, such *stx*-negative variants of EHEC might be potential targets for lysogenization by *stx* phages released, e.g., from other, less virulent Stx-producing *E. coli* strains during infection. Such transduction in vivo has been demonstrated in several animal models including mice (Acheson et al., 1998) and sheep (Cornick et al., 2006) and in ligated porcine ileal loops (Toth et al., 2003).

CONCLUSIONS

Genetic changes in EHEC during infection might influence clinical outcome and have impacts on diagnosis, epidemiology, and evolution. We observed that at the time of microbiological diagnosis a subset of patients with bloody diarrhea or HUS no longer excrete the causative EHEC strains which harbor the Stx-encoding gene (*stx*) but instead excrete Stx-negative derivatives of EHEC that had lost Stx during infection (EHEC-LST). For clinicians, awareness of a potential conversion of the pathotype of the infecting EHEC during infection is essential in making decisions about correct management of the patients and appropriate therapies. Therefore, microbiological laboratories should apply an extended diagnostic scheme to the stool analyses which includes, besides detection of *stx*/Stx (which misses EHEC-LST), a non-*stx* target common to these organisms (e.g., *eae*, which encodes the adhesin intimin), and should report the results to clinicians immediately. In epidemiological investigations of EHEC outbreaks, findings of not only the outbreak EHEC strain but also epidemiologically related EHEC-LST strains should be considered when tracing the source and modes of transmission of the infection. Observations from an outbreak caused by EHEC O157 suggest that loss of *stx* by the outbreak strain might cause milder disease. The possibility of converting EHEC into EHEC-LST during infection could be potentially exploited as a basis for the development of new therapeutic strategies for EHEC infections.

ACKNOWLEDGMENTS

We thank Andreas Bauwens for skillful assistance during the creation of the figures.

Part of the presented research was supported by a grant from the EU Network ERA-NET PathoGenoMics 2 (no. 0315443) and by a grant from the Interdisciplinary Clinical Research Center (IZKF), Münster, Germany (no. Me2/023/08).

REFERENCE

Acheson, D. W., J. Reidl, X. Zhang, G. T. Keusch, J. J. Mekalanos, and M. K. Waldor. 1998. In vivo transduction with Shiga toxin 1-encoding phage. *Infect. Immun.* **66:**4496–4498.

Aldick, T., M. Bielaszewska, W. Zhang, J. Brockmeyer, H. Schmidt, A. W. Friedrich, K. S. Kim, M. A. Schmidt, and H. Karch. 2007. Hemolysin from Shiga toxin-negative *Escherichia coli* O26 strains injures microvascular endothelium. *Microbes Infect.* **9:**282–290.

Alpers, K., D. Werber, C. Frank, J. Koch, A. W. Friedrich, H. Karch, M. An der Heiden, R. Prager, A. Fruth, M. Bielaszewska, G. Morlock, A. Heissenhuber, A. Diedler, A. Gerber, and A. Ammon. 2009. Sorbitol-fermenting enterohaemorrhagic *Escherichia coli* O157:H$^-$ causes another outbreak of haemolytic uraemic syndrome in children. *Epidemiol. Infect.* **137:**389–395.

Anjum, M. F., S. Lucchini, A. Thompson, J. C. D. Hinton, and M. J. Woodward. 2003. Comparative genomic indexing reveals the phylogenomics of *Escherichia coli* pathogens. *Infect. Immun.* **71:**4674–4683.

Banatvala, N., P. M. Griffin, K. D. Greene, T. J. Barrett, W. F. Bibb, J. H. Green, and J. G. Wells. 2001. The United States National Prospective Hemolytic Uremic Syndrome Study: microbiologic, serologic, clinical, and epidemiologic findings. *J. Infect. Dis.* **183:**1063–1070.

Bell, B. P., M. Goldoft, P. M. Griffin, M. A. Davis, D. C. Gordon, P. I. Tarr, C. A. Bartleson, J. H. Lewis, T. J. Barrett, and J. G. Wells. 1994. A multistate outbreak of *Escherichia coli* O157:H7-associated bloody diarrhea and hemolytic uremic syndrome from hamburgers: the Washington experience. *JAMA* **272:**1349–1353.

Beutin, L., G. Krause, S. Zimmermann, S. Kaulfuss, and K. Gleier. 2004. Characterization of Shiga toxin-producing *Escherichia coli* strains isolated from human patients in Germany over a 3-year period. *J. Clin. Microbiol.* **42:**1099–1108.

Bielaszewska, M., B. Middendorf, R. Kock, A. W. Friedrich, A. Fruth, H. Karch, M. A. Schmidt, and A. Mellmann. 2008. Shiga toxin-negative attaching and effacing *Escherichia coli:* distinct clinical associations with bacterial phylogeny and virulence traits and inferred in-host pathogen evolution. *Clin. Infect. Dis.* **47:**208–217.

Bielaszewska, M., B. Sinha, T. Kuczius, and H. Karch. 2005a. Cytolethal distending toxin from Shiga toxin-producing *Escherichia coli* O157 causes irreversible G2/M arrest, inhibition of proliferation, and death of human endothelial cells. *Infect. Immun.* **73:**552–562.

Bielaszewska, M., M. Fell, L. Greune, R. Prager, A. Fruth, H. Tschäpe, M. A. Schmidt, and H. Karch. 2004. Characterization of cytolethal distending toxin genes and expression in Shiga toxin-producing *Escherichia coli* strains of non-O157 serogroups. *Infect. Immun.* **72:**1812–1816.

Bielaszewska, M., R. Köck, A. Friedrich, C. von Eiff, L. Zimmerhackl, H. Karch, and A. Mellmann. 2007a. Shiga toxin-mediated hemolytic uremic syndrome: time to change the diagnostic paradigm? *PLoS One* **2:**e1024.

Bielaszewska, M., R. Prager, L. Vandivinit, A. Müsken, A. Mellmann, N. J. Holt, P. I. Tarr, H. Karch, and W. Zhang. 2009. Detection and characterization of fimbrial *sfp* cluster in enterohemorrhagic *Escherichia coli* O165:H25/NM from humans and cattle. *Appl. Environ. Microbiol.* **75:**64–71.

Bielaszewska, M., R. Prager, R. Köck, A. Mellmann, W. Zhang, H. Tschäpe, P. I. Tarr, and H. Karch. 2007b. Shiga toxin gene loss and transfer in vitro and in vivo during enterohemorrhagic *Escherichia coli* O26 infection in humans. *Appl. Environ. Microbiol.* **73:**3144–3150.

Bielaszewska, M., W. Zhang, P. I. Tarr, A. Sonntag, and H. Karch. 2005b. Molecular profiling and phenotype analysis of *Escherichia coli* O26:H11 and O26:NM: secular and geographic consistency of enterohemorrhagic and enteropathogenic isolates. *J. Clin. Microbiol.* **43:**4225–4228.

Bielaszewska, M., and H. Karch. 2005. Consequences of enterohaemorrhagic *Escherichia coli* infection for the vascular endothelium. *Thromb. Haemost.* **94:**312-318.

Bono, J. L., J. E. Keen, M. L. Clawson, L. M. Durso, M. P. Heaton, and W. W. Laegreid. 2007. Association of *Escherichia coli* O157:H7 *tir* polymorphisms with human infection. *BMC Infect. Dis.* **7:**98.

Brockmeyer, J., M. Bielaszewska, A. Fruth, M. L. Bonn, A. Mellmann, H. Humpf, and H. Karch. 2007. Subtypes of the plasmid-encoded serine protease EspP in Shiga toxin-producing *Escherichia coli:* distribution, secretion, and proteolytic activity. *Appl. Environ. Microbiol.* **73:**6351–6359.

Brooks, J. T., E. G. Sowers, J. G. Wells, K. D. Greene, P. M. Griffin, R. M. Hoekstra, and N. A. Strockbine. 2005. Non-O157 Shiga toxin-producing *Escherichia coli* infections in the United States, 1983–2002. *J. Infect. Dis.* **192:**1422–1429.

Brunder, W., H. Karch, and H. Schmidt. 2006. Complete sequence of the large virulence plasmid pSFO157 of the sorbitol-fermenting enterohemorrhagic *Escherichia coli* O157:H$^-$ strain 3072/96. *Int. J. Med. Microbiol.* **296:**467–474.

Brunder, W., H. Schmidt, M. Frosch, and H. Karch. 1999. The large plasmids of Shiga toxin-producing *Escherichia coli* (STEC) are highly variable genetic elements. *Microbiology* **145:**1005–1014.

Brunder, W., H. Schmidt, and H. Karch. 1997. EspP, a novel extracellular serine protease of enterohaemorrhagic *Escherichia coli* O157:H7 cleaves human coagulation factor V. *Mol. Microbiol.* **24:**767–778.

Caprioli, A., S. Morabito, H. Brugere, and E. Oswald. 2005. Enterohaemorrhagic *Escherichia coli:* emerging issues on virulence and modes of transmission. *Vet. Res.* **36:**289–311.

Centers for Disease Control and Prevention. 2006. Ongoing multistate outbreak of *Escherichia coli* serotype O157:H7 infections associated with consumption of fresh spinach—United States, September 2006. *MMWR Morb. Mortal. Wkly. Rep.* **55:**1045–1046.

Cornick, N. A., A. F. Helgerson, V. Mai, J. M. Ritchie, and D. W. K. Acheson. 2006. In vivo transduction of an Stx-encoding phage in ruminants. *Appl. Environ. Microbiol.* **72:**5086–5088.

Creuzburg, K., B. Kohler, H. Hempel, P. Schreier, E. Jacobs, and H. Schmidt. 2005. Genetic structure and chromosomal integration site of the cryptic prophage CP-1639 encoding Shiga toxin 1. *Microbiology* **151:**941–950.

Crump, J. A., A. C. Sulka, A. J. Langer, C. Schaben, A. S. Crielly, R. Gage, M. Baysinger, M. Moll, G. Withers, D. M. Toney, S. B. Hunter, R. M. Hoekstra, S. K. Wong, P. M. Griffin, and T. J. Van Gilder. 2002. An outbreak of *Escherichia coli* O157:H7 infections among visitors to a dairy farm. *N. Engl. J. Med.* **347:**555–560.

Elliott, E. J., R. M. Robins-Browne, E. V. O'Loughlin, V. Bennett-Wood, J. Bourke, P. Henning, G. G. Hogg, J. Knight, H. Powell, and D. Redmond. 2001. Nationwide study of haemolytic uraemic syndrome: clinical, microbiological, and epidemiological features. *Arch. Dis. Child.* **85:**125–131.

Feng, P., M. Dey, A. Abe, and T. Takeda. 2001. Isogenic strain of *Escherichia coli* O157:H7 that has lost both Shiga toxin 1 and 2 genes. *Clin. Diagn. Lab. Immunol.* **8:**711–717.

Friedrich, A. W., K. V. Nierhoff, M. Bielaszewska, A. Mellmann, and H. Karch. 2004. Phylogeny, clinical associations, and diagnostic utility of the pilin subunit gene (*sfpA)* of sorbitol-fermenting, enterohemorrhagic *Escherichia coli* O157:H$^-$. *J. Clin. Microbiol.* **42:**4697–4701.

Friedrich, A. W., M. Bielaszewska, W. Zhang, M. Pulz, T. Kuczius, A. Ammon, and H. Karch. 2002. *Escherichia coli* harboring Shiga toxin 2 gene variants: frequency and association with clinical symptoms. *J. Infect. Dis.* **185:**74–84.

Friedrich, A. W., S. Lu, M. Bielaszewska, R. Prager, P. Bruns, J. Xu, H. Tschäpe, and H. Karch. 2006. Cytolethal distending toxin in *Escherichia coli* O157:H7: spectrum of conservation, structure, and endothelial toxicity. *J. Clin. Microbiol.* **44:**1844–1846.

Friedrich, A. W., W. Zhang, M. Bielaszewska, A. Mellmann, R. Köck, A. Fruth, H. Tschäpe, and H. Karch. 2007. Prevalence, virulence profiles, and clinical significance of Shiga toxin-negative variants of enterohemorrhagic *Escherichia coli* O157 infection in humans. *Clin. Infect. Dis.* **45:**39–45.

Garg, A. X., R. S. Suri, N. Barrowman, F. Rehman, D. Matsell, M. P. Rosas-Arellano, M. Salvadori, R. B. Haynes, and W. F. Clark. 2003. Long-term renal prognosis of diarrhea-associated hemolytic uremic syndrome: a systematic review, meta-analysis, and meta-regression. *JAMA* **290:**1360–1370.

Gerber, A., H. Karch, F. Allerberger, H. M. Verweyen, and L. B. Zimmerhackl. 2002. Clinical course and the role of Shiga toxin-producing *Escherichia coli* infection in the hemolytic-uremic syndrome in pediatric patients, 1997-2000, in

Germany and Austria: a prospective study. *J. Infect. Dis.* **186:**493–500.

Hayashi, T., K. Makino, M. Ohnishi, K. Kurokawa, K. Ishii, K. Yokoyama, C. G. Han, E. Ohtsubo, K. Nakayama, T. Murata, M. Tanaka, T. Tobe, T. Iida, H. Takami, T. Honda, C. Sasakawa, N. Ogasawara, T. Yasunaga, S. Kuhara, T. Shiba, M. Hattori, and M, Shinagawa. 2001. Complete genome sequence of enterohemorrhagic *Escherichia coli* O157:H7 and genomic comparison with a laboratory strain K-12. *DNA Res.* **8:**11–22.

Hilborn, E. D., J. H. Mermin, P. A. Mshar, J. L. Hadler, A. Voetsch, C. Wojtkunski, M. Swartz, R. Mshar, M. A. Lambert-Fair, J. A. Farrar, M. K. Glynn, and L. Slutsker. 1999. A multistate outbreak of *Escherichia coli* O157:H7 infections associated with consumption of mesclun lettuce. *Arch. Intern. Med.* **159:**1758–1764.

Holme, R. 2003. Drinking water contamination in Walkerton, Ontario: positive resolutions from a tragic event. *Water Sci. Technol.* **47:**1–6.

Janka, A., M. Bielaszewska, U. Dobrindt, L. Greune, M. A. Schmidt, and H. Karch. 2003. Cytolethal distending toxin gene cluster in enterohemorrhagic *Escherichia coli* O157:H$^-$ and O157:H7: characterization and evolutionary considerations. *Infect. Immun.* **71:**3634–3638.

Jelacic, J. K., T. Damrow, G. S. Chen, S. Jelacic, M. Bielaszewska, M. Ciol, H. M. Carvalho, A. R. Melton-Celsa, A. D. O'Brien, and P. I. Tarr. 2003. Shiga toxin-producing *Escherichia coli* in Montana: bacterial genotypes and clinical profiles. *J. Infect. Dis.* **188:**719–729.

Johnson, K. E., C. M. Thorpe, and C. L. Sears. 2006. The emerging clinical importance of non-O157 Shiga toxin-producing *Escherichia coli. Clin. Infect. Dis.* **43:**1587–1595.

Karch, H., P. I. Tarr, and M. Bielaszewska. 2005. Enterohaemorrhagic *Escherichia coli* in human medicine. *Int. J. Med. Microbiol.* **295:**405–418.

Klein, E. J., J. R. Stapp, C. R. Clausen, D. R. Boster, J. G. Wells, X. Qin, D. L. Swerdlow, and P. I. Tarr. 2002. Shiga toxin-producing *Escherichia coli* in children with diarrhea: a prospective point-of-care study. *J. Pediatr.* **141:**172–177.

Kudva, I. T., P. S. Evans, N. T. Perna, T. J. Barrett, F. M. Ausubel, F. R. Blattner, and S. B. Calderwood. 2002. Strains of *Escherichia coli* O157:H7 differ primarily by insertions or deletions, not single-nucleotide polymorphisms. *J. Bacteriol.* **184:**1873–1879.

Lee, J. H., and S. Choi. 2006. Isolation and characteristics of sorbitol-fermenting *Escherichia coli* O157 strains from cattle. *Microbes Infect.* **8:**2021–2026.

Leopold, S. R., V. Magrini, N. J. Holt, N. Shaikh, E. R. Mardis, J. Cagno, Y. Ogura, A. Iguchi, T. Hayashi, A. Mellmann, H. Karch, T. E. Besser, S. A. Sawyer, T. S. Whittam, and P. I. Tarr. 2009. A precise reconstruction of the emergence and constrained radiations of *Escherichia coli* O157 portrayed by backbone concatenomic analysis. *Proc. Natl. Acad. Sci. USA* **106:**8713–8718.

Levine, M. M., J. G. Xu, J. B. Kaper, H. Lior, V. Prado, B. Tall, J. Nataro, H. Karch, and K. Wachsmuth. 1987. A DNA probe to identify enterohemorrhagic *Escherichia coli* of O157:H7 and other serotypes that cause hemorrhagic colitis and hemolytic uremic syndrome. *J. Infect. Dis.* **156:**175–182.

Manning, S. D., A. S. Motiwala, A. C. Springman, W. Qi, D. W. Lacher, L. M. Ouellette, J. M. Mladonicky, P. Somsel, J. T. Rudrik, S. E. Dietrich, W. Zhang, B. Swaminathan, D. Alland, and T. Whittam. 2008. Variation in virulence among clades of *Escherichia coli* O157:H7 associated with disease outbreaks. *Proc. Natl. Acad. Sci. USA* **105:**4868–4873.

Mellmann, A., M. Bielaszewska, L. B. Zimmerhackl, R. Prager, D. Harmsen, H. Tschäpe, and H. Karch. 2005. Enterohemorrhagic *Escherichia coli* in human infection: in vivo evolution of a bacterial pathogen. *Clin. Infect. Dis.* **41:**785–792.

Mellmann, A., S. Lu, H. Karch, J. Xu, D. Harmsen, M. A. Schmidt, and M. Bielaszewska. 2008. Recycling of Shiga toxin 2 genes in sorbitol-fermenting enterohemorrhagic *Escherichia coli* O157:NM. *Appl. Environ. Microbiol.* **74:**67–72.

Michino, H., K. Araki, S. Minami, S. Takaya, N. Sakai, M. Miyazaki, A. Ono, and H. Yanagawa. 1999. Massive outbreak of *Escherichia coli* O157:H7 infection in schoolchildren in Sakai City, Japan, associated with consumption of white radish sprouts. *Am. J. Epidemiol.* **150:**787–796.

Müller, D., L. Greune, G. Heusipp, H. Karch, A. Fruth, H. Tschäpe, and M. A. Schmidt. 2007. Identification of unconventional intestinal pathogenic *Escherichia coli* isolates expressing intermediate virulence factor profiles by using a novel single-step multiplex PCR. *Appl. Environ. Microbiol.* **73:**3380–3390.

Muniesa, M., M. de Simon, G. Prats, D. Ferrer, H. Panella, and J. Jofre. 2003. Shiga toxin 2-converting bacteriophages associated with clonal variability in *Escherichia coli* O157:H7 strains of human origin isolated from a single outbreak. *Infect. Immun.* **71:**4554–4562.

Murase, T., S. Yamai, and H. Watanabe. 1999. Changes in pulsed-field gel electrophoresis patterns in clinical isolates of enterohemorrhagic *Escherichia coli* O157:H7 associated with loss of Shiga toxin genes. *Curr. Microbiol.* **38:**48–50.

Müsken, A., M. Bielaszewska, L. Greune, C. H. Schweppe, J. Müthing, H. Schmidt, M. A. Schmidt, H. Karch, and W. Zhang. 2008.

Anaerobic conditions promote expression of Sfp fimbriae and adherence of sorbitol-fermenting enterohemorrhagic *Escherichia coli* O157:NM to human intestinal epithelial cells. *Appl. Environ. Microbiol.* **74:**1087–1093.

Müthing, J., and U. Distler. 2010. Advances on the compositional analysis of glycosphingolipids combining thin-layer chromatography with mass spectrometry. *Mass. Spectrom. Rev.* **29:**425–479.

Ogura, Y., T. Ooka, A. Iguchi, H. Toh, M. Asadulghani, K. Oshima, T. Kodama, H. Abe, K. Nakayama, K. Kurokawa, T. Tobe, M. Hattori, and T. Hayashi. 2009. Comparative genomics reveal the mechanism of the parallel evolution of O157 and non-O157 enterohemorrhagic *Escherichia coli*. *Proc. Natl. Acad. Sci. USA* **106:**17939–17944.

Paros, M., P. I. Tarr, H. Kim, T. E. Besser, and D. D. Hancock. 1993. A comparison of human and bovine *Escherichia coli* O157:H7 isolates by toxin genotype, plasmid profile, and bacteriophage lambda-restriction fragment length polymorphism profile. *J. Infect. Dis.* **168:**1300–1303.

Paton, A. W., P. Srimanote, U. M. Talbot, H. Wang, and J. C. Paton. 2004. A new family of potent AB(5) cytotoxins produced by Shiga toxigenic *Escherichia coli*. *J. Exp. Med.* **200:**35–46.

Perna, N. T., G. Plunkett, V. Burland, B. Mau, J. D. Glasner, D. J. Rose, G. F. Mayhew, P. S. Evans, J. Gregor, H. A. Kirkpatrick, G. Posfai, J. Hackett, S. Klink, A. Boutin, Y. Shao, L. Miller, E. J. Grotbeck, N. W. Davis, A. Lim, E. T. Dimalanta, K. D. Potamousis, J. Apodaca, T. S. Anantharaman, J. Lin, G. Yen, D. C. Schwartz, R. A. Welch, and F. R. Blattner. 2001. Genome sequence of enterohaemorrhagic *Escherichia coli* O157:H7. *Nature* **409:**529–533.

Richardson, S. E., M. A. Karmali, L. E. Becker, and C. R. Smith. 1988. The histopathology of the hemolytic uremic syndrome associated with verocytotoxin-producing *Escherichia coli* infections. *Hum. Pathol.* **19:**1102–1108.

Riley, L. W., R. S. Remis, S. D. Helgerson, H. B. McGee, J. G. Wells, B. R. Davis, R. J. Hebert, E. S. Olcott, L. M. Johnson, N. T. Hargrett, P. A. Blake, and M. L. Cohen. 1983. Hemorrhagic colitis associated with a rare *Escherichia coli* serotype. *N. Engl. J. Med.* **308:**681–685.

Schimmer, B., K. Nygard, H. Eriksen, J. Lassen, B. Lindstedt, L. T. Brandal, G. Kapperud, and P. Aavitsland. 2008. Outbreak of haemolytic uraemic syndrome in Norway caused by *stx2* positive *Escherichia coli* O103:H25 traced to cured mutton sausages. *BMC Infect. Dis.* **8:**41.

Schmidt, H., L. Beutin, and H. Karch. 1995. Molecular analysis of the plasmid-encoded hemolysin of *Escherichia coli* O157:H7 strain EDL 933. *Infect. Immun.* **63:**1055–1061.

Sonntag, A., R. Prager, M. Bielaszewska, W. Zhang, A. Fruth, H. Tschäpe, and H. Karch. 2004. Phenotypic and genotypic analyses of enterohemorrhagic *Escherichia coli* O145 strains from patients in Germany. *J. Clin. Microbiol.* **42:**954–962.

Tarr, P. I., C. A. Gordon, and W. L. Chandler. 2005. Shiga-toxin-producing *Escherichia coli* and haemolytic uraemic syndrome. *Lancet* **365:**1073–1086.

Toth, I., H. Schmidt, M. Dow, A. Malik, E. Oswald, and B. Nagy. 2003. Transduction of porcine enteropathogenic *Escherichia coli* with a derivative of a Shiga toxin 2-encoding bacteriophage in a porcine ligated ileal loop system. *Appl. Environ. Microbiol.* **69:**7242–7247.

Waddell, T., S. Head, M. Petric, A. Cohen, and C. Lingwood. 1988. Globotriosyl ceramide is specifically recognized by the *Escherichia coli* verocytotoxin 2. *Biochem. Biophys. Res. Commun.* **152:**674–679.

Wagner, P. L., and M. K. Waldor. 2002. Bacteriophage control of bacterial virulence. *Infect. Immun.* **70:**3985–3993.

Werber, D., B. W. Mason, M. R. Evans, and R. L. Salmon. 2008. Preventing household transmission of Shiga toxin-producing *Escherichia coli* O157 infection: promptly separating siblings might be the key. *Clin. Infect. Dis.* **46:**1189–1196.

Yu, J., and J. B. Kaper. 1992. Cloning and characterization of the *eae* gene of enterohaemorrhagic *Escherichia coli* O157:H7. *Mol. Microbiol.* **6:**411–417.

Zhang, W., A. Mellmann, A. Sonntag, L. Wieler, M. Bielaszewska, H. Tschäpe, H. Karch, and A. W. Friedrich. 2007. Structural and functional differences between disease-associated genes of enterohaemorrhagic *Escherichia coli* O111. *Int. J. Med. Microbiol.* **297:**17–26.

GENOMIC FLUIDITY OF THE HUMAN GASTRIC PATHOGEN *Helicobacter pylori*

Niyaz Ahmed, Singamaneni Haritha Devi, Shivendra Tenguria, Mohammad Majid, Syed Asad Rahman, and Seyed E. Hasnain

3

Helicobacter pylori is a gram-negative, spiral-shaped, microaerophilic bacterium that colonizes the gastric mucosa of humans, chronically infecting almost half of the world's population. Infection with this pathogen causes diseases and syndromes that show different histological signs ranging from chronic gastritis in a majority of infected people to peptic ulcer in a small fraction, and rarely leading to adenocarcinoma and mucosa-associated lymphoid tissue lymphoma (Ahmed et al., 2009; Huang et al., 1998; Ikeno et al., 1999). It is not known what determines the varied clinical outcome; however, it is likely that a complex interplay of strain virulence, host genetics, and environmental factors might serve as an underlying cause. The extensive genetic diversity among the clinical isolates from different patient populations is a distinctive feature of *H. pylori* (Fig. 1).

Niyaz Ahmed, Pathogen Biology Laboratory, School of Life Sciences, University of Hyderabad, and Institute of Life Sciences, University of Hyderabad Campus, Hyderabad, India. *Singamaneni Haritha Devi, Shivendra Tenguria, and Mohammad Majid,* Pathogen Biology Laboratory, School of Life Sciences, University of Hyderabad, Hyderabad, India. *Syed Asad Rahman,* EMBL-European Bioinformatics Institute, Wellcome Trust Genome Campus, Hinxton, Cambridge, United Kingdom. *Seyed E. Hasnain,* Institute of Life Sciences, University of Hyderabad Campus, Hyderabad, and School of Biological Sciences, Indian Institute of Technology Delhi, New Delhi, India.

It has been found that ~7% of the genes are strain specific that might influence the pathogenicity of *H. pylori* (Alm et al., 1999; Janssen et al., 2001). Genomic fluidity associated with *H. pylori* has important consequences for clinical management of the gastroduodenal diseases caused by colonization with this significant pathogen. In this chapter, we discuss attributes of the genomes of different *Helicobacter* strains and the roles of strain-specific genes from the genomic plasticity region.

THE *HELICOBACTER* GENOMES

Like many other pathogenic bacteria, *H. pylori* is being sequenced to generate replicate, whole-genome sequences. Such replicate genomes (Ahmed, 2009; Lapierre and Gogarten, 2009) are likely to yield novel "backup" functions encoded from within the "dockyard" of accessory genes called the plasticity region cluster (Yamaoka, 2008). Previous studies point to such a pool of strain-specific genes in pathogens such as *H. pylori*, which could be useful in adaptation to a particular host population (Yamaoka, 2008; Ge and Taylor, 1999; Ahmed et al., 2008; Romo-González et al., 2009). Another important reason to sequence replicate genomes of *H. pylori* entails the need to study chronological evolution within

Genome Plasticity and Infectious Diseases,
Edited by J. Hacker, U. Dobrindt, and R. Kurth,

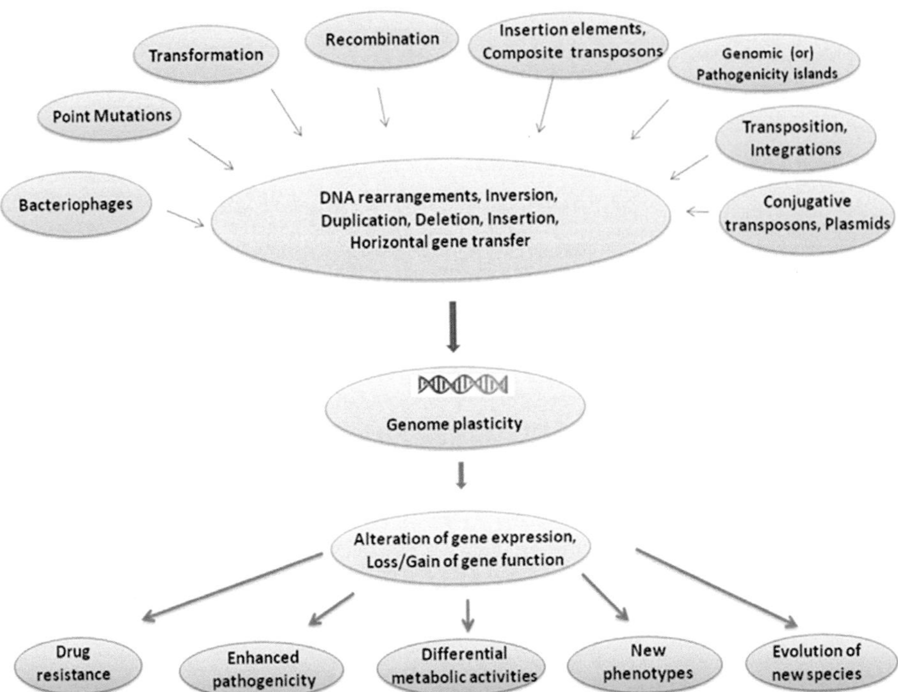

FIGURE 1 Schema showing the origins of genetic heterogeneity among bacteria and its implications. The genetic diversity among microbial pathogens is possibly due to the acquisition or loss of DNA. Mechanisms such as mutation, transformation, recombination, transposition, transduction, and horizontal gene transfer, and genetic elements such as genomic or pathogenic islands, plasmids, etc., result in DNA rearrangements, inversions, duplications, deletions, and insertions that lead to alteration of gene expression and to loss or gain of gene function. These alterations in the genome are responsible for novel phenotypes, varied drug resistance, enhanced pathogenicity, and bacterial fitness in diverse environments.

a single host. The nature and extent of genetic rearrangement accumulated by the chronically inhabiting pathogens such as *H. pylori* (on long timescales) during colonization of different host niches are not known; determination of the advantages of polymorphisms that impart needed fitness to pathogens or commensals to colonize and inhabit their preferred hosts (niches) needs additional in-depth studies (Ahmed, 2009). While some experiments have been conducted to explore chronological strain diversity through multilocus genotyping (Prouzet-Mauléon et al., 2005), microarrays (Israel et al., 2001), and limited sequencing (Alvi et al., 2007), whole-genome profiling of such isolates has not been performed. This needs to be done as early as possible, especially for strains which are obtained at different intervals and from different sites of individual patients, to investigate the occurrence of possible insertions, deletions, and substitutions (and mechanisms thereof) including their functional significance related to host adaptation and gain of niche. Apart from this, geographically distinct strains and their multiple representatives could be sequenced to explore local advantages that prevail in certain geographical regions in terms of host adaptation or disease outcome; for example, *H. pylori* infection in the Indian population (despite a very high colonization rate of up to 90%) rarely leads to serious consequences such as gastric cancer in a significant majority of patients who test positive for *H. pylori* infection (Akhter et al., 2007). Biological coordinates of such "protection," if any, should be studied with the help of bacterial genome sequence data obtained from a number of strains. This appears to be a possibility in the not too distant future, given that the next-generation sequencing methods are becoming increasingly affordable. Also, the costs of whole-genome sequencing should be low, given that the genome sequence is approximately about 1.67 Mb. We analyzed the following complete genome sequences of *Helicobacter* that are available in the public-domain databases, six from *H. pylori* and one each from *H. acinonychis* and *H. hepaticus*. These sequenced strains of *H. pylori* were obtained from individuals of varied clinical backgrounds and different geographic locations: strain 26695 was from an English patient with gastritis (Tomb et al.,1997); strain J99 was from an American patient with a duodenal ulcer (Alm et al., 1999); strain HPAG1 was from a Swedish patient with chronic atrophic gastritis (Oh et al., 2006); strain Shi470 was from an individual from the remote Amazon (unpublished data); strain B38 was from a patient with mucosa-associated lymphoid tissue lymphoma (unpublished data); strain P12 was from a German patient (unpublished data); and strain G27 was from an Italian patient (Baltrus et al., 2009). While strain Sheeba of *H. acinonychis* was found in large felines (Eppinger et al., 2006), strain ATCC 51449 of *H. hepaticus* corresponds to a laboratory mouse with chronic hepatitis and hepatocellular neoplasia (Suerbaum et al., 2003). The genomic features of these strains are presented in Table 1.

Our comparative genomic analysis (unpublished) of the eight complete genomes of *Helicobacter* indicated that the number of coding genes per genome in different strains and species of *Helicobacter* ranges from 1,488 to 1,875. Three different species of *Helicobacter* share only about half of their genes (47.4% for *H. acinonychis*, 41.4% for *H. hepaticus*, and 49.8% for *H. pylori*). The number of genes in common between the different species of *Helicobacter* that make up their core genome was found to be around 750 (Fig. 2). We analyzed two core genome data sets, one at the genus level and the other at the species level. The *Helicobacter* core genome plateaus around 774 genes, and the core genome of *H. pylori* plateaus around 1,244 genes, suggesting the possibility of considering and analyzing a

TABLE 1 Features of the *H. pylori* genomes

Species	*H. pylori*	*H. pylori*	*H. pylori*	*H. pylori*	*H. pylori*	*H. pylori*	*H. acinonychis*	*H. hepaticus*
Strain	26695	J99	HPAG1	Shi470	P12	G27	Sheeba	ATCC 51449
Accession no.	NC_000915	NC_000921	NC_008086	NC_010698	NC_011498	NC_011333	NC_008229	NC_004917
Hosts	Humans	Humans	Humans	Humans	Humans	Humans	Cats	Rodents
Chromosome size (bp)	1,667,867	1,643,831	1,596,366	1,608,548	1,673,813	1,652,982	1,553,927	1,799,146
G+C content (%)	38	39	39	38	38	38	38	35
No. of genes	1,627	1,534	1,574	1,647	1,624	1,570	1,654	1,915
No. of protein-coding genes	1,573	1,488	1,532	1,568	1,568	1,493	1,612	1,875
Coding area (%)	90	90	91	88	89	86	89	93
No. of structural RNAs	43	42	42	42	42	43	42	40
Reference	Tomb et al., 1997	Alm et al., 1999	Oh et al., 2006	Unpublished	Unpublished	Baltrus et al., 2009	Eppinger et al., 2006	Suerbaum et al., 2003

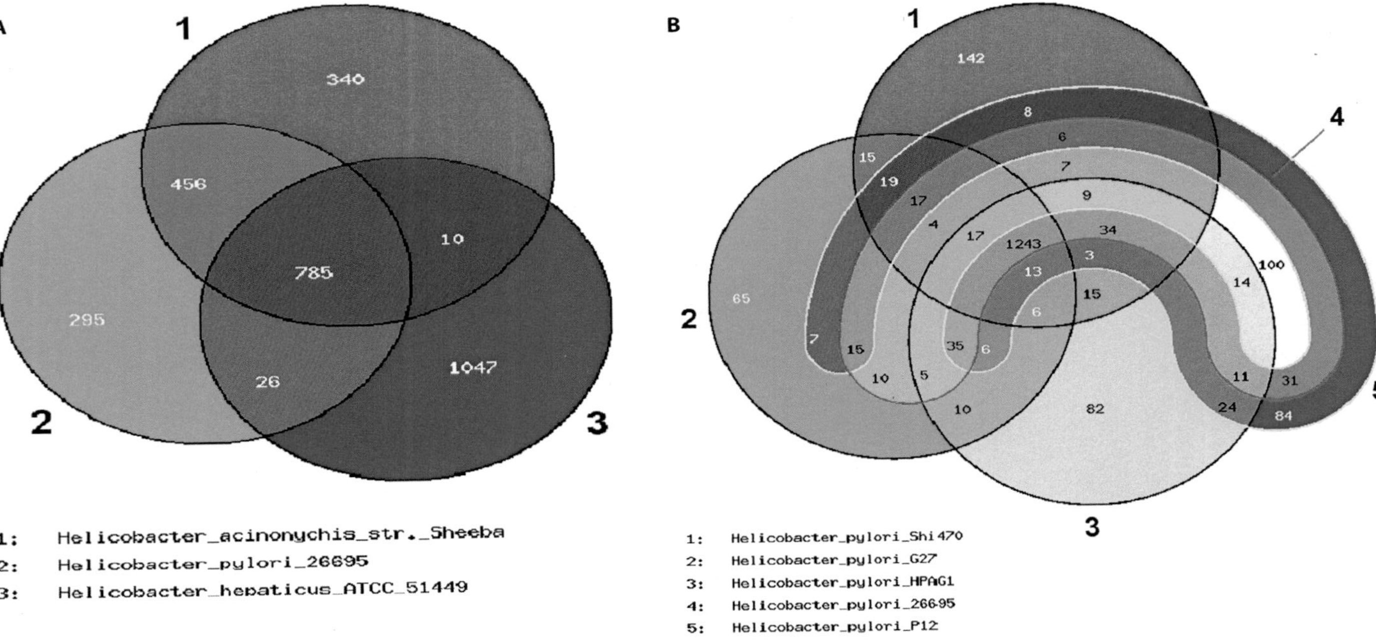

FIGURE 2 Orthologous genes of helicobacters (common gene pools): Every area in the Venn diagram represents a subset of the compared genomes and is labeled with the number of genes in the concerned subset. *Helicobacter* shares about 774 genes at the genome level, and *H. pylori* shares about 1,244 genes, indicating closer connections at species level with conserved functions of genes. The *H. pylori* core genome plateaus around ~1,244 genes with conserved functions, wherein horizontal gene transfer and positive selection are playing key roles in the adaptive evolution of this core genome.

core genome at both genus and species levels. The pangenome of *Helicobacter* consists of 3,575 genes (based on eight genome sequences), and that of *Helicobacter pylori* consists of 2,169 genes (based on six genome sequences). The number of genes that have no orthologs in any other genome of the genus, i.e., singletons, was found to be 110 *(H. acinonychis)*, 1,017 *(H. hepaticus)*, 44 (*H. pylori* 26695), 32 (*H. pylori* G27), 30 (*H. pylori* HPAG1), 14 (*H. pylori* J99), 26 (*H. pylori* P12), and 116 (*H. pylori* Shi470).

We also compared *Helicobacter* genomes at the biochemical level, based on the presence of enzymes in their metabolic pathway (data taken from KEGG [http://www.genome.jp/kegg/catalog/org_list.html]). It is clear from such analysis (Fig. 3) that the genomes of the various *Helicobacter* strains have more enzymes in common with each other than with *Escherichia coli* or *Salmonella enterica* serovar Typhimurium, although the *Helicobacter* genomes appear closest to the *Campylobacter jejuni* genome. An interesting characteristic of the *Helicobacter pylori* genome was made apparent when we zoomed in on the *Helicobacter* genome clusters. The *Helicobacter* genome was found to be subdivided into two clades, highlighting the fact that they have two distinct modes of biochemical transformation. It would be very interesting if such varied metabolic repertoires indeed represent genomic fluidity across these two *Helicobacter* clades.

GENETIC MECHANISMS UNDERLYING GENOME DIVERSITY IN *H. PYLORI*

The spontaneous mutations occur at a very high rate in *H. pylori*. The high frequency of mutations is possibly due to the lack of methyl-directed pathway for recognizing and repairing spontaneous mutations and in turn may be responsible for the high genetic variability between the strains. Kang et al. (2006) described a strategy for generating enhanced diversity of *H. pylori* in stringent environments wherein they exposed the *H. pylori* to reactive nitrogen and oxygen species (RNS/ROS), the natural stress elements present around them due to proinflammatory processes caused by the bacterium. A significant increase in spontaneous mutations was observed, along with intergenomic recombination and rearrangements between DNA direct repetitive elements. Further, in silico analysis of these elements showed that they are located in pathogenicity islands and restriction/modification systems, indicating the occurrence of mutations within specific genetic loci at the time of stress. This (direct DNA damage-induced mutagenesis) might be responsible for the successful colonization and persistence of *H. pylori* within the gastric niches and may be the principal mechanism evolved to allow adaptation to different environments.

Recombination is an important source for both micro- and macrodiversity in *Helicobacter* genomes. The intragenomic and intergenomic recombinations are caused by repetitive elements commonly present in *H. pylori* genomes and by natural transformation, respectively. Frequent recombination within alleles of *H. pylori* results in microdiversity of the genomes (i.e., a high degree of genomic diversity among strains in the sequences of single genes) (Suerbaum et al., 1998). In *H. pylori*, the arrangement of marker genes on the chromosome was also found to be quite variable between strains. The presence of DNA repeats and plasmids with sequence homologies to the chromosome indicates the presence of strong regions of diploidy. This shows that recombination is involved in regulation of macrodiversity too (i.e., the different arrangement of genes across the genomes) (Alm et al., 1999; Tomb et al., 1997). Intragenomic recombination between extensive DNA repeats in *cagA* genes results in addition or insertion of tyrosine phosphorylation sites, which affects the host-bacterium interactions (Aras et al., 2003b). Such variations in antigenic or immunogenic proteins lead to novel phenotypic variants with altered immune responses in the host; this ultimately leads to evolution of new variants in order to increase the bacterial fitness (De Luca and Iaquinto, 2004; Chang et al., 2004).

Natural transformation and other mechanisms of horizontal gene transfer dependent on DNA recombination are significantly involved in shaping the genomic diversity of *H. pylori*.

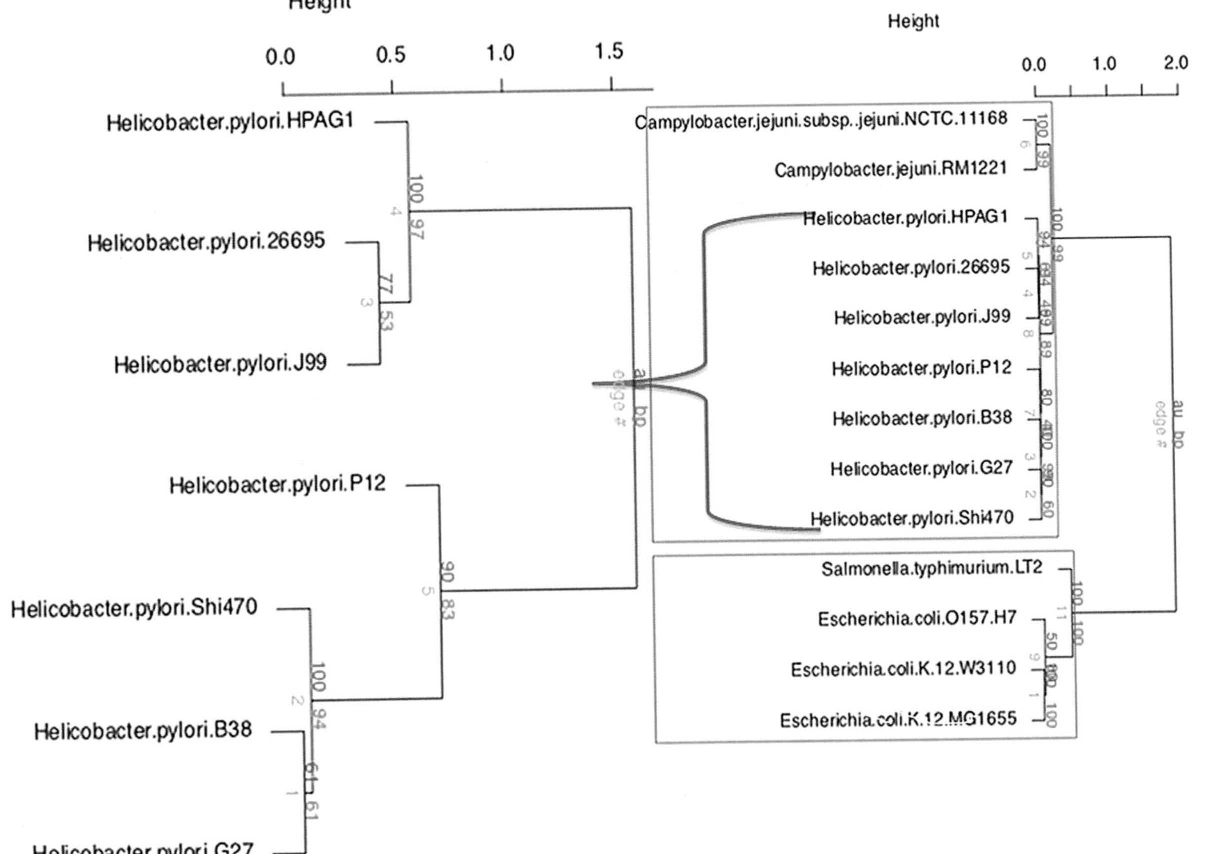

FIGURE 3 Dendrogram based on comparative metabolomics of *Helicobacter* (produced by using KEGG). Organisms which share a larger number of enzymes are clustered together. This highlights the commonality of biochemical transformation between their metabolic pathways.

It is evident from earlier studies that *Helicobacter* lacks type IV pilin-like genes, suggesting the presence of a different system for natural transformation than in other bacteria. Later, the presence of the *comB* operon (which encodes a DNA import system via natural transformation) was identified, and it was found to be necessary but not sufficient for transformation (Hofreuter et al., 2001). Since type IV pilus genes are absent in *H. pylori*, and owing to the homology of *comB* cluster members to the *cagPAI* proteins and to other type IV secretion system components, it can be speculated that they play a role in transformation competence. Determination of the complete genome sequence and functional analysis of different *H. pylori* strains resulted in identification of at least 11 diverse restriction/modification systems and their diversified modification patterns that are important elements in successful transformation (Tomb et al., 1997; Wang et al., 1993; Majewski and Godwin, 1988). Hofreuter et al. (1998) showed the marginal effect of the lipopolysaccharide gene cluster on genetic competence as *comB* was found to cotranscribe with the lipopolysaccharide gene cluster; the pH-regulated operon was more strongly expressed at pH 4 to 5 than at pH 7. In addition, three genes, HP0333, HP1378, and HP1361, which show homology to the transformation competence genes *dprA*, *comL*, and *comEC* were found in *H. pylori strains* 26695 and J99. *recA* is the other gene necessary for transformation competence in *H. pylori* (Schmitt et al., 1995). Besides, many genes such as *recJ*, *recN*, *rep*, *pcrA*, *uvrD*, *xseA*, *recR*, *ssb*, *ruvA*, *ruvB*, *ruvC*, *recG*, *polA*, *lig*, *topA*, *gyrA*, *gyrB*, *priA*, *dnaB*, and *dnaG* were found to be involved in homologous recombination and recombinational repair. In *H. pylori*, however, a *recA*-independent intragenomic deletion of 100 bp was observed, suggesting that *H. pylori* has different mechanisms for intragenomic recombination from *E. coli* (Aras et al., 2003a).

GENOMIC ISLANDS OF *H. PYLORI*

Insertion of genetic elements directly into the genome by horizontal gene transfer results in the formation of genomic islands. It appears that the genes of these genomic islands may be responsible for generation of novel phenotypes with differential bacterial fitness such as enhanced survival ability under extreme environmental conditions and/or ability to fight the host immune system. In *H. pylori*, three types of genomic islands coding for the type IV secretion system were identified: (i) the cytotoxin-associated gene pathogenicity island (*cagPAI*), (ii) the competence island (*comB* gene cluster), and (iii) the plasticity zone.

Cytotoxin-Associated Gene Pathogenicity Island *(cagPAI)*

The *cagPAI* is a 40-kb fragment with 29 genes that produce the principal bacterial virulence factor, CagA, which plays a major role in the invasion of the gastric epithelium during the infection (Censini et al,.1996) .The CagA protein undergoes phosphorylation and gets translocated to the epithelial cells (Asahi et al., 2000; Odenbreit et al., 2000; Stein et al., 2000). The phosphorylated CagA protein elicits growth factor like responses in epithelial cells (hummingbird phenotype) and simultaneously induces the interleukin-8 (IL-8) response that recruits neutrophils. Mutagenesis studies of *cagPAI* showed that mutations interfere with tyrosine phosphorylation and IL-8 induction (Fischer et al., 2001). The *cag* type IV system has been known to show analogy to the structure of type III secretion systems. The *cag* genes are involved mainly in assembly and topological arrangement of the secretory apparatus. The *cag* genes *virD4*, *virB11*, *virB10*, *virB9*, and *virB4/cagE* constitute the core apparatus of the type IV secretory system of *H. pylori* (Censini et al., 1996; Selbach et al., 2002; Covacci et al., 1999; Buhrdorf et al., 2003), in which all are associated with IL-8 production except *virD4*. However, from earlier studies it is known that *cagPAI* is not the only factor linked to IL-8 induction. The acquisition of *cagPAI* has been the subject of many debates, specifically on its origin and the circumstances under which it was imported from a foreign source (Devi et al., 2006). Taking into account the comprehensive genetic analyses that have been performed, it is possible to predict a possible evolutionary scenario (Fig. 4) supporting the contention that the *cagPAI* was acquired by ancestral *H. pylori* populations that arose on different continents before agriculture began in the civilized world. The acquisition of the pathogenicity islands might have occurred in *H. pylori* populations quite recently, possibly due to close contact of humans with domesticated animals, crops, or rodent pests surrounding them. Such an interspecies gene transfer could be partly based on the fact that many constituent genes of the *cagPAI* reveal strong homologies to the type IV system of *Agrobacterium tumifaciens* (Fischer et al., 2001) and that *cagA*-like sequences have been found in some *Aeromonas* isolates (Datta et al., 2003) obtained from environmental samples. Subsequent environmental changes and evolution of the food habits might have led to further continent-specific adaptation of *H. pylori*. Also, the gain of pathogenicity islands might have augmented the fitness of the organism to infect and spread, thus giving rise to modern populations.

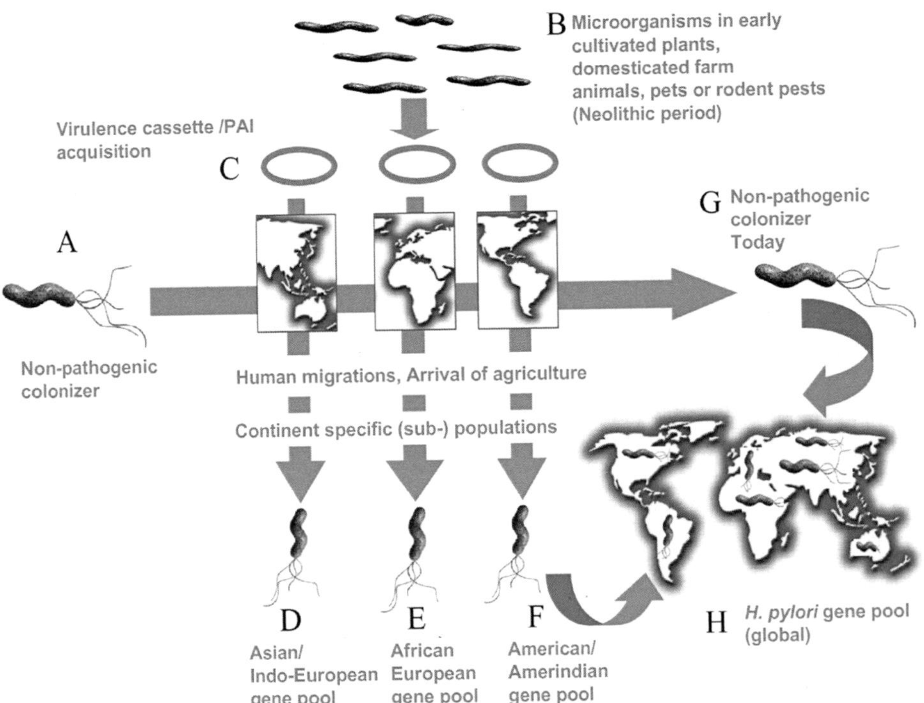

FIGURE 4 Acquisition of virulence, optimization of fitness, and geographically compartmentalized spread of *H. pylori* (sub)populations (Ahmed et al., 2009). Horizontal gene transfer and genome plasticity probably contributed to the evolution of pathogenic variants from nonpathogenic colonizers. Modern *H. pylori* populations thus derived their gene pools from ancestral populations that arose on different continents and can be correlated with different migrations of human populations and other Neolithic events such as the arrival of agriculture. The beginning of agriculture and the domestication of farm animals (which seem to have occurred hand in hand but across multiple domestication events in a continent-specific manner) suggest a scenario, as depicted here, which can be linked to the acquisition of virulence by *H. pylori*. It can be hypothesized that early bacterial communities originating from crop plants, animals, or rodent pests, etc., very common in the vicinity of early human societies, may have served as donors of some of the virulence gene cassettes. Such genetic elements may have been acquired by *H. pylori* either bit by bit or en bloc, at some time, through horizontal gene transfer events. There is indirect evidence to this effect in the form of sequence and structural similarities of some of the *H. pylori* virulence genes to their homologues in plant pathogens and environmental bacteria. Also, we think that the extraneous virulence genes may have conferred some survival advantage upon *H. pylori* strains, making them fitter in different human and animal hosts and, as a result, the pathogen may have spread selectively in a geographically compartmentalized manner.

Similar type IV secretion systems required for pathogenicity have been found in many bacterial pathogens, including *Legionella pneumophila, Bartonella henselae, Brucella suis,* and *Bordetella pertussis*. However, type IV secretion systems of some bacteria, e.g., *A. tumefaciens*, as well as the pR388-encoded system of *E. coli*, enable DNA transfer (Cascales and Christie, 2004). Interestingly, interactions between components of conjugational type IV secretion systems and those responsible for protein translocation have been shown (de Paz et al., 2005). This suggests that corresponding islands coding for type IV secretion systems may also favor the transfer of genetic information including themselves. Accordingly, such selfish DNA regions may also be considered as "evolution genes" or "evolution facilitators" as they encode biological functions that actively contribute to genetic diversity (Arber, 2000).

The Competence Island

Independent of *cagPAI* and other pathogenesis-associated genomic islands, *H. pylori* harbors a dedicated type IV apparatus, the "competence island" or the *comB* gene cluster (Hofreuter et al., 2003), which is linked to horizontal gene transfer and natural transformation due to competence. The *comB* gene cluster is supposed to be indispensable in allowing *H. pylori* uptake of plasmid and chromosomal DNA during natural transformation, especially in the event of mixed infections. The *comB* locus was located by shuttle mutagenesis and was found to consist of *orf2* and *comB1-comB3* (Odenbreit et al., 1996) as important elements of competence which are tandemly arranged as a single transcriptional unit. Subsequently, the *comB* cluster genes, namely, *orf2, comB1, comB2,* and *comB3*, were renamed (in view of their homology to the *A. tumifaciens* type IV secretory system) as *comB7, comB8, comB9,* and *comB10*, respectively (Hofreuter et al., 1998). Another open reading frame (ORF), *HP0017* from the sequenced strain *H. pylori* 26695, was found to be a homologue of the *virB4* gene in the type IV secretory apparatus of *A. tumifaciens* and was named *comB4* (Hofreuter et al., 2003). Similarly, it was also evident that each of the gene products of ORFs *comB8* to *comB10* was absolutely essential for natural transformation competence (Hofreuter et al., 2001). Geneticists think the *comB* transformation apparatus has evolved conservatively in *H. pylori* and is typically present in all the strains. This conservation explains why genomic fluidity in *H. pylori* is so common, especially when the deletions and rearrangements due to natural transformation and transposition are described as frequently occurring phenomena (Falush et al., 2001; Gressmann et al., 2005). It appears that the pathogen needs to keep the gene content flexible and diverse to acclimatize itself to the changing host niche environment during long colonization. Both of these type IV systems, the *cagPAI* and *comB* gene clusters, seem to act completely independently, since the abrogation of one system from the genome of *H. pylori* does not apparently disturb the function of the other. As mentioned above, the DNA regions coding for both of them may be regarded as selfish DNA regions that support evolution as their encoded gene products contribute to genetic diversity.

The Plasticity Zone

The highly heterogeneous *H. pylori* is a model for studying the plastic nature of the genome and its role in the colonization of individual hosts. *H. pylori* has a large number of nonrandomly distributed direct DNA repetitive elements, and the extensive recombination between identical repetitive DNA results in deletion or duplication of intervening sequences, promoting diversity at those loci and variation within individual hosts (Aras et al., 2003).

Based on comparative genome analysis (Alm et al., 1999; Tomb et al ., 1997), it was found that the two genomes of *H. pylori* (strains 26695 and J99) show several regions whose G+C content was lower (35%) than that of the remainder and that the variable region harbored features of a pathogenicity island (Doig et al., 1999; Hacker and Kaper, 1999) as well as the presence of putative virulence genes and the elements suggestive of its acquisition by horizontal gene transfer. It was also found that nearly 48% and 46% of strain-specific genes are present in J99 and

26695, respectively. Based on this variability in the content, this region is called a plasticity zone.

With advanced genome sequencing techniques, it was possible to rapidly sequence the plasticity region of different *Helicobacter* strains; high diversity was found to be present in the plasticity zone gene content among different *Helicobacter* strains (Table 2).

Kersulyte et al. (2003) found a novel type IV secretion apparatus *(tfs3)* in the plasticity region of a Peruvian strain (PeCan18B), a 16.3-kb fragment with lower G+C content, suggesting horizontal gene transfer from other bacteria, whose function is still not known. Kersulyte et al. (2009) subsequently studied in detail the nature of plasticity zones, their acquisition, and their evolution in *Helicobacter* and demonstrated that the "plasticity zones are novel transposons called TnPZs." They also showed that almost 65% of the strains had genes derived from two or more TnPZs. They categorized these TnPZs into three types based on gene arrangement on DNA (Fig. 5), i.e., type 1, type 1b, and type 2. The type 1 TnPZ was identified in strain Shi470 of *H. pylori* and also in 35 of the 44 Shimaa strains. The type 1 TnPZ was characterized by the presence of *xerCD* genes on the left, a tfs3a element on the right, and centrally located type 1- or 1b-specific *virD2* alleles as shown in Fig 3. The type 2 TnPZ was found in urban Peruvian strain PeCan18B, Shi170, and P12. The type 2 TnPZs have type 2-specific *virD2* and *xerT* genes on the left and the *tfs3* gene cluster on the right. The type 1b TnPz was a hybrid element found in strain P12, characterized by the presence of a type 1 TnPZ central region (*orfQ* through *virB9*) flanked by ~8-kb terminal flanking regions, suggesting the recombination of sequences from a type 1 TnPZ to a type 1b TnPZ (Kersulyte et al., 2009).

Seven of the 16 ORFs of *tfs3* were found to be homologous to *virB/D* genes of *Agrobacterium tumefaciens,* i.e., *virB7, virB8, virB9,* and *virB10* (transmembrane pore genes), and *virB4, virB11,* and *virD4* (cytoplasmic membrane-associated ATPase genes). The *H. pylori* strains P12 and Shi170 and *H. cetorum* have type 2 TnPZs, whereby their *tfs3* gene clusters showed 99%, 87%, and 86% identity, respectively, to that of PeCan18B. Strains Shi470 and G27 have type 1 TnPZs with a highly divergent *tfs3* at the level of the DNA sequence; this is named *tfs3a.* Strain P12 also has type 1b TnPZ which is of hybrid ancestry and wherein 97% of its *tfs3* region matches *tfs3a* of type 1 TnPZs and the remaining 3% is not related to either *tfs3* or *tfs3a* fragments of the type 2 or type 1 TnPZs; this is designated *tfs3b.* Almost one-fifth of *H. pylori* strains were found to contain either a full-length or partial *tfs3* element from Spain, Peru, India, and Japan. The complete *tfs3* was found in 8%, 13%, and 33% of the strains from Japan, Korea and Colombia, respectively, but it appears that there is no association between the presence of complete or partial *tfs3* and clinical outcomes (Lu et al., 2005).

In *H. pylori* J99, the plasticity region contains nearly 48 ORFs ranging from *jhp0914* to *jhp0961* present continuously (Alm et al., 1999), which were considered to be J99 strain specific except for ORFs 6 and 10 (of the 48 ORFs), which were found in 26695 and HPAG1, respectively. DNA microarray analysis (Salama et al., 2000; Gressmann et al., 2005) indicated the presence of ORFs *jhp0914* to *jhp0961* at different percentages in as many as 72 different strains,

TABLE 2 Distribution of plasticity zones in the genomes of different *Helicobacter* strains

Strain	Accession no.	Length (bp)	Coordinates
PeCan 18B	AF 487344	56,651	864–53286 Type 1b: 864–3917 Type 2: 3918–53286
HUP-B43	AY487825	33,671	1285–28713
H. cetorum (MIT-00-7128)	EU015081	64,612	3698–58762
Shi470	CP001072 (genome sequence)	Unknown	874704–91386
Shi170	EU807988	47,447	574–47093

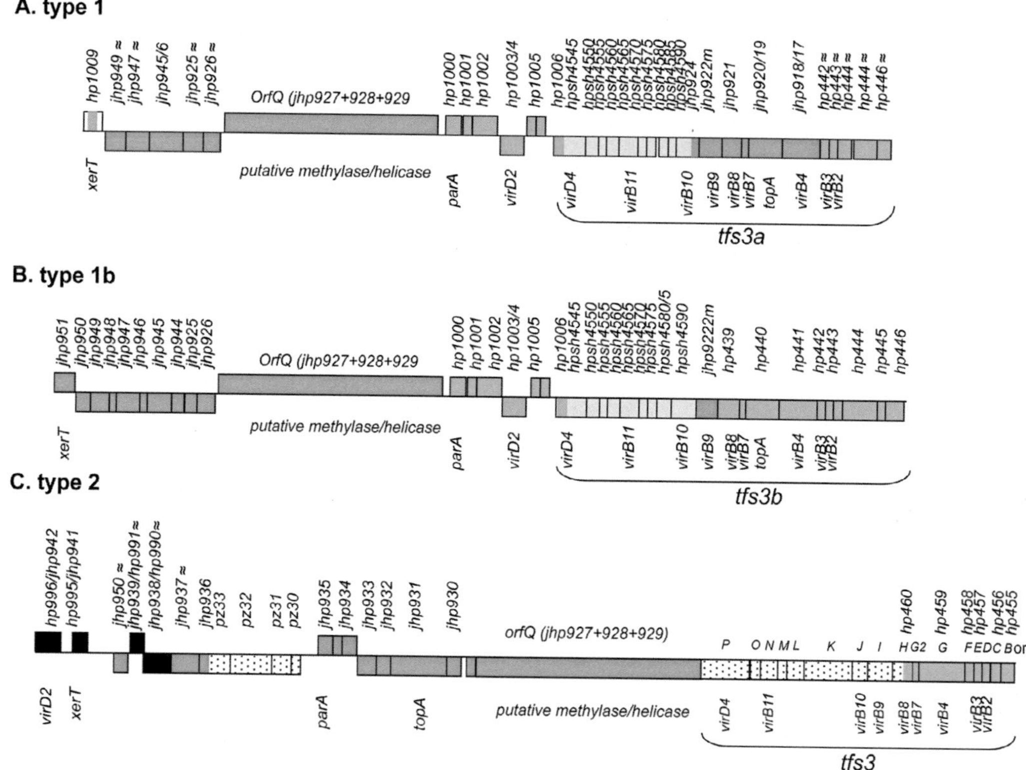

FIGURE 5 Arrangement of ORFs under different types of plasticity zone-encoded transposable elements (TnPZs) in *H. pylori* (from Kersulyte et al., 2009). Different regions/ORFs of the TnPZs have been color coded as per the conventions detailed by Kersulyte et al. (2009).

including strains 26695, J99, and HPAG1, with the exception of *jhp0915*, which was found in all the strains (100%) studied. Genomic analysis revealed that the majority of the plasticity zone ORFs encode putative proteins whose functions are unknown, and some ORFs were found to show protein-level homologies to recombinases, integrases, and topoisomerases (Occhialini et al., 2000), as shown in Table 3.

Occhialini et al. (2000) confirmed the occurrence of plasticity zone ORFs at specific loci based on hybridization methods and demonstrated a varied distribution of ORFs in this region; i.e., all or almost all of the ORFs may be present or some may be deleted from the central part, indicating its real plastic nature. They also found that the genes of the plasticity region do not represent pseudogenes based on their expression profiles; at the same time they cannot be considered pathogenicity islands since an association was not found between specific clinical outcomes or severity of disease and a particular profile of these ORFs in clinical strains.

FUNCTIONAL RELEVANCE OF THE PLASTIC GENOMES OF *H. PYLORI*

H. pylori-induced chronic gastritis is a definitive risk factor for the development of gastric cancer. However, it was found that the statuses of some of the chief virulence factors (CagA and VacA) do not always correlate with particular outcomes of infection, as also discussed previously (Alvi et al., 2007). In view of this, it appears that virulence of *H. pylori* is a complex phenotype that needs to be seen as a function of bacterial strategies aimed at survival and adaptation. However, it is not clear how the bacterium maintains its niches for almost the

TABLE 3 Functional ORFs and homologies of the members of the plasticity region

ORF	Homologous to	Function
jhp0917 and *jhp0918*	*vir* factors	Not fully understood
jhp0919, *jph0920* and *jph0931*	DNA topoisomerase I (*top A*)	Regulation of DNA supercoiling and gene expression
jhp0921, *jhp0922* and *jhp0923*	Competence proteins (*comB8* or *com B9*)	DNA transformation
jhp0928	Methylase	Not studied fully
jhp0935	Partitioning protein A (*par A*)	DNA separation at cell division or preparation for DNA transfer by conjugation
jhp0941 and *jhp0951*	Integrase/recombinase (*xerCD* family)	DNA restriction, modification, recombination, and repair systems

entire life span of its host without being cleared. Perhaps there are highly orchestrated biological interactions between the host and the pathogen, whose nature is not clearly understood. Of late, roles of new virulence determinants are becoming plausible. As mentioned previously, *H. pylori* harbors up to 45% strain-specific genes (Ge and Taylor, 1999), mostly gained through horizontal gene transfer events (Ahmed et al., 2009). Recently, it was proposed that some of the members of the plasticity region cluster were likely to be involved in promoting the proinflammatory capacity of some of the strains (Alvi et al., 2007; Romo-González et al., 2009), thus imparting a survival advantage. We recently tested one such protein from the plasticity region cluster and would like to suggest that some of the members of this cluster encode proinflammatory and/or proapoptotic roles (Alvi et al., 2011). Rizwan et al. (2008) performed genotyping and functional analysis of *jhp0940* in 120 strains from seven countries and found that it is fairly stable and widely prevalent geographically in the majority of the strains but with lowest prevalence in the Spanish and Costa Rican isolates followed by the Japanese and Peruvian isolates. They also found that its geographical prevalence is independent of the presence of *cagA* and the disease status. Recombinant functional studies of *jhp0940* revealed that it codes for a ~36-kDa biologically active protein that induces tumor necrosis factor alpha (TNF-α) and IL-8 in human macrophages and also can induce the translocation of NF-κB in cultured macrophages. This proinflammatory effect of *jhp0940* might be playing a role in chronic gastric inflammation and other clinical outcomes of *H. pylori* infection. In a recent study (Romo-González et al., 2009), 42 isolates of *H. pylori* were profiled, and it was found that 1,319 genes were present in all isolates while 341 (20.5%) genes were variably present among different isolates. Of the variable genes, 127 (37%) were interspersed within the plasticity region cluster. The authors observed the disease association of such genes and found 30 genes to be significantly associated with nonatrophic gastritis, duodenal ulcer, or gastric cancer; 14 (46.6%) of such putative disease-linked genes were operational from within the plasticity region and the *cagPAI* (many of the constituent genes of the *cagPAI* form part of the plasticity region cluster of *H. pylori*). In the earlier observations (Romo-González et al., 2009), two genes (*HP0674* and *JHP0940*) were absent in all gastric cancer isolates. In our observations (S. Tenguria and N. Ahmed, unpublished data), strains representing intestinal metaplasia cases failed to amplify the *JHP0940* gene (data not shown). It is therefore possible that some of the genes are deleted by the pathogen as the disease progresses through intestinal metaplasia to gastric cancer. However, such observations need functional validation and mechanistic explanation. Nevertheless, the disease-linked genes, as discussed above, may be pursued as (putative) biomarkers of the risk for progression of *H. pylori*-induced inflammation towards more serious gastroduodenal illnesses such as atrophic gastritis, intestinal metaplasia, and gastric adenocarcinoma.

Most persistent microbes perhaps actively tend to evolve strategies to counter innate host responses in order to gain niche and to maintain growth fitness. For example, *H. pylori* traditionally harness its chief virulence factors, CagA and VacA, to cause pathology via a two-tier approach: (i) downregulate T-cell responses (through the VacA-mediated cell cycle arrest) and (ii) upregulate mucosal proinflammatory pathways (by *cagPAI*-mediated IL-8 signaling). Surprisingly, in our studies, one of the plasticity region cluster proteins appeared to be able to perform both immune-stimulatory (macrophage proliferation and secretion of IL-8 and TNF-α) and immune evasion (apoptosis of activated macrophages) tasks simultaneously (Alvi et al., 2011). Thus, we conclude that some of the bacterial proinflammatory proteins (such as JHP0940 [Rizwan et al., 2008] and others) are capable of taking up the functions of VacA/CagA, especially in the setting of deficiency of the latter, and probably function as "persistence factors" (Alvi et al., 2011); this, however, awaits validation with appropriate animal models.

The presence of *jhp0917-0918* in all the strains from Japan, Korea, and Colombia was identified; a 1-bp insertion (C or T) in the 3′ region of *jhp0917* led to a frameshift turning *jhp0917* and *jhp0918* into a continuous gene which serves as a marker for duodenal ulcers and as a protective marker against gastric adenocarcinoma; the two genes together were designated the duodenal ulcer-promoting gene (*dupA*); its function is not completely known, but part of its protein is homologous to the *ftsk/Spo IIIE* and *TraG/TraD* family of proteins which have roles in chromosomal DNA transfer. The same was found in 97% of the isolates from Brazilian patients (86 of 89), confirming the presence of *jhp0917-0918* as a continuous gene which is homologous to *virB4* except in strain J99. Further studies of 500 *H. pylori* strains showed 42%, 21%, 27%, and 9% prevalences of *dupA* in duodenal ulcer, gastritis, gastric ulcer, and gastric cancer strains, respectively (Lu et al., 2005). The in vitro experiments (mutation studies) by the same authors demonstrated that the presence of *dupA* increased IL-8 production from gastric epithelial cells by activating the transcription factors that bind to the IL-8 promoter (NF-κB and Ap-1) (Lu et al., 2005). A similar prevalence was reported by Yamaoka et al. (Yamaoka et al., 1998a, 1998b; Yamaoka, 2010) in some *dupA* mutant strains (but not in all of them); they also found that the *dupA* gene in combination with some *vir* homologues of the plasticity zone may be forming a novel type IV secretion system similar to the *cagPAI*, and that it might be involved in gastroduodenal inflammation. The *dupA* gene was more prevalent in strains from patients with duodenal ulcer (38% [36 of 96]) than from those with functional dyspepsia (23% [16 of 70]) in North India (Arachchi et al., 2007). On the other front (Douraghi et al., 2008), no association was found between the presence of *dupA* and clinical outcomes such as duodenal ulcer, gastric ulcer, and gastric cancer in strains from Iran; however, an inverse association of *dupA* was found with the presence of precancerous lesions, gastric dyspepsia, and lymphoid follicles based on histological experiments, thus supporting the finding of *dupA* as a protective marker against gastric cancer.

Gomes et al. (2008) reported that *dupA* was more prevalent in strains from Brazilian children and adults (92% [445 of 482]) independent of the disease status, i.e., gastritis, duodenal ulcer, or gastric cancer. These strains were found at significantly higher frequencies in children, in whom *H. pylori* may persist for life if not treated and *dupA* may be deleted during long-term colonization, leading perhaps to the development of gastric cancer and chronic atrophic gastritis. In view of the above, it seems that there are variations in the prevalence of *dupA* with respect to geographical distribution, and the association between *dupA* and duodenal ulcers seems to be present in some populations but not all.

GENOMIC FLUIDITY OF *H. PYLORI*: CLINICAL IMPLICATIONS

Earlier, in our opinion article, we discussed the development of genetic markers associated with bacterial genome fluidity and their application for diagnostics, molecular epidemiology, and vaccine production (Ahmed et al., 2008). The *cagA* antigen is the universally accepted

TABLE 4 Exploitation of genomic fluidity of *H. pylori* for diagnostic and health care applications[a]

Genetic lesion	Type of change	Application
Indel of the *cag* right junction	Small-scale insertions and deletions at the right junction of the *cag*PAI	Markers of human migration and *H. pylori* lineage identification
cagA	Presence or absence of the locus; expression of functional toxin	Diagnostic markers and antigens; markers of invasive gastric inflammation
cagA EPIYA motif	Strain specificity tyrosine phosphorylation of *cagA*	Geographical markers of gastric-cancer predisposition
Plasticity region cluster	Presence or absence of loci	Putative virulence genes; possible interventional targets

[a]Based on Ahmed et al., 2008.

virulence marker that is linked to gastric and peptic ulcer disease and gastric cancer (Argent et al., 2004; Hatakeyama, 2004; Saadat et al., 2007). It can also be determined whether the *H. pylori* strains are carcinogenic or ulcerogenic based on the presence or absence of a particular motif (EPIYA motif; type C or D) of *cagPAI*, involved in phosphorylation of *cagA*, which is linked to the severity of atrophic gastritis and gastric carcinoma in patients infected with *cagA*-positive strains of *H. pylori*. Besides this, certain ORFs from the plasticity region can be used as diagnostic markers, as mentioned above (Table 4).

PERSPECTIVES

H. pylori is a unique bacterium which shows extensive genomic diversity among strains. Strains obtained from different individuals are also diverse at the metabolic levels. Point mutations, recombination, horizontal gene transfer, genomic islands, repetitive elements, insertion elements, bacteriophages, etc., contribute to genome plasticity. The acquisition of foreign DNA in the form of genomic islands by *H. pylori* is responsible for the evolution of pathogens with novel phenotypes and virulence characters. Similarly, the loss or deletion of DNA results in reductive genome evolution, imparting parasitic advantages. The plastic nature of *H. pylori* and acquisition of genes by horizontal transfer from other bacteria may be responsible for the ability of this organism to adapt to different environmental conditions within and between hosts and thus give rise to varied clinical outcomes in patients. The natural competence, which facilitates conjugation, results in the formation of more recombinants and in turn reflects the varied distribution of genes in a flexible gene pool. Flexibility and diversity of the genetic repertoire might impart fitness to the strains for survival in different members of varied human populations. Further investigation at the biochemical level is likely to reveal the cross talk between different pathways and their impact on the host. Since *H. pylori* is highly heterogeneous, further studies are needed to focus on multiple strains obtained across the world. Also, investigation of the genome sequences in serial isolates obtained from a single individual over long timescales might provide a much needed handle on studying evolutionary forces that operate on the genome over different timescales and how fast or slowly the genome evolves over years and decades and in different host backgrounds. Further studies on the regulation of genomic fluidity as well as the role of environmental factors in inducing the genomic fluidity or plasticity are clearly needed. Such studies will be able to explain the exact roles of the variable genomic repertoire of *H. pylori* in its evolution and adaptation and the significance of the latter in pathogen survival tactics and in the development of accurate diagnostics and timely therapeutic interventions.

REFERENCES

Ahmed, N. 2009. A flood of microbial genomes—do we need more? *PLoS One* **4:**e5831.

Ahmed, N., U. Dobrindt, J. Hacker, and S. E. Hasnain. 2008. Genomic fluidity and pathogenic bacteria: applications in diagnostics, epidemiology and intervention. *Nat. Rev. Microbiol.* **6:**387–394.

Ahmed, N., S. Tenguria, and N. Nandanwar. 2009. *Helicobacter pylori*—a seasoned pathogen by any other name. *Gut Pathog.* **1:**24. doi:10.1186/1757-4749-1-24.

Akhter, Y., I. Ahmed, S. M. Devi, and N. Ahmed. 2007. The co-evolved *Helicobacter pylori* and gastric cancer: trinity of bacterial virulence, host susceptibility and lifestyle. *Infect. Agents Cancer* **2:**2.

Alm, R. A., L. S. Ling, D. T. Moir, B. L. King, E. D. Brown, P. C. Doig, D. R. Smith, B. Noonan, B. C. Guild, B. L. deJonge, G. Carmel, P. J. Tummino, A. Caruso, M. Uria-Nickelsen, D. M. Mills, C. Ives, R. Gibson, D. Merberg, S. D. Mills, Q. Jiang, D. E. Taylor, G. F. Vovis, and T. J. Trust. 1999. Genomic-sequence comparison of two unrelated isolates of the human gastric pathogen *Helicobacter pylori. Nature* **397:**176–180.

Alvi, A., S. A. Ansari, N. Z. Ehtesham, M. Rizwan, S. Devi, L. A. Sechi, I. A. Qureshi, S. E. Hasnain, and N. Ahmed. 2011. Concurrent proinflammatory and apoptotic activity of a Helicobacter pylori protein (HP986) points to its role in chronic persistence. *PLoS One* **64:**e22530.

Alvi, A., S. M. Devi, I. Ahmed, M. A. Hussain, M. Rizwan, H. Lamouliatte, F. Mégraud, and N. Ahmed. 2007. Microevolution of *Helicobacter pylori* type IV secretion systems in an ulcer disease patient over a ten-year period. *J. Clin. Microbiol.* **45:**4039–4043.

Arachchi, H. S., V. Kalra, B. Lal, V. Bhatia, C. S. Baba, S. Chakravarthy, S. Rohatgi, P. M. Sarma, V. Mishra, B. Das, and V. Ahuja. 2007. Prevalence of duodenal ulcer-promoting gene (dupA) of Helicobacter pylori in patients with duodenal ulcer in North Indian population. *Helicobacter* **12:**591–597.

Aras, R. A., J. Kang, A. I. Tschumi, Y. Harasaki, and M. J. Blaser. 2003a. Extensive repetitive DNA facilitates prokaryotic genome plasticity. *Proc. Natl. Acad. Sci. USA* **100:**13579–13584.

Aras, R. A., Y. Lee, S. K. Kim, D. Israel, R. M. Peek, Jr., and M. J. Blaser. 2003b. Natural variation in populations of persistently colonizing bacteria affect human host cell phenotype. *J. Infect. Dis.* **188:**486–496.

Arber, W. 2000. Genetic variation: molecular mechanisms and impact on microbial evolution. *FEMS Microbiol Rev.* **24:**1–7.

Argent, R. H., M. Kidd, R. J. Owen, R. J. Thomas, M. C. Limb, and J. C. Atherton. 2004. Determinants and consequences of different levels of *CagA* phosphorylation for clinical isolates of *Helicobacter pylori. Gastroenterology* **127:**514–523.

Asahi, M., T. Azuma, S. Ito, Y. Ito, H. Suto, Y. Nagai, M. Tsubokawa, Y. Tohyama, S. Maeda, M. Omata, T. Suzuki, and C. Sasakawa. 2000. *Helicobacter pylori CagA* protein can be tyrosine phosphorylated in gastric epithelial cells. *J. Exp. Med.* **191:**593–602.

Baltrus, D. A., M. R. Amieva, A. Covacci, T. M. Lowe, D. S. Merrell, K. M. Ottemann, M. Stein, N. R. Salama, and K. Guillemin. 2009. The complete genome sequence of *Helicobacter pylori* strain G27. *J. Bacteriol.* **191:**447–448.

Buhrdorf, R., C. Forster, R. Haas, and W. Fischer. 2003. Topological analysis of a putative *virB8* homologue essential for the *cag* type IV secretion system in *Helicobacter pylori. Int. J. Med. Microbiol.* **293:**213–217.

Cascales, E., and P. J. Christie. 2004. Definition of a bacterial type IV secretion pathway for a DNA substrate. *Science* **304:**1170–1173.

Censini, S., C. Lange, Z. Y. Xiang, J. E. Crabtree, P. Ghiara, and M. Borodovsky. 1996. *Cag*, a pathogenicity island of *Helicobacter pylori*, encodes type I-specific and disease-associated virulence factors. *Proc. Natl. Acad. Sci. USA* **93:** 14648–14653.

Chang, C. S., W. N. Chen, H. H. Lin, C. C. Wu, and C. J. Wang. 2004. Increased oxidative DNA damage, inducible nitric oxide synthase, nuclear factor kappa B expression and enhanced antiapoptosis-related proteins in Helicobacter pylori-infected noncardiac gastric adenocarcinoma. *World J. Gastroenterol.* **10:**2232–2240.

Covacci, A., J. L. Telford, G. G. Del, J. Parsonnet, and R. Rappuoli. 1999. *Helicobacter pylori* virulence and genetic geography. *Science* **284:**1328–1333.

Datta, S., A. Khan, R. K. Nandy, M. Rehman, S. Sinha, S. Chattopadhyay, S. C. Das, and G. B. Nair. 2003. Environmental isolates of *Aeromonas* spp. harboring the *cagA*-like gene of *Helicobacter pylori. Appl. Environ. Microbiol.* **69:**4291–4295.

De Luca, A., and G. Iaquinto. 2004. Helicobacter pylori and gastric diseases: a dangerous association. *Cancer Lett.* **213:**1–10.

de Paz, H. D., F. J. Sangari, S. Bolland, J. M. Garcia-Lobo, C. Dehio, F. de la Cruz, and M. Llosa. 2005. Functional interactions between type IV secretion systems involved in DNA transfer and virulence. *Microbiology* **151:**3505–3516.

Devi, S. M., I. Ahmed, A. A. Khan, S. A. Rahman, A. Alvi, L. A. Sechi, and N. Ahmed. 2006. Genomes of Helicobacter pylori from native Peruvians suggest admixture of ancestral and modern lineages and reveal a western type cag-pathogenicity island. *BMC Genomics* **7:**191.

Doig, P., B. L. De Jonge, R. A. Alm, E. D. Brown, M. Uria-Nickelsen, B. Noonan, S. D. Mills, P. Tummino, G. Carmel, B. C. Guild, D. T. Moir, G. F. Vovis, and T. J. Trust. 1999. *Helicobacter* *pylori* physiology predicted from genomic comparison of two strains. *Microbiol. Mol. Biol. Rev.* **63:**675–707.

Douraghi, M., M. Mohammadi, A. Oghalaie, A. Abdirad, M. A. Mohagheghi, M. Eshagh Hosseini, H. Zeraati, A. Ghasemi, M. Esmaieli, and N. Mohajerani. 2008. *dupA* as a risk determinant in Helicobacter pylori infection. *J. Med. Microbiol.* **57:**554–562.

Eppinger, M., C. Baar, B. Linz, G. Raddatz, C. Lanz, H. Keller, G. Morelli, H. Gressmann, M. Achtman, and S. C. Schuster. 2006. Who ate whom? Adaptive Helicobacter genomic changes that accompanied a host jump from early humans to large felines. *PLoS Genet.* **2:**e120.

Falush, D., C. Kraft, N. S. Taylor, P. Correa, J. G. Fox, M. Achtman, and S. Suerbaum. 2001. Recombination and mutation during long-term gastric colonization by *Helicobacter pylori*: estimates of clock rates, recombination size, and minimal age. *Proc. Natl. Acad. Sci. USA* **98:**15056–15061.

Fischer, W., J. Püls, R. Buhrdorf, B. Gebert, S. Odenbreit, and R. Haas. 2001. Systematic mutagenesis of the *Helicobacter pylori cag* pathogenicity island: essential genes for *CagA* translocation in host cells and induction of interleukin-8. *Mol. Microbiol.* **42:**1337–1348.

Ge, Z., and D. E. Taylor. 1999. Contributions of genome sequencing to understanding the biology of *Helicobacter pylori*. *Annu. Rev. Microbiol.* **53:**353–387.

Gomes, L. I., G. A. Rocha, A. M. Rocha, T. F. Soares, C. A. Oliveira, P. F. Bittencourt, and D. M. Queiroz. 2008. Lack of association between *Helicobacter pylori* infection with dupA-positive strains and gastroduodenal diseases in Brazilian patients. *Int. J. Med. Microbiol.* **298:**223–230.

Gressmann, H., B. Linz, R. Ghai, K. P. Pleissner, R. Schlapbach, Y. Yamaoka, C. Kraft, S. Suerbaum, T. F. Meyer, and M. Achtman. 2005. Gain and loss of multiple genes during the evolution of *Helicobacter pylori*. *PLoS Genet.* **1:**e43.

Hacker, J., and J. Kaper. 1999. The concept of pathogenicity islands, p. 1–11. *In* J. B. Kaper and J. Hacker (ed.), *Pathogenicity Islands and Other Mobile Virulence Elements*. ASM Press, Washington, DC.

Hatakeyama, M. 2004. Oncogenic mechanisms of the *Helicobacter pylori CagA* protein. *Nat. Rev. Cancer* **4:**688–694.

Hofreuter, D., A. Karnholz, and R. Haas. 2003. Topology and membrane interaction of *Helicobacter pylori ComB* proteins involved in natural transformation competence. *Int. J. Med. Microbiol.* **293:**153–165.

Hofreuter, D., S. Odenbreit, and R. Haas. 2001. Natural transformation competence in *Helicobacter pylori* is mediated by the basic components of a type IV secretion system. *Mol. Microbiol.* **41:**379–391.

Hofreuter, D., S. Odenbreit, G. Henke, and R. Haas. 1998. Natural competence for DNA transformation in *Helicobacter pylori*: identification and genetic characterization of the *comB* locus. *Mol. Microbiol.* **28:**1027–1038.

Huang, J. Q., S. Sridhar, Y. Chen, and R. H. Hunt. 1998. Meta-analysis of the relationship between *Helicobacter pylori* seropositivity and gastric cancer. *Gastroenterology* **114:**1169–1179.

Ikeno, T., H. Ota, A. Sugiyama, K. Ishida, T. Katsuyama, R. M. Genta, and S. Kawasaki. 1999. *Helicobacter pylori*-induced chronic active gastritis, intestinal metaplasia, and gastric ulcer in Mongolian gerbils. *Am. J. Pathol.* **154:**951–960.

Israel, D. A., N. Salama, U. Krishna, M. Rieger, J. C. Atherton, S. Falkow, and M. Peek. 2001. *Helicobacter pylori* genetic diversity within the gastric niche of a single human host. *Proc. Natl. Acad. Sci. USA* **98:**14625–14630.

Janssen, P. J., B. Audit, and C. A. Ouzounis. 2001. Strain-specific genes of *Helicobacter pylori*, distribution, function and dynamics. *Nucleic Acids Res.* **29:**4395–4404.

Kang, J. M., N. M. Iovine, and M. J. Blaser. 2006. A paradigm for direct stress-induced mutation in prokaryotes. *FASEB J.* **20:**2476–2485.

Kersulyte, D., W. Lee, D. Subramaniam, S. Anant, P. Herrera, L. Cabrera, J. Balqui, O. Barabas, A. Kalia, R. H. Gilman, and D. E. Berg. 2009. *Helicobacter pylori's* plasticity zones are novel transposable elements. *PLoS One* **4**(9)**:**e6859. doi:10.1371/journal.pone.0006859.

Kersulyte, D., B. Velapatiño, A. K. Mukhopadhyay, L. Cahuayme, A. Bussalleu, J. Combe, R. H. Gilman, and D. E. Berg. 2003. Cluster of type IV secretion genes in *Helicobacter pylori*'s plasticity zone. *J. Bacteriol.* **185:**3764–3772.

Lapierre, P., and J. P. Gogarten. 2009. Estimating the size of the bacterial pan-genome. *Trends Genet.* **25:**107–110.

Lu, H., P. I. Hsu, D. Y. Graham, and Y. Yamaoka. 2005. Duodenal ulcer promoting gene of *Helicobacter pylori*. *Gastroenterology* **128:**833–848.

Majewski, S. I. H., and C. S. Goodwin. 1988. Restriction endonuclease analysis of the genome of *Campylobacter pylori* with a rapid extraction method: evidence for considerable genomic variation. *J. Infect. Dis.* **157:**465–471.

Occhialini, A., A. Marais, R. Alm, F. Garcia, R. Sierra, and F. Megraud. 2000. Links of open reading frames of plasticity region of strain J99 in *Helicobacter pylori* strains isolated from gastric carcinoma and gastritis patients in Costa Rica. *Infect. Immun.* **68:**6240–6249.

Odenbreit, S., J. Püls, B. Sedlmaier, E. Gerland, W. Fischer, and R. Haas. 2000. Translocation of *Helicobacter pylori CagA* into gastric epithelial cells by type IV secretion. *Science* **287:**1497–1500.

Odenbreit, S., M. Till, and R. Haas. 1996. Optimized BlaM-transposon shuttle mutagenesis of *Helicobacter pylori* allows the identification of novel genetic loci involved in bacterial virulence. *Mol. Microbiol.* **20:**361–373.

Oh, J. D., H. Kling-Bäckhed, M. Giannakis, J. Xu, R. S. Fulton, L. A. Fulton, H. S. Cordum, C. Wang, G. Elliott, J. Edwards, E. R. Mardis, L. G. Engstrand, and J. I. Gordon. 2006. The complete genome sequence of a chronic atrophic gastritis Helicobacter pylori strain: evolution during disease progression. *Proc. Natl. Acad. Sci. USA* **103:**9999–10004.

Prouzet-Mauléon, V., M. A. Hussain, H. Lamouliatte, F. Kauser, F. Mégraud, and N. Ahmed. 2005. Pathogen evolution in vivo: genome dynamics of two isolates obtained 9 years apart from a duodenal ulcer patient infected with a single *Helicobacter pylori* strain. *J. Clin. Microbiol.* **43:**4237–4241.

Rizwan, M., A. Alvi, and N. Ahmed. 2008. Novel protein antigen (JHP940) from the genomic plasticity region of *Helicobacter pylori* induces tumor necrosis factor alpha and interleukin-8 secretion by human macrophages. *J. Bacteriol.* **190:**1146–1151.

Romo-González, C., N. R. Salama, J. Burgeño-Ferreira, V. Ponce-Castañeda, E. Lazcano-Ponce, M. Camorlinga-Ponce, and J. Torres. 2009. Differences in the genome content between *Helicobacter pylori* isolates from gastritis, duodenal ulcer or gastric cancer reveal novel disease associated genes. *Infect. Immun.* **77:**2201–2211.

Saadat, I., H. Higashi, C. Obuse, M. Umeda, N. Murata-Kamiya, Y. Saito, H. Lu, N. Ohnishi, T. Azuma, A. Suzuki, S. Ohno, and M. Hatakeyama. 2007. *Helicobacter pylori* CagA targets PAR1/MARK kinase to disrupt epithelial cell polarity. *Nature* **447:**330–333.

Salama, N., K. Guillemin, T. K. McDaniel, G. Sherlock, L. Tompkins, and S. Falkow. 2000. A whole-genome microarray reveals genetic diversity among Helicobacter pylori strains. *Proc. Natl. Acad. Sci. USA* **97:**14668–14673.

Schmitt, W., S. Odenbreit, D. Heuermann, and R. Haas. 1995. Cloning of the *Helicobacter pylori recA* gene and functional characterization of its product. *Mol. Gen. Genet.* **248:**563–572.

Selbach, M., S. Moese, T. F. Meyer, and S. Backert. 2002. Functional analysis of the *Helicobacter pylori cag* pathogenicity island reveals both VirD4-CagA-dependent and VirD4-CagA-independent mechanisms. *Infect. Immun.* **70:**665–671.

Stein, M., R. Rappuoli, and A. Covacci. 2000. Tyrosine phosphorylation of the *Helicobacter pylori CagA* antigen after *cag*-driven host cell translocation. *Proc. Natl. Acad. Sci. USA* **97:**1263–1268.

Suerbaum, S., C. Josenhans, T. Sterzenbach, B. Drescher, P. Brandt, M. Bell, M. Droge, B. Fartmann, H. P. Fischer, Z. GeZ, A. Horster, R. Holland, K. Klein, J. Konig, L. Macko, G. L. Mendz, G. Nyakatura, D. B. Schauer, Z. Shen, J. Weber, M. Frosch, and J. G. Fox. 2003. The complete genome sequence of the carcinogenic bacterium *Helicobacter hepaticus. Proc. Natl. Acad. Sci. USA* **100:**7901–7906.

Suerbaum, S., J. M. Smith, K. Bapumia, G. Morelli, N. H. Smith, E. Kunstmann, I. Dyrek, and M. Achtman. 1998. Free recombination within *Helicobacter pylori. Proc. Natl. Acad. Sci. USA* **95:**12619–12624.

Tomb, J. F., O. White, A. R. Kerlavage, R. A. Clayton, G. G. Sutton, R. D. Fleischmann, K. A. Ketchum, H. P. Klenk, S. Gill, B. A. Dougherty, K. Nelson, J. Quackenbush, L. Zhou, E. F. Kirkness, S. Peterson, B. Loftus, D. Richardson, R. Dodson, H. G. Khalak, A. Glodek, K. McKenney, L. M. Fitzegerald, N. Lee, M. D. Adams, E. K. Hickey, D. E. Berg, J. D. Gocayne, T. R. Utterback, J. D. Peterson, J. M. Kelley, M. D. Cotton, J. M. Weidman, C. Fujii, C. Bowman, L. Watthey, E. Wallin, W. S. Hayes, M. Borodovsky, P. D. Karp, H. O. Smith, C. M. Fraser, and J. C. Venter. 1997. The complete genome sequence of the gastric pathogen *Helicobacter pylori. Nature* **388:**539–547.

Wang, Y., K. P. Roos, and D. E. Taylor. 1993. Transformation of *Helicobacter pylori* by chromosomal metronidazole resistance and by a plasmid with a selectable chloramphenicol resistance marker. *J. Gen. Microbiol.* **139:**2485–2493.

Yamaoka, Y. 2008. Roles of the plasticity regions of *Helicobacter pylori* in gastroduodenal pathogenesis. *J. Med. Microbiol.* **57:**545–553.

Yamaoka, Y. 2010. Mechanisms of disease: Helicobacter pylori virulence factors. *Nat. Rev. Gastroenterol. Hepatol.* **7:**629–641.

Yamaoka, Y., M. Kita, T. Kodama, N. Sawai, T. Tanahashi, K. Kashima, and J. Imanishi. 1998a. Chemokines in the gastric mucosa in Helicobacter pylori infection. *Gut* **42:**609–617.

Yamaoka, Y., T. Kodama, K. Kashima, D. Y. Graham, and A. R. Sepulveda. 1998b. Variants of the 3′ region of the *cagA* gene in *Helicobacter pylori* isolates from patients with different *H. pylori*-associated diseases. *J. Clin. Microbiol.* **36:**2258–2263.

GENOME STRUCTURE AND VARIABILITY IN COAGULASE-NEGATIVE STAPHYLOCOCCI

Wilma Ziebuhr

4

Coagulase-negative staphylococci (CoNS) are primarily commensals residing on the skin and mucosa of humans and animals. In contrast to their highly pathogenic cousin *Staphylococcus aureus*, CoNS have a low pathogenic potential, typically causing opportunistic infections in immunocompromised individuals. CoNS are pathogens associated with medical progress as the vast majority of infections are linked to the use of indwelling medical devices such as intravascular and intrathecal catheter systems, pacemaker electrodes, arthroplasties, as well as urinary tract catheters and a range of other polymer and metal implants (Rupp and Archer, 1994). Also, the increasing number of immunocompromised patients favors the emergence of CoNS as pathogens. Although in the 1970s CoNS did not play any significant role as infectious agents, from the 1980s onward this situation changed considerably, with CoNS now being among the most common health care-associated pathogens. Thus, CoNS rank first in line-associated bloodstream infections and are the second most common cause of surgical-site infections (Dettenkofer et al., 2005; Edmond et al., 1999; Hugonnet et al., 2004; Richards et al., 2000; Wisplinghoff et al., 2004).

Nosocomial isolates of CoNS exhibit alarmingly high antibiotic resistance rates. In the United States, 89.1% of CoNS in intensive care units were found to be methicillin resistant, and similar figures have been reported for other countries as well (NNIS System Report, 2004; Goossens, 2005; Hope et al., 2008; Kresken et al., 2009). Because methicillin resistance is often associated with resistance to other groups of antibiotics, CoNS infections are extremely difficult to treat. Thus, CoNS increase morbidity and mortality rates and contribute significantly to the overall economic burden of health care-associated infections (Hope et al., 2008; Lauria and Angeletti, 2003; Rice, 2006). Despite their importance as pathogens, diagnosis of CoNS infections is still ambigous and challenging, mainly due to the lifestyle of CoNS as ubiquitous skin and mucosa colonizers. For this reason it is often difficult to decide whether an isolate represents the causative agent of an infection or a nonspecific contamination of a clinical specimen. In comparison to many other bacterial pathogens, knowledge of virulence-associated factors, pathogenesis, genome evolution, and

Wilma Ziebuhr, Universität Würzburg, Institut für Molekulare Infektionsbiologie, Josef-Schneider Str. 2, 97080 Würzburg, Germany.

Genome Plasticity and Infectious Diseases,
Edited by J. Hacker, U. Dobrindt, and R. Kurth,

epidemiology of CoNS was limited for a very long time.

Recent progress in genome research and molecular epidemiology has provided exciting novel insights into the biology of these bacteria. Thus, CoNS have proved to be extremely versatile and flexible microorganisms that can adapt very rapidly to changing environmental conditions on both the genetic and regulatory levels. This flexibility occurs in vitro and in vivo and is obviously influenced by the endowment of strains with certain virulence-associated factors and mobile genetic elements, the latter keeping the genome on the move. Interestingly, the majority of nosocomial infections with *Staphylococcus epidermidis* were found to be caused by a limited number of well-adapted clonal lineages that have become established in hospital settings as resident, potentially pathogenic bacteria. In these strains two putative virulence-associated determinants were identified. One is the *ica* gene cluster, mediating polysaccharide-dependent biofilm formation, and the other is IS*256*, an IS element thought to influence genome flexibility and adaptation of gene expression during an infection (Cho et al., 2002; Frebourg et al., 2000; Galdbart et al., 2000; Gu et al., 2005; Kozitskaya et al., 2004; Ziebuhr et al., 1997, 2006). This chapter summarizes the most recent findings in the genomics of CoNS and discusses the mechanisms and factors contributing to the extraordinary flexibility of these pathogens.

FITNESS AND VIRULENCE-ASSOCIATED FACTORS OF CoNS

Genome sequencing of microbes has become widely available and is currently revolutionizing the field of bacteriology and the understanding of infectious diseases in general. So far, representatives of all notable human bacterial pathogens have been sequenced, and the genome sequences of a number of strains of some species have been identified (Fournier et al., 2007). Genome sequencing projects are complete for the most common CoNS pathogens *S. epidermidis*, *S. haemolyticus*, and *S. saprophyticus*, as well as for the nonpathogenic species *S. carnosus*, and incomplete or provisional genome sequences exist for *S. hominis*, *S. capitis*, *S. warneri*, and *S. lugdunensis* (Tse et al., 2010). Most strikingly, all CoNS were found to be devoid of superantigen and toxin genes, but a number of genes and factors were identified which are obviously associated with the commensal lifestyle and also the virulence of CoNS.

S. epidermidis was the first CoNS genome to be sequenced and analyzed, and to date, two finished and another five incomplete genomes of the species are available (Gill et al., 2005; Zhang et al., 2003). The two completely sequenced strains are *S. epidermidis* ATCC 12228, a commensal isolate widely used as a reference strain for antibiotic susceptibility testing, and *S. epidermidis* RP62A, a strong biofilm-forming and pathogenic isolate originally obtained from a blood culture associated with a catheter-associated septicemia (Christensen et al., 1985). Direct comparison of the two genomes demonstrated a very uniform overall organization, except in a region around the origin of replication. This DNA region is inverted in RP62A and harbors a number of genes involved in adhesion and biofilm formation. Most strikingly, the *ica* gene complex, involved in polysaccharide intercellular adhesin (PIA)-mediated biofilm formation, is present in the RP62A strain but is missing in ATCC 12228. In both genomes, a number of genomic islands were detected (Table 1). Genomic islands are genetic elements on the bacterial chromosome which have been acquired by horizontal gene transfer. They often differ in their G+C content from the surrounding DNA, carry mobility genes, and are inserted in highly conserved regions of the chromosome such as tRNA loci. Most genomic islands are derived from mobile genetic elements, and in *S. epidermidis* they carry, among others, surface-associated proteins, heavy-metal resistance genes, or genes coding for phenol-soluble modulins, which are known to interact with the human innate immune system (Vuong et al., 2004) (Table 1).

From the genome analysis it is reasonable to suggest that both *S. epidermidis* strains are capable of maintaining an association with

TABLE 1 Genomic islands detected in coagulase-negative staphylococcal genomes

Genomic island	Prominent features encoded on island	Strain	Reference
S. epidermidis			
νSe1	Cadmium efflux	RP62A ATCC 1228	Gill et al., 2005
νSe2	Sortase, 2 LPXTG surface proteins	ATCC 1228	Zhang et al., 2003
νSeγ	Phenol-soluble modulin (β subunit)	RP62A ATCC 1228	Gill et al., 2005
ϕSPβ	*Bacillus subtilis* prophage	RP62A	Gill et al., 2005
S. haemolyticus			
νSh1	Sporulation control protein Spo0M	JCSC1435	Takeuchi et al., 2005
νSh2	Unknown		
νSh3	Na^+-transporting ATPase		
πSh1	Integrated plasmid carrying macrolide and cadmium resistance genes		
πSh2	Integrated plasmid encoding ABC transporters (mutidrug efflux pump)		
ϕSh1	Prophage carrying Tn*552* (conferring β-lactam resistance)		
ϕSh2	Truncated mercuric resistance gene		
S. saprophyticus			
νSs_{15305}	Streptomycin and fosfomycin resistance	ATCC 15305	Kuroda et al., 2005
ϕSs	39.3-kb prophage remnant		
S. carnosus			
νSCA1	Putative IgG-binding protein	TM300	Rosenstein et al., 2009
ϕTM300	45.7-kb prophage		

their host and thriving as commensals on the skin by interacting with matrix proteins and withstanding the action of the innate immune system. However, only *S. epidermidis* RP62A seems to have the potential to cause device-associated infections through its capcity to form a strong biofilm on inert surfaces by PIA/poly-*N*-acetylglucosamine (PNAG) production. In the other sequenced CoNS genomes, factors were also identified which are characteristic of the occurrence of a species in a certain ecological niche or are likely to be involved in pathogenesis. Thus, *S. saprophyticus*, a common uropathogen in young women, has additional sets of genes coding for transporter systems involved in osmoprotection, which probably help the species to survive under the high-ion-strength conditions in urine (Kuroda et al., 2005). Moreover, the presence of an adhesin mediating adherence to human bladder cells along with a highly active urease gene is likely to have shaped the species as a uropathogen (Gatermann et al., 1992a,1992b; Meyer et al., 1996; Szabados et al., 2008). In *S. haemolyticus*, the second most common cause of CoNS bloodstream infections, species-specific adaptive and virulence-associated factors include certain metabolic pathways, a typical hemolysin gene, a number of cell wall-associated adhesin genes, and genes encoding poly-γ-glutamate (PGA) capsule synthesis enzymes (Takeuchi et al., 2005). In contrast to other CoNS, *S. carnosus* is a completely apathogenic species which is used in the food industry (Götz, 1990), and the species was found to encode a series of metabolic pathways which obviously play a role when the bacterium is employed as a meat starter culture (e.g. nitrate/nitrite reduction, various sugar degradation pathways, and osmoprotection systems) (Rosenstein et al., 2009).

THE *oriC* ENVIRON OF CoNS GENOMES: A HOT SPOT FOR GENOME REARRANGEMENTS

An interesting finding of the CoNS sequencing projects was that many of the species- and virulence-specific genes described above are located in a certain region of the staphylococcal genome around the chromosomal origin of replication. This so-called *oriC* environ is defined as the region around *oriC* in which fewer than 45% of the genes encode common staphylococcal genes, and, indeed, most of the species-specific as well as accessory genes of CoNS are localized in this region. It seems to be the most dynamic part of the staphylococcal chromosome, in which the establishment of genetic diversity and delineation of strains and species are most likely to occur, including the incorporation of DNA that has been acquired by horizontal gene transfer. Thus, the region harbors not only biofilm and adhesion-associated genes but also many genomic islands and antibiotic resistance genes such as SCC elements. SCC cassettes represent large chromosomal DNA fragments which may harbor, in addition to the methicillin resistance-conferring *mecA* gene, a great variety of accessory genes, such as restriction modification systems, metabolic genes, integrated plasmids, transposons, insertion sequence elements, and many more. A characteristic feature of SCC cassettes is the presence of recombinase genes that confer mobility and mediate the site-specific integration of these elements into a highly conserved locus in the *oriC* environ (e.g., *orfX*). SCC elements are highly dynamic structures that readily undergo rearrangements, and a number of SCCs have been identified which are devoid of *mecA* but carry other genes instead (Katayama et al., 2003; Mongkolrattanothai et al., 2004). Therefore, SCCs are regarded as effective vectors for spreading useful genes among staphylococci (Hanssen and Ericson Sollid, 2006).

CoNS HAVE AN UNBALANCED GENOME STRUCTURE

When analyzing the general organization of various staphylococcal genomes, it became obvious that, in contrast to *S. aureus*, CoNS have unbalanced genomes in which, again, the *oriC* environ seems to play a role (Rosenstein et al., 2009). All circular bacterial chromosomes exhibit two replicores: replicore 1 is the DNA strand spanning clockwise from the origin of replication *oriC* to *terC*, the terminus of replication, while replicore 2 spans the rest of the genome counterclockwise from *oriC* to *terC*. Replication of bacterial circular chromosomes initiates at *oriC* and runs in both directions. It terminates at *terC*, where the two replication forks meet. In all *S. aureus* genomes sequenced so far and in many other bacterial genomes, *terC* is located exactly 180° from *oriC*, ensuring that the two replication forks have to cover an equal distance until termination. Such genomes are called balanced genomes. In contrast, in all sequenced CoNS genomes, *terC* significantly deviates from the 180° position. The biological consequences of this imbalance for CoNS are currently poorly understood. However, it is hypothesized that genome imbalance is a result of the accumulation of exogenous DNA by horizontal gene transfer and its incorporation mainly into the *oriC* environ of the staphylococcal chromosome. Frequent DNA inversions, deletions, and rearrangements detectable in this region are understood as mechanisms to (re)establish the physical balance of the genome (Rosenstein et al., 2009).

CoNS GENOMES AND MOBILE GENETIC ELEMENTS

CoNS harbor a great diversity of mobile genetic elements which comprise, in addition to plasmids, mainly bacteriophages, genomic islands, transposons, and insertion sequence elements (IS). Prophages and chromosomally integrated plasmids may lose their replicative function and become stable and integral parts of the chromosome to form genomic islands. Genomic islands often become hot spots for recombination events and the further uptake and integration of foreign DNA. The evolution of novel SCC elements, which obviously takes place preferentially within the CoNS population, is a good example of the ongoing evolution of genomic islands in these bacteria (Hanssen et al., 2004; Hanssen and Ericson Sollid, 2006). Other important players in shaping staphyloccal genomes are transposons and IS elements. Transposons and IS are DNA sequences capable of moving from one site within a genome to another. IS exclusively encode genes necessary for their own mobility, whereas transposons encode additional factors as well, usually antibiotic resistance genes.

While complex mobile genetic elements (i.e., plasmids, phages, and transposons) represent a clear benefit for the recipient cell through the acquisition of useful traits, the function of IS in bacterial genomes is not that obvious. IS can be found in all three kingdoms of life, and there is hardly any organism that is devoid of these elements (Filee et al., 2007; Mahillon and Chandler, 1998). With the notable exception of *S. carnosus*, CoNS harbor a large number of various IS in their genomes. IS exert a significant influence on expression of the genetic material and are important elements in genome organization (Siguier et al., 2006). Thus, IS are capable of inactivating genes by active transposition to new insertion sites, but they can also trigger gene expression of neighboring genes through intrinsic promoter structures (Maki et al., 2004; Maki and Murakami, 1997; Ziebuhr et al., 1999). IS often occur in multiple copies within a bacterial genome, thereby influencing the genome structure more passively by their mere presence. Thus, multiple copies of the same IS form repetitive DNA sequence stretches which serve as crossover points for homologous recombination events. The number of IS within a bacterial genome therefore also reflects the dynamics of the genetic material and its capacity for rearrangements and the generation of genetic diversity (Siguier et al., 2006). *Staphylococcus* species differ to some degree with respect to the number and nature of IS residing in their genomes. Thus, *S. aureus* strains contain on average 10 to 20 IS, while this number is considerably larger in coagulase-negative species involved in infections. The largest number (i.e., 82 IS) can be found in *S. haemolyticus*, and the two *S. epidermidis* genomes sequenced so far harbor up to 54 IS copies (Gill et al., 2005; Takeuchi et al., 2005; Zhang et al., 2003).

IS-mediated genome flexibility was recently suggested to play a role in the infection process; in particular, the IS*256* element detected in *S. epidermidis* RP62A and in other biofilm-forming clinical isolates was shown to be involved in the generation of phenotypic and genotypic diversity (Cho et al., 2002; Conlon et al., 2004; Gu et al., 2005; Kozitskaya et al., 2004; Ziebuhr et al., 1999). In contrast, the *S. carnosus* genome does not contain intact mobile genetic elements such as plasmids, transposons, SCCs, IS, or any other repetitive sequence stretches (Rosenstein et al., 2009). Lack of these elements is attributed to a relative stability of the *S. carnosus* genome and a low tendency for horizontal gene exchange with other bacteria as well as the apathogenicity of the species (Rosenstein et al., 2009).

EXTENSIVE HORIZONTAL GENE TRANSFER AMONG CoNS AND MECHANISMS OF ITS LIMITATION

A surprising result of the genome-sequencing projects was the strong evidence for an ongoing horizontal gene transfer across staphylococcal species and even genus borders. Thus, *S. epidermidis* RP62A was found to contain the *cap* operon, which encodes a PGA capsule and represents a major virulence factor in *Bacillus anthracis* (Gill et al., 2005). The presence of the *Bacillus* phage SPβ and detection of SCCmec cassettes, conferring methicillin resistance, that had been detected before in *S. aureus* are further hints that CoNS genomes are shaped by the uptake and incorporation of foreign DNA which often encodes antibiotic resistance genes or metabolic and virulence-associated genes whose acquisition might be of benefit for the recipient bacterium (Hanssen and Ericson Sollid, 2006). Therefore, horizontal gene transfer by mobile genetic elements has a major impact on enhancing the biological fitness of CoNS, but also contributes to the generation of genetic diversity within a species and the evolution and adaptation of the genome. However, from the evolutionary point of view, intensive exchange of genetic material may also represent an element of risk when nonbeneficial DNA is acquired and less fit or even nonviable variants are generated. Bacteria have evolved various mechanisms of self-protection against invading foreign DNA, of which restriction modification systems are the most widespread and best known systems (Kobayashi et al., 1999).

More recently it was discovered that *S. epidermidis* has adopted another fascinating mechanism to limit horizontal gene transfer and to specifically prevent the repeated uptake of elements that have already been acquired. So-called clustered, regularly interspaced, short palindromic repeat (CRISPR) loci were detected in the multiresistant clinical strain *S. epidermidis* RP62A (Marraffini and Sontheimer, 2008, 2010). CRISPR loci are known to be widespread in bacteria and archaea (Deveau et al., 2010; Horvath and Barrangou, 2010; Rousseau et al., 2009). In *S. epidermidis* they confer acquired immunity against the invasion of phages and conjugative plasmids (Marraffini and Sontheimer, 2008, 2010). CRISPR-mediated immunity is based on sequence matches between the invading mobile DNA element and short spacer DNA stretches that separate the CRISPR repeats. These spacer regions are highly dynamic and evolve rapidly upon contact with a novel mobile genetic element. The CRISPR repeats are regularly linked to a cluster of genes, *cas* (CRISPR-associated genes), encoding a sophisticated machinery of proteins involved in CRISPR adaptation and interference with invading DNA. The spacers, along with parts of the conserved CRISPR sequence, encode small untranslated RNAs that target the invading DNA in a sequence-specific manner by blocking it by direct base pairing (Karginov and Hannon, 2010). The mechanism is regarded as a kind of adaptive immune system of bacteria which acts as an important factor in limiting the spread of antibiotic resistance traits.

BIOFILM FORMATION ON MEDICAL DEVICES AND EVASION OF HOST DEFENSES BY CoNS

The vast majority of CoNS infections occur in immunocompromised patients carrying indwelling or implanted medical devices on which the bacteria form biofilms (Mack et al., 2006). Biofilms are understood to be bacterial communities which are engulfed in a self-produced extracellular matrix and which adhere to surfaces and/or to each other (Costerton et al., 1999). Biofilm formation is a major pathomechanism of CoNS, notably in *S. epidermidis*, the species causing most of the device-related infections in hospitalized patients (O'Gara, 2007). *S. epidermidis* employs various mechanisms to ensure biofilm formation. Thus, the biofilm matrix can consist of a PIA, which is also known, according to its structure, as poly-*N*-acetylglucosamine (PNAG) (Mack et al., 1996). The enzyme complex responsible for PIA/PNAG synthesis is encoded by the *icaADBC* operon (Heilmann et al., 1996), a gene cluster preferentially found in epidemic, health care-associated clonal lineages (Cho et al., 2002; Frebourg et al., 2000; Galdbart et al., 2000; Kozitskaya et al., 2004; Kozitskaya et al., 2005; Ziebuhr et al., 1997, 2006). However, *S. epidermidis* biofilm formation can also be mediated by proteins such as the accumulation-associated protein Aap and the biofilm-associated protein Bap/Bhp, respectively (Hussain et al., 1997; Lasa and Penades, 2006; Rohde et al., 2005; Tormo et al., 2005). Bacteria organized within a biofilm exhibit higher resistance to antibiotics than do their planktonically living peers, and biofilms are therefore regarded as one strategy to evade host defenses and to protect the bacteria from unfavorable external conditions. Moreover, PIA/PNAG itself was also shown to have direct effects on the innate immune system by inhibiting phagocytosis and killing through polymorphonuclear leukocytes as well as by increasing resistance to host-derived antimicrobial peptides (AMPs) and to the action of the complement system (Kristian et al., 2008; Vuong et al., 2004).

Another mechanism to evade the host defense is the PGA capsule of *S. epidermidis*, which was demonstrated to protect the organism from major components of the innate immune system and which is obviously present in many CoNS genomes (Kocianova et al., 2005). Also, *S. epidermidis* is able to sense AMPs in the environment by dedicated signaling systems (Bader et al., 2005; Li et al., 2007; Otto, 2009). AMPs are produced by eukaryotes and are in the first line of defense against many pathogens (Hancock and Sahl, 2006; Peschel and Sahl, 2006). Staphylococci, notably CoNS, are notoriously resistant to AMPs as a result of upregulation of genes that decrease susceptibiliy to these peptides or facilitate their export from the staphylococcal cell (Peschel et al., 1999, 2001). Other small molecules interacting with the immune system are the phenol-soluble modulins (PSMs), which are encoded by genomic islands or the *agr* quorum-sensing system (Vuong et al., 2004). PSMs were demonstrated to have proinflammatory and cytolytic effects on eukaryotes, and one compound, PSMδ (delta-toxin), is supposed to play a role in biofilm detachment and reinitiation of the process at other sites (Kong et al., 2006; Mehlin et al., 1999; Wang et al., 2007).

PHENOTYPIC AND GENETIC INSTABILITY OF CoNS

Clinical isolates of CoNS exhibit a pronounced heterogeneity which affects their phenotypic appearance on agar plates as well as their metabolic, antibiotic resistance, and virulence-associated traits. Thus, primary cultures from clinical specimens may differ in colony morphology, size, color, hemolysis, and other properties, suggesting, at first glance, a mixed bacterial population (Christensen et al., 1990; Deighton et al., 1992). Often this colony polymorphism disappears upon subcultivation in the laboratory, but some variations in biofilm formation and antibiotic resistance may be permanently detectable. Thus, early studies of *Staphylococcus* biofilm formation reported a high variability of biofilm expression, with the regular and spontaneous generation of biofilm-negative variants arising from a biofilm-forming population (Christensen et al., 1990; Ziebuhr et al., 1997).

In addition to biofilm formation, methicillin resistance was often found to be affected, and there is growing evidence to suggest that IS*256* plays a crucial role in these processes (Gu et al., 2005; Koskela et al., 2009; Kozitskaya et al., 2005; Mempel et al., 1994). IS*256* is present in multiple copies in the genomes of certain *icaADBC*-positive *S. epidermidis* clonal lineages preferentially associated with nosocomial infections, and the element is therefore regarded as a marker for invasive isolates (Kozitskaya et al., 2004, 2005; Petrelli et al., 2006; Ziebuhr et al., 1999, 2000). As IS*256* also forms the ends of composite transposon Tn*4001*, conferring aminoglycoside resistance, the element is detected in other multiresistant CoNS strains and species (e.g., *S. haemolyticus*) as well (Byrne et al., 1989). When active, IS transpose from one insertion site within a genome to another, and IS*256* was shown to insert spontaneously into biofilm-associated genes and global regulators of staphylococcal gene expression (Cho et al., 2002; Conlon et al., 2004; Gu et al., 2005; Kozitskaya et al., 2004; Ziebuhr et al., 1999). IS*256* also has the capacity to activate the expression of genes through the formation of strong hybrid promoters when the element inserts into the neighborhood of genes and operons (Couto et al., 2003; Maki et al., 2004; Maki and Murakami, 1997). As a result, a heterogeneous bacterial population is generated in which virulence, metabolic, and antibiotic resistance genes are differentially expressed. It is tempting to speculate that the presence of IS*256* confers an advantage to the infection process by facilitating the emergence of a variety of well-adapted variants that can readily cope with the very different environments on the skin and within the bloodstream, respectively. Thus, IS*256* was shown to impair *S. epidermidis* PIA expression by insertion into the *icaADBC* operon (Ziebuhr et al., 1999). The process is reversible, and precise IS*256* excision from an insertion site is due to an illegitimate recombination event which is independent of the element's transposase (Hennig and Ziebuhr, 2008). Interestingly, it was demonstrated that strains with a dysfunctional *ica* operon are able to induce biofilm formation, after repeated passages, by proteins, suggesting that the biofilm lifestyle is crucial for *S. epidermidis* and is ensured by more than one mechanism (Hennig et al., 2007). In addition to active transposition, multiple genomic IS*256* copies are supposed to trigger genome rearrangements. Thus, during the course of an infection, spontaneous IS*256*-mediated chromosomal DNA fragment deletions which encompass, among many metabolic genes, the *ica* operon and large parts of the methicillin/oxacillin resistance-conferring SCC*mec* elements may occur (Weisser et al., 2010; Ziebuhr et al., 2000).

S. epidermidis genome analyses indicate that both the *ica* genes and SCC*mec* elements are co-located in the *oriC* environ of the chromosome, suggesting a joint genetic instability of these traits (Ohlsen et al., 2006). This phenomenon is obviously not restricted to *S. epidermidis* but has also been found in *S. haemolyticus*, a species which typically harbors a large number of IS in its genome (Watanabe et al., 2007). Thus, upon drug-free passage of the multiresistant clinical isolate *S. haemolyticus* JCSC1435, large chromosomal rearrangements and deletions occurred as a result of the action of multiple copies of IS*Sha1*, an IS that forms composite transposons and mediates the excision and self-integration of large chromosomal fragments in the *oriC* environ (Watanabe et al., 2007).

CLINICAL IMPACT OF CoNS HETEROGENEOUS GENE EXPRESSION AND GENOME VARIABILITY

During the last decade, evidence has accumulated to suggest that heterogeneous gene expression and genome instability might play a crucial role in CoNS pathogenesis. Notably, the different mechanisms discussed above to modulate biofilm formation are indeed detectable during CoNS infections, and the process is therefore supposed to be critically involved in the establishment of device-associated *S. epidermidis* infections (Hennig et al., 2007). Thus, in a recently described clinical case of a fatal *S. epidermidis* septicemia, a number of consecutive isogenic isolates were obtained which differed with respect to biofilm formation and oxacillin resistance (Weisser et al., 2010). Isolates from the beginning of the infection produced a weak protein-mediated biofilm, while isogenic isolates from a later stage of the infection were strong PIA-expressing biofilm formers (Weisser et al., 2010). Moreover, in the same infection, a subpopulation of *S. epidermidis* was identified in which large chromosomal deletions had occurred in the *oriC* environ (Weisser et al., 2010). The deletions affected the *ica* operon along with the *mecA* gene, rendering the variants biofilm negative and oxacillin susceptible.

Similar observations have been made in the past in a number of other *S. epidermidis* infections such as cerebrospinal shunt-associated meningitis, native and prosthetic valve endocarditis, and joint prosthesis infections (Deighton et al., 1992; Galdbart et al., 1999; Van Eldere et al., 2000; Ziebuhr et al., 2000). In most cases, hypervariability of biofilm formation was detected which was also accompanied by genome rearrangements, reflecting a significant flexibility of the staphylococcal genome during the infection process. From these data it is reasonable to suggest that biofilm switching is of biological relevance in the highly dynamic course of a device-associated infection (illustrated in Fig. 1). PIA synthesis is a costly, energy- and resource-consuming process which was recently shown to be unnecessary and even detrimental when the bacteria live as commensals on the skin (Rogers et al., 2008). These data explain why, in numerous studies, the vast majority of *S. epidermidis* skin isolates were found to be PIA negative, either by downregulation or complete lack of the *icaADBC* operon or by the formation of protein-mediated biofilms (Cho et al., 2002; Frebourg et al., 2000; Galdbart et al., 2000; Kozitskaya et al., 2004, 2005; Ziebuhr et al., 1997, 2006).

In contrast, when the bacteria are translocated into the bloodstream, PIA production was demonstrated to be required and indispensable for survival as the polysaccharide protects the bacteria efficiently from antibiotics and the action of the host immune system (Flückiger et al., 2005). Therefore, *S. epidermidis* isolates recovered from bloodstream infections are likely to be *ica* positive and strong PIA producers (Cho et al., 2002; Frebourg et al., 2000; Galdbart et al., 2000; Kozitskaya et al., 2004, 2005; Ziebuhr et al., 1997, 2006). Thus, given the very different environments that *S. epidermidis*

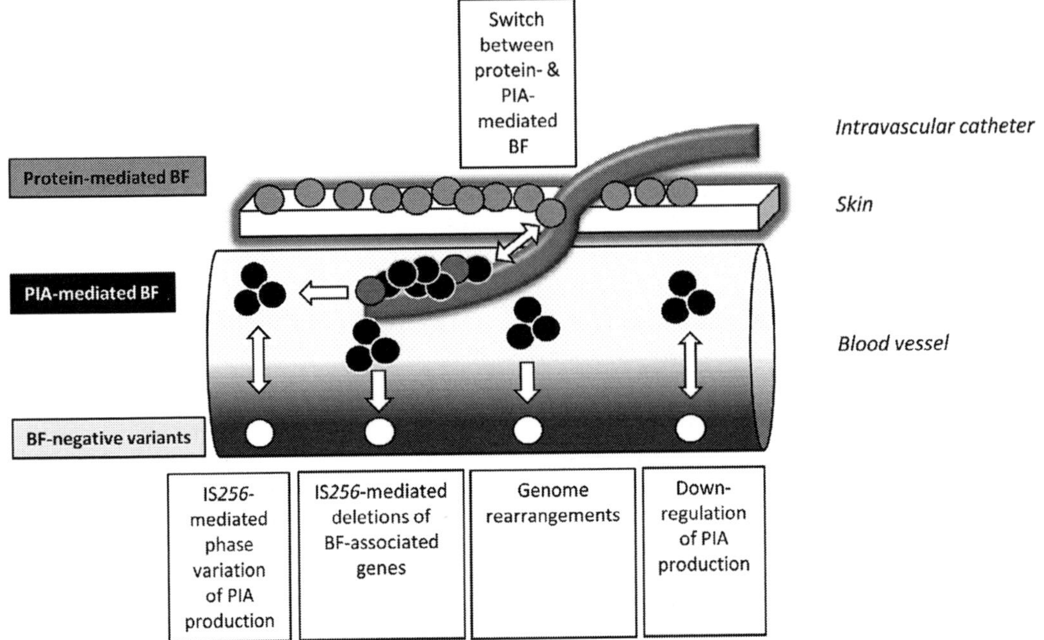

FIGURE 1 Dynamics of *S. epidermidis* biofilm formation (BF) during device-related infections.

encounters during a device-related infection (i.e., skin, inert implant surface, or bloodstream), biofilm formation needs to be highly adaptable; the species has indeed evolved various reversible and nonreversible mechanisms to switch off PIA production. Reversible mechanisms comprise (i) the regulatory control of *icaADBC* operon expression in response to external conditions such as subinhibitory concentrations of antibiotics (Rachid et al., 2000), (ii) the switch between protein- and PIA-mediated biofilm formation (Hennig et al., 2007; Weisser et al., 2010), and eventually (iii) the IS*256*-mediated phase variations of PIA production (Ziebuhr et al., 1999; Conlon et al., 2004). These mechanisms guarantee the reversion to a PIA-producing phenotype when needed. In contrast, other variants which have irreversibly lost their ability to form a biofilm occur regularly (Fig. 1). In such variants the biofilm-negative phenotype is mostly due to (IS-mediated) deletions of biofilm-associated genes and/or chromosomal rearrangements that occur preferentially in the *oriC* environ of the genome and that also affect antibiotic resistance genes (Ziebuhr et al., 2000; Weisser et al., 2010). Such permanently biofilm-negative and antibiotic-susceptible variants were found to be readily outcompeted by their strongly PIA-producing and antibiotic-resistant peers in the bloodstream (Weisser et al. 2010).

However, it is tempting to speculate that these variants might have an advantage and thrive when translocated again into another environment. The colocalization of biofilm and resistance genes within the unstable *oriC* environ of the genome certainly favors the loss of these traits. Moreover, this highly dynamic region is likely to be a hot spot for the integration of horizontally acquired DNA, giving rise to the generation of novel well-adapted variants and the clonal divergence of the species.

CONCLUSIONS

CoNS are now recognized as highly versatile bacteria that can adapt their gene expression patterns and genome very efficiently to rapidly changing environmental conditions. This flexibility is particularly pronounced in clinical isolates, and recent research suggests that the number and activity of mobile genetic elements present in the genomes of CoNS play a crucial role in this process, which may also determine pathogenesis, disease progression, and outcome of CoNS infections. Interestingly, this heterogeneity obviously not only influences the course of individual infections, but also favors the generation of novel genetic variants which have now adapted to and established in the hospital environment. High recombination rates and the unanticipated strong capacity for executing horizontal gene transfer even across species and genus borders make CoNS populations a significant reservoir for the evolution of novel resistance and virulence traits which might be passed on to more pathogenic species such as *S. aureus*.

REFERENCES

Bader, M. W., S. Sanowar, M. E. Daley, A. R. Schneider, U. Cho, W. Xu, R. E. Klevit, H. Le Moual, and S. I. Miller. 2005. Recognition of antimicrobial peptides by a bacterial sensor kinase. *Cell* **122:**461–472.

Byrne, M. E., D. A. Rouch, and R. A. Skurray. 1989. Nucleotide sequence analysis of IS*256* from the *Staphylococcus aureus* gentamicin-tobramycin-kanamycin-resistance transposon Tn*4001*. *Gene* **81:**361–367.

Cho, S. H., K. Naber, J. Hacker, and W. Ziebuhr. 2002. Detection of the *icaADBC* gene cluster and biofilm formation in *Staphylococcus epidermidis* isolates from catheter-related urinary tract infections. *Int. J. Antimicrob. Agents* **19:**570–575.

Christensen, G. D., L. M. Baddour, B. M. Madison, J. T. Parisi, S. N. Abraham, D. L. Hasty, J. H. Lowrance, J. A. Josephs, and W. A. Simpson. 1990. Colonial morphology of staphylococci on Memphis agar: phase variation of slime production, resistance to beta-lactam antibiotics, and virulence. *J. Infect. Dis.* **161:**1153–1169.

Christensen, G. D., W. A. Simpson, J. J. Younger, L. M. Baddour, F. F. Barrett, D. M. Melton, and E. H. Beachey. 1985. Adherence of coagulase-negative staphylococci to plastic tissue culture plates: a quantitative model for the adherence of staphylococci to medical devices. *J. Clin. Microbiol.* **22:**996–1006.

Conlon, K., H. Humphreys, and J. O'Gara. 2004. Inactivations of *rsbU* and *sarA* by IS*256* represent novel mechanisms of biofilm phenotypic variation in *Staphylococcus epidermidis*. *J. Bacteriol.* **186:**6208–6219.

Costerton, J. W., P. S. Stewart, and E. P. Greenberg. 1999. Bacterial biofilms: a common cause of persistent infections. *Science* **284:**1318–1322.

Couto, I., S. W. Wu, A. Tomasz, and H. de Lencastre. 2003. Development of methicillin resistance in clinical isolates of *Staphylococcus sciuri* by transcriptional activation of the *mecA* homologue native to the species. *J. Bacteriol.* **185:**645–653.

Deighton, M., S. Pearson, J. Capstick, D. Spelman, and R. Borland. 1992. Phenotypic variation of *Staphylococcus epidermidis* isolated from a patient with native valve endocarditis. *J. Clin. Microbiol.* **30:**2385–2390.

Dettenkofer, M., S. Wenzler-Rottele, R. Babikir, H. Bertz, W. Ebner, E. Meyer, H. Ruden, P. Gastmeier, and F. D. Daschner. 2005. Surveillance of nosocomial sepsis and pneumonia in patients with a bone marrow or peripheral blood stem cell transplant: a multicenter project. *Clin. Infect. Dis.* **40:**926–931.

Deveau, H., J. E. Garneau, and S. Moineau. 2010. CRISPR/Cas system and its role in phage-bacteria interactions. *Annu. Rev. Microbiol.* **64:**475–493.

Edmond, M. B., S. E. Wallace, D. K. McClish, M. A. Pfaller, R. N. Jones, and R. P. Wenzel. 1999. Nosocomial bloodstream infections in United States hospitals: a three-year analysis. *Clin. Infect. Dis.* **29:**239–244.

Filee, J., P. Siguier, and M. Chandler. 2007. Insertion sequence diversity in archaea. *Microbiol. Mol. Biol. Rev.* **71:**121–157.

Flückiger, U., M. Ulrich, A. Steinhuber, G. Döring, D. Mack, R. Landmann, C. Goerke, and C. Wolz. 2005. Biofilm formation, *icaADBC* transcription, and polysaccharide intercellular adhesin synthesis by staphylococci in a device-related infection model. *Infect. Immun.* **73:**1811–1819.

Fournier, P. E., M. Drancourt, and D. Raoult. 2007. Bacterial genome sequencing and its use in infectious diseases. *Lancet Infect. Dis.* **7:**711–723.

Frebourg, N. B., S. Lefebvre, S. Baert, and J. F. Lemeland. 2000. PCR-based assay for discrimination between invasive and contaminating *Staphylococcus epidermidis* strains. *J. Clin. Microbiol.* **38:**877–880.

Galdbart, J. O., J. Allignet, H. S. Tung, C. Ryden, and N. El Solh. 2000. Screening for *Staphylococcus epidermidis* markers discriminating between skin-flora strains and those responsible for infections of joint prostheses. *J. Infect. Dis.* **182:**351–355.

Galdbart, J. O., A. Morvan, N. Desplaces, and N. el Solh. 1999. Phenotypic and genomic variation among *Staphylococcus epidermidis* strains infecting joint prostheses. *J. Clin. Microbiol.* **37:**1306–1312.

Gatermann, S., B. Kreft, R. Marre, and G. Wanner. 1992a. Identification and characterization of a surface-associated protein (Ssp) of *Staphylococcus saprophyticus*. *Infect. Immun.* **60:**1055–1060.

Gatermann, S., H. G. Meyer, and G. Wanner. 1992b. *Staphylococcus saprophyticus* hemagglutinin is a 160-kilodalton surface polypeptide. *Infect. Immun.* **60:**4127–4132.

Gill, S. R., D. E. Fouts, G. L. Archer, E. F. Mongodin, R. T. Deboy, J. Ravel, I. T. Paulsen, J. F. Kolonay, L. Brinkac, M. Beanan, R. J. Dodson, S. C. Daugherty, R. Madupu, S. V. Angiuoli, A. S. Durkin, D. H. Haft, J. Vamathevan, H. Khouri, T. Utterback, C. Lee, G. Dimitrov, L. Jiang, H. Qin, J. Weidman, K. Tran, K. Kang, I. R. Hance, K. E. Nelson, and C. M. Fraser. 2005. Insights on evolution of virulence and resistance from the complete genome analysis of an early methicillin-resistant *Staphylococcus aureus* strain and a biofilm-producing methicillin-resistant *Staphylococcus epidermidis* strain. *J. Bacteriol.* **187:**2426–2438.

Goossens, H. 2005. European status of resistance in nosocomial infections. *Chemotherapy* **51:**177–181.

Götz, F. 1990. *Staphylococcus carnosus*: a new host organism for gene cloning and protein production. *Soc. Appl. Bacteriol. Symp. Ser.* **19:**49S–53S.

Gu, J., H. Li, M. Li, C. Vuong, M. Otto, Y. Wen, and Q. Gao. 2005. Bacterial insertion sequence IS*256* as a potential molecular marker to discriminate invasive strains from commensal strains of *Staphylococcus epidermidis*. *J. Hosp. Infect.* **61:**342–348.

Hancock, R. E., and H. G. Sahl. 2006. Antimicrobial and host-defense peptides as new anti-infective therapeutic strategies. *Nat. Biotechnol.* **24:**1551–1557.

Hanssen, A. M., and J. U. Ericson Sollid. 2006. SCCmec in staphylococci: genes on the move. *FEMS Immunol. Med. Microbiol.* **46:**8–20.

Hanssen, A. M., G. Kjeldsen, and J. U. Sollid. 2004. Local variants of staphylococcal cassette chromosome *mec* in sporadic methicillin-resistant *Staphylococcus aureus* and methicillin-resistant coagulase-negative staphylococci: evidence of horizontal gene transfer? *Antimicrob. Agents Chemother.* **48:**285–296.

Heilmann, C., O. Schweitzer, C. Gerke, N. Vanittanakom, D. Mack, and F. Götz. 1996. Molecular basis of intercellular adhesion in the biofilm-forming *Staphylococcus epidermidis*. *Mol. Microbiol.* **20:**1083–1091.

Hennig, S., S. Nyunt Wai, and W. Ziebuhr. 2007. Spontaneous switch to PIA-independent biofilm formation in an *ica*-positive *Staphylococcus epidermidis* isolate. *Int. J. Med. Microbiol.* **297:**117–122.

Hennig, S., and W. Ziebuhr. 2008. A transposase-independent mechanism gives rise to precise excision of IS*256* from insertion sites in *Staphylococcus epidermidis*. *J. Bacteriol.* **190:**1488–1490.

Hope, R., D. M. Livermore, G. Brick, M. Lillie, and R. Reynolds. 2008. Non-susceptibility trends among staphylococci from bacteraemias in the UK and Ireland, 2001–06. *J. Antimicrob. Chemother.* **62**(Suppl. 2)**:**ii65–ii74.

Horvath, P., and R. Barrangou. 2010. CRISPR/Cas, the immune system of bacteria and archaea. *Science* **327:**167–170.

Hugonnet, S., H. Sax, P. Eggimann, J. C. Chevrolet, and D. Pittet. 2004. Nosocomial bloodstream infection and clinical sepsis. *Emerg. Infect. Dis.* **10:**76–81.

Hussain, M., M. Herrmann, C. von Eiff, F. Perdreau-Remington, and G. Peters. 1997. A 140-kilodalton extracellular protein is essential for the accumulation of *Staphylococcus epidermidis* strains on surfaces. *Infect. Immun.* **65:**519–524.

Karginov, F. V., and G. J. Hannon. 2010. The CRISPR system: small RNA-guided defense in bacteria and archaea. *Mol. Cell* **37:**7–19.

Katayama, Y., F. Takeuchi, T. Ito, X. X. Ma, Y. Ui-Mizutani, I. Kobayashi, and K. Hiramatsu. 2003. Identification in methicillin-susceptible *Staphylococcus hominis* of an active primordial mobile genetic element for the staphylococcal cassette chromosome *mec* of methicillin-resistant *Staphylococcus aureus*. *J. Bacteriol.* **185:**2711–2722.

Kobayashi, I., A. Nobusato, N. Kobayashi-Takahashi, and I. Uchiyama. 1999. Shaping the genome—restriction-modification systems as mobile genetic elements. *Curr. Opin. Genet. Dev.* **9:**649–656.

Kocianova, S., C. Vuong, Y. Yao, J. M. Voyich, E. R. Fischer, F. R. DeLeo, and M. Otto. 2005. Key role of poly-gamma-DL-glutamic acid in immune evasion and virulence of *Staphylococcus epidermidis*. *J. Clin. Investig.* **115:**688–694.

Kong, K. F., C. Vuong, and M. Otto. 2006. *Staphylococcus* quorum sensing in biofilm formation and infection. *Int. J. Med. Microbiol.* **296:**133–139.

Koskela, A., A. Nilsdotter-Augustinsson, L. Persson, and B. Soderquist. 2009. Prevalence of the *ica* operon and insertion sequence IS*256* among *Staphylococcus epidermidis* prosthetic joint infection isolates. *Eur. J. Clin. Microbiol. Infect. Dis.* **28:**655–660.

Kozitskaya, S., S. H. Cho, K. Dietrich, R. Marre, K. Naber, and W. Ziebuhr. 2004. The bacterial insertion sequence element IS*256* occurs preferentially in nosocomial *Staphylococcus epidermidis* isolates: association with biofilm formation and resistance to aminoglycosides. *Infect. Immun.* **72:**1210–1215.

Kozitskaya, S., M. E. Olson, P. D. Fey, W. Witte, K. Ohlsen, and W. Ziebuhr. 2005. Clonal analysis of *Staphylococcus epidermidis* isolates carrying or lacking biofilm-mediating genes by multilocus sequence typing. *J. Clin. Microbiol.* **43:**4751–4757.

Kresken, M., D. Hafner, F.-J. Schmitz, and T. A. Wichelhaus. 2009. *Resistenzsituation bei klinisch wichtigen Infektionserregern gegenüber Antibiotika in Deutschland und im mitteleuropäischen Raum.*

Antiinfectives Intelligence, Rheinbach, Germany. http://www.p-e-g.org/ag_resistenz/PEG-Studie-2007.pdf.

Kristian, S. A., T. A. Birkenstock, U. Sauder, D. Mack, F. Götz, and R. Landmann. 2008. Biofilm formation induces C3a release and protects *Staphylococcus epidermidis* from IgG and complement deposition and from neutrophil-dependent killing. *J. Infect. Dis.* **197:**1028–1035.

Kuroda, M., A. Yamashita, H. Hirakawa, M. Kumano, K. Morikawa, M. Higashide, A. Maruyama, Y. Inose, K. Matoba, H. Toh, S. Kuhara, M. Hattori, and T. Ohta. 2005. Whole genome sequence of *Staphylococcus saprophyticus* reveals the pathogenesis of uncomplicated urinary tract infection. *Proc. Natl. Acad. Sci. USA* **102:**13272–13277.

Lasa, I., and J. R. Penades. 2006. Bap: a family of surface proteins involved in biofilm formation. *Res. Microbiol.* **157:**99–107.

Lauria, F. N., and C. Angeletti. 2003. The impact of nosocomial infections on hospital care costs. *Infection* **31**(Suppl. 2):35–43.

Li, M., Y. Lai, A. E. Villaruz, D. J. Cha, D. E. Sturdevant, and M. Otto. 2007. Gram-positive three-component antimicrobial peptide-sensing system. *Proc. Natl. Acad. Sci. USA* **104:**9469–9474.

Mack, D., W. Fischer, A. Krokotsch, K. Leopold, R. Hartmann, H. Egge, and R. Laufs. 1996. The intercellular adhesin involved in biofilm accumulation of *Staphylococcus epidermidis* is a linear beta-1,6-linked glucosaminoglycan: purification and structural analysis. *J. Bacteriol.* **178:**175–183.

Mack, D., H. Rohde, L. G. Harris, A. P. Davies, M. A. Horstkotte, and J. K. Knobloch. 2006. Biofilm formation in medical device-related infection. *Int. J. Artif. Organs* **29:**343–359.

Mahillon, J., and M. Chandler. 1998. Insertion sequences. *Microbiol. Mol. Biol. Rev.* **62:**725–774.

Maki, H., N. McCallum, M. Bischoff, A. Wada, and B. Berger-Bächi. 2004. *tcaA* inactivation increases glycopeptide resistance in *Staphylococcus aureus*. Antimicrob. Agents Chemother. **48:**1953–1959.

Maki, H., and K. Murakami. 1997. Formation of potent hybrid promoters of the mutant *llm* gene by IS*256* transposition in methicillin-resistant *Staphylococcus aureus*. *J. Bacteriol.* **179:**6944–6948.

Marraffini, L. A., and E. J. Sontheimer. 2008. CRISPR interference limits horizontal gene transfer in staphylococci by targeting DNA. *Science* **322:**1843–1845.

Marraffini, L. A., and E. J. Sontheimer. 2010. Self versus non-self discrimination during CRISPR RNA-directed immunity. *Nature* **463:**568–571.

Mehlin, C., C. M. Headley, and S. J. Klebanoff. 1999. An inflammatory polypeptide complex from *Staphylococcus epidermidis*: isolation and characterization. *J. Exp. Med.* **189:**907–918.

Mempel, M., H. Feucht, W. Ziebuhr, M. Endres, R. Laufs, and L. Grüter. 1994. Lack of *mecA* transcription in slime-negative phase variants of methicillin-resistant *Staphylococcus epidermidis*. *Antimicrob. Agents Chemother.* **38:**1251–1255.

Meyer, H. G., U. Wengler-Becker, and S. G. Gatermann. 1996. The hemagglutinin of *Staphylococcus saprophyticus* is a major adhesin for uroepithelial cells. *Infect. Immun.* **64:**3893–3896.

Mongkolrattanothai, K., S. Boyle, T. V. Murphy, and R. S. Daum. 2004. Novel non-*mecA*-containing staphylococcal chromosomal cassette composite island containing *pbp4* and *tagF* genes in a commensal staphylococcal species: a possible reservoir for antibiotic resistance islands in *Staphylococcus aureus*. *Antimicrob. Agents Chemother.* **48:**1823–1836.

National Nosocomial Infections Surveillance System. 2004. National Nosocomial Infections Surveillance (NNIS) System Report, data summary from January 1992 through June 2004, issued October 2004. *Am. J. Infect. Control* **32:**470-485.

O'Gara, J. P. 2007. *ica* and beyond: biofilm mechanisms and regulation in *Staphylococcus epidermidis* and *Staphylococcus aureus*. *FEMS Microbiol. Lett.* **270:**179–188.

Ohlsen, K., M. Eckart, C. Hüttinger, and W. Ziebuhr. 2006. Pathogenic staphylococci: lessons from comparative genomics, p. 175–210. *In* J. Hacker and U. Dobrindt (ed.), *Pathogenomics: Genome Analysis of Pathogenic Microbes*. Wiley-VCH, Weinheim, Germany.

Otto, M. 2009. Bacterial sensing of antimicrobial peptides. *Contrib. Microbiol.* **16:**136–149.

Peschel, A., R. W. Jack, M. Otto, L. V. Collins, P. Staubitz, G. Nicholson, H. Kalbacher, W. F. Nieuwenhuizen, G. Jung, A. Tarkowski, K. P. van Kessel, and J. A. van Strijp. 2001. *Staphylococcus aureus* resistance to human defensins and evasion of neutrophil killing via the novel virulence factor MprF is based on modification of membrane lipids with l-lysine. *J. Exp. Med.* **193:**1067–1076.

Peschel, A., M. Otto, R. W. Jack, H. Kalbacher, G. Jung, and F. Götz. 1999. Inactivation of the *dlt* operon in *Staphylococcus aureus* confers sensitivity to defensins, protegrins, and other antimicrobial peptides. J. Biol. Chem. **274:**8405–8410.

Peschel, A., and H. G. Sahl. 2006. The co-evolution of host cationic antimicrobial peptides and microbial resistance. *Nat. Rev. Microbiol.* **4:**529–536.

Petrelli, D., C. Zampaloni, S. D'Ercole, M. Prenna, P. Ballarini, S. Ripa, and L. A. Vitali. 2006. Analysis of different genetic traits and their association with biofilm formation in *Staphylococcus epidermidis* isolates from central venous catheter infections. *Eur. J. Clin. Microbiol. Infect. Dis.* **25:**773–781.

Rachid, S., K. Ohlsen, W. Witte, J. Hacker, and W. Ziebuhr. 2000. Effect of subinhibitory antibiotic concentrations on polysaccharide intercellular adhesin expression in biofilm-forming *Staphylococcus epidermidis. Antimicrob. Agents Chemother.* **44:**3357–3363.

Rice, L. B. 2006. Antimicrobial resistance in gram-positive bacteria. *Am. J. Med.* **119:**S11–S19, discussion S62–S70.

Richards, M. J., J. R. Edwards, D. H. Culver, and R. P. Gaynes. 2000. Nosocomial infections in combined medical-surgical intensive care units in the United States. *Infect. Control Hosp. Epidemiol.* **21:**510–515.

Rogers, K. L., M. E. Rupp, and P. D. Fey. 2008. The presence of *icaADBC* is detrimental to the colonization of human skin by *Staphylococcus epidermidis. Appl. Environ. Microbiol.* **74:**6155–6157.

Rohde, H., C. Burdelski, K. Bartscht, M. Hussain, F. Buck, M. A. Horstkotte, J. K. Knobloch, C. Heilmann, M. Herrmann, and D. Mack. 2005. Induction of *Staphylococcus epidermidis* biofilm formation via proteolytic processing of the accumulation-associated protein by staphylococcal and host proteases. *Mol. Microbiol.* **55:**1883–1895.

Rosenstein, R., C. Nerz, L. Biswas, A. Resch, G. Raddatz, S. C. Schuster, and F. Götz. 2009. Genome analysis of the meat starter culture bacterium *Staphylococcus carnosus* TM300. *Appl. Environ. Microbiol.* **75:**811–822.

Rousseau, C., M. Gonnet, M. Le Romancer, and J. Nicolas. 2009. CRISPI: a CRISPR interactive database. *Bioinformatics* **25:**3317–3318.

Rupp, M. E., and G. L. Archer. 1994. Coagulase-negative staphylococci: pathogens associated with medical progress. *Clin. Infect. Dis.* **19:**231–243.

Siguier, P., J. Filee, and M. Chandler. 2006. Insertion sequences in prokaryotic genomes. *Curr. Opin. Microbiol.* **9:**526–531.

Szabados, F., B. Kleine, A. Anders, M. Kaase, T. Sakinc, I. Schmitz, and S. Gatermann. 2008. *Staphylococcus saprophyticus* ATCC 15305 is internalized into human urinary bladder carcinoma cell line 5637. *FEMS Microbiol. Lett.* **285:**163–169.

Takeuchi, F., S. Watanabe, T. Baba, H. Yuzawa, T. Ito, Y. Morimoto, M. Kuroda, L. Cui, M. Takahashi, A. Ankai, S. Baba, S. Fukui, J. C. Lee, and K. Hiramatsu. 2005. Whole-genome sequencing of *Staphylococcus haemolyticus* uncovers the extreme plasticity of its genome and the evolution of human-colonizing staphylococcal species. *J. Bacteriol.* **187:**7292–7308.

Tormo, M. A., E. Knecht, F. Götz, I. Lasa, and J. R. Penades. 2005. Bap-dependent biofilm formation by pathogenic species of *Staphylococcus*: evidence of horizontal gene transfer? *Microbiology* **151:**2465–2475.

Tse, H., H. W. Tsoi, S. P. Leung, S. K. Lau, P. C. Woo, and K. Y. Yuen. 2010. Complete genome sequence of *Staphylococcus lugdunensis* strain HKU09-01. *J. Bacteriol.* **192:**1471–1472.

Van Eldere, J., W. E. Peetermans, M. Struelens, A. Deplano, and H. Bobbaers. 2000. Polyclonal staphylococcal endocarditis caused by genetic variability. *Clin. Infect. Dis.* **31:**24–30.

Vuong, C., M. Durr, A. B. Carmody, A. Peschel, S. J. Klebanoff, and M. Otto. 2004. Regulated expression of pathogen-associated molecular pattern molecules in *Staphylococcus epidermidis*: quorum-sensing determines pro-inflammatory capacity and production of phenol-soluble modulins. *Cell. Microbiol.* **6:**753–759.

Vuong, C., J. M. Voyich, E. R. Fischer, K. R. Braughton, A. R. Whitney, F. R. DeLeo, and M. Otto. 2004. Polysaccharide intercellular adhesin (PIA) protects *Staphylococcus epidermidis* against major components of the human innate immune system. *Cell. Microbiol.* **6:**269–275.

Wang, R., K. R. Braughton, D. Kretschmer, T. H. Bach, S. Y. Queck, M. Li, A. D. Kennedy, D. W. Dorward, S. J. Klebanoff, A. Peschel, F. R. DeLeo, and M. Otto. 2007. Identification of novel cytolytic peptides as key virulence determinants for community-associated MRSA. *Nat. Med.* **13:**1510–1514.

Watanabe, S., T. Ito, Y. Morimoto, F. Takeuchi, and K. Hiramatsu. 2007. Precise excision and self-integration of a composite transposon as a model for spontaneous large-scale chromosome inversion/deletion of the *Staphylococcus haemolyticus* clinical strain JCSC1435. *J. Bacteriol.* **189:**2921–2925.

Weisser, M., S. M. Schoenfelder, C. Orasch, C. Arber, A. Gratwohl, R. Frei, M. Eckart, U. Flückiger, and W. Ziebuhr. 2010. Hypervariability of biofilm formation and oxacillin resistance in a *Staphylococcus epidermidis* strain causing persistent severe infection in an immunocompromised patient. *J. Clin. Microbiol.* **48:**2407–2412.

Wisplinghoff, H., T. Bischoff, S. M. Tallent, H. Seifert, R. P. Wenzel, and M. B. Edmond. 2004. Nosocomial bloodstream infections in US hospitals: analysis of 24,179 cases from a prospective nationwide surveillance study. *Clin. Infect. Dis.* **39:**309–317.

Zhang, Y. Q., S. X. Ren, H. L. Li, Y. X. Wang, G. Fu, J. Yang, Z. Q. Qin, Y. G. Miao, W. Y. Wang, R. S. Chen, Y. Shen, Z. Chen, Z. H. Yuan, G. P. Zhao, D. Qu, A. Danchin, and Y. M. Wen. 2003. Genome-based analysis of virulence genes in a non-biofilm-forming *Staphylococcus epidermidis* strain (ATCC 12228). *Mol. Microbiol.* **49:**1577–1593.

Ziebuhr, W., K. Dietrich, M. Trautmann, and M. Wilhelm. 2000. Chromosomal rearrangements affecting biofilm production and antibiotic resistance in a *Staphylococcus epidermidis* strain causing shunt-associated ventriculitis. *Int. J. Med. Microbiol.* **290:**115–120.

Ziebuhr, W., C. Heilmann, F. Götz, P. Meyer, K. Wilms, E. Straube, and J. Hacker. 1997. Detection of the intercellular adhesion gene cluster (*ica*) and phase variation in *Staphylococcus epidermidis* blood culture strains and mucosal isolates. *Infect. Immun.* **65:**890–896.

Ziebuhr, W., S. Hennig, M. Eckart, H. Kraenzler, C. Batzilla, and S. Kozitskaya. 2006. Nosocomial infections by *Staphylococcus epidermidis*: how a commensal bacterium turns into a pathogen. *Int. J. Antimicrob. Agents* **28**(Suppl. 1)**:**S14–S20.

Ziebuhr, W., V. Krimmer, S. Rachid, I. Loessner, F. Götz, and J. Hacker. 1999. A novel mechanism of phase variation of virulence in *Staphylococcus epidermidis*: evidence for control of the polysaccharide intercellular adhesin synthesis by alternating insertion and excision of the insertion sequence element IS*256*. *Mol. Microbiol.* **32:**345–356.

GENOME PLASTICITY IN *Legionella pneumophila* AND *Legionella longbeachae*: IMPACT ON HOST CELL EXPLOITATION

L. Gomez Valero, C. Rusniok, and C. Buchrieser

5

The genus *Legionella* comprises gram-negative bacilli belonging to the gamma subgroup of the proteobacteria. At present 56 species and subspecies and 70 serogroups (http://www.dsmz.de/bactnom/bactname.htm) have been described (Fields et al., 2002; Gomez-Valero et al., 2009; Steinert et al., 2002). *Legionella* species are ubiquitous in aquatic environments, in moist soil, and in mud. The fastidious nature of *Legionella* in axenic cultures (a high requirement of L-cysteine and ferric iron in laboratory media) contrasts with the nutritionally poor environments in which *Legionella* species are commonly detected. However, it is assumed that dense microbial communities, as occurring in sediments and biofilms—but not likely in surface and drinking water—may provide the necessary growth requirements for *Legionella*. In fact, in its natural environment *Legionella* seems to replicate only intracellularly in protozoan hosts (e.g., amoebas like *Acanthamoeba castellanii*) (Fields, 1993, 2008; Rowbotham, 1986).

L. Gomez Valero, C. Rusniok, and C. Buchrieser, Institut Pasteur, Unité de Biologie des Bactéries Intracellulaires and CNRS URA 2171, 28, rue du Dr. Roux, 75724 Paris Cedex 15, France.

Although *Legionella* are mainly environmental bacteria, important human pathogens are present within this genus, of which the most prominent are *Legionella pneumophila* (Fraser et al., 1977; McDade et al., 1977) and *Legionella longbeachae* (McKinney et al., 1981). Legionellosis has emerged in the second half of the 20th century partly due to human alterations of the environment. The development of artificial water systems like air conditioning systems, cooling towers, showers, and other aerosolizing devices in recent decades has allowed *Legionella* to gain access to the human respiratory system. When inhaled in contaminated aerosols, pathogenic *Legionella* organisms can reach the alveoli of the lung, where they are subsequently engulfed by macrophages. In contrast to most bacteria, which are destroyed, some *Legionella* species can multiply within the phagosome and eventually kill the macrophage, resulting in a severe, often fatal pneumonia called legionellosis or Legionnaires' disease (mortality rate of 5% to 20%, up to 50% in nosocomial infections) (Marrie, 2008; Steinert et al., 2002). Treatment of infections by *Legionella* necessitates the use of antibiotics that penetrate well into macrophages, the host cells in human infection (Pedro-Botet and Yu, 2009). Delay in the onset of adequate therapy is a key

Genome Plasticity and Infectious Diseases,
Edited by J. Hacker, U. Dobrindt, and R. Kurth,

factor associated with a poor outcome of the treatment. Therefore, the development of rapid and efficient methods of detection is critical for an optimal result.

An interesting epidemiological observation is that among the over 50 *Legionella* species described today, strains belonging to the species *L. pneumophila* are responsible for over 90% of legionellosis cases worldwide and strains belonging to the species *L. longbeachae* are responsible for about 5% of human legionellosis cases worldwide (Yu et al., 2002). Surprisingly, this distribution is very different in Australia and New Zealand, where *L. pneumophila* accounts for only 45.7% of human cases but *L. longbeachae* is implicated in 30.4% of human cases. Furthermore, among the strains causing Legionnaires' disease, *L. pneumophila* Sg1 alone is responsible for 85% of cases (Doleans et al., 2004; Yu et al., 2002) despite the description of 15 different serogroups within this species. In addition, the characterization of more than 400 different *L. pneumophila* Sg1 strains has shown that only a minority among them are responsible for causing most of the human disease (Edelstein and Metlay, 2009). Some of these clones are distributed worldwide like *L. pneumophila* strain Paris (Cazalet et al., 2008), while others have a more restricted geographical distribution, like the recently described endemic clone prevalent in Ontario, Canada (Tijet et al., 2010).

Despite the fact that the main human pathogenic *Legionella* species, *L. pneumophila* and *L. longbeachae*, cause the same disease and symptoms in humans (Amodeo et al., 2010), there exist major differences between the two species in niche adaptation and host susceptibility.

1. They are found in different environmental niches, as *L. pneumophila* is found mainly in natural and artificial water circuits and *L. longbeachae* is found mainly in soil and is therefore associated with gardening and use of potting compost (O'Connor et al., 2007). However, although less common, the isolation of *L. pneumophila* from potting soil in Europe has also been reported (Velonakis et al., 2009; Casati et al., 2009). Human infection due to *L. longbeachae* is particularly common in Australia, but cases have also been documented in other countries, such as the United States, Japan, Spain, England, and Germany (CDC, 2000; Kubota et al., 2007; Kumpers et al., 2008; Garcia et al., 2004; Pravinkumar et al., 2010).
2. Like other *Legionella* species, person-to-person transmission has not been documented; however, for *L. longbeachae*, the primary transmission mode seems to be inhalation of dust from contaminated compost or soil that contains the organism and not contaminated water droplets as for *L. pneumophila* (CDC, 2000; O'Connor et al., 2007; Steele et al., 1990).
3. Furthermore, for *L. pneumophila* a biphasic life cycle was observed in vitro and in vivo as exponential-phase bacteria do not express virulence factors and are unable to replicate intracellularly. The ability of *L. pneumophila* to replicate intracellularly is triggered at the postexponential phase together with other virulence traits. In contrast, less is known about the *L. longbeachae* intracellular life cycle and its virulence factors. It was recently shown that, unlike *L. pneumophila*, the ability of *L. longbeachae* to replicate intracellularly is independent of the bacterial growth phase (Asare and Abu Kwaik, 2007) and that phagosome biogenesis is different. Like *L. pneumophila*, the *L. longbeachae* phagosome is surrounded by endoplasmic reticulum and does not mature to a phagolysosome; however, it acquires early and late endosomal markers (Asare and Abu Kwaik, 2007).
4. Another interesting difference between these two species is their ability to colonize the lungs of mice. While only A/J mice are permissive for replication of *L. pneumophila*, A/J, C57BL/6, and BALB/c mice are all permissive for replication of *L. longbeachae* (Asare et al., 2007; Gobin et al., 2009). Resistance of C57BL/6 and BALB/c mice to *L. pneumophila* has been attributed to polymorphisms in the Nod-like receptor apoptosis inhibitory protein

5 (*naip5*) allele (Molofsky et al., 2006; Ren et al., 2006; Wright et al., 2003). The current model is that *L. pneumophila* replication is restricted due to flagellin-dependent caspase-1 activation through Naip5-Ipaf and early macrophage cell death by pyroptosis. Why *L. longbeachae*, in contrast to *L. pneumophila*, is able to replicate in macrophages of all three different mouse strains is still not understood.

Differences in the ecological niches, probable differences in the mode of transmission, and differences in the host susceptibility to these two *Legionella* species suggest differences in the genetic makeup of these species, leading in part to the differences in disease prevalence of the *Legionella* species. Genomics has the potential to decipher the genetic basis underlying these differences and to uncover potential virulence genes. Genome plasticity allowing acquisition or loss of specific genes, genomic regions, or plasmids plays a major role leading to these differences. In the last few years, four genomes of different *L. pneumophila* strains (Paris, Lens, Philadelphia, and Corby) (Cazalet et al., 2004; Chien et al., 2004; Steinert et al., 2007) have been completely sequenced, analyzed, and published. Recently the sequencing and analysis of four genomes of *L. longbeachae* has also been carried out (Cazalet et al., 2010). *L. longbeachae* strain NSW150 was sequenced completely, and three draft genome sequences, two belonging to Sg1 and two to Sg2, were reported. A fifth *L. longbeachae* strain isolated in the United States was recently sequenced by pyrosequencing, and the analysis of the draft genome sequences published in 13 contigs was reported (Kozak et al., 2010). Thus, we now have for the first time the unique possibility to compare and analyze four *L. pneumophila* and five *L. longbeachae* isolates of different origins.

This chapter starts with a description of the general characteristics of the genome sequences of *L. pneumophila* and *L. longbeachae* and then highlights the characteristic features and common traits of the two main human-pathogenic *Legionella* species. Emphasis is given to putative virulence and *Legionella* life cycle-related functions. In the second part, we focus on the comparison of these genome sequences, in order to learn about the plasticity of the *Legionella* genomes and the possible mechanisms involved. In the third part we analyze and discuss the possible evolution of the identified virulence factors. Finally, future perspectives in *Legionella* genomics are presented.

GENERAL FEATURES OF THE *L. PNEUMOPHILA* AND *L. LONGBEACHAE* GENOMES

The complete genome sequences of four *L. pneumophila* strains (Paris, Lens, Corby, and Philadelphia-1) are available at the time of writing (Cazalet et al., 2004; Chien et al., 2004; Steinert et al., 2007). These strains were all isolated from humans, two in France (Paris and Lens), one in the United States (Philadelphia-1), and one in Great Britain (Corby), and are members of Sg1 (Jepras et al., 1985; Lawrence et al., 1999; McDade et al., 1977; Nhu Nguyen et al., 2006).

L. pneumophila has a single, circular chromosome, 3,503,610 bp (Paris), 3,345,687 bp (Lens), 3,576,470 bp (Corby), or 3,397,754 bp (Philadelphia-1) in size, with an average G+C content of 38.9% (Table 1). Strains Paris and Lens each contain a plasmid, 131.9 and 59.8 kb, respectively. In strains Philadelphia-1 and Corby, no plasmid was identified. The genomes each contain ~3,000 genes distributed fairly evenly between the two strands (~57% on the leading strand) and accounting for ~88% of the potential coding capacity. No function could be predicted for about 40% of the *L. pneumophila* genes, and about 20% of the genes are unique to the genus *Legionella*. Comparative analysis of the genome structure of the four *L. pneumophila* genomes showed high colinearity, with only a few translocations, duplications, deletions, or inversions (Fig. 1) and identified between 6.3 and 11.3% of the genes as specific to each *L. pneumophila* strain (Fig. 2). Principally, the genomes contain three large plasticity zones, where the synteny is disrupted: a 26-kb inversion in strain Lens with respect to strains Paris and Philadelphia-1; a 13-kb fragment which is partly similar

TABLE 1 Complete *L. pneumophila* genomes obtained by classical Sanger sequencing

Feature	Paris	Lens	Philadelphia-1	Corby
Chromosome size (kb)[a]	3,504 (131.8)	3,345 (59.8)	3,397	3,576
G+C content (%)	38.3 (37.4)	38.4 (38)	38.27	38
G+C content of CDS[b] (%)	39.1	39.4	38.6	38.6
No. of genes[a]	3,136 (142)	3,001 (60)	3,002	3,259
No. of protein-coding genes[a]	2,878 (140)	2,878 (60)	2,942	3,206
% of CDS[b]	87.9	88	90.2	86.8
No. of specific genes	200	198	241	368
No. of 16S/23S/5S	3/3/3	3/3/3	3/3/3	3/3/3
No. of tRNAs	44	43	43	43
No. of plasmids	1	1	0	0

[a]Updated annotation. Data from plasmids are given in parentheses.
[b]CDS coding sequence.

and partly different and which is inserted in a different genomic location in strains Paris and Philadelphia-1 but is truncated in strain Lens; and the chromosomal region carrying the Lvh type IV secretion system. The Lvh type IV secretion system, previously described in strain Philadelphia (Segal et al., 1999), is encoded by a 36-kb region (strain Paris) or a 45-kb region (strain Philadelphia-1) that can be either carried on a multi-copy plasmid or integrated into the

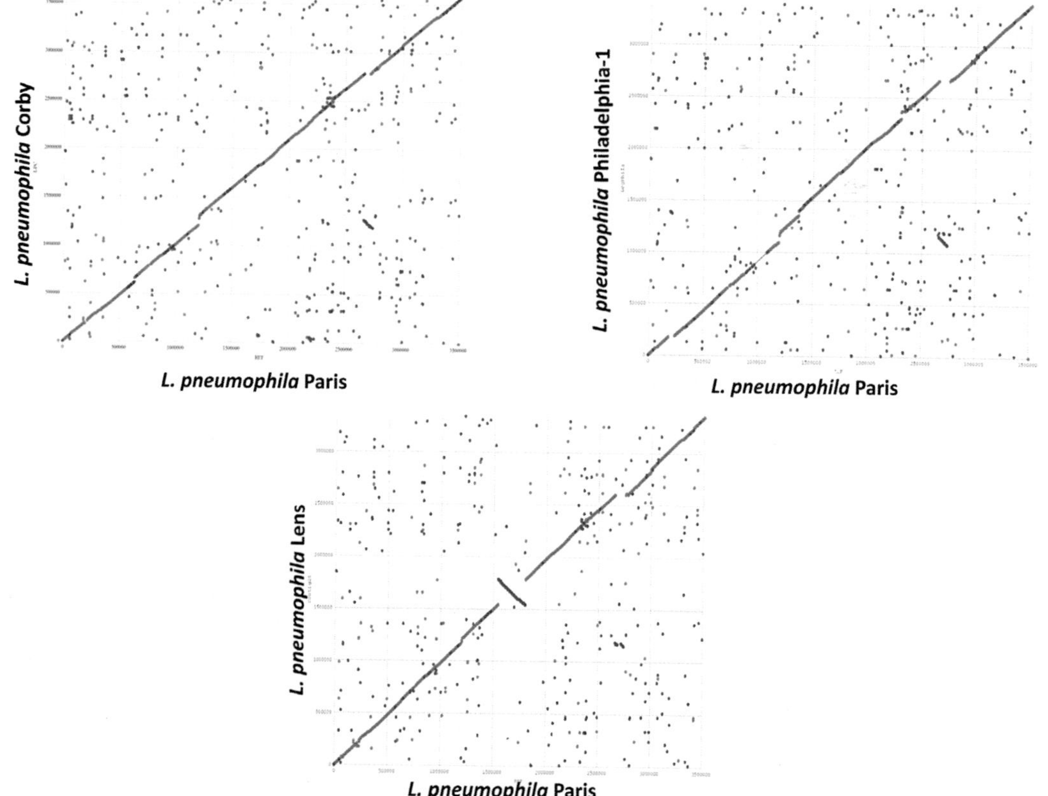

FIGURE 1 Synteny plot of the chromosomes of *L. pneumophila* Paris, Lens, Corby, and Philadelphia-1. The plot was created with the MUMmer software package.

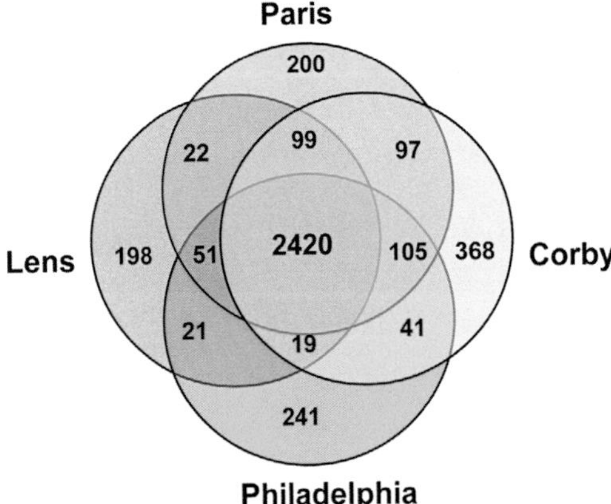

FIGURE 2 Diagram showing the core genome and the unique gene complement of *L. pneumophila* Paris, Lens, Philadelphia-1, and Corby. Orthologous genes were defined by reciprocal best-match FASTA comparisons. The threshold was set to a minimum of 80% sequence identities and a ratio of the length of 0.75 to 1.33.

chromosome. Further diversity on the genome level is present, as deletions and insertions of several smaller regions were identified in each strain, as well as regions where the gene content is variable, as discussed later.

The *L. longbeachae* genomes also consist of a circular chromosome of 4,077,332 bp (NSW 150), 4,086,210 bp (D-4968), 4,096,903 bp (ATCC 39462), 4,018,631 bp (98072), and 3,979,481 bp (C-4E7) with an average G+C content of 38 % (Table 2). Strains NSW 10 and D-4986 carry a highly similar plasmid of about 70-kb and DNA identity of 99%; strains C-4E7 and 98072 also contain a highly similar plasmid of 138 kb. This indicates that similar plasmids circulate among *L. longbeachae* strains. A total of 3,500 protein-encoding genes are predicted in the two completely annotated genomes, 58% of which have been assigned a putative function. The *L. longbeachae* chromosomes are about 500 kb larger than those of *L. pneumophila* and have a significantly different organization, as seen in the synteny plot in Fig.3. Moreover, only about 65% of the *L. longbeachae* genes are orthologous to *L. pneumophila* genes, whereas about 34% of all genes are *L. longbeachae* specific with respect to *L. pneumophila* Paris, Lens, Philadelphia-1, and Corby (defined by less than 30% amino acid identity over 80% of the length of the smallest protein).

Analysis of the draft genome sequences of three additional *L. longbeachae* strains sequenced using Illumina technology allowed further analysis of diversity among the genomes by determining single-nucleotide polymorphisms (SNP). High-quality SNPs were detected by mapping the Illumina reads on the finished NSW 150 genome sequence. This revealed a high conservation in genome size, content, and organization and a low SNP number among the four *L. longbeachae* genomes (Table 2). Interestingly, in contrast to *L. pneumophila*, where strains of the same serogroup may have very different gene content (Cazalet et al., 2008, Cazalet et al., 2004), the *L. longbeachae* genomes belonging to Sg1 or Sg2,

TABLE 2 Complete and draft genomes of *L. longbeachae* obtained by classical sequencing and new generation sequencing

Feature	NSW 150	D-4968	ATCC 39462	98072	C-4E7
Chromosome size (kb)	4,077 (71)	4,016 (70)[a]	4,096	4,018 (133.8)	3,979 (133.8)
G+C content (%)	37.1 (38.2)	37.0	37.0	37.0 (37.8)	37 (37.8)
No. of genes	3,660 (75)	3,557 (61)[a]	ND[d]	ND	ND
No. of 16S/23S/5S	4/4/4	4/4/4	4/4/4	4/4/4	4/4/4
No. of contigs >0.5–300 kb	Complete	13	64	65	63
N50 contig size (kb)[b]	Complete	ND	138	129	134
% of coverage[c]	100	96.3	96.3	93.4	93.1
No. of SNPs with NSW 150	ND	1,900	1,611	16,853	16,820
No. of plasmids	1	1	0	1	1

[a]Updated annotation according to the criteria used to annotate NSW 150 to allow comparisons.
[b]N50 contig size, calculated by ordering all contig sizes and then adding the lengths (starting from the longest contig) until the summed length exceeds 50% of the total length of all contigs (half of all bases reside in a contiguous sequence of the given size or more).
[c]For SNP detection.
[d]ND, no data.

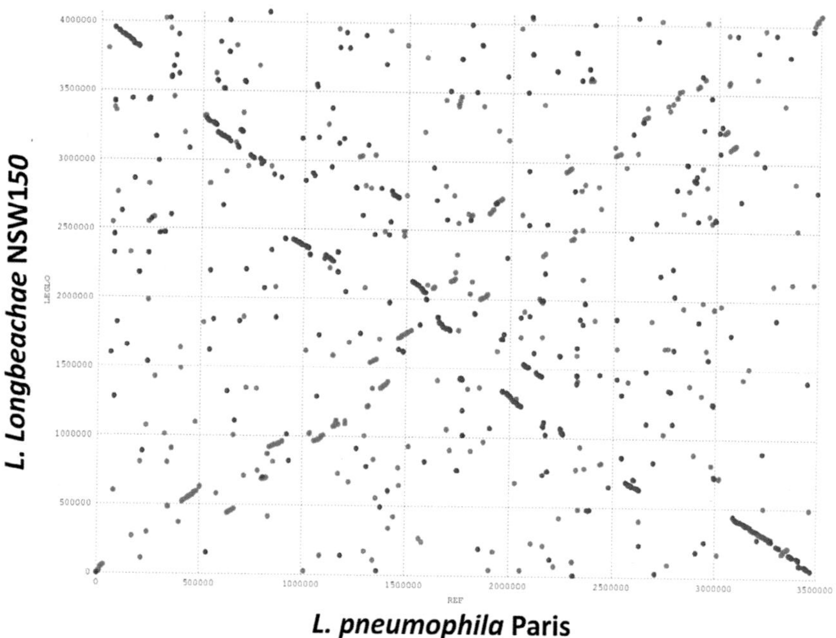

FIGURE 3 Synteny plot of the chromosomes of *L. pneumophila* Paris and *L. longbeachae* NSW 150. The plot was created with the MUMmer software package.

respectively, showed highly conserved genomes. Comparison of the two Sg1 genomes (NSW 150 and ATCC 39462) identified 1,611 SNPs, of which 1,426 are located in only seven chromosomal regions, mainly encoding putative mobile elements, whereas the remaining 185 SNPs were evenly distributed around the chromosome. A similar number of SNPs (about 1,900) were identified when strains NSW 150 and D-4968 were compared (Table 2). In contrast, the SNP number between two strains of different serogroups was higher, with about 16,000 SNPs present between Sg1 and Sg2 strains (Table 2). This represents an overall polymorphism of less than 0.4%, which is significantly lower than the polymorphism of about 2% between *L. pneumophila* Sg1 strains. The low SNP number and relatively homogeneous distribution of the SNPs around the chromosome suggest recent expansion for the species *L. longbeachae*.

Investigation of the phylogenetic relationship among the *L. pneumophila* and *L. longbeachae* strains was undertaken based on the nucleotide sequence of *recN* (recombination and repair protein-encoding gene) aligned with respect to the protein alignment (Gomez-Valero et al., 2009). RecN was chosen as it has been described, based on an analysis of 32 protein-encoding genes widely distributed among bacterial genomes, as the gene with the greatest potential for predicting genome relatedness at the genus or subgenus level (Zeigler, 2003). The phylogenetic relationship among the four *L. pneumophila* strains is very close while *L. longbeachae* is clearly more distant, as shown in Fig. 4. The sequences and their analysis are accessible at http://genolist.pasteur.fr/LegioList/.

HOST-PATHOGEN INTERACTION: SPECIFICITIES AND COMMON FEATURES OF *L. PNEUMOPHILA* AND *L. LONGBEACHAE*

Secretion Systems: an Exceptional Number and Wide Variety

A particular feature of *Legionella* is its dual host system, allowing intracellular growth in protozoa and, during infection, in human alveolar macrophages. The capacity of pathogens like

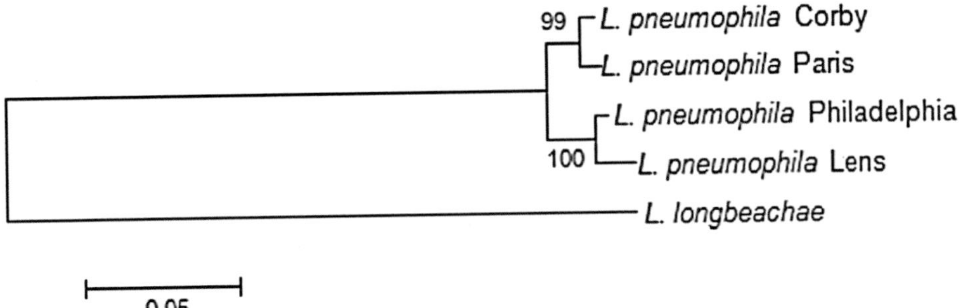

FIGURE 4 Phylogenetic tree showing the relationship of the four sequenced *L. pneumophila* strains based on the *recN* sequence. The tree was constructed using the neighbor-joining method in MEGA. Numbers at branching nodes are percentages of 1,000 bootstrap replications.

Legionella to infect eukaryotic cells is intimately linked to the ability to manipulate host cell functions to establish an intracellular niche for their replication. Upon internalization into the eukaryotic cell, *Legionella* guarantees its survival by manipulating host cell functions such as vesicle trafficking, thereby reprogramming the endosomal-lysosomal degradation pathway of the phagocytic cell. Essential for the ability of *Legionella* to subvert host functions are its different secretion systems. The two major systems known to be involved in virulence of *L. pneumophila* are the Dot/Icm type IV secretion system (T4SS) and the Lsp type II secretion system (T2SS) (Berger and Isberg, 1993; Marra et al., 1992; Rossier and Cianciotto, 2001), which translocates a large repertoire of bacterial effectors into the host cell. These effectors modulate multiple host cell processes and, in particular, redirect trafficking of the *L. pneumophila* phagosome and mediate its conversion into an endoplasmic reticulum-derived organelle competent for intracellular bacterial replication (Shin and Roy, 2008; Cianciotto, 2009).

Analysis and comparison of the *L. pneumophila* and *L. longbeachae* genomes showed that *L. longbeachae*, like *L. pneumophila*, encodes a Lsp T2SS machinery since its genome includes all 12 *lsp* (*Legionella* secretion pathway) genes described in *L. pneumophila*, which are organized in five loci that encode the core components of the T2SS apparatus (Cazalet et al., 2010; Kozak et al., 2010). However, 45% of the T2SS substrates described for *L. pneumophila* (Cianciotto, 2009; DebRoy et al., 2006) are absent from *L. longbeachae;* these include a *chiA*-encoded chitinase, which was shown to promote *L. pneumophila* persistence in the lungs of A/J mice (DebRoy et al., 2006). Thus, the number and type of T2SS substrates vary depending on the ecological niche occupied by the species. Furthermore, the twin arginine translocation systems and three putative type I secretion systems (T1SS) are present in *L. longbeachae*. However, the Lss T1SS might not be functional in *L. longbeachae*, since only LssXYZA are conserved (55 to 82% identity to strain Paris) and the two essential components LssB (ABC transporter-ATP binding) and LssD (HlyD family secretion protein) are missing. In contrast, the two additional putative T1SS, encoded by the genes *llo2283-llo2288* and *llo0441-llo0444* in strain NSW 150, appeared to be functional. Furthermore, two HlyD-like proteins localized next to ABC transporters are present, but no contiguous outer membrane protein was found. However, these proteins could also be part of T1SS and function together with a genetically unlinked outer membrane component, similar to what is seen for the Hly T1SS of *Escherichia coli*, and may thus constitute two additional T1SS. This organization is conserved in strains NSW 150 and D-4968.

Finally, *L. longbeachae* NSW 150 encodes four T4SS, a rather exceptional number (Cazalet et al., 2010), and *L. longbeachae* D-4968 encodes two T4SS (Kozak et al., 2010). *L. pneumophila* strains Paris, Lens, and Philadelphia-1 express a T4ASS called Lvh (*Legionella vir homologues*) (Cazalet et al., 2004; Chien et al., 2004). *L. pneumophila* strain Corby lacks Lvh, but it contains two novel T4ASSs, Trb-1 and Trb-2 (Glöckner et al., 2007), whose roles are not known. The Lvh T4ASS of *L. pneumophila* is absent from *L. longbeachae* NSW 150 (Cazalet et al., 2010) but present in *L. longbeachae* D-4968 (Kozak et al., 2010). The three additional T4ASS present in *L. longbeachae* NSW 150 might have been acquired by horizontal gene transfer as one T4ASS is present on the plasmid and the other two are embedded on putative mobile genomic islands (GIs) in the chromosome. *llo1819-llo1929* (GI-1), with a size of around 120 kb, is bordered by Ser and Arg tRNAs and carries a gene coding for a phage integrase (*llo1819*). The second cluster (GI-2), of 106 kb, spans from the integrase coding gene *llo2859* to *llo2960ab* and is also bordered by a Met tRNA. Most of the proteins encoded on GI-2 are of unknown function. However, both islands code for several proteins, which may be dedicated to the stress response.

Central to the establishment of the intracellular replicative niche and to *L. pneumophila* virulence is the Dot/Icm T4SS. This T4BSS is also present in *L. longbeachae*, and the general organization of the genomic region encoding it is conserved, with protein identities of 47 to 92% with respect to that of *L. pneumophila* (Fig. 5). This is similar to what has been reported previously for other *Legionella* species (Morozova et al., 2004). In *L. longbeachae* the

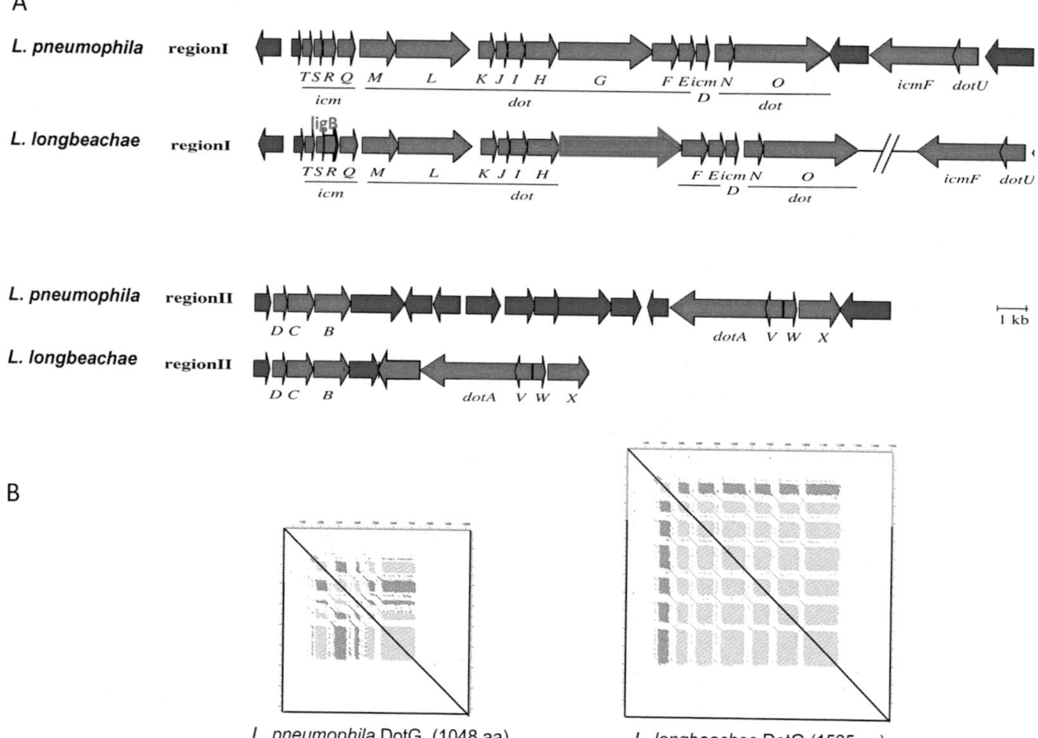

FIGURE 5 Alignment of the chromosomal regions of *L. pneumophila* and *L. longbeachae* encoding the Dot/Icm type 4 secretion system genes. (A) The comparison shows that all genes are highly conserved (47% to 92% identity) between *L. pneumophila* Paris and *L. longbeachae*. Red, conserved genes; blue, specific genes; green arrows, *L. longbeachae*-specific genes. (B) Self matrix of DotG of *L. pneumophila* and *L. longbeachae*.

icmR gene is replaced by the *ligB* gene; however, the encoded proteins have been shown to perform similar functions (Feldman et al., 2004, 2005). Here we found that IcmE/DotG of *L. longbeachae* (1,525 amino acids) is 477 amino acids larger than that of *L. pneumophila* (1,048 amino acids). DotG of *L. pneumophila* is part of the core transmembrane complex of the secretion system and is composed of three domains: a transmembrane N-terminal domain, a central region of 42 repeats of 10 amino acids, and a C-terminal region homologous to VirB10. In contrast, the central region of *L. longbeachae* DotG is composed of approximately 90 repeats. These multiple repeats of 10 amino acids are not found in any other VirB10 homolog except in *Coxiella* (Fig. 5B). It will be challenging to understand the possible impact of this modification on the function of the T4SS.

Thus, some of the secretion systems are common between *L. pneumophila* and *L. longbeachae* whereas others are specific. Most of the T4SS are located on regions of genome plasticity; some even show plasticity on the gene/protein level, as shown above for DotG. This indicates that genes necessary for niche adaptation may have been acquired through horizontal gene transfer by phages or plasmid-like elements carrying secretion systems and that exchange of genetic information between *Legionella* species is a common feature.

Eukaryotic Proteins and Effectors: Molecular Mimicry is a Major Virulence Strategy of *L. pneumophila* and *L. longbeachae*

From the analysis of the genome sequence of *L. pneumophila*, it was clear that *L. pneumophila* encodes specific virulence factors that have evolved during its evolution with eukaryotic host cells such as freshwater amoebas. These constitute a multitude of proteins similar to eukaryotic proteins or containing motifs found mainly or only in eukaryotic proteins (Brüggemann et al., 2006a; Cazalet et al., 2004; de Felipe et al., 2005; Nora et al., 2009). Protein motifs found predominantly in eukaryotes, which were identified in the *L. pneumophila* genomes, are ankyrin repeats, Sel-1 (TPR), Set domain, Sec7, serine threonine kinase domains, and U-box and F-box motifs. Examples of eukaryotic-like proteins of *L. pneumophila* are two secreted apyrases, a sphingosine-1 phosphate lyase and sphingosine kinase, eukaryotic-like glycoamylase, cytokinin oxidase, zinc metalloprotease, and an RNA binding precursor (Brüggemann et al., 2006b; Cazalet et al., 2004). Function prediction based on similarity searches suggested that many of these proteins are implicated in modulating host cell functions to the pathogen's advantage (Cazalet et al., 2004). Recent functional studies confirm these predictions. Eukaryotic-like proteins of *L. pneumophila* are virulence factors involved in host cell adhesion, formation of the *Legionella*-containing vacuole, modulation of host cell functions, induction of apoptosis, and egress of *Legionella*. Most of these effector proteins are expressed at different stages of the intracellular life cycle of *L. pneumophila* (Brüggemann et al., 2006b) and are delivered to the host cell by the Dot/Icm T4SS (Burstein et al., 2009; de Felipe et al., 2005, 2008). The question now arises whether the presence of eukaryotic-like proteins is a common feature of the *Legionella* genomes, whether these proteins are conserved among the different species, and whether plasticity and diversity in the different effectors may explain differences in host and niche adaptation.

Comparison of the genome sequences of *L. pneumophila* and *L. longbeachae* sheds light on this question. Indeed, many eukaryotic-like proteins and protein-encoding domains found mainly in eukaryotic proteins are indeed present in the *L. longbeachae* genomes, confirming that molecular mimicry is also a virulence strategy of *L. longbeachae*. However, there is a considerable diversity between the two species in the repertoire of these proteins. For example, a homologue of sphingosine-1 phosphate lyase is missing in all sequenced *L. longbeachae* genomes and the homologue of only one (Lpp1880) of the two apyrases encoded in the *L. pneumophila* genomes is present in the *L. longbeachae* genomes. In contrast, a glycoamylase and uridine kinase homologue is also present in *L. longbeachae* (Cazalet et al., 2010; Kozak et al., 2010). Furthermore, despite the high degree of conservation of the Dot/Icm T4SS components between *L. pneumophila* and *L. longbeachae*, the Dot/Icm substrates were not highly conserved. When comparing the substrates identified for *L. pneumophila* with those encoded in the *L. longbeachae* NSW 150 genome, it becomes clear that 66% of the reported *L. pneumophila* Dot/Icm substrates are absent from *L. longbeachae* (Table 3). However, 51 new putative Dot/Icm substrates specific for *L. longbeachae* were predicted, all of which encode eukaryotic-like domains, all but one of which contain the secretion signal described by Nagai and colleagues (2005), and many of which also meet the additional criteria defined by Kubori and colleagues (2008) (Table 4). Both *L. pneumophila* and *L. longbeachae* replicate within a vacuole that recruits endoplasmic reticulum. Several effector proteins contribute to the ability of *L. pneumophila* to manipulate host cell trafficking events resulting in this association. The effector proteins SidJ, RalF, VipA, VipF, SidC, YlfA, and LepB, which contribute to trafficking or recruitment and retention of vesicles to *L. pneumophila* vacuoles, are conserved in *L. longbeachae*, but VipD, SidM/DrrA, and LidA, which also interfere in these events, are absent from the *L. longbeachae* genome; however, VipD and SidM/DrrA are also not present in all the *L. pneumophila* genomes sequenced, indicating heterogeneity in the repertoire of effectors not only between *L. pneumophila* and *L. longbeachae* but also among different *L. pneumophila* strains. Another example that genome plasticity is playing a role in effector diversity is the region of the *L. pneumophila* genomes encoding seven putative effectors (PieABCDEFG), which has been found in *L. pneumophila* Philadelphia-1 (Ninio et al., 2009). Only some of these effectors are present in all sequenced *L. pneumophila* strains, and only PieE is present in *L. longbeachae*.

Although *L. pneumophila* also communicates with early and late endosomal vesicle trafficking pathways (Shevchuk et al., 2009; Urwyler et al., 2009a, 2009b), a major difference in the phagosome maturation of the two species is that the *L. longbeachae* phagosome acquires early and late endocytic markers. Several proteins identified specifically in the genome of *L. longbeachae* may contribute to these differences. First, *L. longbeachae* encodes a family of Ras-related small GTPases (Llo3288, Llo2329, Llo1716, and Llo2249), which may also be involved in vesicular trafficking and may account for the specificities of the *L. longbeachae* life cycle. Remarkably, Llo3288, Llo2329, and Llo1716 are the first small GTPases of the Rab subfamily found in a prokaryote. *L. pneumophila* is also known to exploit monophosphorylated host phosphoinositides (PIs) to anchor the effector proteins SidC, SidM/DrrA, LpnE, and LidA to the membrane of the replication vacuole (Machner et al., 2006; Murata et al., 2006; Newton et al., 2007; Weber et al., 2006, 2009; Brombacher et al., 2009). *L. longbeachae* may employ an additional strategy to interfere with the host PI, since Llo0793 is homologous to a mammalian PI-metabolizing enzyme, phosphatidylinositol-4-phosphate 5-kinase, and it is tempting to speculate that this protein allows direct modulation of the host cell PI levels.

As another strategy to alter host trafficking pathways, *L. pneumophila* is able to target microtubule-dependent vesicular transport. AnkX/AnkN, for example, prevents microtubule-dependent vesicular transport from interfering with the fusion of the *L. pneumophila*-containing vacuole with late endosomes (Pan et al., 2008). AnkX/AnkN is absent from *L. longbeachae*; however, *L. longbeachae* does encode a putative tubulin-tyrosine ligase (TTL), Llo2200, which adds to the 19 bacterial TTL identified to date. TTL catalyzes the ATP-dependent posttranslational addition of a tyrosine to the carboxy-terminal end of detyrosinated α-tubulin. Although the exact physiological function of α-tubulin has so far not been established, it has been linked to altered microtubule structure and function (Eiserich et al., 1999). Besides AnkX/AnkN, a large family of ankyrin repeat proteins is secreted into host cells through the *L. pneumophila* Dot/Icm secretion system. Interestingly, 23 of the 29 ankyrin proteins identified in the *L. pneumophila* strains are absent from the *L. longbeachae* genome; however,

TABLE 3 Distribution of known and predicted Dot/Icm substrates of *L. pneumophila* in *L. longbeachae*[a]

L. pneumophila				*L. longbeachae*				Name	Product
Philadelphia-1	Paris	Lens	Corby	NSW 150	ATCC 39462	98072	C-4E7		
lpg0012	*lpp0012*	*lpl0012*	*lpc0013*	*llo0432*	+	+	+	*cegC1*	Ankyrin repeat
lpg0038	*lpp0037*	*lpl0038*	*lpc0039*	–	–	–	–	*ankQ/legA10*	Unknown
lpg0045	*lpp0046*	*lpl0044*	*lpc0047*	–	–	–	–		Unknown
lpg0080	*lpp0094*	*lpl2046*	*lpc1561*	–	–	–	–		Unknown
lpg0081	*lpp0095*	–	–	–	–	–	–		Unknown
lpg0090	*lpp0104*	*lpl0089*	*lpc0109*	–	–	–	–		Unknown
lpg0096	*lpp0110*	*lpl0096*	*lpc0115*	*llo1322*	+	+	+		Unknown
lpg0103	*lpp0117*	*lpl0103*	*lpc0122*	*llo3312*	+	+	+	*vipF*	N-terminal acetyltransferase, GNAT family
lpg0126	*lpp0140*	*lpl0125*	*lpc0146*	–	–	–	–	*cegC2*	Ninein
lpg0171	*lpp0233*	*lpl0234*	–	–	–	–	–	*legU1*	F-box motif
lpg0191	*lpp0251*	–	–	–	–	–	–		Unknown
lpg0227	*lpp0286*	*lpl0281*	*lpc0303*	*llo2491*	+	+	+	*ceg7*	Unknown
lpg0234	*lpp0304*	*lpl0288*	*lpc0309*	*llo0425*	+	+	+	*sidE/laiD*	Unknown
lpg0240	*lpp0310*	*lpl0294*	*lpc0316*	*llo1601*	+	+	+		Unknown
lpg0246	*lpp0316*	*lpl0300*	*lpc0323*	–	–	–	–	*ceg9*	Unknown
lpg0257	*lpp0327*	*lpl0310*	*lpc0334*	*llo2362*	+	+	+	*sdeA*	Multidrug resistance protein
lpg0276	*lpp0350*	*lpl0328*	*lpc0353*	*llo0327*	+	+	+	*legG2*	Ras guanine nucleotide exchange factor
lpg0284	*lpp0360*	*lpl0336*	*lpc0361*	–	–	–	–	*ceg10*	Unknown
lpg0285	*lpp0361*	*lpl0337*	*lpc0362*	–	–	–	–		Unknown
lpg0294	*lpp0372*	*lpl0347*	*lpc0373*	*llo0464*	+	+	+		Unknown
lpg0365	*lpp0430*	*lpl0406*	*lpc2979*	*llo0525*	+	+	+		Unknown
lpg0376	*lpp0443*	*lpl0419*	*lpc2967*	–	–	–	–	*sdhA*	GRIP, coiled-coil
lpg0390	*lpp0457*	*lpl0433*	*lpc2954*	*llo2824*	+	+	+	*vipA*	Unknown
lpg0401	*lpp0468*	*lpl0444*	*lpc2942*	*llo2582*	+	+	+	*ceg11*	Unknown
lpg0402	–	–	–	–	–	–	–	*ankY/legA9*	Ankyrin, STPK
lpg0403	*lpp0469*	*lpl0445*	*lpc2941*	–	–	–	–	*ankG/ankZ/ legA7*	Ankyrin
lpg0436	*lpp0503*	*lpl0479*	*lpc2906*	–	–	–	–	*ankJ/legA11*	Ankyrin
lpg0437	*lpp0504*	*lpl0480*	*lpc2905*	–	–	–	–		Unknown
lpg0483	*lpp0547*	*lpl0523*	*lpc2861*	*llo2705*	+	+	+	*ankC/legA12*	Ankyrin
lpg0518	*lpp0581*	*lpl0557*	*lpc2826*	–	–	–	–		Unknown
lpg0519	–	–	–	*llo1222*	+	+	+		Unknown
lpg0621	*lpp0675*	*lpl0658*	*lpc2673*	–	–	–	–	*sidA*	Unknown
lpg0634	*lpp0688*	*lpl0671*	*lpc2660*	*llo2574*	+	+	+		Unknown
lpg0642	*lpp0696*	*lpl0679*	*lpc2651*	–	–	–	–	*wipB*	

lpg0695	*lpp0750*	*lpl0732*	*lpc2599*	–	–	–	–	*ankN/ankX/legA8*	Ankyrin
lpg0696	*lpp0751*	*lpl0733*	*lpc2598*	–	–	–	–		
lpg0898	*lpp0959*	*lpl0929*	*lpc2395*	–	–	–	–	*ceg18*	
lpg0940	*lpp1002*	*lpl0971*	*lpc2349*	–	–	–	–	*lidA*	
lpg0945	*lpp1007*	*lpl1579*	*lpc2344*	–	–	–	–	*legL1*	LRR
lpg0963	*lpp1025*	*lpl0992*	*lpc2324*	*llo0934*	+	+	+		
lpg1101	*lpp1101*	*lpl1100*	*lpc2154*	–	–	–	–		
lpg1120	–	–	–	*llo2959*	+	+	+		
lpg1121	*lpp1121*	*lpl1126*	*lpc0578*	*llo1321*	+	+	+	*ceg19*	
lpg1144	*lpp1146*	*lpl1150*	*lpc0607*	*llo1019*	+	+	+	*cegC3*	
lpg1145	*lpp1147*	*lpl1151*	*lpc0608*	–	–	–	–		
lpg1148	*lpp1150*	*lpl1154*	*lpc0611*	–	–	–	–		
lpg1158	*lpp1160*	*lpl1165*	*lpc0621*	–	–	–	–		
lpg1227	*lpp1235*	*lpl1235*	*lpc0696*	–	–	–	–	*vpdB*	
lpg1273	*lpp1236*	*lpl1236*	*lpc0698*	–	–	–	–		Unknown
lpg1290	*lpp1253*	–	–	–	–	–	–		Unknown
lpg1328	*lpp1283*	*lpl1282*	*lpc0743*	–	–	–	–	*legT*	Thaumatin domain
lpg1355	*lpp1309*	–	–	–	–	–	–	*sidG*	Coiled-coil
lpg1426	*lpp1381*	*lpl1377*	*lpc0842*	*llo1791*	+	+	+		
lpg1488	*lpp1444*	*lpl1540*	*lpc0903*	–	–	–	–	*lgt3/legc5*	Coiled-coil
lpg1491	*lpp1447*	–	–	–	–	–	–		
lpg1496	*lpp1453*	*lpl1530*	*lpc0915*	–	–	–	–		
lpg1588	*lpp1546*	*lpl1437*	*lpc1013*	–	–	–	–	*legC6*	Coiled-coil
lpg1598	*lpp1556*	*lpl1427*	*lpc1025*	–	–	–	–		
lpg1602	*lpp1567*	*lpl1423*	*lpc1028*	–	–	–	–	*legL2*	LRR
lpg1621	*lpp1591*	*lpl1402*	*lpc1048*	*llo1014*	+	+	+	*ceg23*	
lpg1625	*lpp1595*	*lpl1398*	*lpc1052*	*llo0719*	+	+	+		
lpg1642	*lpp1612a/b*	*lpl1384*	*lpc1071*	*llo1144*	+	+	+	*sidB*	Rtx toxin, lipase
lpg1660	*lpp1631*	*lpl1625*	*lpc1090*	–	–	–	–	*legL3*	LRR protein
lpg1689	*lpp1658*	*lpl1652*	*lpc1120*	*llo1697*	+	+	+		
lpg1701	*lpp1666*	*lpl1660*	*lpc1130*	–	–	–	–	*ppeA/legC3*	Coiled-coil
lpg1702	*lpp1667*	*lpl1661*	*lpc1131*	–	–	–	–	*ppeB*	
lpg1717	*lpp1682*	–	–	–	–	–	–		
lpg1718	*lpp1683*	*lpl1682*	*lpc1152*	–	–	–	–	*ankI/legAS4*	Ankyrin
lpg1751	*lpp1715*	*lpl1715*	*lpc1191*	*llo2314*	+	+	+		
lpg1851	*lpp1818*	*lpl1817*	*lpc1296*	*llo1047*	+	+	+		
lpg1884	*lpp1848*	*lpl1845*	*lpc1331*	–	–	–	–	*ylfB/legC2*	Coiled-coil
lpg1890	–	*lpl1852*	*lpc1338*	–	–	–	–	*legLC8*	LRR, coiled-coil

(continued)

TABLE 3 Distribution of known and predicted Dot/Icm substrates of *L. pneumophila* in *L. longbeachae*[a] (*continued*)

L. pneumophila				*L. longbeachae*				Name	Product
Philadelphia-1	Paris	Lens	Corby	NSW 150	ATCC 39462	98072	C-4E7		
lpg1933	*lpp1914*	*lpl1903*	*lpc1406*	–	–	–	–		
lpg1947	*lpp1930*	–	–	–	–	–	–		
lpg1948	–	–	–	–	–	–	–	legLC4	LRR, coiled-coil
lpg1949	*lpp1931*	*lpl1918*	*lpc1422*	–	–	–	–		
lpg1950	*lpp1932*	*lpl1919*	*lpc1423*	*llo1397*	+	+	+	*ralF*	
lpg1953	*lpp1935*	*lpl1922*	*lpc1426*	–	–	–	–	*legC4*	Coiled-coil
lpg1958	*lpp1940*	–	–	–	–	–	–	*legL5*	LRR
lpg1960	*lpp1942*	–	*lpc1437*	*llo0565*	+	+	+	*lirA*	
lpg1962	*lpp1946*	*lpl1936*	*lpc1440*	–	–	–	–	*lirB*	
lpg1963	–	–	*lpc1442*	–	–	–	–	*pieA/lirC*	
lpg1964	–	–	–	–	–	–	–	*pieB/lirD*	
lpg1965	–	–	*lpc1443*	–	–	–	–	*pieC/lirE*	
lpg1966	*lpp1947*	–	*lpc1446*	–	–	–	–	*pieD/lirF*	
lpg1969	*lpp1952*	*lpl1941*	*lpc1452*	*llo3131*	+	+	+	*pieE*	
lpg1972	*lpp1955*	*lpl1950*	*lpc1459*	–	–	–	–	*pieF*	
lpg1975	*lpp1959*	*lpl1953*	*lpc1462*	–	–	–	–		
lpg1976	*lpp1959*	*lpl1953*	*lpc1462*	–	–	–	–	*pieG/legG1*	
lpg1978	*lpp1961*	*lpl1955*	*lpc1464*	–	–	–	–	*setA*	Putative glycosyltransferase
lpg2137	*lpp2076*	*lpl2066*	*lpc1586*	–	–	–	–	*legK2*	STPK
lpg2144	*lpp2082*	*lpl2072*	*lpc1593*	–	–	–	–	*ankB/legAU13, ceg27*	Ankyrin, F-box
lpg2155	*lpp2094*	*lpl2083*	*lpc1604*	*llo3096*	+	+	+	*sidJ*	
lpg2157	*lpp2096*	*lpl2085*	*lpc1618*	–	–	–	–	*sdeC*	
lpg2166	*lpp2104*	*lpl2093*	*lpc1626*	*llo2398*	+	+	+		
lpg2176	*lpp2128*	*lpl2102*	*lpc1635*	–	–	–	–	*legS2*	
lpg2200	*lpp2150*	*lpl2124*	*lpc1664*	*llo0140*	+	+	+	*cegC4*	
lpg2215	*lpp2166*	*lpl2140*	*lpc1680*	–	–	–	–	*legA2*	
lpg2216	*lpp2167*	*lpl2141*	*lpc1681*	–	–	–	–		
lpg2222	*lpp2174*	*lpl2147*	*lpc1689*	–	–	–	–	*lpnE*	Putative β-lactamase
lpg2224	–	–	–	–	–	–	–	*ppgA*	Regulator of chromosome condensation
lpg2248	*lpp2202*	*lpl2174*	*lpc1717*	–	–	–	–		
lpg2298	*lpp2246*	*lpl2217*	*lpc1763*	*llo1707*	+	+	+	*ylfA/legC7*	Coiled-coil
lpg2300	*lpp2248*	*lpl2219*	*lpc1765*	*llo0584*	+	+	+	*ankH/legA3, ankW*	Ankyrin, NF-κB inhibitor
lpg2322	*lpp2270*	*lpl2242*	*lpc1789*	*llo0570*	+	+	+	*ankK/legA5*	Ankyrin

lpg2327	*lpp2275*	*lpl2247*	*lpc1794*	–	–	–	–		
lpg2328	*lpp2276*	*lpl2248*	*lpc1795*	–	–	–	–		
lpg2392	*lpp2459*	*lpl2316*	*lpc2085*	–	–	–	–	*legL6*	LLR-containing protein
lpg2400	–	*lpl2323*	–	–	–	–	–	*legL6*	LLR-containing protein
lpg2406	*lpp2472*	*lpl2329*	*lpc2070*	*llo2172*	+	+	+		
lpg2407	*lpp2474*	–	*lpc2069*	–	–	–	–		
lpg2409	*lpp2476*	*lpl2332*	*lpc2067*	–	–	–	–	*ceg29*	
lpg2410	*lpp2479*	*lpl2334*	*lpc2065*	–	–	–	–	*vpdA*	
lpg2411	*lpp2480*	*lpl2335*	*lpc2064*	*llo2227*	+	+	+		
lpg2422	*lpp2487*	*lpl2345*	*lpc2055*	*llo1650*	+	+	+		
lpg2433	*lpp2500*	*lpl2353*	*lpc2043*	–	–	–	–		
lpg2452	*lpp2517*	*lpl2370*	*lpc2026*	–	–	–	–	*ankF/legA14/ceg31*	Ankyrin
lpg2456	*lpp2522*	*lpl2375*	*lpc2020*	*llo0365*	+	+	+	*ankD/legA15*	Ankyrin
lpg2464	–	*lpl2384*	–	–	–	–	–	*sidM/drrA*	
lpg2465	–	*lpl2385*	–	–	–	–	–	*sidD*	
lpg2490	*lpp2555*	*lpl2411*	*lpc1987*	*llo0796*	+	+	+	*lepB*	Coiled-coil, Rab1 GAP
lpg2504	*lpp2572*	*lpl2426*	*lpc1967*	*llo2525*	+	+	+		
lpg2508	*lpp2576*	*lpl2430*	*lpc1963*	–	–	–	–	*sdjA*	
lpg2511	*lpp2579*	*lpl2433*	*lpc1959*	*llo3098*	+	+	+	*sidC*	PI(4)P binding domain
lpg2523	–	–	–	–	–	–	–		
lpg2527	*lpp2592*	*lpl2447*	*lpc1944*	*llo3335*	+	+	+		
lpg2529	*lpp2594*	*lpl2449*	*lpc1942*	*llo2238*	+	+	+		
lpg2556	*lpp2626*	*lpl2481*	*lpc1906*	*llo2218*	+	+	+	*legK3*	STPK
lpg2584	*lpp2637*	*lpl2507*	*lpc0561*	–	–	–	–	*sidF*	
lpg2591	*lpp2644*	*lpl2514*	*lpc0551*	*llo0626*	+	+	+	*ceg33*	
lpg2603	*lpp2656*	*lpl2526*	*lpc0539*	–	–	–	–		
lpg2718	*lpp2775*	*lpl2646*	*lpc0415*	–	–	–	–	*wipA*	
lpg2744	*lpp2800*	*lpl2669*	*lpc0386*	–	–	–	–		
lpg2793	*lpp2839*	*ipl2708*	*lpc3079*	–	–	–	–	*lepA*	Coiled-coil
lpg2804	*lpp2850*	*lpl2719*	*lpc3090*	*llo0267*	+	+	+		
lpg2826	–	*lpl2741*	*lpc3113*	–	–	–	–		
lpg2829	*lpp2883*	–	–	–	–	–	–	*sidH*	
lpg2830	*lpp2887*	–	–	–	–	–	–	*lubX/legU2*	U box motif
lpg2831	*lpp2888*	*lpl4276*	–	–	–	–	–	*VipD*	Patatin-like phospholipase
lpg2862	–	–	–	–	–	–	–	*Lgt2/legC8*	Coiled-coil
lpg2999	*lpp3071*	*lpl2927*	*lpc3315*	–	–	–	–	*legP*	Astacin protease

[a]The list of substrates is based on Isberg et al. (2009), de Felipe et al. (2008), and Ninio et al. (2009). +, gene is present; −, gene is absent; STPK, serine-threonine protein kinase.

TABLE 4 Putative new type IV secretion substrates specific for *L. longbeachae*

NSW 150	ATCC 39462	98072	c-4E7	Motif	Hydrophobic residue or proline[a]	% Enrichment[b]	% Flavored polar amino acids[c]
llo0037	+	+	+	Ankyrin	+	42.86	60.00
llo0087	+	+	+	Ankyrin	+	57.14	53.33
llo0115	+	+	+	Ankyrin	+	28.57	53.33
llo0246	+	+	+	Ankyrin	+	28.57	66.67
llo0990	+	–	–	Ankyrin	+	28.57	46.67
llo1043	+	+	+	Ankyrin	+	28.57	46.67
llo1142	+	+	+	Ankyrin	+	28.57	53.33
llo1168	+	+	+	Ankyrin	+	28.57	53.33
llo1371	+	+	+	Ankyrin, coiled-coil	+	28.57	66.67
llo1395	+	+	+	Ankyrin	+	42.86	53.33
llo1618	+	+	+	Ankyrin	+	28.57	66.67
llo1646	+	+	+	Ankyrin	+	28.57	40.00
llo1651	+	+	+	Ankyrin	+	14.29	60.00
llo1715	+	+[d]	+[d]	Ankyrin	+	28.57	40.00
llo1742	+	+	+	Ankyrin	+	57.14	46.67
llo1894	+	+	+	Ankyrin	+	28.57	66.67
llo2133[d]	+	+	+	Ankyrin	+	0.00	33.33
llo2476	+	+	+	Ankyrin	+	14.29	46.67
llo2668	+	+	+	Ankyrin	+	14.29	46.67
llo3081	+	+	+	Ankyrin, patatin-like phospholipase	+	28.57	60.00
llo3093	+	+	+	Ankyrin, STPK	+	0.00	66.67
llo3343	+	+	+	Ankyrin	+	14.29	33.33
llo3353	+	+	+	Ankyrin, NUDIX hydrolase	+	28.57	53.33
llo0114	+	+	+	LRR	+	14.29	40.00
llo1314	+	+	+	LRR	+	0.00	40.00
llo2165	+	+	+	LRR	+	42.86	66.67
llo2494	+	+	+	LRR	+	28.57	66.67
llo3116	–	–	–	LRR	+	57.14	26.67
llo3118	–	–	–	LRR	+	28.57	66.67
llo1139	+	+	+	STPK	+	14.29	33.33
llo1681	+	+	+	STPK	+	42.86	73.33
llo2132	+	+	+	STPK, coiled-coil	–	14.29	73.33
llo2984	+	+	+	STPK	+	14.29	53.33
llo3049	+	+	+	STPK	+	14.29	66.67

llo1984	+	+	+	STPK	+	14.29	33.33
llo1427	+	+	+	F-box	+	14.29	66.67
llo2109	+	+	+	F-box	+	28.57	60.00
llo0448	+	+	+	U-box	+	28.57	73.33
llo1404	+	+	+	PPR	+	28.57	20.00
llo2643	+	+	+	PPR, coiled-coil	+	28.57	46.67
llo2200	+	+	+	TTL	+	14.29	53.33
llo2327	+	+	+	SH2	+	28.57	73.33
llo2352	+	+	+	PAM2	+	42.86	60.00
llo1196	+	+	+	Snare	+	0.00	73.33
llo2381	+	+	+	Snare	+	42.86	60.00
llo0793	+	+	+	Putative phosphatidylinositol-4-phosphate 5-kinase	+	28.57	66.67
llo3288	+	+	+	Ras-related small GTPase domain	+	14.29	60.00
llo2329	+	+	+	Ras-related small GTPase + Miro-like domains	+	28.57	60.00
llo2249	+	+	+	Miro-like domains	+	57.14	80.00
llo1716	+	+	+	Ras-related small GTPase + Miro-like domains	+	28.57	73.33
llo1892	+	+	+	Putative immunoglobulin I-set domain	+	14.29	40.00

[a]Presence of a hydrophobic residue or a proline in position −3 or −4 according to Nagai et al. (2005).
[b]Enrichment in amino acids that have small side chains (alanine, glycine, serine, and threonine) at positions −8 to −2 according to Kubori et al. (2008).
[c]Percentage of polar amino acids that are favored at positions −13 to −1 according to Kubori et al. (2008).
[d]Pseudogene.

L. longbeachae encodes 23 specific ankyrin repeat proteins (Table 4).

L. pneumophila is also able to interfere with the host ubiquitination pathway. The U-box protein LubX, which possesses an in vitro ubiquitin ligase activity specific for the eukarytotic Cdc2-like kinase Clk1 (Kubori et al., 2008), is absent from *L. longbeachae*. However, *llo0448* encodes a predicted U-box protein. *L. pneumophila* also encodes three F-box proteins of which one, AnkB, was shown to be a T4SS effector that is implicated in virulence of *L. pneumophila* and in recruiting ubiquitinated proteins to the *Legionella*-containing vacuole (Al-Khodor et al., 2008; Habyarimana et al., 2010; Price et al., 2009). None of the three *L. pneumophila* F-box proteins are conserved in *L. longbeachae*, but two new putative F-box proteins are encoded by its genome (Table 4). Thus, although the specific proteins may not be conserved, the eukaryotic-like protein-protein interaction domains found in *L. pneumophila* are also present in *L. longbeachae*.

L. longbeachae also contains several proteins with eukaryotic domains that are not present in *L. pneumophila*. One is the above-mentioned protein Llo2200, which contains a TTL domain. A second is Llo2327, the first bacterial protein found to contain a Src homology 2 (SH2) domain. SH2 domains in eukaryotes have regulatory functions in various intracellular signaling cascades. Furthermore, *L. longbeachae* contains two proteins with pentatricopeptide repeat (PPR) domains. This family seems to be greatly expanded in plants, where they appear to play essential roles in organellar RNA metabolism (Lurin et al., 2004; Nakamura et al., 2004; Schmitz-Linneweber and Small, 2008). Only 12 bacterial PPR domain proteins have been identified to date, all encoded by two species, the plant pathogen *Ralstonia solanacearum* and the facultative photosynthetic bacterium *Rhodobacter sphaeroides*. Thus, genome analysis revealed a particular feature of the *Legionella* genomes, the presence of many eukaryotic-like proteins, several of which mimic host proteins to allow intracellular replication of *Legionella*.

Surface Structures: a Clue to Mouse Susceptibility to Infection with *Legionella*

Despite the presence of many different species of *Legionella* in aquatic reservoirs, the vast majority of human disease is caused by a single serogroup of a single species, namely, *L. pneumophila* Sg1, which is responsible for about 84% of all cases worldwide (Yu et al., 2002). Similar results are obtained for *L. longbeachae*. Two serogroups are described, but *L. longbeachae* Sg1 is predominant in human disease. Lipopolysaccharide (LPS) is the basis for the classification of serogroups but is also a major immunodominant antigen of *L. pneumophila* and *L. longbeachae*. Interestingly, it has also been shown that membrane vesicles shed by virulent *L. pneumophila* containing LPS are sufficient to inhibit phagosome-lysosome fusion (Fernandez-Moreira et al., 2006). Results obtained from large-scale genome comparisons of *L. pneumophila* suggested that LPS of Sg1 itself might be implicated in the predominance of Sg1 strains in human disease compared to other serogroups of *L. pneumophila* and other *Legionella* species (Cazalet et al., 2008). A comparative search for LPS coding regions in the genome of *L. longbeachae* NSW 150 identified two gene clusters encoding proteins that could be involved in production of LPS and/or capsule. Neither of these gene clusters shared homology to the *L. pneumophila* LPS biosynthesis gene cluster, suggesting considerable differences in this major immunodominant antigen between the two *Legionella* species. However, homologs of *L. pneumophila* lipid A biosynthesis genes (LpxA, LpxB, LpxD, and WaaM) are present. Electron microscopy also clearly suggested that *L. longbeachae*, unlike *L. pneumophila*, encodes a capsule-like structure, further suggesting that one region codes the LPS cluster and the second region encodes the capsule structure, which can be visualized by electron microscopy (Cazalet et al., 2010).

Another important surface structure of *L. pneumophila* is its flagella. Cytosolic flagellin of *L. pneumophila* triggers Naip5-dependent caspase-1 activation and subsequent proinflammatory cell death by pyroptosis in C57BL/6 mice, rendering these mice resistant to infection with *L. pneumophila* (Diez et al., 2003; Lamkanfi et al., 2007; Lightfield et al., 2008; Molofsky et al., 2006; Ren et al., 2006; Wright et al., 2003; Zamboni et al., 2006). In contrast, caspase-1 activation does not occur upon infection of C57BL/6 and A/J mouse macrophages with *L. longbeachae*, which is then able to replicate. Genome analysis allowed elucidation of these differences. *L. longbeachae* does not carry any flagellar biosynthesis genes except those encoding the sigma factor FliA, the regulator FleN, the two-component system FleR/FleS, and the flagellar basal body rod modification protein FlgD. Interestingly, all genes bordering flagellar gene clusters are conserved between *L. longbeachae* and *L. pneumophila*, suggesting deletion of these regions from the *L. longbeachae* genome. Analysis of the genome sequences of *L. longbeachae* D-4968, ATCC 39642, 98072, and C-4E7, as well as a PCR-based screening of 50 *L. longbeachae* isolates belonging to both serogroups by Kozak and colleagues (2010) and of 15 additional isolates by Cazalet and colleagues (2010), did not detect flagellar genes in any isolate, confirming that *L. longbeachae*, in contrast to *L. pneumophila*, does not synthesize flagella. This result suggests that *L. longbeachae* fails to activate caspase-1 due to the lack of flagellin, which may also partly explain the differences in mouse susceptibility to *L. pneumophila* and *L. longbeachae* infection. The putative *L. longbeachae* capsule may also contribute to this difference.

Quite interestingly, although *L. longbeachae* does not encode flagella, it encodes a putative chemotaxis system. Chemotaxis enables bacteria to find favorable conditions by migrating toward higher concentrations of attractants. The chemotactic response is mediated by a two-component signal transduction pathway, with the histidine kinase CheA and the response regulator CheY, putatively encoded by the genes *llo3302* and *llo3303*, respectively, in the *L. longbeachae* genome. Furthermore, two homologues of the "adaptor" protein CheW (encoded by *llo3298* and *llo3300*) that associate with CheA or cytoplasmic chemosensory receptors are present. Ligand-binding to receptors regulate the autophosphorylation activity of CheA in these complexes. The CheA phosphoryl group is subsequently transferred to CheY, which then diffuses away to the flagellum, where it modulates motor rotation. Adaptation to continuous stimulation is mediated by a methyltransferase CheR encoded by *llo3299* in *L. longbeachae*. Together, these proteins represent an evolutionarily conserved core of the chemotaxis pathway, common to many bacteria and archaea (Kentner and Sourjik, 2006; Hazelbauer et al., 2008). A similar chemotaxis system is also present in *Legionella drancourtii* LLAP12 (La Scola et al., 2004) but is absent from *L. pneumophila*. The flanking genomic regions are highly conserved among *L. longbeachae* and all *L. pneumophila* strains sequenced, suggesting that although *L. pneumophila* encodes flagella, it has lost the chemotaxis system-encoding genes.

Thus, these two species differ markedly in their surface structures. *L. longbeachae* encodes a capsule-like structure, synthesizes a very different LPS, and does not synthesize flagella but encodes a chemotaxis system. These differences in surface structures seem to be due to deletion events leading to the loss of flagella in *L. longbeachae* and the loss of chemotaxis in *L. pneumophila*, in part explaining the adaptation of these two species to their different main niches, soil and water, respectively.

EVOLUTION OF EUKARYOTIC EFFECTORS: ACQUISITION BY HORIZONTAL GENE TRANSFER

Human-to-human transmission of *Legionella* has never been reported. Thus, humans have been inconsequential in the evolution of these bacteria. However, *Legionella* species have coevolved with freshwater protozoa, allowing their adaptation to eukaryotic cells. The idea that protozoa are training grounds for intracellular pathogens was born with the finding by Rowbotham (1980) that *Legionella* has the ability to multiply intracellularly. This led to a new insight in microbiology: bacteria parasitize protozoa and can utilize the same process to infect humans. Indeed, the long coevolution of *Legionella* with protozoa is reflected in its genome by the presence of eukaryotic-like genes, many of which are clearly virulence factors used by *L. pneumophila* to subvert host functions. These genes may have been acquired through horizontal gene transfer from the host cells (e.g., aquatic protozoa) or from bacteria or may have evolved by convergent evolution. Recently it has been reported that *L. drancourtii*, a relative of *L. pneumophila*, has acquired a sterol reductase gene from the genome of *Acanthamoeba polyphaga mimivirus*, a virus that grows in amoebas (Moliner et al., 2009). Thus, the acquisition of some of the eukaryotic-like genes of *L. pneumophila* by HGT from protozoa is plausible. *ralF* was the first gene suggested to have been acquired by *L. pneumophila* from eukaryotes by HGT. RalF carries a eukaryotic Sec7 domain and is probably derived from a eukaryotic host (Nagai et al., 2002). To study the evolutionary origin of eukaryotic *L. pneumophila* genes, we have undertaken a phylogenetic analysis of the eukaryote-like sphingosine-1-phosphate lyase (SPL) of *L. pneumophila* that is encoded by *lpp2128*. In eukaryotes, SPL is an enzyme that catalyzes the irreversible cleavage of sphingosine-1 phosphate (S1P). S1P is implicated in various physiological processes such as cell survival, apoptosis, proliferation, migration, differentiation, platelet aggregation, angiogenesis, lymphocyte trafficking, and development. Although the function of the *L. pneumophila* sphingosine-1-phosphate lyase remains unknown, the hypothesis is that it plays a role in autophagy and/or apoptosis (Brüggemann et al., 2006b; Cazalet et al., 2004). Recently it has been shown that the *Legionella* SPL is able to complement the sphingosine-sensitive phenotype of *Saccharomyces cervisiae* and that it colocalizes to the host cell mitochondria (Degtyar et al., 2009). In our phylogenetic analysis we included homologous sequences, representative of the main groups of organisms according to the best BlastP result of Lpp2128 against the NCBI database. Sequences were aligned using CLUSTALX2, and maximum likelihood was used as the tree reconstruction method according to ProtTest results. For phylogenetic reconstruction, the program Phyml was used. Figure 6 shows the result of our analysis. The Lpp2128 protein sequence of *L. pneumophila* clearly falls into the eukaryotic clade of SPL sequences, suggesting acquisition of this gene by horizontal gene transfer from eukaryotes.

Similarly, we tested the hypothesis that *L. longbeachae* might also have acquired genes from plants, which is conceivable as it is found in soil. We thus undertook a phylogenetic analysis similar to that described above for the *L. longbeachae* protein Llo2643, which contains PPR repeats, a protein family typically present in plants. Figure 7 shows the phylogenetic tree we obtained. The Llo2634 protein of *L. longbeachae* does not appear embedded in the eukaryotic clade but is closer to plant proteins than to prokaryotic ones, which suggests that *L. longbeachae* may have acquired genes from protozoa and plants.

Legionella is not the only prokaryote whose genome shows an enrichment of proteins with eukaryotic domains. Analysis of different amoeba-associated genomes suggests that bacteria thriving within amoebas use similar mechanisms for host cell interaction to facilitate survival in the host cell and have thus evolved proteins containing similar domains. Recently the genome sequence of "*Candidatus* Amoebophilus asiaticus," a gram-negative, obligate intracellular amoeba symbiont belonging to the *Bacteroidetes*, which was discovered within an amoeba isolated from lake sediment (Schmitz-Esser et al., 2008) has been reported (Schmitz-Esser et al., 2010). This genome also encodes an arsenal of proteins with eukaryotic domains. To further investigate the distribution of these protein domains in other bacteria, the authors have undertaken an enrichment analysis, comparing the fraction of all functional protein domains among 514 bacterial proteomes (Schmitz-Esser et al., 2010). This showed that the genomes of bacteria for which the replication in amoebas has been demonstrated were enriched in protein domains that are found predominantly in eukaryotic proteins.

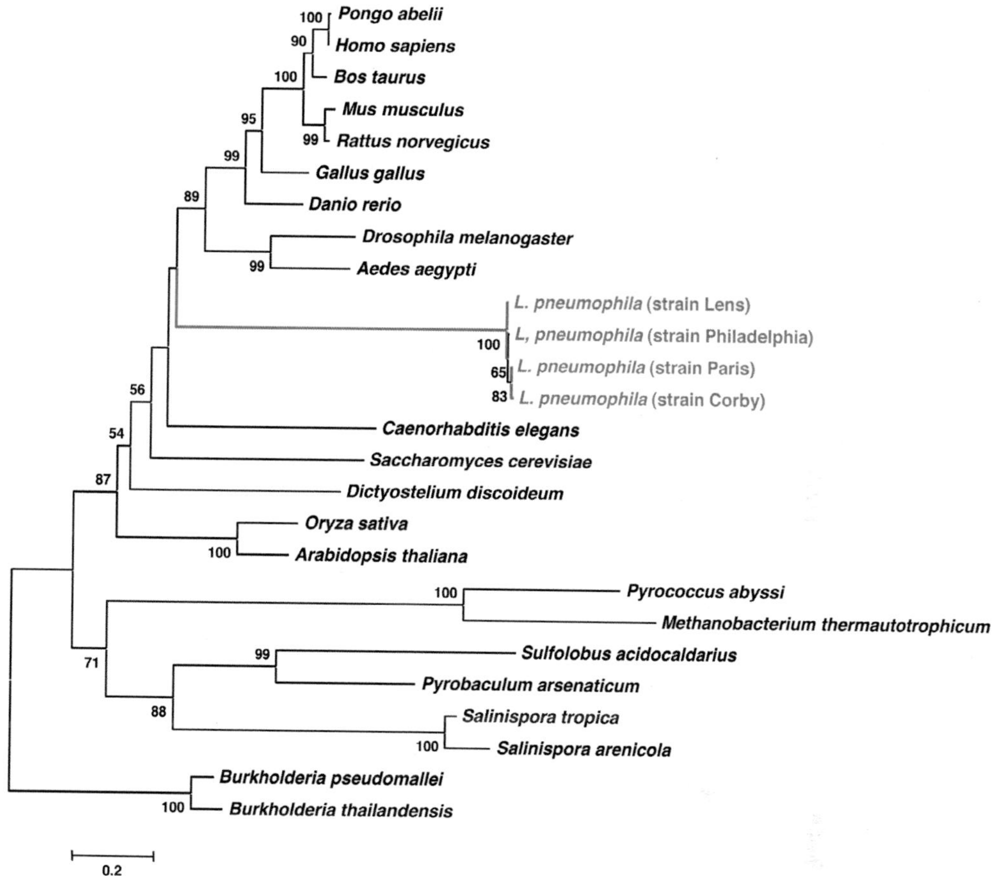

FIGURE 6 Phylogenetic tree of a multiple-sequence comparison of SPL proteins present in eukaryotic and prokaryotic genomes. Phylogenetic reconstruction was done with MEGA, using the neighbor-joining method. Numbers indicate bootstrap values after 1,000 bootstrap replicates. The red lines indicate the *L. pneumophila* sequences that are embedded in the eukaryotic clade. The bar at the bottom represents the estimated evolutionary distance.

Interestingly, the domains potentially involved in host cell interaction described above, such as ANK repeats, leucine-rich repeats (LRRs), SEL1 repeats, and F- and U-box domains, are among the most highly enriched domains in proteomes of amoeba-associated bacteria. Bacteria that can exploit amoebas as hosts thus share a set of eukaryotic domains important for host cell interaction despite their different lifestyles and their high phylogenetic diversity. This suggests that bacteria thriving within amoebas use similar mechanisms for host cell interaction to facilitate survival in the host cell. Due to the phylogenetic diversity of these bacteria, it is most parsimonious that these traits were acquired independently during early evolutionary interaction with ancient protozoa.

CONCLUSIONS

L. pneumophila and *L. longbeachae* are two human pathogens that are able to modulate, manipulate, and subvert many eukaryotic host cell functions to their advantage in order to enter, replicate in, and evade protozoa or human alveolar macrophages during disease. In the last few years, genome analyses, as well as comparative and functional genomics, have demonstrated that genome plasticity plays a major

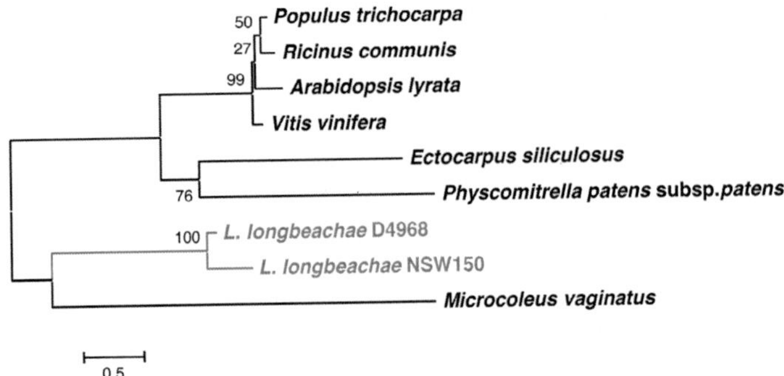

FIGURE 7 Phylogenetic tree of the protein Llo2643 and its homologues after a BlastP search. The tree was constructed by the neighbor-joining method using the program MEGA. The red lines indicate the *L. longbeachae* sequences that are close to sequences derived from plant genomes. Numbers indicate bootstrap support for nodes from 1,000 neighbor-joining bootstrap replicates. The bar at the bottom represents the estimated evolutionary distance.

role in differences in host cell exploitation and niche adaptation of *Legionella*. The genomes of these environmental pathogens are shaped by horizontal gene transfer between eukaryotes and prokaryotes, allowing them to mimic host cell functions and to exploit host cell pathways. Genome plasticity and horizontal gene transfer lead in each strain and species to a different repertoire of secreted effectors that may allow subtle adaptations to, e.g., different protozoan hosts. Plasmids can be exchanged among strains and circulate even between different species of *Legionella*. Phages and/or plasmids seem to play a role in acquisition of T4SS, and deletion of surface structures like flagella or chemotaxis systems may help the adaptation to different niches.

Access to genomic data has revealed many potential virulence factors of *L. pneumophila* and *L. longbeachae*, as well as the metabolic capacities of these bacteria. The increasing amount of information in the genomic database will allow a better identification of the origin and similarity of eukaryotic-like proteins or eukaryotic protein domains and other virulence factors. New eukaryotic genome sequencing projects such as that of the natural host of *Legionella*, *Acanthamoeba castellanii*, are in progress. These additional data will allow a better understanding of possible transfer events of genes from the eukaryotic host to *Legionella*. Taken together, the progressive increase of information on *Legionella* as well as on protozoa will lead to more complete comparative and phylogenetic studies that should shed light on the evolution of virulence in *Legionella*. However, much work remains to be done to translate the basic findings from genomics research into an improved understanding of the biology of this organism. As data are accumulating, new fields of investigation will emerge. Without doubt, the investigation and characterization of regulatory noncoding RNAs will be one such field. Manipulation of host-epigenetic information and investigation of host susceptibility to disease will be another. In particular, the development of high-throughput techniques for comparative and functional genomics as well as more and more powerful imaging techniques will accelerate the pace of knowledge acquisition.

ACKNOWLEDGMENTS

We thank many of our colleagues who have contributed in different ways to this research.

This work received financial support from the Institut Pasteur, the Centre National de la Recherche Scientifique (CNRS), the EuroPathoGenomics Network of Excellence (LSHB-CT-2005-512061), and the Institut Carnot. L. Gomez-Valero is holder of a

Fondation pour la Recherche Médicale (FRM) postdoctoral research fellowship financed by the Institut Pasteur.

REFERENCES

Al-Khodor, S., C. T. Price, F. Habyarimana, A. Kalia, and Y. Abu Kwaik. 2008. A Dot/Icm-translocated ankyrin protein of *Legionella pneumophila* is required for intracellular proliferation within human macrophages and protozoa. *Mol. Microbiol.* **70:**908–923.

Amodeo, M. R., D. R. Murdoch, and A. D. Pithie. 2010. Legionnaires' disease caused by *Legionella longbeachae* and *Legionella pneumophila*: comparison of clinical features, host-related risk factors, and outcomes. *Clin. Microbiol. Infect.* **16:**1405–1407.

Asare, R., and Y. Abu Kwaik. 2007. Early trafficking and intracellular replication of *Legionella longbeachae* within an ER-derived late endosome-like phagosome. *Cell. Microbiol.* **9:**1571–1587.

Asare, R., M. Santic, I. Gobin, M. Doric, J. Suttles, J. E. Graham, C. D. Price, and Y. Abu Kwaik. 2007. Genetic susceptibility and caspase activation in mouse and human macrophages are distinct for *Legionella longbeachae* and *L. pneumophila*. *Infect. Immun.* **75:**1933–1945.

Berger, K. H., and R. R. Isberg. 1993. Two distinct defects in intracellular growth complemented by a single genetic locus in *Legionella pneumophila*. *Mol. Microbiol.* **7:**7–19.

Brombacher, E., S. Urwyler, C. Ragaz, S. S. Weber, K. Kami, M. Overduin, and H. Hilbi. 2009. Rab1 guanine nucleotide exchange factor SidM is a major phosphatidylinositol 4-phosphate-binding effector protein of *Legionella pneumophila*. J. Biol. Chem. **284:**4846–4856.

Brüggemann, H., C. Cazalet, and C. Buchrieser. 2006a. Adaptation of *Legionella pneumophila* to the host environment: role of protein secretion, effectors and eukaryotic-like proteins. *Curr. Opin. Microbiol.* **9:**86–94. Epub 6 January 2006.

Brüggemann, H., A. Hagman, M. Jules, O. Sismeiro, M. Dillies, C. Gouyette, F. Kunst, M. Steinert, K. Heuner, J. Coppée, and C. Buchrieser. 2006b. Virulence strategies for infecting phagocytes deduced from the *in vivo* transcriptional program of *Legionella pneumophila*. *Cell. Microbiol.* **8:**1228–1240.

Burstein, D., T. Zusman, E. Degtyar, R. Viner, G. Segal, and T. Pupko. 2009. Genome-scale identification of *Legionella pneumophila* effectors using a machine learning approach. *PLoS Pathog* **5:**e1000508.

Casati, S., A. Gioria-Martinoni, and V. Gaia. 2009. Commercial potting soils as an alternative infection source of *Legionella pneumophila* and other *Legionella* species in Switzerland. *Clin. Microbiol. Infect.* **15:**571–575.

Cazalet, C., L. Gomez-Valero, C. Rusniok, M. Lomma, D. Dervins-Ravault, H. J. Newton, F. M. Sansom, S. Jarraud, N. Zidane, L. Ma, C. Bouchier, J. Etienne, E. L. Hartland, and C. Buchrieser. 2010. The *Legionella longbeachae* genome and transcriptome uncovers unique strategies to cause Legionnaires' disease. *PLoS Genet.* **6:**e1000851.

Cazalet, C., S. Jarraud, Y. Ghavi-Helm, F. Kunst, P. Glaser, J. Etienne, and C. Buchrieser. 2008. Multigenome analysis identifies a worldwide distributed epidemic *Legionella pneumophila* clone that emerged within a highly diverse species. *Genome Res.* **18:**431–441.

Cazalet, C., C. Rusniok, H. Bruggemann, N. Zidane, A. Magnier, L. Ma, M. Tichit, S. Jarraud, C. Bouchier, F. Vandenesch, F. Kunst, J. Etienne, P. Glaser, and C. Buchrieser. 2004. Evidence in the *Legionella pneumophila* genome for exploitation of host cell functions and high genome plasticity. *Nat. Genet.* **36:**1165–1173.

CDC. 2000. Legionnaires' disease associated with potting soil—California, Oregon, and Washington, May–June 2000. *MMWR Morb. Mortal. Wkly. Rep.* **49:**777–778.

Chien, M., I. Morozova, S. Shi, H. Sheng, J. Chen, S. M. Gomez, G. Asamani, K. Hill, J. Nuara, M. Feder, J. Rineer, J. J. Greenberg, V. Steshenko, S. H. Park, B. Zhao, E. Teplitskaya, J. R. Edwards, S. Pampou, A. Georghiou, I. C. Chou, W. Iannuccilli, M. E. Ulz, D. H. Kim, A. Geringer-Sameth, C. Goldsberry, P. Morozov, S. G. Fischer, G. Segal, X. Qu, A. Rzhetsky, P. Zhang, E. Cayanis, P. J. De Jong, J. Ju, S. Kalachikov, H. A. Shuman, and J. J. Russo. 2004. The genomic sequence of the accidental pathogen *Legionella pneumophila*. *Science* **305:**1966–1968.

Cianciotto, N. P. 2009. Many substrates and functions of type II secretion: lessons learned from *Legionella pneumophila*. *Future Microbiol.* **4:**797–805.

DebRoy, S., J. Dao, M. Soderberg, O. Rossier, and N. P. Cianciotto. 2006. *Legionella pneumophila* type II secretome reveals unique exoproteins and a chitinase that promotes bacterial persistence in the lung. *Proc. Natl. Acad. Sci. USA* **103:**19146–19151.

de Felipe, K. S., R. T. Glover, X. Charpentier, O. R. Anderson, M. Reyes, C. D. Pericone, and H. A. Shuman. 2008. *Legionella* eukaryotic-like type IV substrates interfere with organelle trafficking. *PLoS Pathog.* **4:**e1000117.

de Felipe, K. S., S. Pampou, O. S. Jovanovic, C. D. Pericone, S. F. Ye, S. Kalachikov, and H. A. Shuman. 2005. Evidence for acquisition of *Legionella* type IV secretion substrates via interdomain horizontal gene transfer. *J. Bacteriol.* **187:**7716–7726.

Degtyar, E., T. Zusman, M. Ehrlich, and G. Segal. 2009. A *Legionella* effector acquired from protozoa is involved in sphingolipids metabolism and is targeted to the host cell mitochondria. *Cell. Microbiol.* **11:**1219–1235.

Diez, E., S. H. Lee, S. Gauthier, Z. Yaraghi, M. Tremblay, S. Vidal, and P. Gros. 2003. Birc1e is the gene within the Lgn1 locus associated with resistance to *Legionella pneumophila. Nat. Genet.* **33:**55–60.

Doleans, A., H. Aurell, M. Reyrolle, G. Lina, J. Freney, F. Vandenesch, J. Etienne, and S. Jarraud. 2004. Clinical and environmental distributions of *Legionella* strains in France are different. *J. Clin. Microbiol.* **42:**458–460.

Edelstein, P. H., and J. P. Metlay. 2009. *Legionella pneumophila* goes clonal—Paris and Lorraine strain-specific risk factors. *Clin. Infect. Dis.* **49:** 192–194.

Eiserich, J. P., A. G. Estévez, T. V. Bamberg, Y. Z. Ye, P. H. Chumley, J. S. Beckman, and B. A. Freeman. 1999. Microtubule dysfunction by posttranslational nitrotyrosination of alpha-tubulin: a nitric oxide-dependent mechanism of cellular injury. *Proc. Natl. Acad. Sci. USA* **96:**6365–6370.

Feldman, M., and G. Segal. 2004. A specific genomic location within the *icm/dot* pathogenesis region of different *Legionella* species encodes functionally similar but nonhomologous virulence proteins. *Infect. Immun.* **72:**4503–4511.

Feldman, M., T. Zusman, S. Hagag, and G. Segal. 2005. Coevolution between nonhomologous but functionally similar proteins and their conserved partners in the *Legionella* pathogenesis system. *Proc. Natl. Acad. Sci. USA* **102:**12206–12211.

Fernandez-Moreira, E., J. H. Helbig, and M. S. Swanson. 2006. Membrane vesicles shed by *Legionella pneumophila* inhibit fusion of phagosomes with lysosomes. *Infect. Immun.* **74:**3285–3295.

Fields, B. S. 1993. *Legionella* and protozoa: interaction of a pathogen and its natural host,.p. 129–136. *In* J. M. Barbaree, R. F. Breiman, and A. P. Dufour (ed.), Legionella: *Current Status and Emerging Perspectives.* American Society for Microbiology, Washington, DC.

Fields, B. S. 2008. *Legionella* in the environment, p. 85–91. *In* P. Hoffmann, H. Friedman, and M. Bendinelli (ed.), Legionella pneumophila: *Pathogenesis and Immunity.* Springer, New York, NY.

Fields, B. S., R. F. Benson, and R. E. Besser. 2002. *Legionella* and Legionnaires' disease: 25 years of investigation. *Clin. Microbiol. Rev.* **15:**506–526.

Fraser, D. W., T. R. Tsai, W. Orenstein, W. E. Parkin, H. J. Beecham, R. G. Sharrar, J. Harris, G. F. Mallison, S. M. Martin, J. E. McDade, C. C. Shepard, and P. S. Brachman. 1977. Legionnaires' disease: description of an epidemic of pneumonia. *N. Engl. J. Med.* **297:**1189–1197.

Garcia, C., E. Ugalde, A. B. Campo, E. Minambres, and N. Kovacs. 2004. Fatal case of community-acquired pneumonia caused by *Legionella longbeachae* in a patient with systemic lupus erythematosus. *Eur. J. Clin. Microbiol. Infect. Dis.* **23:**116–118.

Glöckner, G., C. Albert-Weissenberger, E. Weinmann, S. Jacobi, E. Schunder, M. Steinert, J. Hacker, and K. Heuner. 2007. Identification and characterization of a new conjugation/type IVA secretion system (trb/tra) of Legionella pneumophila Corby localized on a mobile genomic island. *Int. J. Med. Microbiol.* **298:**411–428.

Gobin, I., M. Susa, G. Begic, E. L. Hartland, and M. Doric. 2009. Experimental *Legionella longbeachae* infection in intratracheally inoculated mice. *J. Med. Microbiol.* **58:**723–730.

Gomez-Valero, L., C. Rusniok, and C. Buchrieser. 2009. *Legionella pneumophila*: population genetics, phylogeny and genomics. Infect. Genet. Evol. **9:**727–739.

Habyarimana, F., C. T. Price, M. Santic, S. Al-Khodor, and Y. A. Kwaik. 2010. Molecular characterization of the Dot/Icm-translocated AnkH and AnkJ eukaryotic-like effectors of *Legionella pneumophila. Infect. Immun.* **78:**1123–1134.

Hazelbauer, G. L., J. J. Falke, and J. S. Parkinson. 2008. Bacterial chemoreceptors: high-performance signaling in networked arrays. *Trends Biochem. Sci.* **33:**9–19.

Isberg, R. R., T. J. O'Connor, and M. Heidtman. 2009. The *Legionella pneumophila* replication vacuole: making a cosy niche inside host cells. *Nat. Rev. Microbiol.* **7:**13–24.

Jepras, R. I., R. B. Fitzgeorge, and A. Baskerville. 1985. A comparison of virulence of two strains of *Legionella pneumophila* based on experimental aerosol infection of guinea pigs. *J. Hyg.* **95:**29–38.

Kentner, D., and V. Sourjik. 2006. Spatial organization of the bacterial chemotaxis system. *Curr. Opin. Microbiol.* **9:**619–624.

Kozak, N. A., M. Buss, C. E. Lucas, M. Frace, D. Govil, T. Travis, M. Olsen-Rasmussen, R. F. Benson, and B. S. Fields. 2010. Virulence factors encoded by *Legionella longbeachae* identified on the basis of the genome sequence analysis of clinical isolate D-4968. *J. Bacteriol.* **192:**1030–1044.

Kubori, T., A. Hyakutake, and H. Nagai. 2008. *Legionella* translocates an E3 ubiquitin ligase that has multiple U-boxes with distinct functions. *Mol. Microbiol.* **67:**1307–1319.

Kubota, M., K. Tomii, R. Tachikawa, Y. Harada, R. Seo, R. Kaji, Y. Takeshima, M. Hayashi, T.

Nishimura, and K. Ishihara. 2007. *Legionella longbeachae* pneumonia infection from home garden soil. *Nihon Kokyuki Gakkai Zasshi* **45:**698–703. (In Japanese.)

Kumpers, P., A. Tiede, P. Kirschner, J. Girke, A. Ganser, and D. Peest. 2008. Legionnaires' disease in immunocompromised patients: a case report of *Legionella longbeachae* pneumonia and review of the literature. *J. Med. Microbiol.* **57:**384–387.

Lamkanfi, M., A. Amer, T. D. Kanneganti, R. Munoz-Planillo, G. Chen, P. Vandenabeele, A. Fortier, P. Gros, and G. Nunez. 2007. The Nod-like receptor family member Naip5/Birc1e restricts *Legionella pneumophila* growth independently of caspase-1 activation. *J. Immunol.* **178:**8022–8027.

La Scola, B., R. J. Birtles, G. Greub, T. J. Harrison, R. M. Ratcliff, and D. Raoult. 2004. *Legionella drancourtii* sp. nov., a strictly intracellular amoebal pathogen. *Int. J. Syst. Evol. Microbiol.* **54:**699–703.

Lawrence, C., M. Reyrolle, S. Dubrou, F. Forey, B. Decludt, C. Goulvestre, P. Matsiota-Bernard, J. Etienne, and C. Nauciel. 1999. Single clonal origin of a high proportion of *Legionella pneumophila* serogroup 1 isolates from patients and the environment in the area of Paris, France, over a 10-year period. *J. Clin. Microbiol.* **37:**2652–2655.

Lightfield, K. L., J. Persson, S. W. Brubaker, C. E. Witte, J. von Moltke, E. A. Dunipace, T. Henry, Y. H. Sun, D. Cado, W. F. Dietrich, D. M. Monack, R. M. Tsolis, and R. E. Vance. 2008. Critical function for Naip5 in inflammasome activation by a conserved carboxy-terminal domain of flagellin. *Nat. Immunol.* **9:**1171–1178.

Lurin, C., C. Andrés, S. Aubourg, M. Bellaoui, F. Bitton, C. Bruyère, M. Caboche, C. Debast, J. Gualberto, B. Hoffmann, A. Lecharny, M. Le Ret, M. L. Martin-Magniette, H. Mireau, N. Peeters, J. P. Renou, B. Szurek, L. Taconnat, and I. Small. 2004. Genome-wide analysis of *Arabidopsis* pentatricopeptide repeat proteins reveals their essential role in organelle biogenesis. *Plant Cell* **16:**2089–2103.

Machner, M. P., and R. R. Isberg. 2006. Targeting of host Rab GTPase function by the intravacuolar pathogen *Legionella pneumophila*. *Dev. Cell* **11:**47–56.

Marra, A., S. J. Blander, M. A. Horwitz, and H. A. Shuman. 1992. Identification of a *Legionella pneumophila* locus required for intracellular multiplication in human macrophages. *Proc. Natl. Acad. Sci. USA* **89:**9607–9611.

Marrie, T. J. 2008. Legionnaires' disease—clinical picture, p. 133–150. *In* P. Hoffmann, H. Friedman, and M. Bendinelli (ed.), Legionella pneumophila: *Pathogenesis and Immunity.* Springer, New York, NY.

McDade, J. E., C. C. Shepard, D. W. Fraser, T. R. Tsai, M. A. Redus, and W. R. Dowdle. 1977. Legionnaires' disease: isolation of a bacterium and demonstration of its role in other respiratory disease. *N. Engl. J. Med.* **297:**1197–1203.

McKinney, R. M., R. K. Porschen, P. H. Edelstein, M. L. Bissett, P. P. Harris, S. P. Bondell, A. G. Steigerwalt, R. E. Weaver, M. E. Ein, D. S. Lindquist, R. S. Kops, and D. J. Brenner. 1981. *Legionella longbeachae* species nova, another etiologic agent of human pneumonia. *Ann. Intern. Med.* **94:**739–743.

Moliner, C., C. Ginevra, S. Jarraud, C. Flaudrops, M. Bedotto, C. Couderc, J. Etienne, and P. E. Fournier. 2009. Rapid identification of *Legionella* species by mass spectrometry. *J. Med. Microbiol.* **59:**273–284.

Molofsky, A. B., B. G. Byrne, N. N. Whitfield, C. A. Madigan, E. T. Fuse, K. Tateda, and M. S. Swanson. 2006. Cytosolic recognition of flagellin by mouse macrophages restricts *Legionella pneumophila* infection. *J. Exp. Med.* **17:**1093–1104.

Morozova, I., X. Qu, S. Shi, G. Asamani, J. E. Greenberg, H. A. Shuman, and J. J. Russo. 2004. Comparative sequence analysis of the *icm/dot* genes in *Legionella*. *Plasmid* **51:**127–147.

Murata, T., A. Delprato, A. Ingmundson, D. K. Toomre, D. G. Lambright, and C. R. Roy. 2006. The *Legionella pneumophila* effector protein DrrA is a Rab1 guanine nucleotide-exchange factor. *Nat. Cell Biol.* **8:**971–977.

Nagai, H., E. D. Cambronne, J. C. Kagan, J. C. Amor, R. A. Kahn, and C. R. Roy. 2005. A C-terminal translocation signal required for Dot/Icm-dependent delivery of the *Legionella* RalF protein to host cells. *Proc. Natl. Acad. Sci. USA* **102:** 826–831.

Nagai, H., J. C. Kagan, X. Zhu, R. A. Kahn, and C. R. Roy. 2002. A bacterial guanine nucleotide exchange factor activates ARF on *Legionella* phagosomes. *Science* **295:**679–682.

Nagai, H., E. D. Cambronne, J. C. Kagan, J. C. Amor, R. A. Kahn, and C. R. Roy. 2005. A C-terminal translocation signal required for Dot/Icm-dependent delivery of the *Legionella* RalF protein to host cells. *Proc. Natl. Acad. Sci. USA* **102:** 826–831.

Nakamura, T., G. Schuster, M. Sugiura, and M. Sugita. 2004. Chloroplast RNA-binding and pentatricopeptide repeat proteins. *Biochem. Soc. Trans.* **32:**571–574.

Newton, H. J., F. M. Sansom, J. Dao, A. D. McAlister, J. Sloan, N. P. Cianciotto, and E. L. Hartland. 2007. Sel1 repeat protein LpnE is a *Legionella pneumophila* virulence determinant that influences vacuolar trafficking. *Infect. Immun.* **75:**5575–5585.

Nhu Nguyen, T. M., D. Ilef, S. Jarraud, Rouil L, C. Campese, D. Che, S. Haeghebaert, F. Ganiayre, F. Marcel, J. Etienne, and J. C. Desenclos. 2006. A community-wide outbreak of Legionnaires disease linked to industrial cooling towers—how far can contaminated aerosols spread? *J. Infect. Dis.* **193:**102–111.

Ninio, S., J. Celli, and C. R. Roy. 2009. A Legionella pneumophila effector protein encoded in a region of genomic plasticity binds to Dot/Icm-modified vacuoles. *PLoS Pathog.* **5:**e1000278.

Nora, T., M. Lomma, L. Gomez-Valero, and C. Buchrieser. 2009. Molecular mimicry: an important virulence strategy employed by *Legionella pneumophila* to subvert host functions. *Future Microbiol.* **4:**691–701.

O'Connor, B. A., J. Carman, K. Eckert, G. Tucker, R. Givney, and S. Cameron. 2007. Does using potting mix make you sick? Results from a *Legionella longbeachae* case-control study in South Australia. *Epidemiol. Infect.* **135:**34–39.

Pan, X., A. Lührmann, A. Satoh, M. A. Laskowski-Arce, and C. R. Roy. 2008. Ankyrin repeat proteins comprise a diverse family of bacterial type IV effectors. *Science* **320:**1651–1654.

Pedro-Botet, M. L., and V. L. Yu. 2009. Treatment strategies for *Legionella* infection. *Expert Opin. Pharmacother.* **10:**1109–1121.

Pravinkumar, S., G. Edwards, D. Lindsay, S. Redmond, J. Stirling, R. House, J. Kerr, E. Anderson, D. Breen, O. Blatchford, E. McDonald, and A. Brown. 2010. A cluster of Legionnaires' disease caused by *Legionella longbeachae* linked to potting compost in Scotland, 2008–2009. *Euro Surveill.* **15:**19496.

Price, C. T., S. Al-Khodor, T. Al-Quadan, M. Santic, F. Habyarimana, A. Kalia, and Y. A. Kwaik. 2009. Molecular mimicry by an F-Box effector of *Legionella pneumophila* hijacks a conserved polyubiquitination machinery within macrophages and protozoa. *PLoS Pathog.* **5:**e1000704.

Ren, T., D. S. Zamboni, C. R. Roy, W. F. Dietrich, and R. E. Vance. 2006. Flagellin-deficient *Legionella* mutants evade caspase-1- and Naip5-mediated macrophage immunity. *PLoS Pathog.* **2:**e18.

Rossier, O., and N. P. Cianciotto. 2001. Type II protein secretion is a subset of the PilD-dependent processes that facilitate intracellular infection by *Legionella pneumophila. Infect. Immun.* **69:**2092–2098.

Rowbotham, T. J. 1986. Current views on the relationships between *amoebae, legionellae* and man. *Isr. J. Med. Sci.* **22:**678–689.

Rowbotham, T. J. 1980. Preliminary report on the pathogenicity of *Legionella pneumophila* for freshwater and soil amoebae. *J. Clin. Pathol.* **33:**1179–1183.

Schmitz-Esser, S., P. Tischler, R. Arnold, J. Montanaro, M. Wagner, T. Rattei, and M. Horn. 2010. The genome of the amoeba symbiont "*Candidatus* Amoebophilus asiaticus" reveals common mechanisms for host cell interaction among amoeba-associated bacteria. *J. Bacteriol.* **192:**1045–1057.

Schmitz-Esser, S., E. R. Toenshoff, S. Haider, E. Heinz, V. M. Hoenninger, M. Wagner, and M. Horn. 2008. Diversity of bacterial endosymbionts of environmental *Acanthamoeba* isolates. *Appl. Environ. Microbiol.* **74:**5822–5831.

Schmitz-Linneweber, C., and I. Small. 2008. Pentatricopeptide repeat proteins: a socket set for organelle gene expression. *Trends Plant Sci.* **13:**663–670.

Segal, G., J. J. Russo, and H. A. Shuman. 1999. Relationships between a new type IV secretion system and the *icm/dot* virulence system of *Legionella pneumophila. Mol. Microbiol.* **34:**799–809.

Shevchuk, O., C. Batzilla, S. Hagele, H. Kusch, S. Engelmann, M. Hecker, A. Haas, K. Heuner, G. Glockner, and M. Steinert. 2009. Proteomic analysis of *Legionella*-containing phagosomes isolated from Dictyostelium. *Int. J. Med. Microbiol.* **299:**489–508.

Shin, S., and C. R. Roy. 2008. Host cell processes that influence the intracellular survival of *Legionella pneumophila. Cell. Microbiol.* **10:**1209–1220.

Steele, T. W., C. V. Moore, and N. Sangster. 1990. Distribution of *Legionella longbeachae* serogroup 1 and other legionellae in potting soils in Australia. *Appl. Environ. Microbiol.* **56:**2984–2988.

Steinert, M., U. Hentschel, and J. Hacker. 2002. *Legionella pneumophila*: an aquatic microbe goes astray. *FEMS Microbiol. Rev.* **26:**149–162.

Steinert, M., K. Heuner, C. Buchrieser, C. Albert-Weissenberger, and G. Glöckner. 2007. *Legionella* pathogenicity: genome structure, regulatory networks and the host cell response. *Int. J. Med. Microbiol.* **297:**577–587.

Tijet, N., P. Tang, M. Romilowych, C. Duncan, V. Ng, D. N. Fisman, F. Jamieson, D. E. Low, and C. Guyard. 2010. New Endemic *Legionella pneumophila* serogroup I clones, Ontario, Canada. *Emerg. Infect. Dis.* **16:**447–454.

Urwyler, S., E. Brombacher, and H. Hilbi. 2009a. Endosomal and secretory markers of the Legionella-containing vacuole. *Commun. Integr. Biol.* **2:**107–109.

Urwyler, S., Y. Nyfeler, C. Ragaz, H. Lee, L. N. Mueller, R. Aebersold, and H. Hilbi. 2009b. Proteome analysis of *Legionella* vacuoles purified by magnetic immunoseparation reveals secretory and endosomal GTPases. *Traffic* **10:**76–87.

Velonakis, E. N., I. M. Kiousi, C. Koutis, E. Papadogiannakis, F. Babatsikou, and A. Vatopoulos. 2009. First isolation of *Legionella* species, including *L. pneumophila* serogroup 1, in Greek potting soils: possible importance for public health. *Clin. Microbiol. Infect.* **16:**763–766.

Weber, S. S., C. Ragaz, and H. Hilbi. 2009. The inositol polyphosphate 5-phosphatase OCRL1 restricts intracellular growth of *Legionella*, localizes to the replicative vacuole and binds to the bacterial effector LpnE. *Cell. Microbiol.* **11:**442–460.

Weber, S. S., C. Ragaz, K. Reus, Y. Nyfeler, and H. Hilbi. 2006. *Legionella pneumophila* exploits PI(4)P to anchor secreted effector proteins to the replicative vacuole. *PLoS Pathog.* **2:**e46.

Wright, E. K., S. A. Goodart, J. D. Growney, V. Hadinoto, M. G. Endrizzi, E. M. Long, K. Sadigh, A. L. Abney, I. Bernstein-Hanley, and W. F. Dietrich. 2003. Naip5 affects host susceptibility to the intracellular pathogen Legionella pneumophila. *Curr. Biol.* **13:**27–36.

Yu, V. L., J. F. Plouffe, M. C. Pastoris, J. E. Stout, M. Schousboe, A. Widmer, J. Summersgill, T. File, C. M. Heath, D. L. Paterson, and A. Chereshsky. 2002. Distribution of *Legionella* species and serogroups isolated by culture in patients with sporadic community-acquired legionellosis: an international collaborative survey. *J. Infect. Dis.* **186:**127–128.

Zamboni, D. S., K. S. Kobayashi, T. Kohlsdorf, Y. Ogura, E. M. Long, R. E. Vance, K. Kuida, S. Mariathasan, V. M. Dixit, R. A. Flavell, W. F. Dietrich, and C. R. Roy. 2006. The Birc1e cytosolic pattern-recognition receptor contributes to the detection and control of *Legionella pneumophila* infection. *Nat. Immunol.* **7:**318–325.

Zeigler, D. R. 2003. Gene sequences useful for predicting relatedness of whole genomes in bacteria. *Int. J. Syst. Evol. Microbiol.* **53:**1893–1900.

GENOME PLASTICITY IN *Salmonella enterica* AND ITS RELEVANCE TO HOST-PATHOGEN INTERACTIONS

Rosana B. Ferreira, Michelle M. Buckner, and B. Brett Finlay

6

Genome plasticity is defined as the different genome structures that occur among the same bacterial species. It is a poorly understood phenomenon caused by frequent rearrangement of the bacterial genome. Over the years, comparative genomic data have highlighted the importance of genetic variation on genome evolution and the effect of gene organization on the bacterial lifestyle.

Salmonella is a genus of the large *Enterobacteriaceae* family, which comprises a distinct phylogenetic cluster that shares a common ancestor with other gamma-proteobacteria (Garrity, 2001). Like other members of this group, *Salmonella* lives in close association with its host as an intestinal pathogen. Over 2,500 serovars have been identified over the years, each with a different host spectrum of infections (Popoff et al., 2004). These serovars are classified according to the Kauffmann-White serotyping scheme, based on antigenic variation in the outer membrane lipopolysaccharide (O) and phase 1 (H1) and phase 2 (H2) flagella (Ewing, 1986; Le Minor and Bockemuhl, 1984, 1988).

Genome plasticity in *Salmonella* was first detected in *S. enterica* serovar Typhi (Liu and Sanderson, 1995a, 1995b, 1996), and it has been observed in a number of *Salmonella* serovars since then (Chan et al., 2003; Holt et al., 2009; Liu et al., 2007; McClelland et al., 2004). A number of genetic events are responsible for the genomic make-up of *Salmonella* serovars. Variability in the genetic composition and organization plays an important role in the growth and development of all organisms, leading to biodiversity in nature. Genetic rearrangements may also be important in creating a pathogen, defining its host specificity, its niche of infection, and the virulence it develops. The way these events affect the interactions between *Salmonella* and its hosts is the main focus of this chapter.

GENETIC MECHANISMS LEADING TO PLASTICITY AND HOST ADAPTATION IN *SALMONELLA*

Bacterial evolution can occur as a result of alterations to the bacterial genome. Therefore, evolution can be achieved by the modification and erosion of existing genes or the acquisition

Rosana B. Ferreira, Michael Smith Laboratories, The University of British Columbia, Vancouver, British Columbia, Canada. *Michelle M. Buckner and B. Brett Finlay*, Michael Smith Laboratories and Department of Microbiology and Immunology, The University of British Columbia, Vancouver, British Columbia, Canada.

Genome Plasticity and Infectious Diseases,
Edited by J. Hacker, U. Dobrindt, and R. Kurth,

of new genes (Brussow et al., 2004; Pallen and Wren, 2007). The acquisition of new genes is a major factor contributing to bacterial evolution. The proportion of the genome that is common within a taxonomic classification such as *Salmonella* is often smaller than the proportion of genes that vary between serovars (Pallen and Wren, 2007). This indicates the importance of the acquisition of new genes and the alteration of existing genes in the creation of serovars. This section, therefore, focuses on lateral gene transfer (LGT) and other mechanisms that lead to evolution and genome plasticity.

Lateral Gene Transfer

Horizontal gene transfer (HGT) and LGT are significant sources of gene acquisition in bacteria (Kado, 2009; Pallen and Wren, 2007). HGT is the transfer of genes between organisms of different domains, whereas LGT is the transfer of genes within a domain (Kado, 2009). Some confusion exists within the literature about the use of these two terms. In this section LGT is the main focus. LGT mediates the transfer of foreign genetic material into a new recipient cell (Porwollik and McClelland, 2003). For LGT to result in the successful acquisition of new traits and therefore in enhanced evolution of the bacterium, three requirements must be fulfilled. The DNA must be delivered, it must be incorporated into the chromosome or replicate autonomously, and the encoded protein must be beneficial to the new host (Ochman et al., 2000).

LGT events can be identified and classified based on a few different criteria (Ochman et al., 2000). First, the G+C content of the gene of interest and the core genome of the bacteria can be compared; if a difference is seen, the gene of interest may have originated in a different organism. Second, differences in codon usage may indicate LGT events. The codon and the dinucleotide and trinucleotide usage within the gene of interest can be compared with that in the core or constant regions of the genome. Third, the sequence for the gene of interest can be compared between organisms; if a high degree of similarity is seen between relatively distant organisms, an LGT event may have taken place. When using these criteria to identify genes of LGT origin, it is important to consider whether the gene may have simply arisen as a result of convergent evolution. The complete genome sequences of many bacteria have been immensely useful in the identification of genes originating in different organisms.

LGT occurs via three main routes: conjugation, transformation, and transduction (Kado, 2009; Ochman et al., 2000; Porwollik and McClelland, 2003). Conjugation occurs when physical contact between two cells allows the direct transfer of DNA (Ochman et al., 2000; Porwollik and McClelland, 2003). It is usually mediated by a self-transmissible/mobilizable plasmid or a conjugative transposon (Ochman et al., 2000; Porwollik and McClelland, 2003). Transformation, on the other hand, involves the uptake of naked DNA by the cell. Some bacteria are naturally competent for the uptake of foreign DNA (Ochman et al., 2000), and because no direct contact is required, transformation has the potential for transmission between organisms of distant taxonomy or organisms at different times (Ochman et al., 2000). Lastly, transduction involves the use of a bacteriophage (Ochman et al., 2000; Porwollik and McClelland, 2003). There are two types of transduction, generalized transduction and specialized transduction. Generalized transduction involves the packaging of random portions of DNA into phage particles from the donor cell. Specialized transduction occurs when phage excision occurs and includes DNA segments adjacent to the phage. The fragment size varies substantially but can be upwards of 100 kb (Ochman et al., 2000).

Insertion elements, transposons, bacteriophages, plasmids, and pathogenicity islands can all act as vectors of DNA transfer in LGT (Pallen and Wren, 2007; Porwollik and McClelland, 2003). Mediation of the integration of transferred DNA can occur via a few methods: homologous recombination may occur between closely related bacteria at regions of homology, the mobile elements transferred may have their own sequences mediating integration (integrases or transposases), the DNA may persist as an episome, or it may be incorporated during double-strand break repair (Ochman et al., 2000). If the DNA is not stably maintained, it will be degraded and the potential for evolution will be thwarted (Kado, 2009).

The acquisition of genetic material from other organisms by LGT or HGT is a major contributor to bacterial diversity and genome structure (Kado, 2009; Ochman et al., 2000). Gene transfer has contributed to such a great extent to the development of bacterial species that it has been suggested that bacteria should not be considered to reside within a phylogenetic tree but, instead, a phylogenetic web may be a more accurate analogy (Brussow et al., 2004). This demonstrates the extent to which gene transfer is vital to the evolution and diversification of bacterial species. The importance of LGT can be seen by the improvement of overall bacterial fitness by the spread of antibiotic resistance, virulence attributes, and metabolic properties (Kado, 2009; Ochman et al., 2000).

Other Mechanisms

Other mechanisms that can lead to alterations in the genome include changes at the single-nucleotide level, gene loss, and genome rearrangements. Nucleotide exchange, insertions, deletions, and single-nucleotide polymorphisms are very common in *Salmonella*; however, they represent the smallest scale of variation (Brussow et al., 2004; Pallen and Wren, 2007). Their contribution to genome plasticity consists of the potential to modify the encoded protein or prevent the transcription of the gene.

In general, the size of a bacterial genome remains relatively constant; therefore, gene gain must be balanced by gene loss (Pallen and Wren, 2007). The loss of genes is important for evolution (Pallen and Wren, 2007). Genes that do not provide a selective advantage are less likely to be maintained over generations (Ochman et al., 2000); therefore, natural selection can provide pressure for the loss of specific genes (Pallen and Wren, 2007). Positive selection for gene loss is an important component of pathoadaptation, a process by which virulence mechanisms are refined (Pallen and Wren, 2007). One of the mechanisms that can lead to gene loss is phage integration (Brussow et al., 2004). Some bacteriophages may integrate into the coding region of a gene, leading to disruption and loss (Brussow et al., 2004). *S. enterica* serovar Typhi has a large quantity of pseudogenes, which are thought to be the remnants of genes (Dobrindt and Hacker, 2001; Pallen and Wren, 2007). These losses are thought to be associated with the change in lifestyle of the bacterium.

Genome rearrangement can also lead to evolution and genome plasticity. Large-scale chromosomal rearrangements can occur as a result of homologous recombination within the bacterial genome (Pallen and Wren, 2007). Homologous recombination can lead to deletion, duplication, and inversions of segments of the genome (Dobrindt and Hacker, 2001). Inversion of DNA can affect the expression of the inverted gene, which is normally flanked by inverted repeats (Craig, 1985). In serovar Typhimurium, the Hin recombinase catalyzes a reversible site-specific recombination event occurring at *hixL* and *hixR* (Nanassy and Hughes, 1998). This inversion results in flagellar-phase variation, which is the expression of different flagella antigens (Nanassy and Hughes, 1998). To accomplish this inversion an invertasome, a nucleoprotein complex composed of the *Salmonella* proteins Hin, Fis, and HU conducts the strand exchange (Nanassy and Hughes, 1998). Thus, genome rearrangements including inversions and translocations can lead to genome plasticity, contributing to the divergence of *Salmonella* strains. For example, in *S. enterica* serovar Agona, a map of the genome found a 1,000-kb inversion, seven deletions, and seven insertions compared to serovar Typhimurium strain LT2 (Chen et al., 2009). In serovar Paratyphi C, a genome map found a 1,602-kb inversion, four insertions totaling 176 kb, and seven deletions totaling 165 kb compared to strain LT2 (Liu et al., 2007). These changes exemplify the changes that may occur within and contribute to the plasticity of the bacterial genome.

In summary, LGT is a mechanism that many bacteria, including *Salmonella*, use to transfer and obtain entire gene sequences, allowing the transfer of blocks of genetic information from one organism to another. This process is very important in the evolution and diversification of *Salmonella* strains, as they are able to evolve in quantum leaps, transferring genes for metabolism, pathogenicity, or general improvements to bacterial fitness. Additional mechanisms that contribute to the plasticity and evolution of the *Salmonella* genome include gene loss, single-nucleotide alterations, and genome rearrangements including inversions and translocations.

GENOME ORGANIZATION IN *SALMONELLA*

Salmonella Genomic Islands

Genomic islands are distinct regions within the bacterial genome, which are thought to originate from gene transfer. Genomic islands are classified based on a few characteristics: a G+C content unique from the rest of the genome, alternative codon preferences, and mobility genes (Kelly et al., 2009). Pathogenicity islands are a subset of genomic islands; genomic islands contribute to bacterial fitness, while pathogenicity islands more specifically contribute to bacterial virulence (Kelly et al., 2009). Genomic islands are associated with symbiosis, fitness, metabolism, antimicrobial resistance, and pathogenicity (Dobrindt et al., 2004).

Salmonella contains a genomic island (*Salmonella* genomic island) called SGI1, which is an integrative mobilizable element associated with multiple drug resistance (MDR) (Doublet et al, 2009; Kelly et al., 2009; Yang et al., 2009). SGI1 is a complex class 1 integron found at the 3′ end of the *thdF* gene in serovar Typhimurium (Mulvey et al., 2006). It is a 43-kb region flanked by 18-bp imperfect direct repeats, with 44 open reading frames (ORFs), containing a 13-kb cluster of genes associated with MDR (Boyd et al., 2001; Doublet et al., 2005, 2009; Kelly et al., 2009; Mulvey et al., 2006). The ORFs have been classified based on homology as involved in DNA recombination, DNA replication, conjugal transfer, regulation, drug resistance, or other/unknown functions (Mulvey et al., 2006). SGI1 is able to conjugate and integrate in a site-specific manner into other *S. enterica* strains or *Escherichia coli* strains in vitro (Doublet et al., 2005). SGI1 has been found in many serovars of *S. enterica* including serovars Agona, Albany, Paratyphi B, Meleagridis, Newport, Kentucky, Kingston, Virchow, Derby, Ceero, Kiambu, Emek, Dusseldorf, Haifa, and Infantis (Boyd et al., 2001; Doublet et al., 2009; Mulvey et al., 2006). In addition, *Proteus mirabilis* strains have been found to contain SGI1 (Ahmed et al., 2007).

The increasing emergence of MDR *Salmonella* strains is of great concern, as these strains pose serious problems for clinical treatment (Hensel, 2005; Mulvey et al., 2006; Varma et al., 2005; Yang et al., 2009). In serovar Typhimurium strain DT104, SGI1 is associated with resistance to ampicillin, chloramphenicol, streptomycin, sulfonamides, and tetracycline (Boyd et al., 2001; Mulvey et al., 2006). *S. enterica* serovar Albany has a trimethoprim resistance cassette in place of the streptomycin resistance cassette (Hensel, 2005). A great deal of variability exists between strains, as the SGI1 region is considered a hot spot for antibiotic resistance genes (Doublet et al., 2008, 2009; Kelly et al., 2009). There is evidence for recent changes and acquisitions of antibiotic resistance genes implying continual evolution of the pathogen (Doublet et al., 2003; Hensel, 2005). These genes are thought to be acquired via transposition of In4-type integrons and IS26-composite transposons (Doublet et al., 2009). The variants of SGI1 are categorized as SGI1-A through SGI1-O, depending on the cassettes present (Doublet et al., 2008). In summary, SGI1 is a mobile genetic element, found in an increasing number of serovars and containing multiple genes including MDR cassettes.

Salmonella Pathogenicity Islands

As mentioned earlier, included on the *Salmonella* genome are *Salmonella* pathogenicity islands (SPI). These SPIs are large regions of DNA, which were most likely acquired as a result of HGT and are often associated with virulence (Bishop et al., 2005). SPIs are often found in a mosaic-like structure, indicating that multiple insertion events have led to their formation (Bishop et al., 2005). Some SPIs are highly conserved among *Salmonella*, such as SPI1, while other SPIs are found only in some *Salmonella* serovars (Bishop et al., 2005). SPI1 through SPI5 have been fairly well characterized in serovar Typhimurium, even though a large number of SPIs have been identified in various *Salmonella* serovars (Table 1). In this section we focus on SPI1 through SPI10.

SPI1 is around 40 kb long, with 29 or 30 genes and a G+C content of 47% (the *Salmonella* core genome G+C content averages around 52%) (Ellermeier and Slauch, 2007; Hensel, 2005; Marcus et al., 2000). It is found in nearly all *S. bongori* and *S. enterica* strains (Hensel, 2005; Hu et al., 2008). There are two main components to SPI1; the first encodes the type 3 secretion system (T3SS)-associated proteins, the second, *sitABCD*, is found at the flank of SPI1 and encodes an iron uptake system (Hensel, 2005; Zhou et al., 1999). SPI1-encoded T3SS-associated proteins include the T3SS apparatus, some of the proteins that are translocated via the T3SS (termed effectors), and regulators (Ellermeier and Slauch, 2007; Kelly et al., 2009). Some effectors are encoded outside of SPI1 but are secreted by the SPI1-encoded T3SS. These genes include *sopA, sopB, sopD, sopE*, and *sopE2* (*sopE* is encoded by a phage which is not present in all strains) (Hensel, 2005). This T3SS plays an important role during infection (Ellermeier and Slauch, 2007; Galan, 2001; Kelly et al., 2009). The importance of SPI1 lies in its mediation of bacterial uptake by non-phagocytic cells (Galan, 2001; Hensel, 2005; Schmidt and Hensel, 2004). SPI1 is very stable and has no evidence of genes associated with DNA mobility; because of its wide distribution, it is considered an element acquired very early in *Salmonella* development (Ginocchio et al., 1997; Hensel, 2005; Kingsley and Baumler, 2002b; Schmidt and Hensel, 2004). However, in serovars Senftenberg and Litchfield, some deletions from within SPI1 have been detected (Ginocchio et al., 1997).

SPI2 encodes the apparatus for a different T3SS, a two-component regulatory system, and some effectors; it is required for systemic

TABLE 1 Genetic regions found within *Salmonella* genomes

Region	Species	Serovar(s)
SPI1	*S. bongori* and *S. enterica*	Broad
SPI2	*S. enterica*	Broad
SPI3	*S. enterica*	Typhi, Typhimurium
SPI4	*S. enterica*	Different organization among serovars
SPI5	*S. enterica*	Broad[a]
SPI6	*S. enterica*	Typhimurium, Typhi
SPI7	*S. enterica*	Typhi, Dublin, Paratyphi C
SPI8	*S. enterica*	Typhi
SPI9	*S. enterica*	Typhi, Typhimurium
SPI10	*S. enterica*	Typhi, Enteritidis
SGI1	*S. enterica*	Agona, Albany, Cerro, Derby, Dusseldorf, Emek, Haifa, Infantis, Kentucky, Kiambu, Kingston, Meleagridis, Newport, Paratyphi B, Virchow
Gifsy 1	*S. enterica*	Typhimurium
Gifsy 2	*S. enterica*	Typhimurium
Gifsy 3	*S. enterica*	Typhimurium
Fels1	*S. enterica*	Typhimurium
Fels2	*S. enterica*	Typhimurium, Typhi, Sendai, Enteritidis
pSLT	*S. enterica*	Typhimurium, Dublin, Paratyphi C
Virulence plasmid[b]	*S. enterica*	Abortusovis, Abortusequi, Choleraesuis, Dublin, Enteritidis, Gallinarum, Pullorum, Sendai, Typhimurium

[a]*sopB* found in *S. enterica* and *S. bongori*, *pipAB* not found in *S. enterica* subspecies II.
[b]serovar specific.

infection (Bishop et al., 2005; Ellermeier and Slauch, 2007; Hensel, 2005; Kelly et al., 2009). The SPI1- and SPI2-encoded T3SS are different from each other and are thought to have arisen from separate gene transfer events, as opposed to duplication of a single T3SS (Hensel, 2005; Kelly et al., 2009). SPI2 is around 40 kb, contains 42 ORFs, and is inserted next to the *valV* tRNA gene (Hensel et al., 1997; Kelly et al., 2009). Similar to SPI1, SPI2 is divided into two components. The first one is 14.5 kb long and contains five *ttr* genes, which encode for tetrathionate respiration proteins (Hensel et al., 1999), with a G+C content of 54%. The second one is 25 kb, with four operons that encode the secretion system regulator *(ssr)*, secretion system chaperone *(ssc)*, secretion system apparatus *(ssa)*, and secretion system effectors *(sse)*, and has a G+C content of 43% (Hensel, 2005; Kelly et al., 2009). Many of the effectors secreted by the SPI2-encoded T3SS are encoded outside of SPI2 and may be associated with bacteriophages (Figueroa-Bossi et al., 2001). SPI2 is found only in *S. enterica*, indicating that it was added to the *Salmonella* genome more recently than SPI1 (Hensel, 2005; Hensel et al., 1997; Ochman and Groisman, 1996). SPI2 has become a part of the core *Salmonella* genome, and evolution and adaptation of SPI2 occur via the loss or acquisition of genes at additional loci (Hensel, 2005). SPI2 is important for the proliferation of the bacteria postinvasion and is required for intracellular survival within murine macrophages (Ellermeier and Slauch, 2007; Kelly et al., 2009; Santos et al., 2003). It enables the bacteria not only to survive in phagocytic cells but also to replicate within a vacuole, termed the *Salmonella*-containing vacuole (SCV) (Hensel, 2005). In general, SPI2 provides the bacteria with protection within the SCV by preventing the colocalization of the phagocyte oxidase and the inducible nitric oxide synthase with the SCV (Chakravortty et al., 2002; Hensel, 2005; Vazquez-Torres et al., 2000).

SPI3 is a 17-kb region inserted at the *selC* tRNA gene for selenocysteine, with a highly variable G+C content (on average 47.5%) (Blanc-Potard et al., 1999; Hensel, 2005; Kelly et al., 2009). This pathogenicity island is found in all serovars (Fierer and Guiney, 2001) but has extensive variation in structure and location (Amavisit et al., 2003; Blanc-Potard et al., 1999; Kelly et al., 2009). SPI3 is flanked by remnants of insertion sequences (Kelly et al., 2009). It contains the genes *mgtCB*, which encodes magnesium transport ATPase accessory proteins. This high-affinity magnesium transport system is important for growth in magnesium-limiting conditions (Hensel, 2005; Kelly et al., 2009). Not surprisingly, these genes have been found to play a role in the survival of the bacteria in macrophages and in systemic disease in a murine model (Blanc-Potard and Groisman, 1997; Hensel, 2005; Marcus et al., 2000; van Asten and van Dijk, 2005). It also contains other genes, including *misL* (an extracellular matrix adhesion protein), and *marT* (a putative transcriptional regulator) (Kelly et al., 2009).

SPI4 is a 25-kb pathogenicity island with a G+C content of 44.8% and 18 potential ORFs (Hensel, 2005; Kelly et al., 2009). It is located adjacent to a tRNA-like sequence and is conserved between *S. enterica* serovars, with some variation in its organization (Amavisit et al., 2003; Hensel, 2005; Wong et al., 1998). It encodes a single-stranded DNA binding protein and contains superoxide response regulatory genes (*soxSR)* (Marcus et al., 2000). It is thought to also encode a T1SS, mediating toxin secretion, and may be important for survival within macrophages (Schmidt and Hensel, 2004; van Asten and van Dijk, 2005). SPI4 also contains *ims98*, which is required for bacterial survival within macrophages (Wong et al., 1998).

SPI5 is a 7.6-kb region with a G+C content of 43.6%, found between the gene for serine tRNA (*serT)* and the gene for a copper-inducible two-component regulatory system (*copSR*) (Hensel, 2005; Kelly et al., 2009). This pathogenicity island is thought to be involved in enteropathogenesis, as mutations in SPI5 can lead to a reduction in enteritis (Marcus et al., 2000). Also encoded in SPI5 are SopB and PipB, two effectors secreted by the SPI1- and SPI2-encoded T3SS, respectively (Schmidt and Hensel, 2004). The *sopB* gene, which triggers fluid secretion leading to diarrhea, is found in both *S. bongori* and *S. enterica* (Knodler et al., 2002). In contrast, *pipAB* are found in *S. enterica* subspecies I, III, IV, and VII but not in *S. bongori* (Knodler et al., 2002). Little is known about the roles of *pipA* and *pipB* (Haraga et al., 2008); however, *pipB2*, a homologue of *pipB*, is associated with the formation of *Salmonella*-induced filaments within macrophages (Knodler and Steele-Mortimer, 2005).

SPI6 is a 59- and 47-kb region in serovars Typhi and Typhimurium, respectively, and is located beside the *aspV* tRNA gene (Hensel, 2005; Kelly et al., 2009). In serovar Typhimurium, SPI6 is sometimes called *Salmonella* centisome 7 genomic island (Hensel, 2005). SPI6 encodes the *Salmonella* atypical fimbriae, which may be involved in virulence; it also contains *pagN*, a gene putatively involved in invasion, and other less well-characterized genes (Kelly et al., 2009). Interestingly, homologues of SPI6 have been identified in *P. aeruginosa* and *Y. pestis* (Hensel, 2005).

SPI7 is a 133-kb region found only in serovars Typhi, Dublin, and Paratyphi C; it is located next to the *pheU* tRNA gene (Hansen-Wester and Hensel, 2002; Kelly et al., 2009). It contains *viaB*, a gene involved in the biosynthesis of VI capsular exopolysaccharide, *sopE* (a phage-encoded SPI1 secreted effector), and a putative type IV pilus gene cluster (Hensel, 2005; Kelly et al., 2009). It is important to the ability of serovar Dublin to invade epithelial cells (Bueno et al., 2004). It is hypothesized that SPI7 originated as a conjugative plasmid or transposon and is composed of individual horizontally acquired elements (Hensel, 2005).

Less is known about SPI8, SPI9, and SPI10. SPI8 is a 6.8-kb region found adjacent to *pheV* tRNA gene in serovar Typhi (Kelly et al., 2009; Parkhill et al., 2001). It encodes a bacteriocin and contains an integrase gene, indicating the possibility of mobility (Hensel, 2005; Kelly et al., 2009). SPI9 is a 16-kb pathogenicity island located next to a lysogenic bacteriophage in serovar Typhi (Kelly et al., 2009; Parkhill et al., 2001). It encodes a T1SS and a RTX (repeats in toxin)-like protein (Hensel, 2005; Kelly et al., 2009). SPI9 is also present in serovar Typhimurium, although in this serovar the RTX-like gene is actually a pseudo-gene (Hensel, 2005). SPI10 is 32.8 kb long and located at the *leuX* tRNA gene (Hensel, 2005; Kelly et al., 2009). This pathogenicity island is found in serovars Typhi and Enteritidis (Hensel, 2005). It contains the serovar Enteritidis fimbriae (*sef*) operon and a cryptic bacteriophage (Hensel, 2005; Kelly et al., 2009).

Salmonella Phages

Temperate bacteriophages are an important source of DNA transfer leading to evolution because of their ability to carry foreign DNA (Figueroa-Bossi et al., 2001). *Salmonella* harbors multiple phages, which contribute to fitness and virulence. *Salmonella* phages are categorized into five groups: P27-like, P2-like, lambdoid, P22-like, and T7-like (Kropinski et al., 2007). Three phages do not fit into these groups: KS7, FelixO1, and ε15 (Kropinski et al., 2007).

Gifsy 1 and Gifsy 2 are two lambdoid prophages discovered in *S. enterica* serovar Typhimurium (Figueroa-Bossi and Bossi, 1999; Slominski et al., 2007). Gifsy 2 contributes directly to systemic virulence (Figueroa-Bossi and Bossi, 1999). This prophage has genes including *sodC, gtgE*, and *gtgB/sseI* (Slominski et al., 2007). Some of the proteins encoded by these genes are secreted by the SPI1- and SPI2-encoded T3SS (Coombes et al., 2005; Ho et al., 2002). SodC is a periplasmic Cu/Zn superoxide dismutase important for bacterial survival within macrophages, as it mediates the production of hydrogen peroxide from superoxide radicals (De Groote, 1997; Figueroa-Bossi et al., 2001). *Salmonella* strains lacking the *sodC* gene had reduced survival within macrophages and reduced virulence in mice (De Groote et al., 1997). Variations of SodC, SodCI, and SodCII, have been identified in serovar Typhimurium strain 14028 (Krishnakumar et al., 2007). Despite some sequence similarities, unlike SodCII, SodCI is protease resistant, dimeric, and tethered to the periplasm, characteristics that may contribute to the virulence and action of SodCI within the phagosome (Krishnakumar et al., 2007). GtgE was also found to contribute to the virulence of *Salmonella* (Ho et al., 2002).

Gifsy 1 also was found to be associated with virulence genes, although this was not apparent in the presence of Gifsy 2, indicating that Gifsy

1 may have genes with functional equivalents in Gifsy 2 (Figueroa-Bossi et al., 2001). Gifsy 1 encodes virulence factors including GipA and GogB (Coombes et al., 2005; Slominski et al., 2007; Stanley et al., 2000). GogB has some sequence similarities to virulence-associated proteins from other bacteria (Coombes et al., 2005). GogB is secreted by both the SPI1- and SPI2-encoded T3SS; however, it is a SPI2-mediated process. The protein was found to localize to the cytoplasm (Coombes et al., 2005). GipA is specifically induced in the small intestine of host animals, and the loss of this protein is associated with a reduction in the growth and survival of *Salmonella* in Peyer's patches, indicating that bacteria may be able to sense and respond to the environment within the Peyer's patches (Stanley et al., 2000).

Other phages have also been identified in the *Salmonella* genome; they include Fels1, Fels2, Gifsy 3, and SopEΦ (Chan et al., 2003; Figueroa-Bossi et al., 2001). Fels1 was found in serovar Typhimurium strain LT2 and encodes NanH and SodCIII (Chan et al., 2003; Figueroa-Bossi et al., 2001). Fels2 is present in serovars Typhimurium, Typhi, Enteritidis, and Sendai (Chan et al., 2003). The Fels2 prophage is 33.7 kb long with a G+C content of 52.5% (Kropinski et al., 2007). Gifsy 3 was found in serovar Typhimurium strain ATCC14028 and carries gene *pagJ*, which is activated by PhoP/PhoQ (Figueroa-Bossi et al., 2001). It also contains the SPI1- and SPI2-secreted effector SspH1 (Figueroa-Bossi et al., 2001). SopEΦ is found in serovar Typhimurium and is around 34.7 kb long with a G+C content of 51.3% (Kropinski et al., 2007). It encodes SopE, a protein secreted by the SPI1-encoded T3SS, which contributes to bacterial invasiveness (Kropinski et al., 2007).

Salmonella Plasmids

Salmonella serovars also contain plasmids. In particular, a virulence plasmid is found in serovars Abortusovis, Abortusequi, Choleraesuis, Dublin, Enteritidis, Gallinarum, Sendai, and Typhimurium (Chu and Chiu, 2006; Porwollik and McClelland, 2003). Frequently located on the virulence plasmid of *Salmonella* is the *spv* operon (Chu and Chiu, 2006; Porwollik and McClelland, 2003). The *spv* operon is found on the chromosome in *S. enterica* subspecies I, II, IIIa, IV, and VII (Chu and Chiu, 2006). This operon contains five genes important for the intracellular replication of the bacteria (Matsui et al., 2001). SpvB is an ADP-ribosylating protein that modifies actin within the host cell (Browne et al., 2008; Hochmann et al., 2006; Matsui et al., 2001). In serovar Typhimurium, the *spv* operon is a major contributor to the virulence attributes conferred by the plasmid (Matsui et al., 2001). The 90-kb virulence plasmid of Typhimurium also contains the *pef* operon, which encodes fimbrial subunits (Porwollik and McClelland, 2003). In addition, the serovar Typhimurium virulence plasmid is self-transferable and associated with drug resistance (Chu and Chiu, 2006). Serovar Enteritidis has a 60-kb virulence plasmid, while serovar Typhi has two plasmids, pHCM1 and pHCM2 (Porwollik and McClelland, 2003). pHCM1 is 218 kb long and contains regions of MDR, and pHCM2 is 107 kb long and has high sequence similarity to the virulence plasmid of *Y. pestis* (Porwollik and McClelland, 2003). Serovar Choleraesuis contains antibiotic resistance genes encoding resistance to ampicillin and sulfonamides, which may be transmissible under some circumstances (Chu and Chiu, 2006). The virulence plasmids of *Salmonella* strains contribute to the adaptation of the organism, and in some cases allow the transfer of genes.

The *Salmonella* genome therefore has some components that are conserved among strains, but it also has many regions that are unique to a group of serovars, a single serovar, or even a single isolate. Progress is continuing on elucidating the presence and function of regions within the *Salmonella* genome.

SALMONELLA SEROVARS AND HOST ADAPTATION

Three species are assigned to the *Salmonella* genus: *S. bongori*, *S. enterica*, and, more recently, *S. subterranea* (Shelobolina et al., 2004; Su and Chiu, 2007). All *S. enterica* serovars are closely related, and comparative genomics studies revealed 96 to 99.5% identity between them (Edwards et al., 2002). Within *S. enterica*, a number of evolutionary subspecies emerged and are classified based on their DNA similarities and phenotypic characteristics, as *S. enterica* subspecies I, II, IIIa, IIIb, IV, and VI (Popoff and Le Minor, 1997). Subspecies VII has also been identified by multilocus enzyme electrophoresis data (Boyd et al., 1996). However, this subspecies did not present a unique biochemical profile.

S. enterica subspecies I is able to colonize a broad range of hosts, from reptiles to warm-blooded animals, whereas serovars belonging to *S. bongori* and *S. enterica* subspecies II to VII are isolated mostly from reptiles (Popoff and Le Minor, 1992). Figure 1 illustrates the wide range of host specificity among *Salmonella* serovars, as well as the different pathologies caused. The adaptation of *S. enterica* subspecies I to warm-blooded animals might have been driven at least in part by the acquisition of a genomic island containing the *shdA* gene (Kingsley et al., 2000), which is absent in other members of the *Salmonella* genus. A mutation of this gene leads to a decrease of the duration of shedding of serovar Typhimurium in mice, affecting the transmission and consequently the ability of *Salmonella* to circulate within a population. Therefore, it appears that expansion of host range is linked to the LGT of genes involved in host-pathogen interactions.

As mentioned above, other genes carried on phages, plasmids, and pathogenicity islands have scattered distribution among *S. enterica* subspecies I serovars, indicative of repeated acquisition and loss (Baumler et al., 1997; Tsolis et al., 1999). It is unknown if the presence or absence of these mobile elements is linked to host adaptation and can play a role in modulating the host range of different *Salmonella* serovars (Kingsley amd Baumler, 2002a).

To date, more than 1,500 serovars have been classified as *S. enterica* subspecies I (Popoff et al., 2004). Although they are very closely related to each other as judged by DNA reassociation rates (Crosa et al., 1973; Le Minor, 1988), these serovars differ greatly in their host range, the degree of host adaptation, and the nature of the disease they cause (Fig. 1).

It is important to note that when a particular serovar is described as host adapted, it means that it is able to cause disease and circulate within a population without having to be reintroduced (Kingsley and Baumler, 2002a). The host specificity of *Salmonella* appears to be very complex and to depend on multiple factors during the multiple stages of infection. Currently, analysis of the correlation between the genetic differences and the phenotypic diversity among *Salmonella* serovars is a major topic of interest.

Broad-Host-Range or Ubiquitous *Salmonella*

S. enterica serovar Typhimurium is a representative of the broad host specificity of *S. enterica* subspecies I. This serovar is frequently associated with disease in a number of hosts, including humans, cattle, pigs, horses, poultry, rodents, and sheep (Edwards and Brunner, 1943; Sojka and Wray, 1975; Wray et al., 1981). As a broad-host-range pathogen, serovar Typhimurium has been used as a tool to determine which genetic regions are important for host specificity. For example, the effect of signature-tagged mutations on virulence in mice and cattle has been compared. Mutations on horizontally acquired virulence factors, including the *spv* operon, SPI1, and SPI2, affect colonization on both animal models (Tsolis et al., 1999). However, some DNA regions were required for the colonization of one but not the other animal. A mutation on a putative fimbrial synthesis gene called *bcfC*, located in a genomic island, was defective only for cattle colonization, whereas a mutation on a pathogenicity islet encoding SlrP, a SPI2 T3SS effector protein, was defective only for colonizing mice. Other T3SS effectors might also be important for host adaptation. *sspH1*, *sspH2*, and *sipA* mutants are defective in colonizing cattle but not mice (Miao et al., 1999; Tsolis et al., 2000).

A serovar Typhimurium strain LT2 microarray slide (PCR based) was used to analyze the presence of homologues in 22 other *Salmonella* members, including strains from all the subspecies and *S. bongori* (Porwollik et al., 2002). With this approach, 56 *Salmonella*-specific genes were identified in all *Salmonella* strains tested,

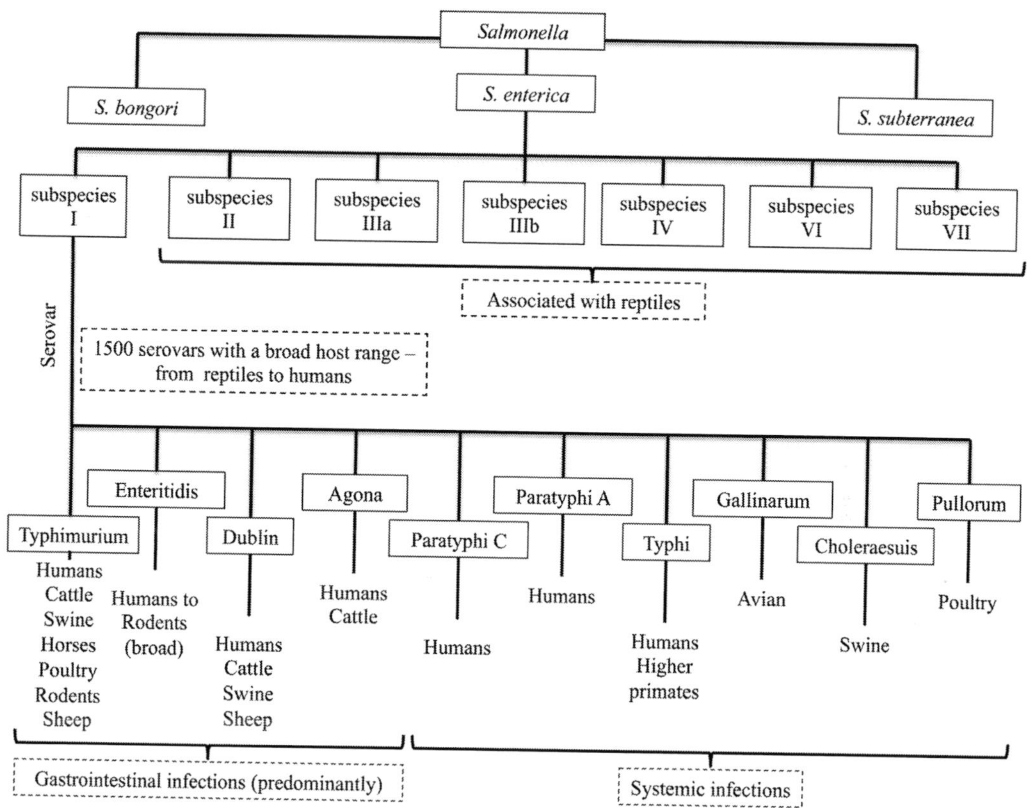

FIGURE 1 Schematic distribution of *Salmonella enterica* serovars, their hosts, and their pathological manifestations.

including 7 SPI1 genes, the DNA helicase gene *(res)*, the tetrathionate reductase complex gene *(ttr)*, the anaerobe sulfide reductase complex gene *(asr)*, and genes involved in hydrogen sulfide production *(phsB* and *phsC)*. The majority of these genes are of unknown function, indicating that genes belonging to this group are largely unstudied. Comparison of different strains showed that the majority of the absent genes are of plasmid or phage origin, illustrating the role of these mobile elements on the development of different *Salmonella* species, subspecies, and serovars. Other than that, some metabolic clusters, like the *eut* cluster, which encodes enzymes involved in the utilization of ethanolamine as a carbon and energy source under aerobic conditions, are missing in *S. bongori* and subspecies VII. A considerable number of sugar transport and metabolism genes are not uniformly distributed among *Salmonella* strains, indicating redundancy of different sugar compounds for adaptation to the environment. Fimbrial operons, which are particularly important for host-pathogen interactions, are also not evenly present in the strains tested. For example, of the 12 fimbrial clusters present in serovar Typhimurium, 7 are present in serovars Paratyphi A and Typhi, and only 2 are present in subspecies IV and VII. Altogether, these data suggest a high level of gene gain and loss among all strains.

In another study, a serovar Typhimurium strain LT2 microarray was used to examine the genome of nine different serovar Dublin isolates, three serovar Agona isolates, and six different serovar Typhimurium strains isolated from four animal species (Reen et al., 2005). Both serovar Dublin and serovar Agona are cattle-adapted serovars that can also infect humans. Genomic regions that are present in one of the serovars but absent in others were detected, and significant intraserovar diversity was limited to one serovar Dublin isolate. In comparison with serovar Typhimurium, serovar Dublin lacked a number of genes, including genes involved in sugar metabolism and transport and in fimbrial and phage biogenesis, as well as putative secreted proteins. Serovar Agona lacked genes that encoded flavoproteins, cytoplasmic and membrane proteins, phage proteins, LysR transcriptional regulators, galactonate metabolic proteins, and a phosphotransferase transport system. Gene clusters containing PhoP-PhoQ-activated genes, phage genes, and integrase genes were absent in all serovar Agona isolates. Moreover, the pSLT plasmid, Gifsy-2, and SPI-3 region were absent in all serovar Agona isolates, as well as one serovar Dublin isolate. Genes that were absent in both serovars in comparison with serovar Typhimurium include a phosphotransferase sugar transport system, glycosyltransferases, Gifsy-1, and several regions involved in sugar metabolism. When different serovar Typhimurium isolates were compared, one region was shown to be absent in all isolates. This region contained genes required for anaerobic assimilation of allantoin. A common theme for the variable regions between serovars was the diversity in sugar metabolism, highlighting the redundancy of these systems. In accordance with this finding, most host-adapted serovars, such as serovars Dublin and Agona, require certain amino acids and vitamins to grow whereas ubiquitous serovars, such as serovar Typhimurium, are able to grow in relatively simple media (Koser, 1968; Virgilio and Cordano, 1981). Furthermore, the scattered distribution of fimbrial operons suggests that deletion and horizontal transfers occurred multiple times within *S. enterica*.

Like serovar Typhimurium, serovar Enteritidis is able to cause gastroenteritis in a broad range of hosts and to cause typhoid-like disease in mice. However, significant phenotype differences exist between these serovars (Thomson et al., 2008). An alignment of the genome of strains from both serovars revealed similar regions except for an inversion at the terminus region in serovar Typhimurium (McClelland et al., 2001). Only 6.4% of the genome of serovar Enteritidis is absent in the genome of serovar Typhimurium, and only 9.6% of the serovar Typhimurium genome is unique, indicating a high similarity of the strains. The majority of coding regions unique to serovar Enteritidis encode prophage-related functions (Thomson et al., 2008). Virulence factors and genes involved in host interactions are among the ones common in both strains, including multiple SPIs and fimbrial operons.

Host-Restricted and Host-Specific *Salmonella*

Host-specific serovars are associated almost exclusively with typhoid fever in a single species; they include serovars Typhi and Gallinarum. Host-restricted serovars are usually associated with one host but are occasionally isolated from other hosts (Uzzau et al., 2000). Serovar Dublin is an example of a host-restricted serovar from *S. enterica* subspecies I, predominantly infecting cattle and occasionally causing disease in sheep and pigs (Sojka and Field, 1970; Sojka and Wray, 1975).

Serovar Typhi is the prototype of a host-restricted *Salmonella* serovar, causing typhoid fever, a systemic and potentially life-threatening disease, in humans and higher primates (Edsall et al., 1960). Serovar Typhi strains show little DNA sequencing diversity, indicating that its adaptation as a human pathogen arose about 50,000 years ago (Kidgell et al., 2002). Compared with serovar Typhimurium, serovar Typhi contains more than 600 unique genes (13% of its genes), some of which are likely involved in its ability to cause typhoid fever (Parkhill et al., 2001). Among those unique genes, serovar Typhi contains large genome insertions including SPI7 when compared to the sequenced strains (Liu et al., 2006). It was found that the acquisition of SPI7 disrupted the physical balance of the bacterial genome between the replication origin and terminus (Liu et al., 2006). Subsequent genome rearrangements occurred to reestablish the balance of the genome structure and consequently provide opportunities for genome stabilization during evolution.

Based on microarray data, serovar Paratyphi A is closely related to serovar Typhi (Chan et al., 2003; Porwollik et al., 2002, 2004). It is also a human-restricted pathogen and is the second most prevalent cause of typhoid fever (Selander et al., 1990; Sood et al., 1999). By sequence analysis, differences and similarities between the genomes of these two serovars were revealed (McClelland et al., 2004). Serovar Paratyphi A has a smaller genome than serovar Typhi, primarily because it has fewer mobile elements, including SPI7 and Vi exopolysaccharide synthesis genes. The order of orthologues is conserved in comparison with serovar Typhimurium except for a recombination between the *rrnH* and *rrnG* operons (Liu and Sanderson, 1995c; McClelland et al., 2004). Interestingly, the number of pseudogenes in serovar Paratyphi A genome is similar to that in serovar Typhi, which is larger than that in serovar Typhimurium. Pseudogenes are usually caused by single-base mutations that lead to a frame shift or a stop codon in genes that are otherwise >98% similar to their orthologs in serovar Typhimurium (McClelland et al., 2004). It seems that genome degradation through pseudogene formation is linked to evolution to a specific niche. This formation sheds genes that are no longer needed in their new niche.

Serovar Paratyphi C also causes typhoid fever and is a human-adapted pathogen (Liu et al., 2007). For a long time, it was unknown if serovars Paratyphi C and Typhi had emerged from a common ancestor or acquired similar pathogenic traits independently. By comparing the sequences of serovar Paratyphi C with those of previously sequenced *Salmonella* strains, it was found that serovars Paratyphi C and Typhi have different ancestors (Liu et al., 2009). Surprisingly, serovar Paratyphi C seems to have a common ancestor with serovar Choleraesuis, a swine pathogen that causes paratyphoid fever. The presence of differential nucleotide substitutions and different sets of pseudogenes between serovars Paratyphi C and Choleraesuis suggests the enormous selective pressure in the adaptation of serovar Paratyphi C to humans. The existence of different typhoid agents causing similar disease manifestations offers a great opportunity to ask questions about the origin of the pathogens, the essential genomic make-up for successful systemic infection, and the molecular mechanisms of host adaptation.

A high-resolution genomic map of serovar Paratyphi C revealed the presence of large insertions, including SPI7, and deletions compared with serovar Typhimurium strain LT2. These deletions might be particularly interesting as they may be involved in host restriction. When a large number of genome maps for serovar Paratyphi C strains were constructed with I-CeuI cleavage, diverse genome structures were revealed between different isolates. Partial or complete cleavage using I-CeuI, an intron-encoded endonuclease with cleavage sites in *rrl* genes that encode 23S rRNA (Liu and Sanderson, 1993), can be used to lay out the overall genome structure of the bacteria. All *Salmonella* serovars contain seven *rrl* genes, generating seven I-CeuI fragments (Liu et al., 1999). The order of the fragments indicates potential genetic rearrangements, including translocations. Intriguingly, a deletion on a region between *rrlA* and *rrlB* was revealed in two serovar Paratyphi C strains. Deletion of this region has never been found in other *Salmonella* strains, indicating considerable genome stability of this region in *Salmonella* that was disrupted in these strains (Liu et al., 2007). Serovars Paratyphi C and Typhi appear to have a similar degree of genome plasticity, suggesting that these serovars went through similar evolutionary steps to become a typhoid agent, acquiring typhoid-related genes, which probably led to disruption of the physical balance of the genome, and, consequently, went through similar genomic rearrangements to restore the balance. However, in this case, their similar plasticity does not indicate a common ancestor.

S. enterica serovar Pullorum is a fowl-adapted bacterial pathogen that causes dysentery (pullorum disease), a systemic infection that affects mostly young birds (Wigley et al., 2001). A genome map of this serovar was constructed to study bacterial evolution and speciation (Liu et al., 2002). Although the genome sequence was found to be very similar to those of other *Salmonella* serovars, the genetic arrangement was significantly different, with three major inversions and one translocation found between strains. By comparison with the serovar Typhimurium genome, seven putative insertions and eight deletions were discovered. It appears that a major insertion disrupted the genome balance and that rebalancing by independent recombination events in individual strains resulted in different structures.

S. enterica serovar Gallinarum is also a host-restricted, avian-adapted pathogen closely related to *S. enterica* serovar Pullorum in its antigenicity, but it causes typhoid fever in chickens, making comparison between these serovars a good model to study bacterial evolution (Wu et al., 2005). Phylogenetic analysis indicated that serovar Gallinarum evolved from a motile ancestor related to serovar Enteritidis, which, as mentioned above, has a broad range of hosts (Li et al., 1993). This lack of motility in serovar Gallinarum has been linked to mutations in *fliC*, a flagellin subunit gene (Kilger and Grimont, 1993). Nonmotility may enhance the ability to invade cells in the gut, avoiding the TLR5-induced proinflammatory response from the host, giving rise to a systemic pathogen (Iqbal et al., 2005; Kaiser, 2000). During its evolution to a poultry-adapted pathogen, serovar Gallinarum may have undergone genetic alterations that caused the loss of adaptation to other hosts, such as rodents. A physical map of serovar Gallinarum was constructed and compared to other sequences. Insertions and deletions were found in the prophage regions of serovar Typhimurium, and some rare rearrangements were also revealed (Wu et al., 2005). Whole-genome sequencing of such serovars also shed light on regions that are dispensable during poultry infections as well as the ones that are necessary for a broad host range of infection. Sequence comparison with serovar Enteritidis showed that serovar Gallinarum is closely related to serovar Enteritidis and may be a direct descendent of this serovar (Thomson et al., 2008), even though they have different host spectra and cause distinct diseases. Compared to serovar Enteritidis, serovar Gallinarum carries significantly fewer tRNA genes, and is colinear except for a single inversion and a translocation of a region between two different rRNA operons. Serovar Gallinarum contains a significantly larger number of pseudogenes, similar to other host-restricted pathogens, serovars Typhi and Paratyphi A (Thomson et al., 2008). The large number of pseudogenes, which carry frame shifts or premature stop codons or that are remnants of genes present in other bacteria, argues for reductive evolution in these host-adapted serovars. Among the pathways lost by serovar Gallinarum are the ones involved in the use of different substrates as a source of carbon and energy, like the ones required for the breakdown of 1,2-propanediol, an important source of energy in serovar Typhimurium (Klumpp and Fuchs, 2007). Mutations in genes of this pathway are also present in the serovar Typhi genome. Moreover, numerous mutations in the glycogen biosynthetic pathway are present in serovar Gallinarum, which may in part explain the poor survival of the bacteria outside the host (Thomson et al., 2008). Unlike serovar Enteritidis, serovar Gallinarum is unable to produce cellulose, probably due to a mutation in *bcsG* (Thomson et al., 2008). Cellulose is a key component of biofilm formation, which is thought to improve gut colonization in serovar Enteritidis (Solano et al., 2002), as well as its resistance to mechanical and chemical stress. The lack of cellulose production in serovar Gallinarum may play a role in its poor colonization of the gut and may also explain its poor survival outside the host. Another similarity of serovars Gallinarum and Typhi is the number of mutations found on fimbrial operons. Both have a higher rate of mutations on these regions than on the rest of the genome (Thomson et al., 2008), suggesting parallel paths towards host adaptation. Mutations in T3SS effector genes, including *sopA*, which is required for serovar Typhimurium enteritis development, are also present in the serovar Gallinarum genome (Zhang et al., 2006). Mutations in *sopA* and other effector-encoding genes may help explain the different pathological effects of these serovars.

The order of I-CeuI fragments in host-specialized *Salmonella* serovars such as serovars Typhi, Paratyphi, Gallinarum, and Pullorum is different from the order in serovars that grow in multiple hosts. These fragments were rearranged mainly due to homologous recombination between the *rrn* operons, resulting in translocations and inversions that would perhaps explain some of the host specificity. Other genetic events, such as inversions on the termination of replication region and lateral transfer of nonhomologous DNA, were also observed in the host-restricted strains (Sanderson and Liu, 1998).

Genome comparisons of host-restricted and adapted *Salmonella* serovars indicate that the loss of gene function may be a common evolutionary mechanism that enables host adaptation and restricted pathology (Thomson et al., 2008). Gene loss can limit the ability of a pathogen to survive outside its host, as well as to target the pathogen to invade particular tissues and evade immune responses. Further characterization of these genetic events can clarify the molecular basis of specific host-pathogen interactions and the genomic evolution that occurs to create a new pathogen.

CONCLUSIONS

The genome of different *S. enterica* serovars bears the potential for ongoing rearrangements, deletions, and insertions that can lead to genomic variability within the species. The large number of *Salmonella enterica* serovars and the wide range of hosts that they can infect may present an opportunity to further study and understand the interrelations of host adaptation and genome variability.

Understanding the phenomenon of genome plasticity in this species is important to characterize the relationship between genetic variation and host adaptation, as well as the ability to cause a relatively minor gastrointestinal disease or a potentially life-threatening systemic fever.

Advances in the detection of genome plasticity will allow new questions to be asked and duly answered, and will give us insights into the mechanisms involved in the changes in genome content, as well as the consequences for the evolutionary bacterial adaptation.

ACKNOWLEDGMENTS

We thank L. C. M. Antunes and other members of the Finlay lab for critical reading of the manuscript.

B.B.F. is an HHMI International Research Scholar and the UBC Peter Wall Distinguished Professor. Work in his lab was supported by operating grants to B.B.F. from the Canadian Institute for Health Research (CIHR), Canadian Crohn's and Colitis Foundation, and Genome Canada. R.B.F. is funded by a CIHR Industrial Fellowship. M.M.B. is funded by NSERCCGS.

REFERENCES

Ahmed, A. M., A. I. Hussein, and T. Shimamoto. 2007. *Proteus mirabilis* clinical isolate harbouring a new variant of *Salmonella* genomic island 1 containing the multiple antibiotic resistance region. *J. Antimicrob. Chemother.* **59:**184–190.

Amavisit, P., D. Lightfoot, G. F. Browning, and P. F. Markham. 2003. Variation between pathogenic serovars within *Salmonella* pathogenicity islands. *J. Bacteriol.* **185:**3624–3635.

Baumler, A. J., A. J. Gilde, R. M. Tsolis, A. W. van der Velden, B. M. Ahmer, and F. Heffron. 1997. Contribution of horizontal gene transfer and deletion events to development of distinctive patterns of fimbrial operons during evolution of *Salmonella* serotypes. *J. Bacteriol.* **179:**317–322.

Bishop, A. L., S. Baker, S. Jenks, M. Fookes, P. O. Gaora, D. Pickard, M. Anjum, J. Farrar, T. T. Hien, A. Ivens, and G. Dougan. 2005. Analysis of the hypervariable region of the *Salmonella enterica* genome associated with tRNA(*leuX*). *J. Bacteriol.* **187:**2469–2482.

Blanc-Potard, A. B., and E. A. Groisman. 1997. The *Salmonella selC* locus contains a pathogenicity island mediating intramacrophage survival. *EMBO J.* **16:**5376–5385.

Blanc-Potard, A. B., F. Solomon, J. Kayser, and E. A. Groisman. 1999. The SPI-3 pathogenicity island of *Salmonella enterica*. *J. Bacteriol.* **181:**998–1004.

Boyd, D., G. A. Peters, A. Cloeckaert, K. S. Boumedine, E. Chaslus-Dancla, H. Imberechts, and M. R. Mulvey. 2001. Complete nucleotide sequence of a 43-kilobase genomic island associated with the multidrug resistance region of *Salmonella enterica* serovar Typhimurium DT104 and its identification in phage type DT120 and serovar Agona. *J. Bacteriol.* **183:**5725–5732.

Boyd, E. F., F. S. Wang, T. S. Whittam, and R. K. Selander. 1996. Molecular genetic relationships of the salmonellae. *Appl. Environ. Microbiol.* **62:**804–808.

Browne, S. H., P. Hasegawa, S. Okamoto, J. Fierer, and D. G. Guiney. 2008. Identification of *Salmonella* SPI-2 secretion system components required for SpvB-mediated cytotoxicity in macrophages and virulence in mice. *FEMS Immunol. Med. Microbiol.* **52:**194–201.

Brussow, H., C. Canchaya, and W. D. Hardt. 2004. Phages and the evolution of bacterial pathogens: from genomic rearrangements to lysogenic conversion. *Microbiol. Mol. Biol. Rev.* **68:**560–602.

Bueno, S. M., C. A. Santiviago, A. A. Murillo, J. A. Fuentes, A. N. Trombert, P. I. Rodas, P. Youderian, and G. C. Mora. 2004. Precise excision of the large pathogenicity island, SPI7, in *Salmonella enterica* serovar Typhi. *J. Bacteriol.* **186:**3202–3213.

Chakravortty, D., I. Hansen-Wester, and M. Hensel. 2002. *Salmonella* pathogenicity island 2 mediates protection of intracellular *Salmonella* from reactive nitrogen intermediates. *J. Exp. Med.* **195:** 1155–1166.

Chan, K., S. Baker, C. C. Kim, C. S. Detweiler, G. Dougan, and S. Falkow. 2003. Genomic comparison of *Salmonella enterica* serovars and *Salmonella bongori* by use of an *S. enterica* serovar Typhimurium DNA microarray. *J. Bacteriol.* **185:**553–563.

Chen, F., C. Poppe, G. R. Liu, Y. G. Li, Y. H. Peng, K. E. Sanderson, R. N. Johnston, and S. L. Liu. 2009. A genome map of *Salmonella enterica* serovar Agona: numerous insertions and deletions reflecting the evolutionary history of a human pathogen. *FEMS Microbiol. Lett.* **293:**188–195.

Chu, C., and C. H. Chiu. 2006. Evolution of the virulence plasmids of non-typhoid *Salmonella* and its association with antimicrobial resistance. *Microbes Infect.* **8:**1931–1936.

Coombes, B. K., M. E. Wickham, N. F. Brown, S. Lemire, L. Bossi, W. W. Hsiao, F. S. Brinkman, and B. B. Finlay. 2005. Genetic and molecular analysis of GogB, a phage-encoded type III-secreted substrate in *Salmonella enterica* serovar typhimurium with autonomous expression from its associated phage. *J. Mol. Biol.* **348:**817–830.

Craig, N. L. 1985. Site-specific inversion: enhancers, recombination proteins, and mechanism. *Cell* **41:**649–650.

Crosa, J. H., D. J. Brenner, W. H. Ewing, and S. Falkow. 1973. Molecular relationships among the Salmonelleae. *J. Bacteriol.* **115:**307–315.

De Groote, M. A., U. A. Ochsner, M. U. Shiloh, C. Nathan, J. M. McCord, M. C. Dinauer, S. J. Libby, A. Vazquez-Torres, Y. Xu, and F. C. Fang. 1997. Periplasmic superoxide dismutase protects *Salmonella* from products of phagocyte NADPH-oxidase and nitric oxide synthase. *Proc. Natl. Acad. Sci. USA* **94:**13997–14001.

Dobrindt, U., and J. Hacker. 2001. Whole genome plasticity in pathogenic bacteria. *Curr. Opin. Microbiol.* **4:**550–557.

Dobrindt, U., B. Hochhut, U. Hentschel, and J. Hacker. 2004. Genomic islands in pathogenic and environmental microorganisms. *Nat. Rev. Microbiol.* **2:**414–424.

Doublet, B., D. Boyd, M. R. Mulvey, and A. Cloeckaert. 2005. The *Salmonella* genomic island 1 is an integrative mobilizable element. *Mol. Microbiol.* **55:**1911–1924.

Doublet, B., G. R. Golding, M. R. Mulvey, and A. Cloeckaert. 2008. Secondary chromosomal attachment site and tandem integration of the mobilizable *Salmonella* genomic island 1. *PLoS One* **3:**e2060.

Doublet, B., R. Lailler, D. Meunier, A. Brisabois, D. Boyd, M. R. Mulvey, E. Chaslus-Dancla, and A. Cloeckaert. 2003. Variant *Salmonella* genomic island 1 antibiotic resistance gene cluster in *Salmonella enterica* serovar Albany. *Emerg. Infect. Dis.* **9:**585–591.

Doublet, B., K. Praud, F. X. Weill, and A. Cloeckaert. 2009. Association of IS26-composite transposons and complex In4-type integrons generates novel multidrug resistance loci in *Salmonella* genomic island 1. *J. Antimicrob. Chemother.* **63:** 282–289.

Edsall, G., S. Gaines, M. Landy, W. D. Tigertt, H. Sprintz, R.-J. Trapani, A. D. Mandel, and A. S. Benenson. 1960. Studies on infection and immunity in experimental typhoid fever: typhoid fever in chimpanzees orally infected with *Salmonella typhosa*. *J. Exp. Med.* **112:**143–166.

Edwards, P. R., and D. W. Brunner. 1943. The occurence and distribution of *Salmonella* types in the United States. *J. Infect. Dis.* **72:**58–67.

Edwards, R. A., G. J. Olsen, and S. R. Maloy. 2002. Comparative genomics of closely related salmonellae. *Trends Microbiol.* **10:**94–99.

Ellermeier, J. R., and J. M. Slauch. 2007. Adaptation to the host environment: regulation of the SPI1 type III secretion system in *Salmonella enterica* serovar Typhimurium. *Curr. Opin. Microbiol.* **10:**24–29.

Ewing, W. H. 1986. *Edwards and Ewing's Identification of the Enterobacteriaceae.* Elsevier Science Publishing Co., Inc., New York, NY.

Fierer, J., and D. G. Guiney. 2001. Diverse virulence traits underlying different clinical outcomes of *Salmonella* infection. *J. Clin. Investig.* **107:**775–780.

Figueroa-Bossi, N., and L. Bossi. 1999. Inducible prophages contribute to *Salmonella* virulence in mice. *Mol. Microbiol.* **33:**167–176.

Figueroa-Bossi, N., S. Uzzau, D. Maloriol, and L. Bossi. 2001. Variable assortment of prophages provides a transferable repertoire of pathogenic determinants in *Salmonella*. *Mol. Microbiol.* **39:**260–271.

Galan, J. E. 2001. *Salmonella* interactions with host cells: type III secretion at work. *Annu. Rev. Cell. Dev. Biol.* **17:**53–86.

Garrity, G. M. 2001. *Bergey's Manual of Systematic Bacteriology*, 2nd ed. Springer-Verlag, New York, NY.

Ginocchio, C. C., K. Rahn, R. C. Clarke, and J. E. Galan. 1997. Naturally occurring deletions in the centisome 63 pathogenicity island of environmental isolates of *Salmonella* spp. *Infect. Immun.* **65:**1267–1272.

Hansen-Wester, I., and M. Hensel. 2002. Genome-based identification of chromosomal regions specific for *Salmonella* spp. *Infect. Immun.* **70:**2351–2360.

Haraga, A., M. B. Ohlson, and S. I. Miller. 2008. Salmonellae interplay with host cells. *Nat. Rev. Microbiol.* **6:**53–66.

Hensel, M. 2005. Pathogenicity islands and virulence of *Salmonella enterica*, p. 146–167. *In* P. Mastroeni and D. Maskell (ed.), *Salmonella Infections: Clinical, Immunological and Molecular Aspects.* Cambridge University Press, Cambridge, United Kingdom.

Hensel, M., T. Nikolaus, and C. Egelseer. 1999. Molecular and functional analysis indicates a mosaic structure of *Salmonella* pathogenicity island 2. *Mol. Microbiol.* **31:**489–498.

Hensel, M., J. E. Shea, A. J. Baumler, C. Gleeson, F. Blattner, and D. W. Holden. 1997. Analysis of the boundaries of *Salmonella* pathogenicity island 2 and the corresponding chromosomal region of *Escherichia coli* K-12. *J. Bacteriol.* **179:**1105–1111.

Ho, T. D., N. Figueroa-Bossi, M. Wang, S. Uzzau, L. Bossi, and J. M. Slauch. 2002. Identification of GtgE, a novel virulence factor encoded on the Gifsy-2 bacteriophage of *Salmonella enterica* serovar Typhimurium. *J. Bacteriol.* **184:**5234–5239.

Hochmann, H., S. Pust, G. von Figura, K. Aktories, and H. Barth. 2006. *Salmonella enterica* SpvB ADP-ribosylates actin at position arginine-177: characterization of the catalytic domain within the SpvB protein and a comparison to binary clostridial actin-ADP-ribosylating toxins. *Biochemistry* **45:**1271–1277.

Holt, K. E., N. R. Thomson, J. Wain, G. C. Langridge, R. Hasan, Z. A. Bhutta, M. A. Quail, H. Norbertczak, D. Walker, M. Simmonds, B. White, N. Bason, K. Mungall, G. Dougan, and J. Parkhill. 2009. Pseudogene accumulation in the evolutionary histories of *Salmonella enterica* serovars Paratyphi A and Typhi. *BMC Genomics* **10:**36.

Hu, Q., B. Coburn, W. Deng, Y. Li, X. Shi, Q. Lan, B. Wang, B. K. Coombes, and B. B. Finlay. 2008. *Salmonella enterica* serovar Senftenberg human clinical isolates lacking SPI-1. *J. Clin. Microbiol.* **46:**1330–1336.

Iqbal, M., V. J. Philbin, G. S. Withanage, P. Wigley, R. K. Beal, M. J. Goodchild, P. Barrow, I. McConnell, D. J. Maskell, J. Young, N. Bumstead, Y. Boyd, and A. L. Smith. 2005. Identification and functional characterization of chicken toll-like receptor 5 reveals a fundamental role in the biology of infection with *Salmonella enterica* serovar Typhimurium. *Infect. Immun.* **73:**2344–2350.

Kado, C. I. 2009. Horizontal gene transfer: sustaining pathogenicity and optimizing host-pathogen interactions. *Mol. Plant Pathol.* **10:**143–150.

Kaiser, D. 2000. Bacterial motility: how do pili pull? *Curr. Biol.* **10:**R777–R780.

Kelly, B. G., A. Vespermann, and D. J. Bolton. 2009. Gene transfer events and their occurrence in selected environments. *Food Chem. Toxicol.* **47:**978–983.

Kidgell, C., U. Reichard, J. Wain, B. Linz, M. Torpdahl, G. Dougan, and M. Achtman. 2002. *Salmonella typhi*, the causative agent of typhoid fever, is approximately 50,000 years old. *Infect. Genet. Evol.* **2:**39–45.

Kilger, G., and P. A. Grimont. 1993. Differentiation of *Salmonella* phase 1 flagellar antigen types by restriction of the amplified *fliC* gene. *J. Clin. Microbiol.* **31:**1108–1110.

Kingsley, R. A., and A. J. Baumler. 2002a. Pathogenicity islands and host adaptation of *Salmonella* serovars. *Curr. Top. Microbiol. Immunol.* **264:**67–87.

Kingsley, R. A., and A. J. Baumler. 2002b. Pathogenicity islands and host adaptation of *Salmonella* serovars, p. 67–87. *In* J. Hacker and J. B. Kaper (ed.), *Pathogenicity Islands and the Evolution of Pathogenic Microbes*, vol. 1. Springer-Verlag, New York, NY.

Kingsley, R. A., K. van Amsterdam, N. Kramer, and A. J. Baumler. 2000. The *shdA* gene is restricted to serotypes of *Salmonella enterica* subspecies I and contributes to efficient and prolonged fecal shedding. *Infect. Immun.* **68:**2720–2727.

Klumpp, J., and T. M. Fuchs. 2007. Identification of novel genes in genomic islands that contribute to *Salmonella typhimurium* replication in macrophages. *Microbiology* **153:**1207–1220.

Knodler, L. A., J. Celli, W. D. Hardt, B. A. Vallance, C. Yip, and B. B. Finlay. 2002. *Salmonella* effectors within a single pathogenicity island are differentially expressed and translocated by separate type III secretion systems. *Mol. Microbiol.* **43:**1089–1103.

Knodler, L. A., and O. Steele-Mortimer. 2005. The *Salmonella* effector PipB2 affects late endosome/lysosome distribution to mediate Sif extension. *Mol. Biol. Cell* **16:**4108–4123.

Koser, S. A. 1968. *Vitamin Requirements of Bacteria and Yeast.* Charles C Thomas, Springfield, IL.

Krishnakumar, R., B. Kim, E. A. Mollo, J. A. Imlay, and J. M. Slauch. 2007. Structural properties of periplasmic SodCI that correlate with virulence in *Salmonella enterica* serovar Typhimurium. *J. Bacteriol.* **189:**4343–4352.

Kropinski, A. M., A. Sulakvelidze, P. Konczy, and C. Poppe. 2007. *Salmonella* phages and prophages—genomics and practical aspects. *Methods Mol. Biol.* **394:**133–175.

Le Minor, L. 1988. Typing of *Salmonella* species. *Eur. J. Clin. Microbiol. Infect. Dis.* **7:**214–218.

Le Minor, L., and J. Bockemuhl. 1988. 1987 supplement (no. 31) to the schema of Kauffmann-White. *Ann. Inst. Pasteur Microbiol.* **139:**331–335. (In French.)

Le Minor, L., and J. Bockemuhl. 1984. Supplement No. XXVII (1983) to the Kauffmann-White scheme. *Ann. Microbiol.* (Paris) **135B:**45–51. (In French.)

Li, J., N. H. Smith, K. Nelson, P. B. Crichton, D. C. Old, T. S. Whittam, and R. K. Selander. 1993. Evolutionary origin and radiation of the avian-adapted non-motile salmonellae. *J. Med. Microbiol.* **38:**129–139.

Liu, G. R., W. Q. Liu, R. N. Johnston, K. E. Sanderson, S. X. Li, and S. L. Liu. 2006. Genome plasticity and ori-ter rebalancing in *Salmonella typhi*. *Mol. Biol. Evol.* **23:**365–371.

Liu, G. R., A. Rahn, W. Q. Liu, K. E. Sanderson, R. N. Johnston, and S. L. Liu. 2002. The evolving genome of *Salmonella enterica* serovar Pullorum. *J. Bacteriol.* **184:**2626–2633.

Liu, S. L., A. Hessel, and K. E. Sanderson. 1993. Genomic mapping with I-Ceu I, an intron-encoded endonuclease specific for genes for ribosomal RNA, in *Salmonella* spp., *Escherichia coli*, and other bacteria. *Proc. Natl. Acad. Sci. USA* **90:**6874–6878.

Liu, S. L., and K. E. Sanderson. 1995a. Genomic cleavage map of *Salmonella typhi* Ty2. *J. Bacteriol.* **177:**5099–5107.

Liu, S. L., and K. E. Sanderson. 1996. Highly plastic chromosomal organization in *Salmonella typhi*. *Proc. Natl. Acad. Sci. USA* **93:**10303–10308.

Liu, S. L., and K. E. Sanderson. 1995b. Rearrangements in the genome of the bacterium *Salmonella typhi*. *Proc. Natl. Acad. Sci. USA* **92:**1018–1022.

Liu, S. L., and K. E. Sanderson. 1995c. The chromosome of *Salmonella paratyphi* A is inverted by recombination between *rrnH* and *rrnG*. *J. Bacteriol.* **177:**6585–6592.

Liu, S. L., A. B. Schryvers, K. E. Sanderson, and R. N. Johnston. 1999. Bacterial phylogenetic clusters revealed by genome structure. *J. Bacteriol.* **181:**6747–6755.

Liu, W. Q., Y. Feng, Y. Wang, Q. H. Zou, F. Chen, J. T. Guo, Y. H. Peng, Y. Jin, Y. G. Li, S. N. Hu, R. N. Johnston, G. R. Liu, and S. L. Liu. 2009. *Salmonella paratyphi* C: genetic divergence from *Salmonella choleraesuis* and pathogenic convergence with *Salmonella typhi*. *PLoS ONE* **4:**e4510.

Liu, W. Q., G. R. Liu, J. Q. Li, G. M. Xu, D. Qi, X. Y. He, J. Deng, F. M. Zhang, R. N. Johnston, and S. L. Liu. 2007. Diverse genome structures of *Salmonella paratyphi* C. *BMC Genomics* **8:**290.

Marcus, S. L., J. H. Brumell, C. G. Pfeifer, and B. B. Finlay. 2000. *Salmonella* pathogenicity islands: big virulence in small packages. *Microbes Infect.* **2:**145–156.

Matsui, H., C. M. Bacot, W. A. Garlington, T. J. Doyle, S. Roberts, and P. A. Gulig. 2001. Virulence plasmid-borne *spvB* and *spvC* genes can replace the 90-kilobase plasmid in conferring virulence to *Salmonella enterica* serovar Typhimurium in subcutaneously inoculated mice. *J. Bacteriol.* **183:**4652–4658.

McClelland, M., K. E. Sanderson, S. W. Clifton, P. Latreille, S. Porwollik, A. Sabo, R. Meyer, T. Bieri, P. Ozersky, M. McLellan, C. R. Harkins, C. Wang, C. Nguyen, A. Berghoff, G. Elliott, S. Kohlberg, C. Strong, F. Du, J. Carter, C. Kremizki, D. Layman, S. Leonard, H. Sun, L. Fulton, W. Nash, T. Miner, P. Minx, K. Delehaunty, C. Fronick, V. Magrini, M. Nhan, W. Warren, L. Florea, J. Spieth, and R. K. Wilson. 2004. Comparison of genome degradation in Paratyphi A and Typhi, human-restricted serovars of *Salmonella enterica* that cause typhoid. *Nat. Genet.* **36:**1268–1274.

McClelland, M., K. E. Sanderson, J. Spieth, S. W. Clifton, P. Latreille, L. Courtney, S. Porwollik, J. Ali, M. Dante, F. Du, S. Hou, D. Layman, S. Leonard, C. Nguyen, K. Scott, A. Holmes, N. Grewal, E. Mulvaney, E. Ryan, H. Sun, L. Florea, W. Miller, T. Stoneking, M. Nhan, R. Waterston, and R. K. Wilson. 2001. Complete genome sequence of *Salmonella enterica* serovar Typhimurium LT2. *Nature* **413:**852–856.

Miao, E. A., C. A. Scherer, R. M. Tsolis, R. A. Kingsley, L. G. Adams, A. J. Baumler, and S. I. Miller. 1999. *Salmonella typhimurium* leucine-rich repeat proteins are targeted to the SPI1 and SPI2 type III secretion systems. *Mol. Microbiol.* **34:**850–864.

Mulvey, M. R., D. A. Boyd, A. B. Olson, B. Doublet, and A. Cloeckaert. 2006. The genetics of *Salmonella* genomic island 1. *Microbes Infect.* **8:**1915–1922.

Nanassy, O. Z., and K. T. Hughes. 1998. *In vivo* identification of intermediate stages of the DNA inversion reaction catalyzed by the *Salmonella* Hin recombinase. *Genetics* **149:**1649–1663.

Ochman, H., and E. A. Groisman. 1996. Distribution of pathogenicity islands in *Salmonella* spp. *Infect. Immun.* **64:**5410–5412.

Ochman, H., J. G. Lawrence, and E. A. Groisman. 2000. Lateral gene transfer and the nature of bacterial innovation. *Nature* **405:**299–304.

Pallen, M. J., and B. W. Wren. 2007. Bacterial pathogenomics. *Nature* **449:**835–842.

**Parkhill, J., G. Dougan, K. D. James, N. R. Thomson, D. Pickard, J. Wain, C. Churcher, K. L. Mungall, S. D. Bentley, M. T. Holden, M. Sebaihia, S. Baker, D. Basham, K. Brooks, T. Chillingworth, P. Connerton, A. Cronin, P. Davis, R. M. Davies, L. Dowd, N. White,

J. Farrar, T. Feltwell, N. Hamlin, A. Haque, T. T. Hien, S. Holroyd, K. Jagels, A. Krogh, T. S. Larsen, S. Leather, S. Moule, P. O'Gaora, C. Parry, M. Quail, K. Rutherford, M. Simmonds, J. Skelton, K. Stevens, S. Whitehead, and B. G. Barrell. 2001. Complete genome sequence of a multiple drug resistant *Salmonella enterica* serovar Typhi CT18. *Nature* **413:**848–852.

Popoff, M. Y., J. Bockemuhl, and L. L. Gheesling. 2004. Supplement 2002 (no. 46) to the Kauffmann-White scheme. *Res. Microbiol.* **155:**568–570.

Popoff, M. Y., and L. Le Minor. 1992. *Antigenic Formulas of the* Salmonella *Serovars.* Institut Pasteur, Paris, France.

Popoff, M. Y., and L. Le Minor. 1997. *Antigenic Formulas of the* Salmonella *Serovars.* WHO Collaborating Center for Reference and Research on Salmonella, Institut Pasteur, Paris, France.

Porwollik, S., E. F. Boyd, C. Choy, P. Cheng, L. Florea, E. Proctor, and M. McClelland. 2004. Characterization of *Salmonella enterica* subspecies I genovars by use of microarrays. *J. Bacteriol.* **186:**5883–5898.

Porwollik, S., and M. McClelland. 2003. Lateral gene transfer in *Salmonella. Microbes Infect.* **5:**977–989.

Porwollik, S., R. M. Wong, and M. McClelland. 2002. Evolutionary genomics of *Salmonella*: gene acquisitions revealed by microarray analysis. *Proc. Natl. Acad. Sci. USA* **99:**8956–8961.

Reen, F. J., E. F. Boyd, S. Porwollik, B. P. Murphy, D. Gilroy, S. Fanning, and M. McClelland. 2005. Genomic comparisons of *Salmonella enterica* serovar Dublin, Agona, and Typhimurium strains recently isolated from milk filters and bovine samples from Ireland, using a *Salmonella* microarray. *Appl. Environ. Microbiol.* **71:**1616–1625.

Sanderson, K. E., and S. L. Liu. 1998. Chromosomal rearrangements in enteric bacteria. *Electrophoresis* **19:**569–572.

Santos, R. L., R. M. Tsolis, A. J. Baumler, and L. G. Adams. 2003. Pathogenesis of *Salmonella*-induced enteritis. *Braz. J. Med. Biol. Res.* **36:**3–12.

Schmidt, H., and M. Hensel. 2004. Pathogenicity islands in bacterial pathogenesis. *Clin. Microbiol. Rev.* **17:**14–56.

Selander, R. K., P. Beltran, N. H. Smith, R. Helmuth, F. A. Rubin, D. J. Kopecko, K. Ferris, B. D. Tall, A. Cravioto, and J. M. Musser. 1990. Evolutionary genetic relationships of clones of *Salmonella* serovars that cause human typhoid and other enteric fevers. *Infect. Immun.* **58:**2262–2275.

Shelobolina, E. S., S. A. Sullivan, K. R. O'Neill, K. P. Nevin, and D. R. Lovley. 2004. Isolation, characterization, and U(VI)-reducing potential of a facultatively anaerobic, acid-resistant bacterium from low-pH, nitrate- and U(VI)-contaminated subsurface sediment and description of *Salmonella subterranea* sp. nov. *Appl. Environ. Microbiol.* **70:**2959–2965.

Slominski, B., J. Calkiewicz, P. Golec, G. Wegrzyn, and B. Wrobel. 2007. Plasmids derived from Gifsy-1/Gifsy-2, lambdoid prophages contributing to the virulence of *Salmonella enterica* serovar Typhimurium: implications for the evolution of replication initiation proteins of lambdoid phages and enterobacteria. *Microbiology* **153:**1884–1896.

Sojka, W. J., and H. I. Field. 1970. Salmonellosis in England and Wales 1958–1967. *Vet. Bull.* **40:**515–531

Sojka, W. J., and C. Wray. 1975. Incidence of *Salmonella* infection in animals in England and Wales 1968–1973. *Vet. Rec.* **96:**280–284.

Solano, C., B. Garcia, J. Valle, C. Berasain, J. M. Ghigo, C. Gamazo, and I. Lasa. 2002. Genetic analysis of *Salmonella enteritidis* biofilm formation: critical role of cellulose. *Mol. Microbiol.* **43:**793–808.

Sood, S., A. Kapil, N. Dash, B. K. Das, V. Goel, and P. Seth. 1999. Paratyphoid fever in India: an emerging problem. *Emerg. Infect. Dis.* **5:**483–484.

Stanley, T. L., C. D. Ellermeier, and J. M. Slauch. 2000. Tissue-specific gene expression identifies a gene in the lysogenic phage Gifsy-1 that affects *Salmonella enterica* serovar Typhimurium survival in Peyer's patches. *J. Bacteriol.* **182:**4406–4413.

Su, L. H., and C. H. Chiu. 2007. *Salmonella*: clinical importance and evolution of nomenclature. *Chang Gung Med. J.* **30:**210–219.

Thomson, N. R., D. J. Clayton, D. Windhorst, G. Vernikos, S. Davidson, C. Churcher, M. A. Quail, M. Stevens, M. A. Jones, M. Watson, A. Barron, A. Layton, D. Pickard, R. A. Kingsley, A. Bignell, L. Clark, B. Harris, D. Ormond, Z. Abdellah, K. Brooks, I. Cherevach, T. Chillingworth, J. Woodward, H. Norberczak, A. Lord, C. Arrowsmith, K. Jagels, S. Moule, K. Mungall, M. Sanders, S. Whitehead, J. A. Chabalgoity, D. Maskell, T. Humphrey, M. Roberts, P. A. Barrow, G. Dougan, and J. Parkhill. 2008. Comparative genome analysis of *Salmonella* Enteritidis PT4 and *Salmonella* Gallinarum 287/91 provides insights into evolutionary and host adaptation pathways. *Genome Res.* **18:**1624–1637.

Tsolis, R. M., L. G. Adams, M. J. Hantman, C. A. Scherer, T. Kimbrough, R. A. Kingsley, T. A. Ficht, S. I. Miller, and A. J. Baumler. 2000. SspA is required for lethal *Salmonella enterica* serovar Typhimurium infections in calves but is not essential for diarrhea. *Infect. Immun.* **68:**3158–3163.

Tsolis, R. M., S. M. Townsend, E. A. Miao, S. I. Miller, T. A. Ficht, L. G. Adams, and A. J. Baumler. 1999. Identification of a putative *Salmonella enterica* serotype typhimurium host range factor with homology to IpaH and YopM by signature-tagged mutagenesis. *Infect. Immun.* **67:** 6385–6393.

Uzzau, S., D. J. Brown, T. Wallis, S. Rubino, G. Leori, S. Bernard, J. Casadesus, D. J. Platt, and J. E. Olsen. 2000. Host adapted serotypes of *Salmonella enterica*. *Epidemiol. Infect.* **125:**229–255.

van Asten, A. J., and J. E. van Dijk. 2005. Distribution of "classic" virulence factors among *Salmonella* spp. *FEMS Immunol. Med. Microbiol.* **44:**251–259.

Varma, J. K., K. D. Greene, J. Ovitt, T. J. Barrett, F. Medalla, and F. J. Angulo. 2005. Hospitalization and antimicrobial resistance in *Salmonella* outbreaks, 1984–2002. *Emerg. Infect. Dis.* **11:**943–946.

Vazquez-Torres, A., J. Jones-Carson, P. Mastroeni, H. Ischiropoulos, and F. C. Fang. 2000. Antimicrobial actions of the NADPH phagocyte oxidase and inducible nitric oxide synthase in experimental salmonellosis. I. Effects on microbial killing by activated peritoneal macrophages *in vitro*. *J. Exp. Med.* **192:**227–236.

Virgilio, R., and A. M. Cordano. 1981. Naturally occurring prototrophic strains of *Salmonella typhi*. *Can. J. Microbiol.* **27:**1272–1275.

Wigley, P., A. Berchieri, Jr., K. L. Page, A. L. Smith, and P. A. Barrow. 2001. *Salmonella enterica* serovar Pullorum persists in splenic macrophages and in the reproductive tract during persistent, disease-free carriage in chickens. *Infect. Immun.* **69:**7873–7879.

Wong, K. K., M. McClelland, L. C. Stillwell, E. C. Sisk, S. J. Thurston, and J. D. Saffer. 1998. Identification and sequence analysis of a 27-kilobase chromosomal fragment containing a *Salmonella* pathogenicity island located at 92 minutes on the chromosome map of *Salmonella enterica* serovar Typhimurium LT2. *Infect. Immun.* **66:**3365–3371.

Wray, C., W. J. Sojka, and J. C. Bell. 1981. *Salmonella* infection in horses in England and Wales, 1973 to 1979. *Vet. Rec.* **109:**398–401.

Wu, K. Y., G. R. Liu, W. Q. Liu, A. Q. Wang, S. Zhan, K. E. Sanderson, R. N. Johnston, and S. L. Liu. 2005. The genome of *Salmonella enterica* serovar Gallinarum: distinct insertions/deletions and rare rearrangements. *J. Bacteriol.* **187:**4720–4727.

Yang, B., J. Zheng, E. W. Brown, S. Zhao, and J. Meng. 2009. Characterisation of antimicrobial resistance-associated integrons and mismatch repair gene mutations in *Salmonella* serotypes. *Int. J. Antimicrob. Agents* **33:**120–124.

Zhang, Y., W. M. Higashide, B. A. McCormick, J. Chen, and D. Zhou. 2006. The inflammation-associated *Salmonella* SopA is a HECT-like E3 ubiquitin ligase. *Mol. Microbiol.* **62:**786–793.

Zhou, D., W. D. Hardt, and J. E. Galan. 1999. *Salmonella typhimurium* encodes a putative iron transport system within the centisome 63 pathogenicity island. *Infect. Immun.* **67:**1974–1981.

MECHANISMS OF GENOME PLASTICITY IN *Neisseria meningitidis*: FIGHTING CHANGE WITH CHANGE

Roland Schwarz, Biju Joseph, Matthias Frosch, and Christoph Schoen

7

Neisseria meningitidis (the meningococcus) is a commensal bacterium exclusively of the human nasopharynx that is carried by ~10% of the human population (Claus et al., 2005; Yazdankhah et al., 2004). Although more than 99% of all meningococcal infections result in asymptomatic nasopharyngeal carriage (Stephens, 1999), for reasons that are still largely unknown the meningococcus sometimes invades the pharyngeal mucosal epithelium, causing septicemia or acute bacterial meningitis (Rosenstein et al., 2001; Stephens et al., 2007). Apart from epidemic outbreaks, approximately 500,000 cases of meningococcal disease are estimated to occur every year on a worldwide basis, placing a heavy burden on public health systems, especially in developing countries (Roberts, 2008). Based on the chemical composition and the immunological characteristics of their capsular polysaccharide, they can be divided into 12 serogroups (Frosch and Vogel, 2006). The most important serogroups associated with disease in humans are A, B, C, W-135, and Y. While serogroups B and C account for sporadic cases and numerous localized outbreaks worldwide and cause the majority of cases in industrialized countries, serogroup A meningococci are the main pathogens involved in major epidemics in China, the Middle East, South America, and especially sub-Saharan Africa (Connolly and Noah, 1999).

However, despite their well-recognized pathogenic potential, evolutionarily disease is nonetheless a dead end for these bacteria: virulence shortens the window of time during which transmission to new hosts can occur, and the subpopulations of bacteria actually responsible for disease, like those in the blood or cerebrospinal fluid, are rarely transmitted to new hosts (Lipsitch and Moxon, 1997). Therefore, *N. meningitidis* is more appropriately considered an accidental than an obligate human pathogen (Moxon and Jansen, 2005), and models of within-host infection dynamics of *N. meningitidis* have shown that genome variability is key for the understanding of the lifestyle and also the pathogenesis of meningococcal diseases (Meyers et al., 2003).

Accordingly, in this chapter we first give a short overview over the genetic variability at the population level and some peculiarities of meningococcal genome organization as revealed by

Roland Schwarz, Cancer Research UK, Cambridge Research Institute, Li Ka Shing Centre, Cambridge CB2 0RE, United Kingdom. *Biju Joseph, Matthias Frosch, and Christoph Schoen*, Institute for Hygiene and Microbiology, University of Würzburg, 97080 Würzburg, Germany.

Genome Plasticity and Infectious Diseases,
Edited by J. Hacker, U. Dobrindt, and R. Kurth,

genome sequencing projects. We then focus on genetic mechanisms and genomic features that are paramount for the generation of genomic flexibility, and finally we give a brief account of the genetic basis of virulence in *N. meningitidis* as far as it is known today. For more information about the infection biology of *N. meningitidis*, the reader is referred to a recent monograph edited by Frosch and Maiden (2006).

GENETIC VARIABILITY AT THE POPULATION LEVEL

The application of population genetic approaches, first multilocus enzyme electrophoresis (MLEE) (Caugant et al., 1986a) and later multilocus sequence typing (MLST) (Maiden et al., 1998) identified a high level of genetic diversity in *N. meningitidis*. In MLST, the sequence of seven housekeeping genes which are assumed to evolve neutrally and which are thus not under any selective pressure are determined and assigned an arbitrary allele number. The allele numbers of all seven loci examined are then combined into an allelic profile known as the sequence type (ST). At the time of writing, the publicly available and curated PubMLST database (www.neisseria.org) (Jolley et al., 2004) contains almost 7,500 different profiles. Nevertheless, this bewildering species diversity in meningococci is highly structured (Maiden and Caugant, 2006). In particular, while a relatively small proportion of STs are repeatedly identified in many data sets, most of them are found only a few times (Claus et al., 2005; Jolley et al., 2000; Yazdankhah et al., 2004). In addition, a number of the most frequent STs have a wide geographical and temporal distribution, often being observed on multiple continents and over decades (Buckee et al., 2008; Zhu et al., 2001). Finally, these persistent STs appear to form the center of clusters of related genotypes referred to as clonal complexes (CCs) (Feil et al., 2004), and currently about 40 CCs account for about 60% of the meningococcal isolates represented in the PubMLST database.

In principle, the two genetic mechanisms that can generate such a high genetic diversity are de novo mutation and (homologous) recombination. In the clonal model of bacterial populations (Milkman, 1973), bacteria are viewed as haploid, asexual organisms in which genetic diversity is generated principally by mutation and there is no sexual stage in the life cycle. In the absence of sexual exchange and recombination, any novel genetic polymorphism is limited to the descendants of the cell in which the mutation first occurred. During clonal population growth and spread, many variants are lost either due to selective events called periodic selection (Selander and Levin, 1980) or due to stochastic events called bottlenecking (Achtman, 1994). Under this scenario, the population becomes structured into a "clonal population" comprising a number of distinct lineages, each of which is characterized by a unique pattern of polymorphisms (Milkman, 1973; Orskov and Orskov, 1983). In clonal populations, a nonrandom association of genetic polymorphisms termed linkage disequilibrium can be observed. Serogroup A meningococcal strains have a clonal population structure consistent with the epidemic life history of these bacteria (Morelli et al., 1997; Suker et al., 1994; Zhu et al., 2001). In contrast to serogroup A, serogroup B and C meningococci do not have a clonal population structure (Feil et al., 1999; Holmes et al., 1999; Jolley et al., 2000), although "clusters" and clonal complexes of genetically related bacteria do exist as indicated by MLST. Accordingly, the presence of allelic variants that showed patterns of polymorphisms most parsimoniously explained by recombination of two genes with distinct evolutionary histories, first in genes encoding antibiotic resistance (Spratt et al., 1992) and surface antigens (Feavers et al., 1992) and later also in housekeeping genes (Zhou and Spratt, 1992), provided clear evidence for recombination in *N. meningitidis*. In fact, the ratio of the probability that an individual nucleotide site will change by recombination or mutation was shown to be about 10:1 in *N. meningitidis*, a value that ranges among the highest so far found for any eubacterial species (Feil et al., 2001; Jolley et al., 2005). This process has been called "localized sex" in contrast to the exchange of larger parts of the genome or even entire chromosomes in fully sexual, diploid species (Smith et al., 1991); in *N. meningitidis* it involves the exchange of relatively small parts (ca. 1 kb) of the chromosome (Jolley et al., 2005). In consequence, *N. meningitidis* strains are neither fully clonal nor nonclonal but rather show evidence for both clonal spread (Caugant et al., 1986b; Morelli et al., 1997; Zhu et al., 2001) and genetic exchange (Feil et al., 2001; Holmes et al., 1999; Jolley et al., 2000, 2005).

To accommodate clonal complex structure in recombining populations, a number of different population genetic explanations have been put forward over recent years (Buckee et al., 2008; Fraser et al., 2005; Gupta et al., 1996; Smith et al., 1993), and there is an intense and still ongoing debate, particularly between "neutralists" and "selectionists," on the genetic and epidemiological factors that shape the meningococcal population and hence the evolution of new strains. Whatever these mechanisms might turn out to be, population genetics has clearly demonstrated that genetic diversity and the forces which structure it are central to the biology and pathogenicity of meningococci.

GENOME PLASTICITY IN THE PREGENOMIC ERA

Although MLST enables very detailed sequence analyses down to the nucleotide level and thus allows for the inference of population genetic parameters such as recombination rates, population substructure, etc., sequencing about 500 bp from seven loci covers less than 0.2% of the meningococcal chromosome. Therefore, to experimentally assess variability at the whole-genome level, complementary approaches targeting the entire chromosomes, such as pulsed-field gel electrophoresis and representational difference analysis, were used in the pregenomics era for the analysis of meningococcal genome variability. For example, in the 1990s investigations of the chromosome structure by pulsed-field gel electrophoresis (Dempsey et al., 1995; Gaher et al., 1996) suggested a remarkable structural variability of the meningococcal chromosome (Bautsch, 1998). In particular, even closely related strains such as those belonging to the electrophoretic type 5 (ET-5) or the ET-15 clonal complex showed detectable differences in their macrorestriction patterns (Froholm et al., 2000; Strathdee et al., 1993). Perhaps even more surprising was the finding that within the course of a single infection the invading strain can undergo large genomic rearrangements such as the deletion of a 40-kb fragment (Vogel et al., 1998). These structural analyses were later complemented by genome-wide gene content comparisons by representational difference analysis (Klee et al., 2000) of strains belonging to, among others, the ET-37 complex (Claus et al., 2001) and MLEE lineage III (Bart et al., 2000), which also indicated a marked variability in gene content within these subgroups. However, the advent of whole-genome sequences of a serogroup A (Parkhill et al., 2000) and a serogroup B (Tettelin et al., 2000) strain in the year 2000 opened new avenues for basic as well as applied research and allowed for whole-genome comparisons down to the nucleotide level.

THE SEQUENCED GENOMES OF *N. MENINGITIDIS*: AN OVERVIEW

Although considered a haploid organism, *N. gonorrhoeae* was recently shown to be homopolyploid with about 4 to 10 genome equivalents per diplococcal cell (Tobiason and Seifert, 2006); this might also to be true for *N. meningitides*, a close relative of *N. gonorrhoeae*. In all six meningococcal strains sequenced as of the time of writing, each (haploid) genome consists of a single circular chromosome (Table 1), and some meningococcal strains were found to harbor cryptic plasmids encoding resistance to β-lactam antibiotics (Backman et al., 2000), sulfonamides (Facinelli and Varaldo, 1987), and tetracycline (Knapp et al., 1987), which has raised some medical concern regarding effective antibiotic treatment of neisserial meningitis (Dillon and Yeung, 1989). However, in contrast to many other gram-negative pathogens, no virulence plasmids have been detected so far in *N. meningitidis* (van Passel et al., 2006).

On average, the genomes are about 2.19 Mb in size and have an average G+C content of approximately 51.6%. Accordingly, all other

TABLE 1 Meningococcal genomes sequenced by September 2009

Strain	Z2491	MC58	FAM18	053442	α14	α153	α275
Molecular typing							
Serogroup	A	B	C	C	cnl	29E	W-135
Sequence type	4	74	11	4821	53	60	22
Clonal complex	ST-4	ST-32	ST-11	ST-4821	ST-53	ST-60	ST-22
Frequency in carriers[a] (%)	0.0	5.0	1.0	0.0	7.2	3.9	4.6
Frequency in cases[b] (%)	0.0	23.8	18.1	0.0	0.0	2.7	0.4
General information							
No. of contigs (>2 kb)	1	1	1	1	1	87	133
Contigs/genome size (bp)	2,184,406	2,272,351	2,194,961	2,153,416	2,145,295	2,134,469	2,266,686
G+C content (%)	51.8	51.5	51.6	51.7	52.0	51.6	51.2
GenBank accession no.	AL157959	AE002098	AM421808	CP000381	AM889136	AM889137	AM889138
Functional RNAs							
No. of tRNAs	58	59	59	59	58	≥50	≥50
No. of rRNA operons	4	4	4	4	4	≥ 1	≥ 1
Selected repeats							
DUS[c]	1,892	1,910	1,888	1,858	1,851	1,831	1,862
dRS3[d]	672	689	656	725	646	710	692
dRS3 (Nf1 subtype)[e]	303	316	283	327	269	322	307
CE[f]	270	261	nd[i]	nd	269	nd	nd
Coding sequences							
Putative no.	1,993	2,063	1,975	2,020	1,987	≥1,814	≥1,947
Avg CDS length (bp)	902	871	918	853	884	899	870
COGs (%)	68	68	nd	nd	78	86	85
Coding area (%)	78.9	79.1	80.2	80.1	81.8	≥76.4	≥74.7
Putative no. of pseudogenes	84	92	58	61	70	≥59	≥75
CDS with low G+C[g]	77	76	70	122	112	≥51	≥52
New genes[h]	57	46	9	12	58	≥2	≥42

[a]Frequency of clonal complexes in 822 carrier isolates as given by Claus et al. (2005).

[b]Frequency of clonal complexes in 525 disease isolates during the period from 2000 to 2002 in Germany, characterized by the European Meningococcal MLST Centre, Oxford, United Kingdom.

[c]The core DNA uptake sequence is GCCGTCTGAA.

[d]The dRS3 repeat sequence pattern is ATTCCC(N_8)GGGAAT.

[e]The dRS3 repeat type targeted by the prophage Nf1 has the sequence ATTCCCRCCTRCGCGGRAAK (Kawai et al., 2005).

[f]Correia repeat elements.

[g]Defined as genes with a G+C content less than the average G+C content of the CDSs in the respective genome minus two standard deviations.

[h]Defined as genes that have no hits in other genomes in TBLASTN comparisons.

[i]ND, not determined.

benchmark data such as G+C content and number of rRNA operons, tRNA genes, and protein-coding sequences (CDSs) are also quite similar for all strains irrespective of their origin (carriage or disease isolate), clonal complex, or serogroup. With respect to the number of CDSs, all sequenced strains contain about 1,971 with an average CDS length of 885 bp, resulting in a coding density of 78.7%. Compared to the genomes of other respiratory tract pathogens, they are, for example, about half the size of the *Bordetella pertussis* genome (4.1 Mb) (Parkhill et al., 2003) and comparable to the *Haemophilus influenzae* (1.9 Mb) (Harrison et al., 2005) and the *Streptococcus pneumoniae* (2.2 Mb) (Tettelin et al., 2001) genomes.

As can be seen in Fig. 1, although the meningococcal genomes are largely colinear, there are a number of translocations and inversions such as the large symmetrical inversions around the origin of replication (Bentley et al., 2007). In strain MC58, almost half of the chromosome is inverted with respect to the other genomes, and it has been proposed that this inversion is associated with the integration of a circular plasmid containing IHT-B as well as IHT-C together with the Nf2-B3 prophage into the ancestor of strain MC58 (Kawai et al., 2006). In addition to these inversions, a thorough computational analysis by Kawai et al. (2006) revealed a number of other genome rearrangements and stressed the role of mobile genetic elements in the formation of complex chromosome polymorphism in *N. meningitidis*. For example, an IS-mediated replicative inversion of a 29-kb region comprising a putative composite transposon (Tn in Fig. 1) was found to be translocated in the genome of strain MC58 relative to the other two genomes.

GENERATION OF GENOME VARIABILITY IN *N. MENINGITIDIS*

As mentioned above, high genomic diversity can in principle be generated by two mechanisms: (i) de novo mutation by processes such as substitution, insertion, and deletion and (ii) recombination, the combination of genes with distinct evolutionary histories. Recombination may be intergenomic, where the recombining genes are acquired from a distinct organisms via horizontal gene transfer (HGT), or intragenomic, where multiple copies of a gene or sequence unit exist in the genome. Accordingly, in this section, the role of high genome-wide mutation and mutators is discussed as well as the contribution of localized hypermutations known as phase variation. Next, the high repeat content of the meningococcal genomes and the central role of homologous as well as site-specific recombination in genome structure as well as gene content variability in *N. meningitides* are discussed.

Mutation, DNA Repair, and Generation of Genome Variability

Exogenous and endogenous stress induces DNA damage in the meningococcal genome that must be repaired, and DNA repair mechanisms are therefore likely to have a key role in meningococcal genome dynamics. So far, *Escherichia coli* has served as the prime model organism for DNA repair systems in other microorganisms such as *N. meningitidis*. According to the *E. coli* paradigm, excision repair pathways include base excision repair (BER), mismatch repair (MMR), and nucleotide excision repair (NER), while other repair strategies encompass recombination repair, reversal of DNA damage, and tolerance of DNA damage. Here, only a very brief overview of the meningococcal DNA repair pathways can be given; for a detailed account of DNA repair pathways in *N. meningitidis*, see the comprehensive review by Davidsen and Tønjum (2006).

THE "CLASSICAL" DNA REPAIR PATHWAYS IN *N. MENINGITIDIS*

The BER pathway is probably the first line of defense against oxidative DNA damage in meningococci (Slupphaug et al., 2003), and analyses of the meningococcal genome have shown that it contains homologues of all steps of the BER pathway (Ambur et al., 2009). However, the DNA glycosylase MutY is the only DNA repair component of the BER pathway that has been fully characterized in *N. meningitidis* so far (Davidsen et al., 2005), and meningococcal

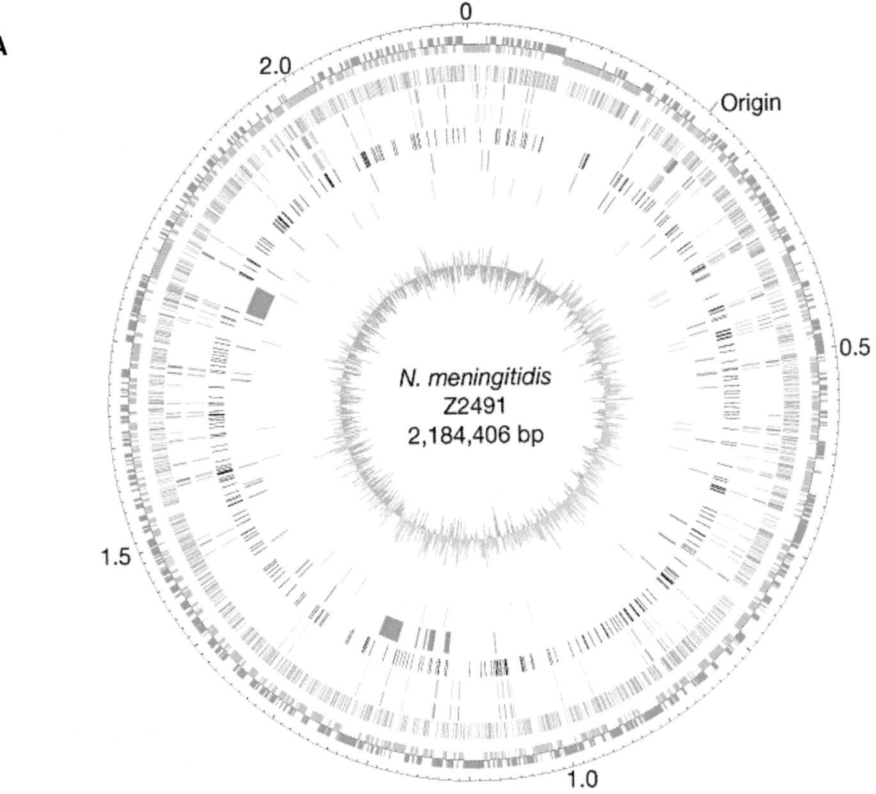

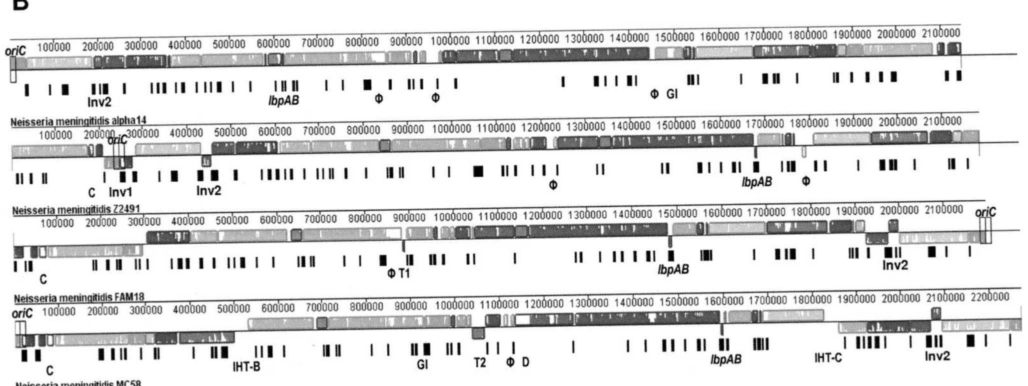

FIGURE 1 The genomes of *Neisseria meningitidis.* (A) Circular representation of the *N. meningitidis* Z2471 genome. The concentric circles show, reading inwards, the scale in megabases, with the origin of replication indicated; predicted coding sequences clockwise (dark green) and counterclockwise (light green); neisserial uptake sequences (red); dRS3 sequences (dark orange); RS elements (light orange); dispersed repeats (Correia, ATR, REP2-5; black); IS elements and phage (narrow ticks and wide bars respectively; turquoise); and tandem repeats (dark blue). The inner histogram shows a plot of (G−C)/(G+C) with values greater than zero in yellow and less than zero in orange. The figure was taken from Parkhill et al. (2000) and is reprinted by permission from Macmillan Publishers Ltd. (*Nature*, copyright 2000). (B) Annotated multiple whole-genome alignment. For each genome, the order of locally colinear blocks (LCBs) is given as a series of colored blocks with the putative origin of replication, designated *oriC*, being indicated by a black rectangle. The genomic locations of dRS3 elements are depicted by short black vertical lines below the corresponding LCB order images. LCBs identically present in the four genomes are given in the same colors, and horizontally flipped LCBs identify chromosomal inversions with respect to the genome of α14

mutY mutants were shown to have high spontaneous mutation rates.

The NER pathway deals with bulky lesions caused by exogenous DNA damage such as ultraviolet (UV) light or polycyclic aromatic hydrocarbons (Hanawalt, 2002). By computational genome comparison, *N. meningitidis* was recently shown to possess the entire set of genes involved in NER (Ambur et al., 2009).

The MMR system controls the fidelity of DNA replication by repairing base mismatches as well as insertion/deletion loops and by participating in processing of DNA lesions during transcription-coupled repair (Schofield and Hsieh, 2003). It therefore allows the degradation of error-containing DNA and resynthesis of unpaired DNA, and defects in MMR consecutively increase mutation rates. Accordingly, the MMR pathway is involved in the maintenance of chromosomal structural integrity and in the control of HGT by preventing recombination between nonidentical DNA sequences (Denamur and Matic, 2006). In *N. meningitidis*, although both the *mutS* and *mutL* genes are present, the *mutH* endonuclease gene is missing. Despite the current lack of experimental data addressing the detailed molecular mechanisms in *N. meningitidis*, *mutS* as well as *mutL* mutants were shown to display an increased rate of phase variation at contingency loci (see below) and a moderate increase in the rate of missense mutations (Richardson and Stojiljkovic, 2001).

In addition to these "traditional" repair pathways, the meningococcus has other means to avoid the mutagenic and cytotoxic effects of DNA damage (reviewed by Davidsen and Tønjum [2006]).

Taken together, although all major DNA pathways are present in *N. meningitidis*, the complexity of genes participating in each pathway is reduced in several cases. This reduced or "streamlined" repertoire of DNA repair enzymes could possibly reflect both a strategy for saving genome space and habitat preferences. In particular, mutations in the DNA repair machinery impact mutation rates, and fine-tuning of mutation rates, either on a genome-wide level or localized only at certain loci, is an important adaptive strategy that is also observed in *N. meningitidis*.

GLOBAL HYPERMUTATION AND THE MUTATOR PHENOTYPE

A state of hypermutation can be achieved either by increasing the misincorporation rate of the DNA polymerization step or by abrogating proofreading as well as by abrogating mismatch correction. This can occur through heritable defects in genes directly responsible for these three processes, and strains that are inherently hypermutable are known as mutator strains (Bridges, 2001). The majority of strong mutators found in a number of bacterial species have a defective MMR pathway due to the inactivation of *mutS* or *mutL* genes. Accordingly, a substantial fraction (22%) of epidemic *N. meningitidis* seroroup A isolates have been shown to harbor defects in MMR genes (Richardson et al., 2002), although 61% of the strains with a mutator phenotype could not be complemented with *mutS* or *mutL*, indicating that other, as yet unknown, mechanisms also influence meningococcal mutability (Davidsen and Tønjum, 2006). Of note, while *mutS* inactivation increased mutation only by around one order of magnitude, *mutY* mutants had mutation frequencies as high as or higher than those of *mutS* mutants. In contrast, in *E. coli* the *mutY* mutation frequency was an order of magnitude

(e.g., the inversion designated Inv1 in the genome of Z2491 composed of two LCBs). Gaps or white spaces in the LCB order image indicate regions not (identically) present in all four genomes such as different prophages (Φ), genomic islands (GI), regions with deviating G+C content termed islands of horizontal transfer (IHT), or a region duplicated only in strain MC58 (D). In addition, the different chromosomal positions of *lbpAB* are shown, as well as some putative composite transposons (T1 in FAM18 and T2 in MC58), the 20-kb region that is inverted in the three disease isolates (Inv2), and the position of the capsule gene locus (C). The figure was taken from Schoen et al. (2008). Copyright 2008 National Academy of Sciences, U.S.A.

lower than that for *mutS* and was similar to the frequency seen for *mutY* in other species (Davidsen et al., 2005; Kim et al., 2003). In an earlier study of serogroup B *N. meningitidis*, elevated mutation frequency also appeared to correlate with an increased rate of capsule variation, although this was measured in only six isolates (Bucci et al., 1999). Both phenotypes were attributed to the absence of DNA methyltransferase (Dam) activity required to identify foreign DNA during mismatch repair, as confirmed by insertional inactivation of *dam*.

LOCALIZED HYPERMUTATION AND PHASE VARIATION

N. meningitidis possesses mechanisms which allow it to permanently maintain high mutation rates at only some loci, thus avoiding fitness costs associated with high genome-wide mutation rates (Moxon et al., 1994). The meningococcal genome is thus compartmentalized into regions of high (contingency) and low (housekeeping) mutation rates. The hypermutability of these loci results from the mutational properties of repetitive DNA sequences located within its controlling elements or within the coding sequence. These so-called simple sequence repeats or "contingency loci" comprise homopolymeric tracts or short tandem sequence repeats either within or 5′ to a coding region and constitute an abundant but heterogeneous class of repeated sequences in the meningococcal genome. The number of these repeated motifs can be modified during replication through slipped-strand mispairing (Lovett, 2004) and can consequently influence translation or transcription, resulting in either a high-frequency, reversible on-off switching of gene expression or an altered function and antigenicity of the encoded protein(s) (Moxon et al., 2006). Computational analyses identified over 80 potentially phase-variable genes in the meningococcal genome (Bentley et al., 2007; Saunders et al., 2000; Snyder et al., 2001), with experimental evidence of phase variation for 15 genes (to date) encoding proteins which are involved mostly in interaction with the host cells (Martin et al., 2003). Examples include (Table 2) the gene encoding the outer membrane protein Opc, which promotes adherence and invasion of epithelial and endothelial cells (Olyhoek et al., 1991), and the *siaD* gene, whose product is involved in capsule biosynthesis (Hammerschmidt et al., 1996a) (Fig. 2). Compared to other bacterial species, *N. meningitidis* seems so far to have the largest repertoire of phase-variable genes, accounting for almost 4% of all CDSs.

In most cases, phase-variable expression mediated by simple tandem repeats has been limited to the gene associated with the repeats. However, *N. meningitidis* also contains potentially phase-variable type III RM systems (Srikhanta et al., 2005), and in some cases more extensive phase variation may be mediated by type III methyltransferases. Individual genes may thus come under the influence of the methyltransferases by point mutations, thereby generating a recognition site in a key position effecting transcriptional control of the gene. Therefore, phase-variable expression of the type III RM system may also influence the expression of multiple genes. Such a phase-variable regulon has been termed a "phasevarion" (Srikhanta et al., 2005).

A number of factors and genes have been shown to influence the rate of phase variation in *N. meningitidis*. For example, defects in the aforementioned MMR genes *mutS* and *mutL* were shown to increase phase variation rates, and likewise the frequency of slippage events in mononucleotide tracts was shown to be increased in DinB-overexpressing strains (Alexander et al., 2004a, 2004b; Martin et al., 2004; Richardson and Stojiljkovic, 2001; Richardson et al., 2002). The observation that DNA derived from various neisserial cocolonizers of the human nasopharynx increased switching frequencies suggests that in *N. meningitidis* transformation is linked to phase variation (Alexander et al., 2004b). The resulting transformation-mediated transient increase in genetic variability was hypothesized to increase the adaptability of *N. meningitidis* to changing environments via "second-order selection"-like phenomenon (Tenaillon et al., 2001). Another layer of complexity to transcriptional control in *N. meningitidis* is added by the finding that

TABLE 2 Phase- and antigen-variable genes in *N. meningitidis*[a]

Functional group and phenotype	Gene	Variation[b]	Mechanism[c]	Reference
Evasins				
Outer membrane protein	*porA*	P	SSM	van der Ende et al., 1995
Capsule	*siaD*	P	SSM	Hammerschmidt et al.; 1996b
LPS biosynthesis	*lgtACDG*	P	SSM	Jennings et al., 1999
Adhesins				
Adhesin	*nadA*	P	SSM	Martin et al., 2003
Opacity protein	*opa*	P+A	SSM	Stern and Meyer, 1987
Outer membrane protein	*opc*	P	SSM	Sarkari et al., 1994
Type IV pilus adhesin	*pilC*	P	SSM	Jonsson et al., 1991
Type IV pili	*pilE, pilS*	P+A	Rec	Segal et al., 1986
Pabulins[d]				
Hemoglobin receptor	*hpuAB, hmbR*	P	SSM	Lewis et al., 1999

[a]Examples were chosen from well-studied systems that together should illustrate the classes of proteins that the phase-varying genes in *N. meningitidis* encode. The table is not meant to be comprehensive.

[b]P, phase variation (reversible switch between on and off expression states); A, antigenic variation (expression of conserved moieties that are antigenically distinct).

[c]The most frequent mechanisms underlying the variation: RecA-dependent recombination (Rec) and slipped-strand mispairing (SSM) mediated by misalignment of repeat tracts during DNA replication or DNA repair.

[d]Molecules involved in scavenging essential nutrients (Moxon and Jansen, 2005).

loss or gain of a tetranucleotide repeat motif affected the binding of integration host factor (IHF) to the promoter of the *nadA* gene encoding a surface adhesion, which provides evidence for an interplay between phase variation (stochastic) and classical (deterministic) mechanisms of gene regulation (Martin et al., 2005). Nonetheless, in contrast to other bacteria such as *E. coli*, meningococcal cells seem to generate a surplus of genetic variants via mutation and phase variation on which selective pressures can act, instead of sensing the environment and responding accordingly.

Repetitive DNA and Recombination

In addition to global mutation and phase variation, intragenomic as well as intergenomic recombination is of pivotal importance for the generation of genome flexibility in *N. meningitidis*, and one of the most striking characteristics of the meningococcal genomes is the abundance and diversity of repetitive DNA serving as potential target sites for homologous recombination or replication slippage (Lovett, 2004). In a recent comparison of 53 complete bacterial chromosomes for repeats, *N. meningitidis* was found to have the fourth highest number, with about 20% of its chromosome consisting of repeated sequence of all kinds (Achaz et al., 2002). Accordingly, by analyzing the loss of gene order conservation in 126 bacterial genomes and deriving an intrinsic measure of genome stability, *N. meningitidis* was assigned rank 121 and thus had the sixth lowest genomic stability (Rocha, 2006).

INTRAGENOMIC RECOMBINATION AND THE GENERATION OF CHROMOSOME STRUCTURE DIVERSITY

Meningococcal repeated sequences belong to a large variety of classes and provide the structural basis for the enormous genomic variability of this bacterium (Table 1) (Bentley et al., 2007; Parkhill et al., 2000).

An important class of repeat sequences consists of the dRS3 elements, which are a family of 20-bp repeats with conserved 6-bp terminal inverted repeats. They occur almost 700 times in the meningococcal genome and, together with the families of 30- to 160-bp RS elements, make up the "neisserial intergenic mosaic elements" (NIME) (Parkhill et al., 2000). These repeat elements in turn are

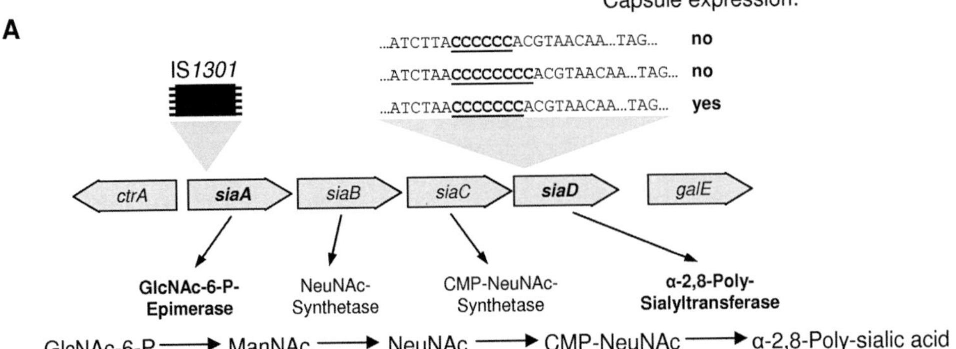

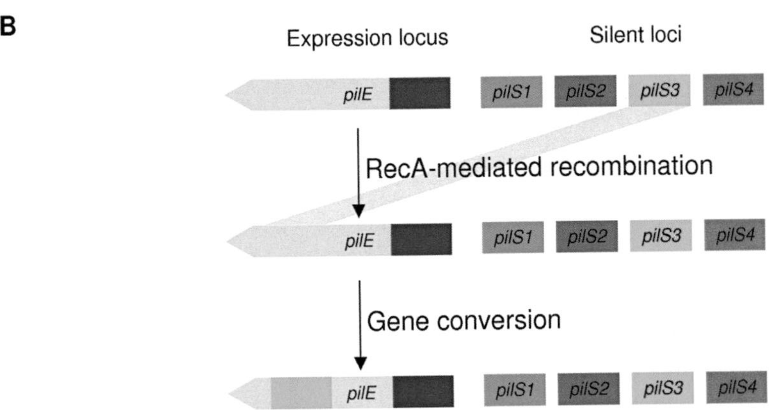

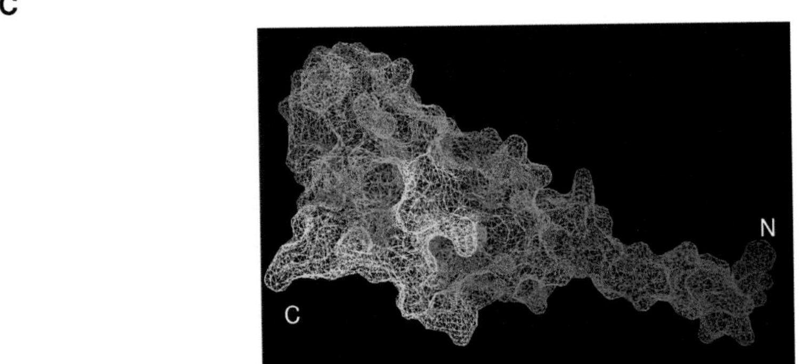

FIGURE 2 Mechanisms of gene variation in *Neisseria meningitidis.* (A) Phase variation at the capsule locus. In serogroup B meningococci starting from *N*-acetylglucosamine-6-phosphate, the synthesis of the capsular polysaccharide, a homopolymer of α-2,8-linked *N*-acetylneuraminic acid, involves four enzymatic steps. The encoding genes are organized into a polycistronic operon, and the last gene in this operon, *siaD*, contains a stretch of seven consecutive cytidines in its 5′ coding region. The molecular mechanism that mediates phase variation at *siaD* is RecA-independent slipped-strand mispairing of the polycytidine tract during DNA replication or repair. The resulting insertion or deletion of a single cytidine leads to a frameshift in the coding sequence and consequently to termination of translation at premature stop codons. As this process is reversible and occurs at a frequency of about 1 in 1,000 to 1 in 10,000 bacterial cells, this allows meningococci a rapid and reversible on/off switch of capsule synthesis (Hammerschmidt et al., 1996b). In addition, capsule

often concentrated within yet larger intergenic repeat arrays of 200 to 2,700 bp. Of note, it has recently been shown that the most abundant member of the dRS3 repeat family serves as target site for the chromosomal integration of a filamentous phage termed Nf1 (Kawai et al., 2005) or meningococcal disease-associated island (MDA) (Bille et al., 2005). Therefore, it was suggested that the phage integrase might also catalyze the recombination between different dRS3 elements, resulting in permanent genomic changes in *N. meningitidis* such as gene insertions and chromosomal rearrangements (Schoen et al., 2008). In addition, these repeat arrays might serve to promote recombination with exogenously acquired DNA, increasing the rate of gene exchange at the adjacent loci. For example, a clear association was demonstrated between repeat arrays and genes encoding cell surface-associated proteins, where increased sequence variation may be an advantage in host interactions (Bentley et al., 2007). The resulting enhanced localized recombination and sequence variation can be seen, for example, in the *lbpAB* locus, encoding a lactoferrin-binding protein, the *tbpAB* locus, encoding a transferring-binding protein, the *porA* locus, encoding a major outer membrane protein, and the *pilC1/pilC2* loci (Bentley et al., 2007).

Also present in such intergenic repeat arrays are larger repeat units including the Correia elements, which represent about 2% of the *N. meningitidis* genome (De Gregorio et al., 2003). Correia elements are apparently mobile elements which are comparable to small insertion sequences (ISs) 100 to155 bp in length with 26-bp inverted repeats and a TA target site duplication, but which, in contrast to conventional IS elements, do not encode a transposase (Buisine et al., 2002; Liu et al., 2002). Such nonautonomous mobile elements are common in eukaryotic genomes, where they are referred to as miniature inverted repeat transposable elements (Delihas, 2008). Correia elements carry transcription initiation signals (Black et al., 1995; Snyder et al., 2003) as well as functional IHF-binding sites (Buisine et al., 2002; Rouquette-Loughlin et al., 2004), and hence may play a role in the regulation of gene expression. Like Correia elements, other repetitive extragenic palindromic sequences called REP2 were found to influence the expression of a set of virulence genes such as *pilC1* and *crgA*, which are necessary for the efficient interaction of *N. meningitidis* with host cells (Morelle et al., 2003).

The meningococcal genomes are also littered with complete IS elements as well as IS remnants, which constitute the largest size class of repeat elements. In particular, a comparative analysis of the distribution of transposases among 80 bacterial genomes revealed that *N. meningitidis* has the fourth highest number of IS elements with respect to genome size (Mahillon and Chandler, 1998), with most of them belonging to the IS*5*, IS*30*, and IS*NCY* families of IS elements. When the sequenced meningococcal genomes are compared, transposed and/or inverted chromosome fragments are often found to be flanked by two IS elements

---

expression can be modulated based on the reversible inactivation of *siaA* by insertion/excision of the insertion sequence element IS*1301* (Hammerschmidt et al., 1996a) (schematic depiction not drawn to scale). (B) Gene conversion at the *pilE/S* locus (Hagblom et al., 1985; Segal et al., 1986). Meningococcal type IV pili consist of thousands of pilin (PilE) subunits polymerized into long fibers. The PilE protein contains a highly conserved N-terminal domain and a variable C-terminal domain, the latter determining the antigenicity of the pili. The variable region is the result of a nonreciprocal transfer of DNA from one of many silent partial *pilS* loci to the single *pilE* expression locus. The silent loci, which are sometimes present several hundred base pairs away from the *pilE* expression locus, can donate a stretch of nucleotides, on the basis of short sequence homology. The genetic mechanism proceeds through a form of gene conversion that requires RecA and several crossover events during recombination (schematic depiction not drawn to scale). (C) Three-dimensional model of the PilE protein. The N and C termini are indicated, and the variable C terminus is highlighted in yellow. The structure was retrieved from the PDB database (2HI2) (Craig et al., 2006) and visualized with the SwissPdb Viewer (http://www.expasy.org/spdbv/) (Guex and Peitsch, 1997).

belonging to the same family, indicating that they have served as target sites for intragenomic homologous recombination (Bentley et al., 2007; Schoen et al., 2007, 2008).

An important recombination-mediated mechanism for the generation of antigenic diversity is silent gene cassette-mediated sequence variation (Hagblom et al., 1985). For example, in the pilin-encoding *pilE/S* system the expressed pilin (PilE) can be altered by incorporation into the *pilE* gene of DNA from 5′-adjacent promoterless *pilS* genes. In *N. meningitidis* the silent *pilS* loci are embedded within NIME arrays (see above), and it is possible that specific dRS3-mediated recombination may contribute to generating silent variation within *pilS* sequences (Bentley et al., 2007). A related yet different mechanism of variation appears to exist for several loci encoding putative hemagglutinins *(fhaB)* and adhesins *(mafB)* (Bentley et al., 2007; Parkhill et al., 2000). Downstream of these genes are what appear to be silent cassettes encoding alternative C termini for the encoded proteins. These cassettes contain short repeats that are identical to sequences only present within the upstream genes. Therefore, the *maf* and *fha* loci show considerable potential for generation of multiple versions of the expressed coding sequence and, together with surface structures such as pilus, capsule and other surface proteins, are likely to be major contributors to cell surface diversity. Likewise, the *N. meningitidis* genomes contain three loci (RTX islands I to III) that code for iron-regulated type I secretion systems belonging to the RTX protein family (van Ulsen and Tommassen, 2006) and that also seem to be involved in adhesion to epithelial cells (Schmitt et al., 2007). In addition to functional and expressed *frpA/C* genes, the RTX islands seem to include partial open reading frames that encode protein cassettes homologous to sequences within the RTX toxins. These RTX cassettes, in contrast to the *maf* and *fha* cassettes, encode protein sequences that differ in their N termini, whereas their C termini are homologous to regions internal in the toxins and are conserved between them, suggesting that they can be exchanged to alter the N-terminal sequence of the secreted proteins (van Ulsen and Tommassen, 2006).

N. meningitidis can thus be taken as a paradigm for genomic variability where the abundance of a diverse set of sequence repeats is exploited via recombination for the generation and maintenance of phenotypic diversity.

INTERGENOMIC RECOMBINATION AND THE MENINGOCOCCAL PAN-GENOME

The meningococci use recombination not only to generate genome structure variability but also to modify their gene repertoire via either homologous or site-specific recombination, and genetic diversity of meningococci is constantly driven more by recombination than by mutation (Feil and Spratt, 2001). Accordingly, comparative genomic analyses revealed that a substantial proportion of the meningococcal chromosome might be imported via HGT, which might therefore play a paramount role in shaping the meningococcal gene content. Although conjugative plasmids have also been found in *N. meningitidis* (Ikeda et al., 1986; Roberts and Knapp, 1988), the main mechanisms contributing to HGT seem to be transduction and, even more important, transformation.

The acquisition of foreign DNA via transformation is particularly facilitated by the fact that *Neisseria* spp. are naturally transformable, being competent for the uptake of DNA throughout their entire life cycle (Koomey, 1998). Efficient neisserial transformation is dependent on the presence of the DNA uptake sequence (DUS) in the exogenous DNA, type IV pilus expression, and homologous recombination mediated by RecA (Davidsen and Tønjum, 2006). There are nearly 2,000 copies of the 12-bp DUS in the meningococcal genome which occur either alone or in inverted repeats as part of a transcriptional terminator (Ambur et al., 2007). Remarkably, the DUS were not equally distributed over the entire genome but were present at a significantly higher density within genes involved in DNA repair, recombination, restriction modification, and replication (Davidsen et al., 2004), indicating that transformation in

Neisseria allows this species to counteract deleterious effects of genome instability in the core genome (Treangen et al., 2008).

Intragenic homologous recombination following transformation can result either in gene conversion of the copy in the recipient genome, as was observed for the *pilE* gene (Seifert et al., 1988), or in exchange of substantial parts of the coding sequence, resulting in mosaic genes, as was observed for, among others, *porA* (encoding a major outer membrane protein) (Feavers et al., 1992), *penA* (conferring penicillin resistance) (Spratt et al., 1992), and housekeeping genes such as *argF, fbp*, and *recA* (Zhou and Spratt, 1992). Likewise, intergenic homologous recombination can result in the acquisition of entire genes by the recipient cell in the form of so-called minimal mobile elements (MMEs) (Saunders and Snyder, 2002). An MME is a region between two conserved genes in which different whole-gene cassettes are found in different strains (Saunders and Snyder, 2002), and comparative analyses of the neisserial genome sequences revealed over 30 potential MME sites, with many of them containing strain-specific genes (Snyder et al., 2007). However, via transformation meningococci rarely take up DNA from bacterial species other than those in their own genus. One notable exception is the introduction of the gene that encodes *Haemophilus influenzae* SodC into the meningococcus by HGT (Kroll et al., 1998).

Still larger entities of laterally transferred DNA called genomic islands (GIs) are frequently found in variable numbers in the genomes of many bacterial species and are often integrated into the chromosomes via site-specific recombination (Hotopp et al., 2006). In general, they are associated with tRNA loci, are flanked by direct repeats, contain genes or pseudogenes coding for genetic mobility, and are often characterized by atypical DNA composition (Dobrindt et al., 2004). They are thought to have originated via reductive evolution from integrated mobile elements such as integrative conjugative plasmids or bacteriophages that have lost their mobile character on inactivation or loss of genes that are required for autonomous replication and mobilization or transfer (Dobrindt et al., 2004). Surprisingly, and in contrast to what has been found in, for example, the *Enterobacteriaceae*, in the *N. meningitidis* genomes sequenced so far only very few regions were found to display the hallmark features of typical GIs. One is present in the genome of strain MC58 and is a degraded form of a λ-like prophage present at the same locus in strains FAM18 and α14, respectively (Hotopp et al., 2006). Another GI present in the genomes of strains α14 and α275 is also a degraded form of a prophage, probably belonging to the family of the P4-like prophages. Finally, a version of the gonococcal genomic island (GGI) (Snyder et al., 2005b) has been found in the genome of strain α275 as well as a number of other serogroup W-135, H, and Z meningococcal strains, presumably representing an integrated conjugative plasmid. It was shown to encode a type IV secretion system that is used for the secretion of chromosomal DNA at least in *N. gonorrhoeae* (Hamilton et al., 2005). More frequently than classical GIs, there are numerous regions in the meningococcal chromosome(s) called islands of horizontally transferred DNA (IHTs) (Tettelin et al., 2000) that do not show the organizational features of typical MMEs or GIs but nonetheless differ in their G+C content and codon usage (Tettelin et al., 2000). For example, in serogroup A strain Z2491 they account for about 5% of the genome, with identification of at least 60 coding regions ranging in size from 224 bp to 11.3 kb (Parkhill et al., 2000). Accordingly, there are also a substantial number of genes in the other meningococcal genomes that show a lower than average G+C content and that might therefore have been acquired via HGT (Table 1). Of note, most of them are also strain specific and some of them code for proteins of paramount importance for interactions with host cells and for pathogenicity features such as the synthesis of a polysaccharide capsule (Frosch et al., 1989). The exact evolutionary origin of most IHTs remains elusive, although the presence of IHT-B and IHT-C has been linked to the integration of a circular phage into the chromosome of strain MC58 (Kawai et al., 2006).

In contrast to GIs or IHTs, so far no uniform criteria have been established for the identification of prophages in bacterial genome sequences (Canchaya et al., 2003). Computational analyses revealed about 10 prophages in *N. meningitidis*, with most of them either being defective mosaic relatives of the Mu-like group of prophages (Bentley et al., 2007; Parkhill et al., 2000; Tettelin et al., 2000) or belonging to the family of the filamentous prophages called Nf (Kawai et al., 2005). The finding that at least the Mu-like prophage NeisMu1 in strain MC58 codes for membrane-associated antigenic proteins suggests that these proteins contribute to the variability in envelope structure and may thus influence virulence and pathogenicity (Masignani et al., 2001). In addition, the presence of a certain subtype of the filamentous prophages called Nf1 or MDA (Bille et al., 2005) is associated with certain hypervirulent meningococcal lineages, although it could not be shown that the phage itself codes for any virulence determinant.

As a consequence of this large variety of mobile DNA elements, about 10% of the genome is strictly strain specific among the seven strains sequenced so far, and only 67% of the genes in each genome belong to the meningococcal core genome, which contains about 1,330 genes. For an increasing number of genomes sequenced, the size of the core genome is expected to approach about 1,300 genes, whereas the number of new genes found in each genome might level off at around 40 new genes per newly sequenced strain (Schoen et al., 2009). This indicates that the size of the meningococcal "pan-genome" (Tettelin et al., 2008), which denotes the set of all genes present in the genomes of *N. meningitidis*, grows slowly with each newly sequenced strain but technically has no limits and thus might be open. This, of course, might not come as a surprise, given that *N. meningitidis* is naturally competent for the uptake of DNA and might accordingly be capable of acquiring a large variety of DNA sequences from different sources via HGT, as outlined above.

GENETIC BASIS OF VIRULENCE IN *N. MENINGITIDIS*

The lack of satisfactory animal models continues to be a frustrating limitation to the experimental study of meningococcal virulence and pathogenesis (Stephens, 2009). Therefore, the search for meningococcal virulence factors has so far been restricted mainly to in vitro cell culture models with their implicit limitations (Bourdoulous and Nassif, 2006; Carbonnelle et al., 2009) and complementarily to population genetic approaches (Bille et al., 2005, 2008; Harrison et al., 2009). In particular, compared to collections of meningococci from the nasopharynx of healthy individuals, meningococci from diseased individuals are typically much less diverse (Jolley et al., 2005; Yazdankhah et al., 2004) and only a limited number of CCs, termed hyperinvasive lineages, dominate worldwide collections of meningococci (Maiden et al., 1998). Epidemiological data indeed lend further support to the hypothesis that outbreaks of meningococcal disease are caused by diversity in the pathogenicity of the meningococcal strains and therefore have a genetic basis (Stollenwerk et al., 2004). The existence of defined genetic types as revealed by MLST with different phenotypes thus allows for the prospect of identifying the genetic traits that are responsible for those phenotypes by genome-wide association studies (Falush and Bowden, 2006) performed with well-defined isolate collections (Maiden, 2008).

However, computational comparisons of whole genomes from strains belonging to three hyperinvasive lineages with the genomes from three carriage strains have so far failed to detect a consistent difference in the distribution of most of the hitherto studied candidate virulence genes (Schoen et al., 2008) between carriage and invasive strains, and comparative genome hybridization studies using microarrays (mCGH) with larger strain collections (Bille et al., 2005; Hotopp et al., 2006; Snyder and Saunders, 2006; Stabler et al., 2005) showed that the majority of genes in pathogenic *Neisseria* species are also present in the nonpathogenic *Neisseria lactamica*. Therefore, most of the *N.*

meningitidis candidate virulence genes studied so far should more appropriately be considered fitness genes being involved in, e.g., colonization of the human nasopharynx and not as virulence factors for the invasion of host tissues. This is in remarkable contrast to the situation in many pathogenic *Enterobacteriaceae* or in streptococci, where the chromosomes of pathogenic isolates often harbor pathogenicity islands or prophages that code for, e.g., adhesins or toxins and that are absent from the chromosomes of nonpathogenic strains.

Instead of a clear-cut difference in gene content between carriage and diseases strains, more detailed statistical analyses of large strain collections revealed a statistically significant although not perfect association between virulence and the presence of phage Nf1 in the genomes of hyperinvasive strains (Bille et al., 2005). In particular, among 1,288 meningococci isolated from patients with disease and asymptomatic carriers, the phage was overrepresented in disease isolates from young adults, indicating that it may contribute to invasive disease in this age group. Further analyses revealed that between 20% and 45% of the pathogenic potential of the five most common disease-causing meningococcal groups was linked to the presence of this phage (Bille et al., 2008). However, it is still unclear how this phage contributes to the pathogenicity of the meningococci since it does not contain genes coding for known virulence factors (Bille et al., 2005). It has been speculated that the prophage Nf1 integrase might affect the expression of certain surface proteins involved in host cell interaction by mediating genomic rearrangements at adjacent dRS3 repeat sequences (Schoen et al., 2008), but this hypothesis still awaits further experimental verification.

Another genetic element that was recently shown to be positively associated with disease was the hemoglobin receptor gene *hmbR*, with isolates of most of the hyperinvasive lineages being exclusively *hmbR* positive (Harrison et al., 2009). Like phage Nf1, it is also probably a mobile genetic element and located on a genomic region with some resemblance to a pathogenicity island. Again, how the *hmbR* gene product contributes to pathogenicity is still not fully understood, although it was shown that a *hmbR* mutant was attenuated in an infant-rat model of meningococcal infection (Stojiljkovic et al., 1995).

In addition to the presence or absence of certain possibly virulence-associated genes, differences in the frequency of phase variation between strains might contribute to the observed epidemiological pattern: if a host population includes sufficient immunological diversity, then, as a consequence of the colonization advantage of strains with high rates of phase variation in contingency genes associated with colonization of novel hosts, natural selection favors fast phase shifters. Virulence of *N. meningitidis* is then a rare consequence of within-host evolution for proliferation into new tissues and other sites of replication (Meyers et al., 2003). In addition, interstrain competition mediated by immune selection would also explain both the persistence of multiple meningococcal lineages and the association of a subset of these with invasive disease (Buckee et al., 2008).

In conclusion, accumulating amounts of genomic and epidemiological data indicate that the propensity to cause disease is probably polygenic, depending on combinations of genes or alleles also present in less invasive meningococci. However, what these meningococcal genes are and how they affect virulence await further experimental elucidation.

CONCLUSIONS

In Lewis Carroll's book *Through the Looking-Glass*, the Red Queen tells Alice, "It takes all the running you can do, to keep in the same place" (Carroll, 2003). For obligate commensals or pathogens, such as *N. meningitidis*, the challenge of coexistence with humans is very stringent and the metaphor of the "Red Queen" race (van Valen, 1973) is especially apt. For organisms existing in such a complex and rapidly fluctuating environment as the human nasopharynx, survival is a race in which the rate of generation of genetic variants is a critical factor (Bayliss et al., 2000). At least one organism must be fit enough to sustain the microbial population in the face of relentless competitive pressures from the host and other members of the resident flora. Not surprisingly, the key messages from meningococcal genome comparisons are therefore ones of flexibility and diversity (Snyder et al., 2005a), and the forces which structure it therefore appear to be central to the biology and pathogenicity of this species.

ACKNOWLEDGMENTS

We thank Gabriele Gerlach for critical reading of the manuscript.

This work was funded by the BMBF funding initiative "PathoGenoMik-Plus" (grant 0313801A).

REFERENCES

Achaz, G., E. P. Rocha, P. Netter, and E. Coissac. 2002. Origin and fate of repeats in bacteria. *Nucleic Acids Res.* **30:**2987–2994.

Achtman, M. 1994. Clonal spread of serogroup A meningococci: a paradigm for the analysis of microevolution in bacteria. *Mol. Microbiol.* **11:**15–22.

Alexander, H. L., A. W. Rasmussen, and I. Stojiljkovic. 2004a. Identification of *Neisseria meningitidis* genetic loci involved in the modulation of phase variation frequencies. *Infect. Immun.* **72:** 6743–6747.

Alexander, H. L., A. R. Richardson, and I. Stojiljkovic. 2004b. Natural transformation and phase variation modulation in Neisseria meningitidis. *Mol. Microbiol.* **52:**771–783.

Ambur, O. H., T. Davidsen, S. A. Frye, S. V. Balasingham, K. Lagesen, T. Rognes, and T. Tønjum. 2009. Genome dynamics in major bacterial pathogens. *FEMS Microbiol. Rev.* **33:**453–470.

Ambur, O. H., S. A. Frye, and T. Tønjum. 2007. New functional identity for the DNA uptake sequence in transformation and its presence in transcriptional terminators. *J. Bacteriol.* **189:**2077–2085.

Backman, A., P. Orvelid, J. A. Vazquez, O. Skold, and P. Olcen. 2000. Complete sequence of a beta—lactamase—encoding plasmid in *Neisseria meningitidis. Antimicrob. Agents Chemother.* **44:**210–212.

Bart, A., J. Dankert, and A. van der Ende. 2000. Representational difference analysis of Neisseria meningitidis identifies sequences that are specific for the hyper—virulent lineage III clone. *FEMS Microbiol. Lett.* **188:**111–114.

Bautsch, W. 1998. Comparison of the genome organization of pathogenic neisseriae. *Electrophoresis* **19:**577–581.

Bayliss, C. D., D. Field, X. de Bolle, and E. R. Moxon. 2000. The generation of diversity by Haemophilus influenzae: response. *Trends Microbiol.* **8:**435–436.

Bentley, S. D., G. S. Vernikos, L. A. Snyder, C. Churcher, C. Arrowsmith, T. Chillingworth, A. Cronin, P. H. Davis, N. E. Holroyd, K. Jagels, M. Maddison, S. Moule, E. Rabbinowitsch, S. Sharp, L. Unwin, S. Whitehead, M. A. Quail, M. Achtman, B. Barrell, N. J. Saunders, and J. Parkhill. 2007. Meningococcal genetic variation mechanisms viewed through comparative analysis of serogroup C strain FAM18. *PLoS Genet.* **3:**e23.

Bille, E., R. Ure, S. J. Gray, E. B. Kaczmarski, N. D. McCarthy, X. Nassif, M. C. Maiden, and C. R. Tinsley. 2008. Association of a bacteriophage with meningococcal disease in young adults. *PLoS One* **3:**e3885.

Bille, E., J. R. Zahar, A. Perrin, S. Morelle, P. Kriz, K. A. Jolley, M. C. Maiden, C. Dervin, X. Nassif, and C. R. Tinsley. 2005. A chromosomally integrated bacteriophage in invasive meningococci. *J. Exp. Med.* **201:**1905–1913.

Black, C., J. Fyfe, and J. Davies. 1995. A promoter associated with the neisserial repeat can be used to transcribe the *uvrB* gene from *Neisseria gonorrhoeae. J. Bacteriol.* **177:**1952–1958.

Bourdoulous, S., and X. Nassif. 2006. Mechanisms of attachment and invasion, p. 257–272. *In* M. Frosch and M. C. Maiden (ed.), *Handbook of Meningococcal Disease.* Wiley—VCH, Weinheim, Germany.

Bridges, B. A. 2001. Hypermutation in bacteria and other cellular systems. *Philos. Trans. R. Soc. Lond.* Ser. B **356:**29–39.

Bucci, C., A. Lavitola, P. Salvatore, L. Del Giudice, D. R. Massardo, C. B. Bruni, and P. Alifano. 1999. Hypermutation in pathogenic bacteria: frequent phase variation in meningococci is a phenotypic trait of a specialized mutator biotype. *Mol. Cell* **3:**435–445.

Buckee, C. O., K. A. Jolley, M. Recker, B. Penman, P. Kriz, S. Gupta, and M. C. Maiden. 2008. Role of selection in the emergence of lineages and the evolution of virulence in *Neisseria meningitidis. Proc. Natl. Acad. Sci. USA* **105:**15082–15087.

Buisine, N., C. M. Tang, and R. Chalmers. 2002. Transposon—like Correia elements: structure, distribution and genetic exchange between pathogenic Neisseria sp. *FEBS Lett* **522:**52–58.

Canchaya, C., C. Proux, G. Fournous, A. Bruttin, and H. Brussow. 2003. Prophage genomics. *Microbiol. Mol. Biol. Rev.* **67:**238–276.

Carbonnelle, E., D. J. Hill, P. Morand, N. J. Griffiths, S. Bourdoulous, I. Murillo, X. Nassif, and M. Virji. 2009. Meningococcal interactions with the host. *Vaccine* **27:**B78–B89.

Carroll, L. 2003. *Alice's Adventures in Wonderland* and *Through the Looking-Glass.* Penguin Books, New York, NY.

Caugant, D. A., K. Bovre, P. Gaustad, K. Bryn, E. Holten, E. A. Hoiby, and L. O. Froholm. 1986a. Multilocus genotypes determined by enzyme electrophoresis of Neisseria meningitidis isolated from patients with systemic disease and from healthy carriers. *J. Gen. Microbiol.* **132:**641–652.

Caugant, D. A., L. O. Froholm, K. Bovre, E. Holten, C. E. Frasch, L. F. Mocca, W. D. Zollinger, and R. K. Selander. 1986b. Intercontinental spread of a genetically distinctive complex of clones of Neisseria meningitidis causing epidemic disease. *Proc. Natl. Acad. Sci. USA* **83:**4927–4931.

Claus, H., M. C. Maiden, D. J. Wilson, N. D. McCarthy, K. A. Jolley, R. Urwin, F. Hessler, M. Frosch, and U. Vogel. 2005. Genetic analysis of meningococci carried by children and young adults. *J. Infect. Dis.* **191:**1263–1271.

Claus, H., J. Stoevesandt, M. Frosch, and U. Vogel. 2001. Genetic isolation of meningococci of the electrophoretic type 37 complex. *J. Bacteriol.* **183:**2570–2575.

Connolly, M., and N. Noah for the European Meningitis Surveillance Group. 1999. Is group C meningococcal disease increasing in Europe? A report of surveillance of meningococcal infection in Europe 1993–6. *Epidemiol. Infect.* **122:**41–49.

Craig, L., N. Volkmann, A. S. Arvai, M. E. Pique, M. Yeager, E. H. Egelman, and J. A. Tainer. 2006. Type IV pilus structure by cryo—electron microscopy and crystallography: implications for pilus assembly and functions. *Mol. Cell* **23:**651–662.

Davidsen, T., M. Bjørås, E. C. Seeberg, and T. Tønjum. 2005. Antimutator role of DNA glycosylase MutY in pathogenic *Neisseria* species. *J. Bacteriol.* **187:**2801–2809.

Davidsen, T., E. A. Rødland, K. Lagesen, E. Seeberg, T. Rognes, and T. Tønjum. 2004. Biased distribution of DNA uptake sequences towards genome maintenance genes. *Nucleic Acids Res.* **32:**1050–1058.

Davidsen, T., and T. Tønjum. 2006. Meningococcal genome dynamics. *Nat. Rev. Microbiol.* **4:**11–22.

De Gregorio, E., C. Abrescia, M. S. Carlomagno, and P. P. Di Nocera. 2003. Asymmetrical distribution of *Neisseria* miniature insertion sequence DNA repeats among pathogenic and nonpathogenic *Neisseria* strains. *Infect. Immun.* **71:**4217–4221.

Delihas, N. 2008. Small mobile sequences in bacteria display diverse structure/function motifs. *Mol. Microbiol.* **67:**475–481.

Dempsey, J. A., A. B. Wallace, and J. G. Cannon. 1995. The physical map of the chromosome of a serogroup A strain of *Neisseria meningitidis* shows complex rearrangements relative to the chromosomes of the two mapped strains of the closely related species *N. gonorrhoeae. J. Bacteriol.* **177:**6390–6400.

Denamur, E., and I. Matic. 2006. Evolution of mutation rates in bacteria. *Mol. Microbiol.* **60:**820–827.

Dillon, J. A., and K. H. Yeung. 1989. Beta—lactamase plasmids and chromosomally mediated antibiotic resistance in pathogenic *Neisseria* species. *Clin. Microbiol. Rev.* **2**(Suppl.)**:**S125–S133.

Dobrindt, U., B. Hochhut, U. Hentschel, and J. Hacker. 2004. Genomic islands in pathogenic and environmental microorganisms. *Nat. Rev. Microbiol.* **2:**414–424.

Facinelli, B., and P. E. Varaldo. 1987. Plasmid—mediated sulfonamide resistance in *Neisseria meningitidis. Antimicrob. Agents Chemother.* **31:**1642–1643.

Falush, D., and R. Bowden. 2006. Genome—wide association mapping in bacteria? *Trends Microbiol.* **14:**353–355.

Feavers, I. M., A. B. Heath, J. A. Bygraves, and M. C. Maiden. 1992. Role of horizontal genetic exchange in the antigenic variation of the class 1 outer membrane protein of Neisseria meningitidis. *Mol. Microbiol.* **6:**489–495.

Feil, E. J., E. C. Holmes, D. E. Bessen, M. S. Chan, N. P. Day, M. C. Enright, R. Goldstein, D. W. Hood, A. Kalia, C. E. Moore, J. Zhou, and B. G. Spratt. 2001. Recombination within natural populations of pathogenic bacteria: short—term empirical estimates and long—term phylogenetic consequences. *Proc. Natl. Acad. Sci. USA* **98:**182–187.

Feil, E. J., B. C. Li, D. M. Aanensen, W. P. Hanage, and B. G. Spratt. 2004. eBURST: inferring patterns of evolutionary descent among clusters of related bacterial genotypes from multilocus sequence typing data. *J. Bacteriol.* **186:**1518–1530.

Feil, E. J., M. C. Maiden, M. Achtman, and B. G. Spratt. 1999. The relative contributions of recombination and mutation to the divergence of clones of Neisseria meningitidis. *Mol. Biol. Evol.* **16:**1496–1502.

Feil, E. J., and B. G. Spratt. 2001. Recombination and the population structures of bacterial pathogens. *Annu. Rev. Microbiol.* **55:**561–590.

Fraser, C., W. P. Hanage, and B. G. Spratt. 2005. Neutral microepidemic evolution of bacterial pathogens. *Proc. Natl. Acad. Sci. USA* **102:**1968–1973.

Froholm, L. O., A. B. Kolsto, J. M. Berner, and D. A. Caugant. 2000. Genomic rearrangements in Neisseria meningitidis strains of the ET—5 complex. *Curr. Microbiol.* **40:**372–379.

Frosch, M., and M. C. Maiden (ed.). 2006. *Handbook of Meningococcal Disease.* Wiley—VCH, Weinheim, Germany.

Frosch, M., and U. Vogel. 2006. Structure and genetics of the meningococcal capsule, p. 145–162. *In*

M. Frosch and M. C. Maiden (ed.), *Handbook of Meningococcal Disease.* Wiley—VCH, Weinheim, Germany.

Frosch, M., C. Weisgerber, and T. F. Meyer. 1989. Molecular characterization and expression in *Escherichia coli* of the gene complex encoding the polysaccharide capsule of *Neisseria meningitidis* group B. *Proc. Natl. Acad. Sci. USA* **86:**1669–1673.

Gaher, M., K. Einsiedler, T. Crass, and W. Bautsch. 1996. A physical and genetic map of Neisseria meningitidis B1940. *Mol. Microbiol.* **19:**249–259.

Guex, N., and M. C. Peitsch. 1997. SWISS—MODEL and the Swiss—PdbViewer: an environment for comparative protein modeling. *Electrophoresis* **18:**2714–2723.

Gupta, S., M. C. Maiden, I. M. Feavers, S. Nee, R. M. May, and R. M. Anderson. 1996. The maintenance of strain structure in populations of recombining infectious agents. *Nat. Med.* **2:**437–442.

Hagblom, P., E. Segal, E. Billyard, and M. So. 1985. Intragenic recombination leads to pilus antigenic variation in Neisseria gonorrhoeae. *Nature* **315:**156–158.

Hamilton, H. L., N. M. Dominguez, K. J. Schwartz, K. T. Hackett, and J. P. Dillard. 2005. Neisseria gonorrhoeae secretes chromosomal DNA via a novel type IV secretion system. *Mol. Microbiol.* **55:**1704–1721.

Hammerschmidt, S., R. Hilse, J. P. van Putten, R. Gerardy-Schahn, A. Unkmeir, and M. Frosch. 1996a. Modulation of cell surface sialic acid expression in Neisseria meningitidis via a transposable genetic element. *EMBO J.* **15:**192–198.

Hammerschmidt, S., A. Muller, H. Sillmann, M. Muhlenhoff, R. Borrow, A. Fox, J. van Putten, W. D. Zollinger, R. Gerardy-Schahn, and M. Frosch. 1996b. Capsule phase variation in Neisseria meningitidis serogroup B by slipped—strand mispairing in the polysialyltransferase gene *(siaD):* correlation with bacterial invasion and the outbreak of meningococcal disease. *Mol. Microbiol.* **20:**1211–1220.

Hanawalt, P. C. 2002. Subpathways of nucleotide excision repair and their regulation. *Oncogene* **21:**8949–8956.

Harrison, A., D. W. Dyer, A. Gillaspy, W. C. Ray, R. Mungur, M. B. Carson, H. Zhong, J. Gipson, M. Gipson, L. S. Johnson, L. Lewis, L. O. Bakaletz, and R. S. Munson, Jr. 2005. Genomic sequence of an otitis media isolate of nontypeable *Haemophilus influenzae*: comparative study with *H. influenzae* serotype d, strain KW20. *J. Bacteriol.* **187:**4627–4636.

Harrison, O. B., N. J. Evans, J. M. Blair, H. S. Grimes, C. R. Tinsley, X. Nassif, P. Kriz, R. Ure, S. J. Gray, J. P. Derrick, M. C. Maiden, and I. M. Feavers. 2009. Epidemiological evidence for the role of the hemoglobin receptor, HmbR, in meningococcal virulence. *J. Infect. Dis.* **200:**94–98.

Holmes, E. C., R. Urwin, and M. C. Maiden. 1999. The influence of recombination on the population structure and evolution of the human pathogen Neisseria meningitidis. *Mol. Biol. Evol.* **16:**741–749.

Hotopp, J. C. D., R. Grifantini, N. Kumar, Y. L. Tzeng, D. Fouts, E. Frigimelica, M. Draghi, M. M. Giuliani, R. Rappuoli, D. S. Stephens, G. Grandi, and H. Tettelin. 2006. Comparative genomics of Neisseria meningitidis: core genome, islands of horizontal transfer and pathogen—specific genes. *Microbiology* **152:**3733–3749.

Ikeda, F., A. Tsuji, Y. Kaneko, M. Nishida, and S. Goto. 1986. Conjugal transfer of beta—lactamase—producing plasmids of Neisseria gonorrhoeae to Neisseria meningitidis. *Microbiol. Immunol.* **30:**737–742.

Jennings, M. P., Y. N. Srikhanta, E. R. Moxon, M. Kramer, J. T. Poolman, B. Kuipers, and P. van der Ley. 1999. The genetic basis of the phase variation repertoire of lipopolysaccharide immunotypes in Neisseria meningitidis. *Microbiology* **145:**3013–3021.

Jolley, K., M.-S. Chan, and M. Maiden. 2004. mlstdbNet—distributed multi—locus sequence typing (MLST) databases. *BMC Bioinformatics* **5:**86.

Jolley, K. A., J. Kalmusova, E. J. Feil, S. Gupta, M. Musilek, P. Kriz, and M. C. Maiden. 2000. Carried meningococci in the Czech Republic: a diverse recombining population. *J. Clin. Microbiol.* **38:**4492–4498.

Jolley, K. A., D. J. Wilson, P. Kriz, G. McVean, and M. C. Maiden. 2005. The influence of mutation, recombination, population history, and selection on patterns of genetic diversity in Neisseria meningitidis. *Mol. Biol. Evol.* **22:**562–569.

Jonsson, A. B., G. Nyberg, and S. Normark. 1991. Phase variation of gonococcal pili by frameshift mutation in *pilC*, a novel gene for pilus assembly. *EMBO J.* **10:**477–488.

Kawai, M., K. Nakao, I. Uchiyama, and I. Kobayashi. 2006. How genomes rearrange: genome comparison within bacteria Neisseria suggests roles for mobile elements in formation of complex genome polymorphisms. *Gene* **383:**52–63.

Kawai, M., I. Uchiyama, and I. Kobayashi. 2005. Genome comparison in silico in Neisseria suggests integration of filamentous bacteriophages by their own transposase. *DNA Res.* **12:**389–401.

Kim, M., T. Huang, and J. H. Miller. 2003. Competition between MutY and mismatch repair at A · C mispairs in vivo. *J. Bacteriol.* **185:**4626–4629.

Klee, S. R., X. Nassif, B. Kusecek, P. Merker, J. L. Beretti, M. Achtman, and C. R. Tinsley. 2000.

Molecular and biological analysis of eight genetic islands that distinguish *Neisseria meningitidis* from the closely related pathogen *Neisseria gonorrhoeae*. *Infect. Immun.* **68:**2082–2095.

Knapp, J. S., J. M. Zenilman, J. W. Biddle, G. H. Perkins, W. E. DeWitt, M. L. Thomas, S. R. Johnson, and S. A. Morse. 1987. Frequency and distribution in the United States of strains of Neisseria gonorrhoeae with plasmid—mediated, high—level resistance to tetracycline. *J. Infect. Dis.* **155:**819–822.

Koomey, M. 1998. Competence for natural transformation in Neisseria gonorrhoeae: a model system for studies of horizontal gene transfer. *APMIS Suppl.* **84:**56–61.

Kroll, J. S., K. E. Wilks, J. L. Farrant, and P. R. Langford. 1998. Natural genetic exchange between *Haemophilus* and *Neisseria*: intergeneric transfer of chromosomal genes between major human pathogens. *Proc. Natl. Acad. Sci. USA* **95:** 12381–12385.

Lewis, L. A., M. Gipson, K. Hartman, T. Ownbey, J. Vaughn, and D. W. Dyer. 1999. Phase variation of HpuAB and HmbR, two distinct haemoglobin receptors of Neisseria meningitidis DNM2. *Mol. Microbiol.* **32:**977–989.

Lipsitch, M., and E. R. Moxon. 1997. Virulence and transmissibility of pathogens: what is the relationship? *Trends Microbiol.* **5:**31–37.

Liu, S. V., N. J. Saunders, A. Jeffries, and R. F. Rest. 2002. Genome analysis and strain comparison of correia repeats and correia repeat—enclosed elements in pathogenic *Neisseria*. *J. Bacteriol.* **184:**6163–6173.

Lovett, S. T. 2004. Encoded errors: mutations and rearrangements mediated by misalignment at repetitive DNA sequences. *Mol. Microbiol.* **52:**1243–1253.

Mahillon, J., and M. Chandler. 1998. Insertion sequences. *Microbiol. Mol. Biol. Rev.* **62:**725–774.

Maiden, M. C. 2008. Population genomics: diversity and virulence in the Neisseria. *Curr. Opin. Microbiol.* **11:**467–471.

Maiden, M. C., J. A. Bygraves, E. Feil, G. Morelli, J. E. Russell, R. Urwin, Q. Zhang, J. Zhou, K. Zurth, D. A. Caugant, I. M. Feavers, M. Achtman, and B. G. Spratt. 1998. Multilocus sequence typing: a portable approach to the identification of clones within populations of pathogenic microorganisms. *Proc. Natl. Acad. Sci. USA* **95:**3140–3145.

Maiden, M. C., and D. A. Caugant. 2006. The population biology of *Neisseria meningitidis*: implications for meningococcal disease, epidemiology and control, p. 17–35. *In* M. Frosch and M. C. Maiden (ed.), *Handbook of Meningococcal Disease*. Wiley—VCH, Weinheim, Germany.

Martin, P., K. Makepeace, S. A. Hill, D. W. Hood, and E. R. Moxon. 2005. Microsatellite instability regulates transcription factor binding and gene expression. *Proc. Natl. Acad. Sci. USA* **102:**3800–3804.

Martin, P., L. Sun, D. W. Hood, and E. R. Moxon. 2004. Involvement of genes of genome maintenance in the regulation of phase variation frequencies in Neisseria meningitidis. *Microbiology* **150:**3001–3012.

Martin, P., T. van de Ven, N. Mouchel, A. C. Jeffries, D. W. Hood, and E. R. Moxon. 2003. Experimentally revised repertoire of putative contingency loci in Neisseria meningitidis strain MC58: evidence for a novel mechanism of phase variation. *Mol. Microbiol.* **50:**245–257.

Masignani, V., M. M. Giuliani, H. Tettelin, M. Comanducci, R. Rappuoli, and V. Scarlato. 2001. Mu—like prophage in serogroup B *Neisseria meningitidis* coding for surface—exposed antigens. *Infect. Immun.* **69:**2580–2588.

Meyers, L. A., B. R. Levin, A. R. Richardson, and I. Stojiljkovic. 2003. Epidemiology, hypermutation, within—host evolution and the virulence of Neisseria meningitidis. *Proc. Biol. Sci.* **270:**1667–1677.

Milkman, R. 1973. Electrophoretic variation in *Escherichia coli* from natural sources. *Science* **182:**1024–1026.

Morelle, S., E. Carbonnelle, and X. Nassif. 2003. The REP2 repeats of the genome of *Neisseria meningitidis* are associated with genes coordinately regulated during bacterial cell interaction. *J. Bacteriol.* **185:**2618–2627.

Morelli, G., B. Malorny, K. Muller, A. Seiler, J. F. Wang, J. del Valle, and M. Achtman. 1997. Clonal descent and microevolution of Neisseria meningitidis during 30 years of epidemic spread. *Mol. Microbiol.* **25:**1047–1064.

Moxon, E. R., and V. A. Jansen. 2005. Phage variation: understanding the behaviour of an accidental pathogen. *Trends Microbiol.* **13:**563–565.

Moxon, E. R., P. B. Rainey, M. A. Nowak, and R. E. Lenski. 1994. Adaptive evolution of highly mutable loci in pathogenic bacteria. *Curr. Biol.* **4:**24–33.

Moxon, R., C. Bayliss, and D. Hood. 2006. Bacterial contingency loci: the role of simple sequence DNA repeats in bacterial adaptation. *Annu. Rev. Genet.* **40:**307–333.

Olyhoek, A. J., J. Sarkari, M. Bopp, G. Morelli, and M. Achtman. 1991. Cloning and expression in Escherichia coli of *opc*, the gene for an unusual class 5 outer membrane protein from Neisseria meningitidis (meningococci/surface antigen). *Microb. Pathog.* **11:**249–257.

Orskov, F., and I. Orskov. 1983. Summary of a workshop on the clone concept in the epidemiology, taxonomy, and evolution of the Enterobacteriaceae and other bacteria. *J. Infect. Dis.* **148:**346–357.

Parkhill, J., M. Achtman, K. D. James, S. D. Bentley, C. Churcher, S. R. Klee, G. Morelli, D. Basham, D. Brown, T. Chillingworth, R. M. Davies, P. Davis, K. Devlin, T. Feltwell, N. Hamlin, S. Holroyd, K. Jagels, S. Leather, S. Moule, K. Mungall, M. A. Quail, M. A. Rajandream, K. M. Rutherford, M. Simmonds, J. Skelton, S. Whitehead, B. G. Spratt, and B. G. Barrell. 2000. Complete DNA sequence of a serogroup A strain of *Neisseria meningitidis* Z2491. *Nature* **404:**502–506.

Parkhill, J., M. Sebaihia, A. Preston, L. D. Murphy, N. Thomson, D. E. Harris, M. T. Holden, C. M. Churcher, S. D. Bentley, K. L. Mungall, A. M. Cerdeno-Tarraga, L. Temple, K. James, B. Harris, M. A. Quail, M. Achtman, R. Atkin, S. Baker, D. Basham, N. Bason, I. Cherevach, T. Chillingworth, M. Collins, A. Cronin, P. Davis, J. Doggett, T. Feltwell, A. Goble, N. Hamlin, H. Hauser, S. Holroyd, K. Jagels, S. Leather, S. Moule, H. Norberczak, S. O'Neil, D. Ormond, C. Price, E. Rabbinowitsch, S. Rutter, M. Sanders, D. Saunders, K. Seeger, S. Sharp, M. Simmonds, J. Skelton, R. Squares, S. Squares, K. Stevens, L. Unwin, S. Whitehead, B. G. Barrell, and D. J. Maskell. 2003. Comparative analysis of the genome sequences of *Bordetella pertussis*, *Bordetella parapertussis* and *Bordetella bronchiseptica*. *Nat. Genet.* **35:**32–40.

Richardson, A. R., and I. Stojiljkovic. 2001. Mismatch repair and the regulation of phase variation in Neisseria meningitidis. *Mol. Microbiol.* **40:**645–655.

Richardson, A. R., Z. Yu, T. Popovic, and I. Stojiljkovic. 2002. Mutator clones of *Neisseria meningitidis* in epidemic serogroup A disease. *Proc. Natl. Acad. Sci. USA* **99:**6103–6107.

Roberts, L. 2008. Infectious disease. An ill wind, bringing meningitis. *Science* **320:**1710–1715.

Roberts, M. C., and J. S. Knapp. 1988. Host range of the conjugative 25.2—megadalton tetracycline resistance plasmid from *Neisseria gonorrhoeae* and related species. *Antimicrob. Agents Chemother.* **32:**488–491.

Rocha, E. P. 2006. Inference and analysis of the relative stability of bacterial chromosomes. *Mol. Biol. Evol.* **23:**513–522.

Rosenstein, N. E., B. A. Perkins, D. S. Stephens, T. Popovic, and J. M. Hughes. 2001. Meningococcal disease. *N. Engl. J. Med.* **344:**1378–1388.

Rouquette-Loughlin, C. E., J. T. Balthazar, S. A. Hill, and W. M. Shafer. 2004. Modulation of the *mtrCDE*—encoded efflux pump gene complex of Neisseria meningitidis due to a Correia element insertion sequence. *Mol. Microbiol.* **54:**731–741.

Sarkari, J., N. Pandit, E. R. Moxon, and M. Achtman. 1994. Variable expression of the Opc outer membrane protein in Neisseria meningitidis is caused by size variation of a promoter containing poly—cytidine. *Mol. Microbiol.* **13:**207–217.

Saunders, N. J., A. C. Jeffries, J. F. Peden, D. W. Hood, H. Tettelin, R. Rappuoli, and E. R. Moxon. 2000. Repeat—associated phase variable genes in the complete genome sequence of Neisseria meningitidis strain MC58. *Mol. Microbiol.* **37:**207–215.

Saunders, N. J., and L. A. Snyder. 2002. The minimal mobile element. *Microbiology* **148:**3756–3760.

Schmitt, C., D. Turner, M. Boesl, M. Abele, M. Frosch, and O. Kurzai. 2007. A functional two—partner secretion system contributes to adhesion of *Neisseria meningitidis* to epithelial cells. *J. Bacteriol.* **189:**7968–7976.

Schoen, C., J. Blom, H. Claus, A. Schramm-Gluck, P. Brandt, T. Muller, A. Goesmann, B. Joseph, S. Konietzny, O. Kurzai, C. Schmitt, T. Friedrich, B. Linke, U. Vogel, and M. Frosch. 2008. Whole—genome comparison of disease and carriage strains provides insights into virulence evolution in *Neisseria meningitidis. Proc. Natl. Acad. Sci. USA* **105:**3473–3478.

Schoen, C., B. Joseph, H. Claus, U. Vogel, and M. Frosch. 2007. Living in a changing environment: insights into host adaptation in Neisseria meningitidis from comparative genomics. *Int. J. Med. Microbiol.* **297:**601–613.

Schoen, C., H. Tettelin, J. Parkhill, and M. Frosch. 2009. Genome flexibility in Neisseria meningitidis. *Vaccine* **27:**B103–B111.

Schofield, M. J., and P. Hsieh. 2003. DNA mismatch repair: molecular mechanisms and biological function. *Annu. Rev. Microbiol.* **57:**579–608.

Segal, E., P. Hagblom, H. S. Seifert, and M. So. 1986. Antigenic variation of gonococcal pilus involves assembly of separated silent gene segments. *Proc. Natl. Acad. Sci. USA* **83:**2177–2181.

Seifert, H. S., R. S. Ajioka, C. Marchal, P. F. Sparling, and M. So. 1988. DNA transformation leads to pilin antigenic variation in Neisseria gonorrhoeae. *Nature* **336:**392–395.

Selander, R. K., and B. R. Levin. 1980. Genetic diversity and structure in *Escherichia coli* populations. *Science* **210:**545–547.

Slupphaug, G., B. Kavli, and H. E. Krokan. 2003. The interacting pathways for prevention and repair of oxidative DNA damage. *Mutat. Res.* **531:**231–251.

Smith, J. M., C. G. Dowson, and B. G. Spratt. 1991. Localized sex in bacteria. *Nature* **349:**29–31.

Smith, J. M., N. H. Smith, M. O'Rourke, and B. G. Spratt. 1993. How clonal are bacteria? *Proc. Natl. Acad. Sci. USA* **90:**4384–4388.

Snyder, L. A., J. K. Davies, C. S. Ryan, and N. J. Saunders. 2005a. Comparative overview of the genomic and genetic differences between the pathogenic Neisseria strains and species. *Plasmid* **54:**191–218.

Snyder, L. A., S. A. Jarvis, and N. J. Saunders. 2005b. Complete and variant forms of the 'gonococcal genetic island' in Neisseria meningitidis. *Microbiology* **151:**4005–4013.

Snyder, L. A., S. McGowan, M. Rogers, E. Duro, E. O'Farrell, and N. J. Saunders. 2007. The repertoire of minimal mobile elements in the Neisseria species and evidence that these are involved in horizontal gene transfer in other bacteria. *Mol. Biol. Evol.* **24:**2802–2815.

Snyder, L. A., and N. J. Saunders. 2006. The majority of genes in the pathogenic Neisseria species are present in non—pathogenic Neisseria lactamica, including those designated as virulence genes. *BMC Genomics* **7:**128.

Snyder, L. A., W. M. Shafer, and N. J. Saunders. 2003. Divergence and transcriptional analysis of the division cell wall *(dcw)* gene cluster in Neisseria spp. *Mol. Microbiol.* **47:**431–442.

Snyder, L. A. S., S. A. Butcher, and N. J. Saunders. 2001. Comparative whole—genome analyses reveal over 100 putative phase—variable genes in the pathogenic Neisseria spp. *Microbiology* **147:**2321–2332.

Spratt, B. G., L. D. Bowler, Q. Y. Zhang, J. Zhou, and J. M. Smith. 1992. Role of interspecies transfer of chromosomal genes in the evolution of penicillin resistance in pathogenic and commensal Neisseria species. *J. Mol. Evol.* **34:**115–125.

Srikhanta, Y. N., T. L. Maguire, K. J. Stacey, S. M. Grimmond, and M. P. Jennings. 2005. The phasevarion: a genetic system controlling coordinated, random switching of expression of multiple genes. *Proc. Natl. Acad. Sci. USA* **102:**5547–5551.

Stabler, R. A., G. L. Marsden, A. A. Witney, Y. Li, S. D. Bentley, C. M. Tang, and J. Hinds. 2005. Identification of pathogen—specific genes through microarray analysis of pathogenic and commensal Neisseria species. *Microbiology* **151:**2907–2922.

Stephens, D. S. 2009. Biology and pathogenesis of the evolutionarily successful, obligate human bacterium Neisseria meningitidis. *Vaccine* **27:**B71–B77.

Stephens, D. S. 1999. Uncloaking the meningococcus: dynamics of carriage and disease. *Lancet* **353:**941–942.

Stephens, D. S., B. Greenwood, and P. Brandtzaeg. 2007. Epidemic meningitis, meningococcaemia, and Neisseria meningitidis. *Lancet* **369:**2196–2210.

Stern, A., and T. F. Meyer. 1987. Common mechanism controlling phase and antigenic variation in pathogenic neisseriae. *Mol. Microbiol.* **1:**5–12.

Stojiljkovic, I., V. Hwa, L. de Saint Martin, P. O'Gaora, X. Nassif, F. Heffron, and M. So. 1995. The Neisseria meningitidis haemoglobin receptor: its role in iron utilization and virulence. *Mol. Microbiol.* **15:**531–541.

Stollenwerk, N., M. C. Maiden, and V. A. Jansen. 2004. Diversity in pathogenicity can cause outbreaks of meningococcal disease. *Proc. Natl. Acad. Sci. USA* **101:**10229–10234.

Strathdee, C. A., S. D. Tyler, J. A. Ryan, W. M. Johnson, and F. E. Ashton. 1993. Genomic fingerprinting of *Neisseria meningitidis* associated with group C meningococcal disease in Canada. *J. Clin. Microbiol.* **31:**2506–2508.

Suker, J., I. M. Feavers, M. Achtman, G. Morelli, J. F. Wang, and M. C. Maiden. 1994. The *porA* gene in serogroup A meningococci: evolutionary stability and mechanism of genetic variation. *Mol. Microbiol.* **12:**253–265.

Tenaillon, O., F. Taddei, M. Radman, and I. Matic. 2001. Second—order selection in bacterial evolution: selection acting on mutation and recombination rates in the course of adaptation. *Res. Microbiol.* **152:**11–16.

Tettelin, H., K. E. Nelson, I. T. Paulsen, J. A. Eisen, T. D. Read, S. Peterson, J. Heidelberg, R. T. DeBoy, D. H. Haft, R. J. Dodson, A. S. Durkin, M. Gwinn, J. F. Kolonay, W. C. Nelson, J. D. Peterson, L. A. Umayam, O. White, S. L. Salzberg, M. R. Lewis, D. Radune, E. Holtzapple, H. Khouri, A. M. Wolf, T. R. Utterback, C. L. Hansen, L. A. McDonald, T. V. Feldblyum, S. Angiuoli, T. Dickinson, E. K. Hickey, I. E. Holt, B. J. Loftus, F. Yang, H. O. Smith, J. C. Venter, B. A. Dougherty, D. A. Morrison, S. K. Hollingshead, and C. M. Fraser. 2001. Complete genome sequence of a virulent isolate of *Streptococcus pneumoniae. Science* **293:**498–506.

Tettelin, H., D. Riley, C. Cattuto, and D. Medini. 2008. Comparative genomics: the bacterial pan—genome. *Curr. Opin. Microbiol.* **11:**472–477.

Tettelin, H., N. J. Saunders, J. Heidelberg, A. C. Jeffries, K. E. Nelson, J. A. Eisen, K. A. Ketchum, D. W. Hood, J. F. Peden, R. J. Dodson, W. C. Nelson, M. L. Gwinn, R. DeBoy, J. D. Peterson, E. K. Hickey, D. H. Haft, S. L. Salzberg, O. White, R. D. Fleischmann, B. A. Dougherty, T. Mason, A. Ciecko, D. S. Parksey, E. Blair, H. Cittone, E. B. Clark, M. D. Cotton, T. R. Utterback, H. Khouri, H. Qin, J. Vamathevan, J. Gill, V. Scarlato, V. Masignani, M. Pizza, G. Grandi, L. Sun, H. O. Smith, C. M. Fraser, E. R. Moxon, R. Rappuoli, and J. C. Venter. 2000. Complete genome sequence of *Neisseria meningitidis* serogroup B strain MC58. *Science* **287:**1809-1815.

Tobiason, D. M., and H. S. Seifert. 2006. The obligate human pathogen, Neisseria gonorrhoeae, is polyploid. *PLoS Biol.* **4:**e185.

Treangen, T. J., O. H. Ambur, T. Tonjum, and E. P. C. Rocha. 2008. The impact of the neisserial

DNA uptake sequences on genome evolution and stability. *Genome Biol.* **9:**R60.

van der Ende, A., C. T. Hopman, S. Zaat, B. B. Essink, B. Berkhout, and J. Dankert. 1995. Variable expression of class 1 outer membrane protein in *Neisseria meningitidis* is caused by variation in the spacing between the _10 and _35 regions of the promoter. *J. Bacteriol.* **177:**2475–2480.

van Passel, M. W., A. van der Ende, and A. Bart. 2006. Plasmid diversity in neisseriae. *Infect. Immun.* **74:**4892–4899.

van Ulsen, P., and J. Tommassen. 2006. Protein secretion and secreted proteins in pathogenic Neisseriaceae. *FEMS Microbiol. Rev.* **30:**292–319.

van Valen, L. 1973. A new evolutionary law. *Evol. Theory* **1:**1–30.

Vogel, U., G. Morelli, K. Zurth, H. Claus, E. Kriener, M. Achtman, and M. Frosch. 1998. Necessity of molecular techniques to distinguish between *Neisseria meningitidis* strains isolated from patients with meningococcal disease and from their healthy contacts. *J. Clin. Microbiol.* **36:**2465–2470.

Yazdankhah, S. P., P. Kriz, G. Tzanakaki, J. Kremastinou, J. Kalmusova, M. Musilek, T. Alvestad, K. A. Jolley, D. J. Wilson, N. D. McCarthy, D. A. Caugant, and M. C. Maiden. 2004. Distribution of serogroups and genotypes among disease—associated and carried isolates of *Neisseria meningitidis* from the Czech Republic, Greece, and Norway. *J. Clin. Microbiol.* **42:**5146–5153.

Zhou, J., and B. G. Spratt. 1992. Sequence diversity within the *argF*, *fbp* and *recA* genes of natural isolates of Neisseria meningitidis: interspecies recombination within the *argF* gene. *Mol. Microbiol.* **6:**2135–2146.

Zhu, P., A. van der Ende, D. Falush, N. Brieske, G. Morelli, B. Linz, T. Popovic, I. G. Schuurman, R. A. Adegbola, K. Zurth, S. Gagneux, A. E. Platonov, J. Y. Riou, D. A. Caugant, P. Nicolas, and M. Achtman. 2001. Fit genotypes and escape variants of subgroup III *Neisseria meningitidis* during three pandemics of epidemic meningitis. *Proc. Natl. Acad. Sci. USA* **98:**5234–5239.

SELFISH ELEMENTS AND SELF-DEFENSE IN THE ENTEROCOCCI

Kelli L. Palmer and Michael S. Gilmore

8

The enterococci are gram-positive lactic acid bacteria, typically found as oral and intestinal colonizers of humans (Tannock and Cook, 2002; DeVriese et al., 2006), and intestinal colonizers of nonhuman mammals, birds, and insects (Aarestrup et al., 2002). Enterococci are of commercial interest because of their use in probiotics (Domann et al., 2007) and fermented food and cheese production (Foulquie Moreno et al., 2006). However, since the 1980s they have emerged as leading causes of hospital-acquired infection (Hidron et al., 2008). Among these infections are device-associated bloodstream and urinary tract infections (Hidron et al., 2008) and surgical-site infections ranging from hospital-acquired endocarditis (Murray, 1990) to endophthalmitis (Callegan et al., 2002; Scott et al., 2003). Enterococci are also the leading cause of surgical-site infections in heart, liver, and kidney transplant patients (Hidron et al., 2008). Most infections are caused by *Enterococcus faecalis* and *E. faecium* (Hidron et al., 2008). Enterococcal species such as *E. gallinarum* (Contreras et al., 2008) and *E. raffinosus* (Samuel et al., 2008) have also been associated with infection, but these are comparatively rare. The recent and alarming trend of increasing antibiotic resistance in the enterococci, especially to last-line antibiotics such as vancomycin, and global hospital infection outbreaks of multidrug-resistant enterococci are of great concern (Kirkpatrick et al., 1999; Kawalec et al., 2000; Pournaras et al., 2000; Handwerger et al., 1993; Valdezate et al., 2009; Zhu et al., 2009; McBride et al., 2007).

Why enterococci in particular emerged from among commensal microorganisms to become leading hospital pathogens is unknown. Their success is due, at least in part, to their propensity to acquire mobile genetic elements that encode novel traits such antibiotic resistance as well as cohorts of other genes that contribute to virulence. It is rapidly becoming apparent that multidrug-resistant, hospital outbreak enterococcal lineages are distinct in genome content from those that stably and benignly inhabit the intestine or are used for probiotic and food production. Further evidence is accumulating that commensal enterococci possess endogenous mechanisms to protect genome integrity and that these mechanisms are absent or have been lost in multidrug-resistant infection isolates. Specific mechanisms implicated in enterococcal genome defense are restriction-modification

Kelli L. Palmer and Michael S. Gilmore, Schepens Eye Research Institute, 20 Staniford St., Boston, MA 02144.

Genome Plasticity and Infectious Diseases,
Edited by J. Hacker, U. Dobrindt, and R. Kurth,

and the recently discovered clustered, regularly interspaced, short palindromic repeats (CRISPR), which are functionally analogous to an acquired immune system (Barrangou et al., 2007). In this chapter, the genome plasticity that has led to distinct subpopulations of enterococci, as well as the evidence for loss of genome defenses as precipitating events in their emergence, is reviewed.

EVIDENCE OF GENOME PLASTICITY

Enterococcal genome plasticity was strikingly revealed when the phylogenetic relatedness within a collection of 106 *E. faecalis* strains was compared to their content of known variable traits, including antibiotic resistances, capsule loci, and elements of the *E. faecalis* pathogenicity island (PAI) (McBride et al., 2007). Strains utilized in the study were isolated over the last century from clinical, commensal, and environmental sites around the world. Relatedness of the *E. faecalis* strains was evaluated by multilocus sequence typing (MLST), an epidemiological tool used to delineate subspecies phylogenetic relationships. MLST relies on amplification, sequencing, and alignment of internal fragments of housekeeping genes (Urwin and Maiden, 2003). It was observed in this study that the capsule locus, which lacks any hallmarks of a mobile element (Hancock and Gilmore, 2002; Hancock et al., 2003), is distributed in a discontinuous manner across the entire MLST-based phylogenetic tree for the *E. faecalis* species (McBride et al., 2007). Portions of the PAI are distributed similarly throughout the species. Interestingly, virulence traits such as cytolytic toxin (cytolysin) production and conjugated bile salt hydrolase production, and the extent of PAI carriage (Shankar et al., 2002), appear to cluster in MLST lineages in which antibiotic resistance traits also cluster (McBride et al., 2007), despite these traits generally being conveyed by separate genetic elements (Fig. 1). Multidrug-resistant lineages of note in which virulence traits appear to have accumulated are the clonal complexes CC2, CC8, and CC9 (Fig. 1). A CC includes single- and double-locus variants of a founder isolate (McBride et al., 2007). Earlier evidence for convergence of virulence traits in certain *E. faecalis* lineages includes the observation that PAI presence is significantly enriched in antibiotic-resistant infection-derived isolates compared to animal and human commensal isolates (Nallapareddy et al., 2005).

Further evidence supporting a high level of plasticity in *E. faecalis* comes from a genomic comparison of the bloodstream infection isolate *E. faecalis* V583 (Sahm et al., 1989; Paulsen et al., 2003), a member of the CC2 lineage, and the human oral isolate *E. faecalis* OG1RF (Gold et al., 1975; Bourgogne et al., 2008), until recently the only two publicly available genome sequences for *E. faecalis*. The V583 genome contains seven predicted prophage, three plasmids, two chromosomally integrated plasmids, the PAI (itself containing another integrated plasmid [Shankar et al., 2002]), a vancomycin resistance transposon, two additional putative genomic islands, and at least 38 insertion sequences (IS) (Paulsen et al., 2003; McBride et al., 2007; Lepage et al., 2006). These elements encode most of the known enterococcal virulence factors, including cytolysin and aggregation substance, antibiotic resistances, and novel metabolic pathways (Paulsen et al., 2003; Shankar et al., 2002). It is estimated that more than one-quarter of the V583 genome is mobile in origin (Paulsen et al., 2003). In contrast, the OG1RF genome possesses only a Tn*916* homologue (Bourgogne et al., 2008) and one prophage that does not appear to be mobile as it has been shown to be a core component of the *E. faecalis* genome (McBride et al., 2007; Solheim et al., 2009).V583 possesses approximately 620 kb of additional coding potential compared to OG1RF, the vast majority of which is predicted to derive from mobile elements.

E. faecalis CC2 strains, such as V583, appear to be well suited for clinical environments and have been associated with hospital infection outbreaks around the world (Huycke et al., 1991; Ruiz-Garbajosa et al., 2006; Nallapareddy et al., 2005; Freitas et al., 2009a; Kawalec et al., 2007). Interestingly, CC2 strains have been been isolated only since 1981 (McBride et al.,

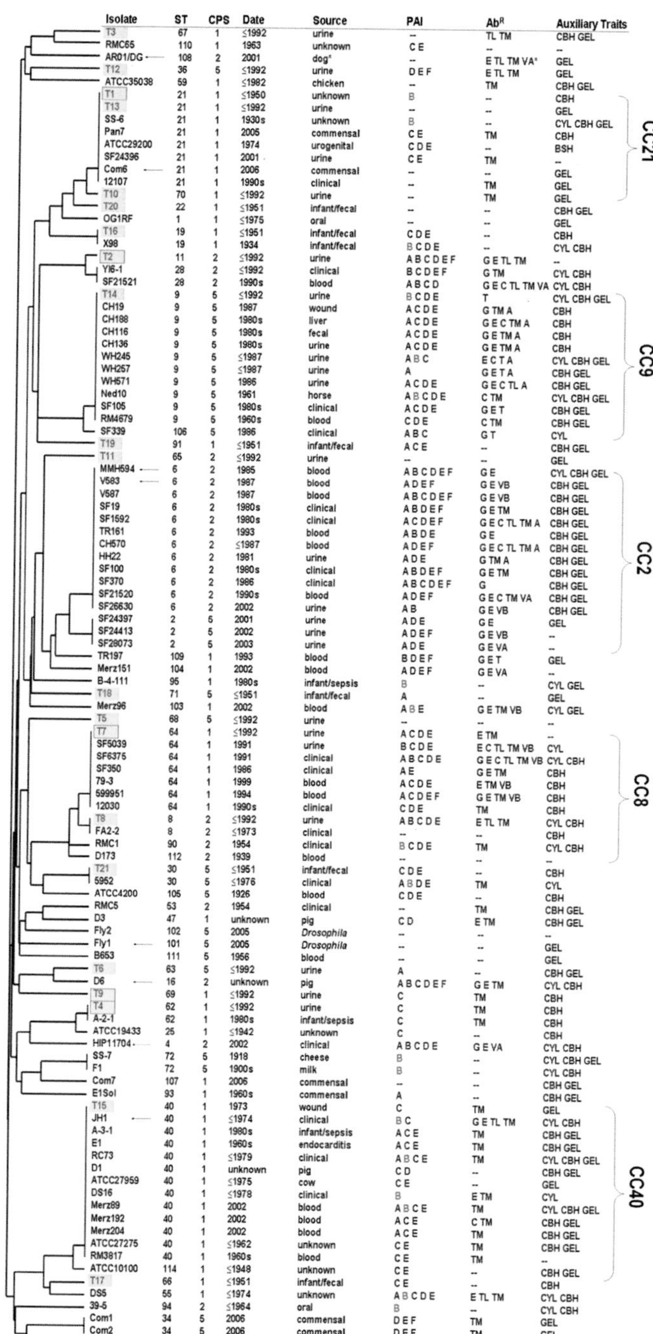

Isolate	ST	CPS	Date	Source	PAI	Ab^R	Auxiliary Traits
T3	67	1	≤1992	urine	--	TL TM	CBH GEL
RMC65	110	1	1963	unknown	C E	--	--
AR01/DG	108	2	2001	dog*	--	E TL TM VA*	GEL
T12	36	5	≤1992	urine	D E F	E TL TM	GEL
ATCC35038	59	1	≤1982	chicken	--	TM	CBH GEL
T1	21	1	≤1950	unknown	B	--	CBH
T13	21	1	≤1992	urine	--	--	GEL
SS-6	21	1	1930s	unknown	B	--	CYL CBH GEL
Pan7	21	1	2005	commensal	C E	TM	CBH
ATCC29200	21	1	1974	urogenital	C D E	--	BSH
SF24396	21	1	2001	urine	C E	TM	--
Com6	21	1	2006	commensal	--	--	GEL
12107	21	1	1990s	clinical	--	TM	GEL
T10	70	1	≤1992	urine	--	TM	GEL
T20	22	1	≤1951	infant/fecal	--	--	CBH GEL
OG1RF	1	1	≤1975	oral	--	--	GEL
T16	19	1	≤1951	infant/fecal	C D E	--	CBH
X98	19	1	1934	infant/fecal	B C D E	--	CYL CBH
T2	11	2	≤1992	urine	A B C D E F	G E TL TM	--
YI6-1	28	2	≤1992	clinical	B C D E F	G TM	CYL CBH
SF21521	28	2	1990s	blood	A B C D	G E C TL TM VA	CYL CBH
T14	9	5	≤1992	urine	B C D E	T	CYL CBH GEL
CH19	9	5	1987	wound	A C D E	G TM A	CBH
CH188	9	5	1980s	liver	A C D E	G E C TM A	CBH
CH116	9	5	1980s	fecal	A C D E	G E TM A	CBH
CH136	9	5	1980s	urine	A C D E	G E TM A	CBH
WH245	9	5	≤1987	urine	A B C	E C T A	CYL CBH GEL
WH257	9	5	≤1987	urine	A	G E T A	CBH GEL
WH571	9	5	1986	urine	A C D E	G E C TL A	CBH GEL
Ned10	9	5	1961	horse	A B C D E	C TM	CYL CBH GEL
SF105	9	5	1980s	clinical	A C D E	G E T	CBH GEL
RM4679	9	5	1960s	blood	C D E	C TM	CBH GEL
SF339	106	5	1986	clinical	A B C	G T	CYL
T19	91	1	≤1951	infant/fecal	A C E	--	CBH GEL
T11	65	2	≤1992	urine	--	--	GEL
MMH594	6	2	1985	blood	A B C D E F	G E	CYL CBH GEL
V583	6	2	1987	blood	A D E F	G E VB	CBH GEL
V587	6	2	1987	blood	A B C D E F	G E VB	CBH GEL
SF19	6	2	1980s	clinical	A B D E F	G E TM	CBH GEL
SF1592	6	2	1980s	clinical	A C D E F	G E C TL TM A	CBH GEL
TR161	6	2	1993	blood	A B D E	G E	CBH GEL
CH570	6	2	≤1987	blood	A D E F	G E C TL TM A	CBH GEL
HH22	6	2	1981	urine	A D E	G TM A	CBH GEL
SF100	6	2	1980s	clinical	A B D E F	G E TM	CBH GEL
SF370	6	2	1986	clinical	A B C D E F	G	CBH GEL
SF21520	6	2	1990s	blood	A D E F	G E C TM VA	CBH GEL
SF26630	6	2	2002	urine	A B	G E VB	CBH GEL
SF24397	2	5	2001	urine	A D E	G E	GEL
SF24413	2	5	2002	urine	A D E F	G E VB	--
SF28073	2	5	2003	urine	A D E	G E VA	--
TR197	109	1	1993	blood	B D E F	G E T	GEL
Merz151	104	1	2002	blood	A D E F	G E VA	--
B-4-111	95	1	1980s	infant/sepsis	B	--	CYL GEL
T18	71	5	≤1951	infant/fecal	A	--	GEL
Merz96	103	1	2002	blood	A B E	G E TM VB	CYL GEL
T5	68	5	≤1992	urine	--	--	--
T7	64	1	≤1992	urine	A C D E	E TM	--
SF5039	64	1	1991	urine	B C D E	E C TL TM VB	CYL
SF6375	64	1	1991	clinical	A B C D E	G E C TL TM VB	CYL CBH
SF350	64	1	1986	clinical	A E	G E TM	CBH
79-3	64	1	1999	blood	A C D E	E TM VB	CBH
599951	64	1	1994	blood	A C D E F	G E TM VB	CBH
12030	64	1	1990s	clinical	C D E	TM	CBH
T8	8	2	≤1992	urine	A B C D E	E TL TM	CYL CBH
FA2-2	8	2	≤1973	clinical	--	--	CBH
RMC1	90	2	1954	clinical	B C D E	TM	CYL CBH
D173	112	2	1939	blood	--	--	--
T21	30	5	≤1951	infant/fecal	C D E	--	CBH
5952	30	5	≤1976	clinical	A B D E	TM	CYL
ATCC4200	105	5	1926	blood	C D E	--	CBH
RMC5	53	2	1954	clinical	--	TM	CBH GEL
D3	47	1	unknown	pig	C D	E TM	CBH GEL
Fly2	102	5	2005	*Drosophila*	--	--	--
Fly1	101	5	2005	*Drosophila*	--	--	GEL
B653	111	5	1956	blood	--	--	GEL
T6	63	5	≤1992	urine	A	--	CBH GEL
D6	16	2	unknown	pig	A B C D E F	G E TM	CYL CBH
T9	69	1	≤1992	urine	C	TM	CBH
T4	62	1	≤1992	urine	C	TM	CBH
A-2-1	62	1	1980s	infant/sepsis	C	TM	CBH
ATCC19433	25	1	≤1942	unknown	C	--	CBH
HIP11704	4	2	2002	clinical	A B C D E	G E VA	CYL CBH
SS-7	72	5	1918	cheese	B	--	CYL CBH GEL
F1	72	5	1900s	milk	B	--	CYL CBH
Com7	107	1	2006	commensal	--	--	CBH GEL
E1Sol	93	1	1960s	commensal	A	--	CBH GEL
T15	40	1	1973	wound	C	TM	GEL
JH1	40	1	≤1974	clinical	B C	G E TL TM	CYL CBH
A-3-1	40	1	1980s	infant/sepsis	A C E	TM	CBH GEL
E1	40	1	1960s	endocarditis	A C E	TM	CBH GEL
RC73	40	1	≤1979	clinical	A B C E	TM	CYL CBH GEL
D1	40	1	unknown	pig	C D	--	CBH GEL
ATCC27959	40	1	≤1975	cow	C E	--	GEL
DS16	40	1	≤1978	clinical	B	E TM	CYL
Merz89	40	1	2002	blood	A B C E	TM	CYL CBH GEL
Merz192	40	1	2002	blood	A C E	C TM	CBH GEL
Merz204	40	1	2002	blood	A C E	TM	CBH GEL
ATCC27275	40	1	≤1962	unknown	C E	TM	CBH GEL
RM3817	40	1	1960s	blood	C E	TM	--
ATCC10100	114	1	≤1948	unknown	C E	--	CBH GEL
T17	66	1	≤1951	infant/fecal	C E	--	CBH
DS5	55	1	≤1974	unknown	A B C D E	E TL TM	CYL CBH
39-5	94	2	≤1964	oral	B	--	CYL CBH
Com1	34	5	2006	commensal	D E F	TM	GEL
Com2	34	5	2006	commensal	D E F	TM	GEL
ATCC6055	113	1	≤1937	milk	--	--	--

FIGURE 1 Phylogenetic relatedness and variable trait profile of diverse *E. faecalis* isolates. Shown is the MLST dendrogram for 106 *E. faecalis* strains, aligned with their capsule type (CPS), date of isolation, isolation source, PAI fragment content, antibiotic resistance profile, and phenotypic auxiliary traits. PAI fragments are designated A through F, and a red letter B indicates that the strain can conjugatively transfer cytolysin to other *E. faecalis* strains. Antibiotic resistance shown includes tetracycline (TL, *tetL*; TM, *tetM*), erythromycin (E, *ermB*), gentamicin (G), chloramphenicol (C, *cat*), ampicillin (A, *blaZ*), and vancomycin (VA, *vanA*; VB, *vanB*) resistance. Auxiliary traits are cytolysin production (CYL), conjugated bile salt hydrolase production (CBH), and gelatinase production (GEL). Reprinted from *PLoS One* (McBride et al., 2007).

2007; Nallapareddy et al., 2005), suggesting that this lineage recently emerged and rapidly expanded. It remains to be determined whether a high level of genome plasticity is a common property of CC2 *E. faecalis*, although the preponderance of acquired antibiotic resistance genes (at least six potentially independently acquired traits in some strains [McBride et al., 2007]), PAI genes (McBride et al., 2007; Nallapareddy et al., 2005), and resistance plasmids

(Freitas et al., 2009a) in CC2 strains strongly suggests that this is so.

Antibiotic resistance determinants have also converged in the *E. faecium* lineage CC17, responsible for hospital infection outbreaks around the world (Willems et al., 2003; Freitas et al., 2009b; Valdezate et al., 2009, Leavis et al., 2006, 2007; Zhu et al., 2009; Libisch et al., 2008). This *E. faecium* lineage appears to be highly adapted for hospital persistence and human infection. Using comparative genomic hybridization of 97 *E. faecium* strains of diverse clinical and nonclinical origins, it was recently shown that mobile element content is a defining feature of *E. faecium* CC17 and other hospital strains (Leavis et al., 2007). Hospital- and outbreak-derived *E. faecium* isolates form a distinct phylogenetic clade enriched in IS and in genes derived from plasmids, phages, and transposons (Leavis et al., 2007). There is also evidence that strains of this hospital clade are more prone to genome rearrangements, potentially resulting from intragenomic recombination between copies of the repetitive mobile element IS*16* (Leavis et al., 2007).

Collectively, studies of *E. faecalis* and *E. faecium* phylogenetic, genotypic, and phenotypic diversity indicate that multidrug-resistant enterococcal outbreaks emerged as a result of the accretion of virulence, antibiotic resistance, and new metabolic properties on mobile elements in specific MLST lineages, generating most of the genome plasticity observed, while commensal enterococcal strains possess smaller, comparatively stable genomes with fewer mobile elements.

RELATIONSHIP OF GENOME PLASTICITY TO VIRULENCE

There are several, non-mutually exclusive scenarios for the success of the *E. faecalis* CC2 and *E. faecium* CC17 lineages in clinical environments (for an extensive model of *E. faecalis* infection, see Pillar and Gilmore [2004]). The multiple antibiotic resistance encoded by these strains could allow them to survive antibiotic treatment, allowing them to proliferate to fill intestinal niches vacated by susceptible microbes. *E. faecalis* V583 contains a number of metabolic pathways that appear to have been conveyed by mobile elements and are absent in OG1RF, suggesting that hospital strains may not compete directly with commensal enterococci for these new niches (Gilmore and Ferretti, 2003). This expansion could be augmented further by genes that promote colonization of new niches, such as bacteriocins for warfare in intermicrobial competition, or adhesins promoting attachment to sites such as the urinary tract and cardiac tissue. All of these are putative or confirmed virulence properties that have been ascribed to the *E. faecalis* PAI (Shankar et al., 2002) and *E. faecium* PAIs (which are distinct from the *E. faecalis* PAI) (Heikens et al., 2008; Leavis et al., 2004). It is also possible that these strains have acquired genes to promote survival on surfaces and hospital persistence. Mobile genetic elements, in combination with core (such as the *E. faecalis* Ace adhesin [Nallapareddy et al., 2000; Lebreton et al., 2009; Singh et al., 2010]) and variable (such as *E. faecalis* gelatinase production [McBride et al., 2007; Engelbert et al., 2004; Suzuki et al., 2008; Sifri et al., 2002]) enterococcal traits, appear to significantly influence the potential for enterococci to cause disease.

Self-mobilizable genetic elements have been well characterized in the enterococci, several for the first time in any microbe, including pheromone-responsive conjugative plasmids and conjugative transposons (reviewed by Weaver et al. [2002] and Clewell and Dunny [2002]). These mobile elements contribute to the influx of new antibiotic resistance genes into enterococci (Weaver et al., 2002) and can mobilize or carry additional elements such as nonconjugative transposons, plasmids, and IS elements into the cell, all of which are likely to contribute to accretion of virulence determinants in genomic islands such as the *E. faecalis* PAI. The PAI itself has been shown to undergo rearrangement at a very high frequency (at rates of ~1 per 1,000 cells in laboratory culture) (Shankar et al., 2002), further adding to genome plasticity. A list of enterococcal plasmids of note and the known virulence or antibiotic resistance traits that they carry are shown in Table 1.

TABLE 1 Examples of enterococcal plasmids that have served as models for understanding their contribution to virulence and antibiotic resistance transmission

Name	Type of element	Virulence traits	Comments and references
pAD1	Pheromone-responsive plasmid	Aggregation substance; cytolysin	Extensively studied *E. faecalis* plasmid (Clewell, 2007)
pCF10	Pheromone-responsive plasmid	Aggregation substance; Tn*925-tetM*	Extensively studied *E. faecalis* plasmid conferring tetracycline resistance (Dunny, 2007)
pMG2200	Pheromone-responsive plasmid	Aggregation substance; Tn*1549-vanB2*	Found in *E. faecalis* isolates from hospitalized patients; confers vancomycin resistance (Zheng et al., 2009)
pMG1	Conjugative broad-host-range plasmid	Tn*4001-aacA-aphD*	From clinical *E. faecium* isolate; confers aminoglycoside resistance (Ike et al., 1998, Tanimoto and Ike, 2008)
pAM830	Conjugative broad-host-range plasmid	Tn*1546-vanA*	Implicated in first documented transfer of vancomycin resistance to methicillin-resistant *S. aureus* (Weigel et al., 2003; Flannagan et al., 2003)

Enterococci have evolved an elaborate system for exchange of mobile DNA. A group of plasmids exploit small peptides (pheromones) extruded by potential recipient cells as signals to induce donor conjugation machinery (for extensive reviews on pheromone-responsive plasmids, see Dunny [2007], Clewell [2007], and Clewell and Dunny [2002]). After successful transfer into a new cell, plasmid-encoded functions quench endogenous pheromone production by interfering with pheromone excretion and directing synthesis of a competitive pheromone inhibitor, turning the cell into a pheromone sensor capable of homing in on plasmid-free cells. Pheromone-responsive plasmids are of clinical concern because of their ability to rapidly shuttle antibiotic resistance genes among enterococcal populations. High-frequency transfers of pheromone-responsive plasmids have been observed during infection (Hirt et al., 2002) and intestinal colonization (Huycke et al.; 1992, Licht et al., 2002). The presence of pheromone-responsive plasmids in enterococci pre-dates the onset of widespread antibiotic therapy. For example, *E. faecalis* X98, isolated in 1934, possesses a pAD1-like pheromone-responsive plasmid lacking antibiotic resistance genes (Jett and Gilmore, 1990 and unpublished observations). The evolutionary and ecological dynamic of enterococci and these plasmids prior to antibiotic selection remains unclear, although it is likely that other beneficial traits, such as the cytolysin genes on the *E. faecalis* X98 pheromone-responsive plasmid (Jett and Gilmore, 1990), promote their maintenance.

The contributions of certain traits encoded by the pheromone-responsive plasmids and the *E. faecalis* PAI to enterococcal virulence have been extensively studied; these include cytolysin, aggregation substance, and the enterococcal surface protein Esp (for reviews of enterococcal virulence factors, see Pillar and Gilmore [2004] and Top et al. [2008]). The cytolysin (referred to historically in enterococcal literature as hemolysin/bacteriocin), encoded by pheromone-responsive plasmids (Clewell and Dunny, 2002) or the *E. faecalis* PAI (Shankar et al., 2002), contributes to the virulence of *E. faecalis* in models of peritoneal infection (Ike et al., 1984; Singh et al., 1998), ocular infection (Jett et al., 1992), and a *Caenorhabditis elegans* infection model (Garsin et al., 2001). In combination with acquired antibiotic resistance, the cytolysin was found to confer a fivefold-increased risk of death from human bacteremia (Huycke et al., 1991). Aggregation substance is an adhesin encoded by pheromone-responsive plasmids (Clewell and Dunny, 2002) that works synergistically with the *E. faecalis* cytolysin to generate lethal endocarditis vegetations (Chow et al., 1993) or by itself to generate larger vegetations (Chow et al., 1993; Chuang et al., 2009; Hirt et al., 2002). It can also be encoded by plasmid remnants inserted into the *E. faecalis* PAI (Shankar et al., 2002). Another virulence trait encoded by mobile elements, the enterococcal surface protein Esp, was first observed in clinical *E. faecalis* isolates (Shankar et al., 1999) and was later found to be encoded on the *E. faecalis* prototypic PAI (Shankar et al., 2002). Esp is also encoded on a putative *E. faecium* PAI, which is distinct from the *E. faecalis* PAI and is associated with clinical and epidemic *E. faecium* isolates (Willems et al., 2001; Leavis et al., 2004). Esp has been shown to promote biofilm formation (Tendolkar et al., 2004) and to contribute to *E. faecalis* and *E. faecium* colonization of the murine urinary tract (Shankar et al., 2001; Leendertse et al., 2009). It is important to note that, while experimental data are available for a handful of novel traits encoded by the pheromone-responsive plasmids and enterococcal PAIs, including cytolysin, aggregation substance, and Esp, there are hundreds of putative open reading frames (ORFs) located on these elements for which a function has not been confirmed or even predicted.

Comparatively little is known about the contributions of elements that generally do not encode antibiotic resistance determinants, such as phages and IS, to enterococcal virulence. Large numbers of phage exist in the gastrointestinal tract and in the environment (Gorski and Weber-Dabrowska, 2005), and the impact of phages on enterococcal ecology could be substantial. Phages capable of infecting enterococci have been isolated from human saliva (Bachrach et al., 2003), the human genitourinary tract (Caprioli et al., 1975), the rat intestinal tract (Rogers and Sarles, 1963), piggery effluent (Mazaheri Nezhad Fard et al., 2010), sewage (Brock, 1964; Caprioli et al., 1975), and water samples (Uchiyama et al., 2008). Further, there is evidence for extensive lysogeny of enterococci. This is apparent from mitomycin C-induced prophage recovery from enterococci isolated from infected root canals (Stevens et al., 2009), piggery effluent (Mazaheri Nezhad Fard et al., 2010), and clinical environments (Yasmin et al., 2010). Seven putative prophage were identified in the *E. faecalis* V583 genome, comprising ~7% of the *E. faecalis* V583 genome (~235 of 3,218 kb) (McBride et al., 2007; Paulsen et al., 2003), and it is possible that novel genes encoded by those elements contributed to V583 bloodstream infection or hospital persistence. Recently published evidence supports a role for prophages in enterococcal virulence (Yasmin et al., 2010). In this study, eight phage isolated by induction of prophage resident in *E. faecalis* clinical isolates were used to lysogenize the *E. faecalis* laboratory strain JH2-2. The virulence of these strains was then evaluated in a *Galleria mellonella* (caterpillar) insect infection model. Effects of lysogeny by individual phages ranged from significant decreases to significant increases in virulence relative to the control strain JH2-2. These results indicate that prophages influence the virulence potential of enterococci; however, further study is necessary to delineate their mechanistic contributions to the cell.

Two ways that IS element insertions could affect enterococcal virulence are by inactivation of chromosomal genes that contribute to stable commensalism and by intragenomic recombination, as multiple IS elements in the same cell provide repetitive homologous sequences at which recombination could occur. To our knowledge, the extent to which IS element inactivation of chromosomal genes contributes to the success of enterococci as pathogens has not been explored. However, there is evidence that intragenomic recombination at IS elements has contributed substantially to genome plasticity of the enterococci. As noted above, recombination at IS*16* elements appears to drive genome rearrangements in *E. faecium* CC17 and other clinical *E. faecium* isolates (Leavis et al., 2007). Further, although it had been inferred since the late 1970s that conjugative plasmids in *E. faecalis* could mobilize chromosomal antibiotic resistance markers, it was recently shown that either of two pheromone-responsive plasmids in *E. faecalis* V583 can mediate the transfer of any marker within the V583 chromosome into *E. faecalis* OG1RF (Manson et al., 2010). This included mobilization of the PAI, a vancomycin resistance transposon, the capsule locus, antibiotic resistance markers inserted into each of the nonessential two-component signaling loci of V583, and even MLST markers. Mobilization involved plasmid integration into the chromosome, which was shown to occur by recombination at IS*256* elements resident on both the chromosome and plasmids, and subsequent conjugative transfer by an Hfr-type mechanism (Manson et al., 2010). Thus, while the roles of IS elements in enterococcal virulence per se are unclear, it is clear that recombination at repetitive IS elements can promote genome diversification of enterococci, and in collusion with conjugative plasmids this process can generate enterococcal strains with "hybrid" genomes.

GENOME DEFENSE MECHANISMS IN THE ENTEROCOCCI

Two competing hypotheses could explain the accretion of plasmids, phages, and other mobile elements conferring novel traits in clinical enterococcal lineages such as *E. faecalis* CC2 and *E. faecium* CC17: either the enterococci are passive, or perhaps even active, receptacles for mobile DNA or the enterococci possess defenses that have become compromised in clinical lineages, perhaps under the pressure of antibiotic selection, allowing facile entry of foreign DNA and leading to rapidly evolving subpopulations. Supporting the second hypothesis is the observation that, of the 228 predicted genes specific to the stable, smaller genome of the non-CC2 strain *E. faecalis* OG1RF compared to the CC2 strain *E. faecalis* V583, several encode potential defense mechanisms (Bourgogne et al., 2008), including a putative restriction modification system and a complete CRISPR-*cas* locus.

Restriction-Modification

Bacterial restriction-modification systems have been extensively studied. These systems were first alluded to in the early 1950s in studies of coliphage infection, where it was noted that phage passaged through one *E. coli* strain could not efficiently infect a different *E. coli* strain (Bertani and Weigle, 1953; Luria and Human, 1952). These studies suggested that the phage had been modified in some way in the original host and that the modification interfered with infection of the new host. We now know that many bacteria modify their genetic material by the addition of chemical moieties such as methyl groups to discriminate self from nonself (Murray, 2002; Tock and Dryden, 2005). Cognate restriction endonucleases cleave unmodified, presumably nonself DNA; thus the system functions as a line of defense against parasitizing foreign DNA (Murray, 2002; Tock and Dryden, 2005). Perhaps not surprisingly, mobile elements have evolved strategies to evade this line of defense (reviewed by Tock and Dryden [2005]; see Serfiotis-Mitsa et al. [2008] for an example relevant to the enterococci). In addition, mobile elements can encode their own restriction modification systems (Jakubauskas et al., 2009; O'Driscoll et al., 2006) for the apparent selective benefit of monopolizing the host. Based on their efficacy at limiting entry of foreign elements, restriction-modification systems have been called a "leaky barrier" to lateral gene transfer (Tock and Dryden, 2005).

Several types of restriction-modification systems have been identified that vary in their subunit composition and number, sequence recognition, and restriction activity (Tock and Dryden [2005] and Murray [2002] are excellent reviews). Of these, type II enzymes are perhaps most familiar because type II restriction endonucleases are commonly utilized for cloning of recombinant DNA. Type II enzymes have two activities typically contained in two subunits: one confers the restriction endonuclease activity, and the other confers methylation (modification) (Tock and Dryden, 2005). Because of the commercial utility of restriction endonucleases, much effort has been devoted to their identification and biochemical characterization. One resource is REBASE, a database of genes and enzymes either predicted or experimentally confirmed to be involved in restriction-modification

(Roberts et al., 2007, 2010). REBASE utilizes GenBank data to predict the presence of restriction-modification systems in prokaryotic genomes (Roberts et al., 2007, 2010). As of January 2010, of the 1,063 prokaryotic genomes analyzed by REBASE, ~93% possess predicted restriction-modification systems. This suggests that restriction-modification is a basic biological property of prokaryotes. The ~7% of prokaryotes lacking predicted restriction-modification systems include intracellular parasites such as *Chlamydia* spp. and insect endosymbionts such as *Wigglesworthia*., *Blochmannia*, and *Blattabacterium* spp., which may have limited exposure to mobile DNA elements (Murray, 2002) and may have lost these activities through genome reduction.

While restriction-modification has been extensively studied for some bacterial species, few biochemical data for restriction-modification in enterococci exist. One type II restriction endonuclease, SfaI, was purified from an *E. faecalis* strain in 1978 (Wu et al., 1978). Interestingly, the authors noted that SfaI activity could not be detected in a different *E. faecalis* strain (Wu et al., 1978), indicating that SfaI production is a variable trait in *E. faecalis*. Two other type II restriction endonucleases, SfaGU and SfaNI, have been characterized in enterococci (Roberts, 1982), as well as the cognate methyltransferase for SfaNI (unpublished data in REBASE).

An analysis of restriction-modification systems encoded in enterococcal genomes has not been published. We utilized the complete genome sequence of *E. faecalis* OG1RF (Bourgogne et al., 2008) and REBASE predictions for restriction-modification components in the complete *E. faecalis* V583 genome to evaluate the potential for restriction-modification in these two strains. The results of this compilation and analysis are shown in Table 2. Our first and most striking observation is that all predicted restriction-modification components of *E. faecalis* V583 reside on mobile genetic elements. In fact, five of the six predicted components code for modification functions only, highlighting a potential subversion tactic. It should be noted that prediction of restriction endonuclease genes is complicated by the divergence of these genes (Roberts et al., 2010); however, initial examination of genes flanking the five predicted type II methyltransferases found no restriction endonuclease candidates. A final predicted component, located on the pTEF3 plasmid, is a potential dual-function restriction-modification enzyme. The lack of chromosomally encoded restriction-modification genes suggests that *E. faecalis* V583 lacks this line of defense and that this may have contributed to the convergence of mobile genetic elements in this strain.

TABLE 2 Putative restriction-modification systems in complete *E. faecalis* genomes

ORF[a]	Annotated function[a]	Predicted function[b]	Genomic location[a]
OG1RF_0043	DNA (cytosine-5-)-MT	Type II M	On Tn*916* homologue
OG1RF_0146	Hypothetical protein	NgoFVII superfamily RE	Chromosomally encoded
OG1RF_0147	DNA (cytosine-5-)-MT	Type II M	Chromosomally encoded
V583 EF1452	Putative adenine MT	Type II M	On prophage 3
V583 EF2114	Putative adenine MT	Type II M	On prophage 5
V583 EF2124	Putative MT	Type II M	On prophage 5
V583 EF2323	Adenine-specific DNA MT-like gene	Type II M	On Tn/*vanB*
V583 EF2340	DNA (cytosine-5-)-MT	Type II M	On putative genomic island
V583 EFC0005	RE related protein	Type II fused RE-M	On pTEF3

[a]*E. faecalis* OG1RF ORFs, annotated functions, and genomic locations are from Bourgogne et al. (2008) supplementary material and GenBank. *E. faecalis* V583 potential restriction-modification ORFs were predicted by REBASE (http://rebase.neb.com/), annotated functions are from GenBank, and genomic locations are described by McBride et al. (2007). MT, methyltransferase; M, modification; RE, restriction endonuclease.

[b]*E. faecalis* V583 predictions were extracted from REBASE. *E. faecalis* OG1RF predictions were obtained by BLASTP of translated ORFs in REBASE. REBASE BLASTP of OG1RF_0146 yielded partial alignments; predicted function is from a conserved protein domain search (http://www.ncbi.nlm.nih.gov/Structure/cdd/wrpsb.cgi).

In contrast to *E. faecalis* V583, *E. faecalis* OG1RF possesses a potential type II restriction-modification system encoded by the ORFs OG1RF_0146 and OG1RF_0147 (Table 2). OG1RF_0147 is a putative type II cytosine-modifying methyltransferase with homology to predicted type II restriction-modification methyltransferases of other gram-positive bacteria including *Bacillus cereus, Thermanaerovibrio acidaminovorans,* and *Clostridium thermocellum*. OG1RF_0146, a putative type II restriction endonuclease, is encoded immediately downstream of OG1RF_0147. Only 18 nucleotides separate these genes, suggesting that they are cotranscribed and thus functionally linked. As discussed above, it has been observed that methyltransferases of restriction-modification pairs are conserved while endonucleases are comparatively divergent (Roberts et al., 2010). As such, alignment of the predicted OG1RF_0146 protein with REBASE proteins yielded only partial alignments; however, a conserved NgoFVII superfamily restriction endonuclease domain is present (Table 2). NgoVII is a type II restriction endonuclease from *Neisseria gonorrhoeae* (Stein et al., 1995). Based on these observations, we propose that OG1RF_0146 and OG1RF_0147 encode a type II restriction-modification pair.

It appears that *E. faecalis* OG1RF possesses a chromosomally encoded restriction modification system while *E. faecalis* V583 does not. Whether lack of a chromosomally encoded restriction-modification system is a general property of CC2 *E. faecalis* remains to be determined. It is also possible that a diverse set of restriction-modification systems exists among different enterococcal strains, as has been discovered for *Helicobacter pylori* (Xu et al., 2000). The distribution of potential restriction-modification systems in draft enterococcal genomes (Palmer et al., 2010), including among CC17 and non-CC17 *E. faecium* strains, is currently being examined by our group. Ultimately, the contribution of restriction-modification systems, such as the putative *E. faecalis* OG1RF type II system, to enterococcal genome stability will have to be explored experimentally.

CRISPR

The term "CRISPR" was first used in 2002 to describe a group of clustered, regularly interspaced, short (21- to 37-bp), roughly palindromic repeats observed in over 40 of the bacterial and archaeal genome sequences available at that time (Jansen et al. [2002] and previously observed by Mojica et al. [2000]). These repeats were found to vary in sequence and number among different prokaryotes and were interspersed by similarly sized novel spacer sequences of unclear origin (Mojica et al., 2000; Jansen et al., 2002). Four genes were found to be associated in some combination with the CRISPR loci, termed the CRISPR-associated genes (*cas1* to *cas4*). Predicted protein products of these genes had homology to enzymes involved in DNA processing and repair (Jansen et al., 2002). The conservation of this phenomenon across prokaryotic phyla, and the association of putative functional genes with these loci, implicated CRISPR in a critical cellular role. Subsequent reports in 2005 demonstrated that CRISPR spacer sequences are derived from extrachromosomal elements such as plasmids and phages, and a role for CRISPR in immunity from mobile genetic elements was proposed (Bolotin et al., 2005; Mojica et al., 2005; Pourcel et al., 2005). Two of these reports suggested that a eukaryote-like RNA interference (RNAi) mechanism could confer immunity (Bolotin et al., 2005; Mojica et al., 2005). The concept that CRISPR loci are part of a eukaryote-like RNAi defense system was later extensively refined (Makarova et al., 2006).

There are now elegant experimental data supporting a role for CRISPR in prokaryotic immunity. *Streptococcus thermophilus*, one of the model organisms for studies of CRISPR function, was found to incorporate pieces of phage DNA as spacers into its CRISPR1 locus during phage challenge. Further, acquisition of a phage-derived spacer, in the presence of functional *cas* genes, was sufficient to confer resistance to future phage challenges (Barrangou et al., 2007). A strain of *Staphylococcus epidermidis* harboring a CRISPR spacer with homology to a nickase gene was found to specifically block uptake of plasmids containing the nickase target sequence. This impediment to plasmid uptake was removed when nucleotide substitutions were introduced into the nickase target (Marraffini and Sontheimer, 2008). Collectively these results demonstrate that CRISPR is a sequence-specific prokaryotic acquired immune system, with spacers acting as a "memory" of past infections, conferring resistance to phage and plasmid attacks.

CRISPR loci appear to be widespread in prokaryotes, with ~94% of archaeal and ~44% of bacterial genomes possessing putative loci (from CRISPRdb [Grissa et al., 2007]). Diverse CRISPR-*cas* loci have been described. These loci vary in the composition of *cas* genes (for which many more than *cas1* to *cas4* have been identified), repeat length and sequence, spacer length, and the presence or absence of repeat-associated mysterious proteins, and have been classified into subtypes based on these structural properties (Haft et al., 2005).

Mechanistic details of CRISPR immunity are currently emerging. Recently it was shown that *Escherichia coli* CRISPR arrays are transcribed and processed by a complex of Cas proteins into small CRISPR RNAs (crRNA), each crRNA containing a spacer putatively capable of targeting a mobile element (Brouns et al., 2008). Because the *E. coli* CRISPR represents only one of eight CRISPR subtypes (Haft et al., 2005), it is unclear how conserved this processing complex is across prokaryotes. Strikingly, there is evidence supporting different modes of interference in different CRISPR subtypes: the *S. epidermidis* CRISPR system has been shown to target foreign DNA for destruction (a crRNA-DNA interaction) (Marraffini and Sontheimer, 2008), while the CRISPR system of *Pyrococcus furiosus* (an archaeon) has been shown to target RNA for destruction (a crRNA-RNA interaction) (Hale et al., 2009). It is clear that many prokaryotes possess elegant and ancient mechanisms, mediated by CRISPR loci, to protect themselves from mobile genetic elements. This is a biological process that we are just beginning to understand.

Supporting the prospect that multidrug-resistant enterococci emerged as a result of a compromise of genome defenses, a CRISPR-*cas* locus was identified in the *E. faecalis* OG1RF genome, and this locus does not occur in the *E. faecalis* V583 genome (Bourgogne et al., 2008) (Fig. 2A). This OG1RF-specific locus possesses 36-bp repeat sequences interspersed with 30-bp spacers and is a member of the Nmeni (for *Neisseria meningitidis*) subtype (Bourgogne et al., 2008). Members of this subtype possess the fewest *cas* genes compared to other subtypes and are found exclusively in pathogens and commensals of vertebrates (Haft et al., 2005). This CRISPR-*cas* locus is accompanied by another CRISPR locus lacking *cas* genes that is located elsewhere on the chromosome. These two loci are termed CRISPR1 and CRISPR2, respectively (Bourgogne et al., 2008). The perfect identity of CRISPR1 and CRISPR2 consensus repeat sequences suggests that these two loci are functionally linked, i.e., that Cas proteins encoded by the CRISPR1-*cas* locus also act upon the CRISPR2 locus. The consensus CRISPR1/CRISPR2 repeat sequence (Bourgogne et al., 2008) is 86% identical to the consensus repeat sequence of the *S. thermophilus* CRISPR3 locus, which has a similar arrangement of *cas* genes (Horvath and Barrangou, 2010) and is of the same subtype. Of the 14 total spacers contained within the *E. faecalis* OG1RF CRISPR1 and CRISPR2 loci, only1, spacer 3 of CRISPR1, has homology to a potential extrachromosomal element (Fig. 2B). This spacer is 93% identical to an intergenic region within a putative integrated plasmid on the *E. faecalis* V583 genome, differing by two nucleotides at the 5′ end. This sequence identity suggests to us that the *E. faecalis* OG1RF CRISPR loci provide immunity from mobile DNA, as has been observed for other bacteria. It is further possible that this immunity is dependent upon crRNA-DNA interactions, given the location of a potential CRISPR target in an intergenic region (Fig. 2B). It also appears that *E. faecalis* OG1RF has been exposed to a mobile

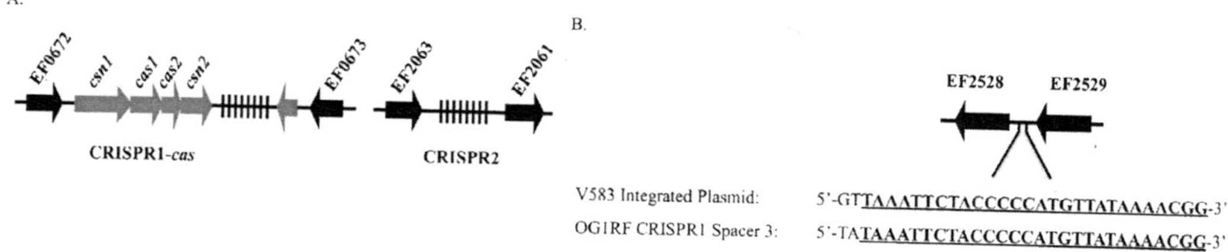

FIGURE 2 *E. faecalis* OG1RF CRISPR loci. (A) Diagram of CRISPR loci identified in the OG1RF genome by Bourgogne et al. (2008). Homologues of *E. faecalis* V583 genes are shown in black with appropriate V583 locus numbers. CRISPR-associated genes (*cas*) genes are specific to OG1RF and are shown in red. An ORF that lacks homology to known *cas* genes and is also specific to OG1RF was predicted to occur downstream of the CRISPR1 repeat-spacer array (Bourgogne et al., 2008). Vertical black lines represent 36-bp repeat sequences of CRISPR repeat-spacer arrays. (B) An OG1RF CRISPR spacer is homologous to a mobile element present in the V583 genome. Shown is the 30-bp OG1RF CRISPR1 spacer 3 sequence aligned with a homologous sequence in V583. Homologous nucleotides are in bold and underlined. The V583 sequence is located in an intergenic region between the ORFs EF2528 and EF2529; this region is found within a predicted integrated plasmid on the V583 genome (EF2512 to EF2545 [McBride et al., 2007]). Components of the figure are not drawn to scale.

element to which it could successfully deny entry, and to which *E. faecalis* V583 could not.

We hypothesize that the presence of a CRISPR-*cas* locus in *E. faecalis* OG1RF has contributed to the paucity of mobile DNA present in this strain compared to *E. faecalis* V583, which lacks a CRISPR-*cas* locus, a hypothesis that was previously advanced in the *E. faecalis* OG1RF genome report (Bourgogne et al., 2008). The role of *E. faecalis* CRISPR loci in mobile DNA defense will have to be proven experimentally and is the subject of ongoing experiments. In addition, the potential for absence of CRISPR loci in hospital-adapted lineages of *E. faecalis*, as well as in *E. faecium*, is of great interest. We speculate that the loss of CRISPR defense in the progenitors of hospital-adapted lineages (such as the progenitor of the *E. faecalis* CC2 lineage) contributed to the accretion of antibiotic resistance determinants and other mobile elements that we observe in these lineages today.

CONCLUSIONS AND FUTURE DIRECTIONS

In this chapter we have presented evidence as it currently exists describing the role of genome plasticity in the virulence and persistence of hospital-adapted, multidrug-resistant enterococcal lineages. We have also highlighted the mechanistic and comparatively unappreciated role that loss of endogenous genome defenses, such as restriction modification and CRISPR systems, may have played in the emergence of these lineages. As is apparent from our discussion, much work remains to be done before we understand whether and how these defense mechanisms influence enterococcal ecology and evolution. Important questions that must be answered experimentally are: Do enterococci possess core genome defense mechanisms? If these mechanisms are disrupted, does this lead to susceptibility to mobile DNA uptake and the potential for long-term genome destabilization? Further, is lack of endogenous genome defenses diagnostic for hospital-adapted lineages, as has been observed for *E. faecalis* V583? These questions drive ongoing work in our research group. We recently deposited a large amount of enterococcal sequence data into GenBank, including draft genome sequences of 16 *E. faecalis* and 8 *E. faecium* strains (Palmer et al., 2010), and these data are being used to catalogue both the diversity of enterococcal genome defenses and the mobile elements that seek to overcome them.

REFERENCES

Aarestrup, F. M., P. Butaye, and W. Witte. 2002. Nonhuman reservoirs of enterococci, p. 55–99. *In* M. S. Gilmore (ed.), *The Enterococci: Pathogenesis, Molecular Biology, and Antibiotic Resistance.* ASM Press, Washington, DC.

Bachrach, G., M. Leizerovici-Zigmond, A. Zlotkin, R. Naor, and D. Steinberg. 2003. Bacteriophage isolation from human saliva. *Lett. Appl. Microbiol.* **36:**50–53.

Barrangou, R., C. Fremaux, H. Deveau, M. Richards, P. Boyaval, S. Moineau, D. A. Romero, and P. Horvath. 2007. CRISPR provides acquired resistance against viruses in prokaryotes. *Science* **315:** 1709–1712.

Bertani, G., and J. J. Weigle. 1953. Host controlled variation in bacterial viruses. *J. Bacteriol.* **65:**113–121.

Bolotin, A., B. Quinquis, A. Sorokin, and S. D. Ehrlich. 2005. Clustered regularly interspaced short palindrome repeats (CRISPRs) have spacers of extrachromosomal origin. *Microbiology* **151:** 2551–2561.

Bourgogne, A., D. A. Garsin, X. Qin, K. V. Singh, J. Sillanpaa, S. Yerrapragada, Y. Ding, S. Dugan-Rocha, C. Buhay, H. Shen, G. Chen, G. Williams, D. Muzny, A. Maadani, K. A. Fox, J. Gioia, L. Chen, Y. Shang, C. A. Arias, S. R. Nallapareddy, M. Zhao, V. P. Prakash, S. Chowdhury, H. Jiang, R. A. Gibbs, B. E. Murray, S. K. Highlander, and G. M. Weinstock. 2008. Large scale variation in *Enterococcus faecalis* illustrated by the genome analysis of strain OG1RF. *Genome Biol.* **9:**R110.

Brock, T. D. 1964. Host range of certain virulent and temperate bacteriophages attacking group D streptococci. *J. Bacteriol.* **88:**165–171.

Brouns, S. J., M. M. Jore, M. Lundgren, E. R. Westra, R. J. Slijkhuis, A. P. Snijders, M. J. Dickman, K. S. Makarova, E. V. Koonin, and J. van der Oost. 2008. Small CRISPR RNAs guide antiviral defense in prokaryotes. *Science* **321:**960–964.

Callegan, M. C., M. Engelbert, D. W. Parke II, B. D. Jett, and M. S. Gilmore. 2002. Bacterial endophthalmitis: epidemiology, therapeutics, and bacterium-host interactions. *Clin. Microbiol. Rev.* **15:**111–124.

Caprioli, T., F. Zaccour, and S. S. Kasatiya. 1975. Phage typing scheme for group D streptococci isolated from human urogenital tract. *J. Clin. Microbiol.* **2:**311–317.

Chow, J. W., L. A. Thal, M. B. Perri, J. A. Vazquez, S. M. Donabedian, D. B. Clewell, and M. J. Zervos. 1993. Plasmid-associated hemolysin and aggregation substance production contribute to virulence in experimental enterococcal endocarditis. *Antimicrob. Agents Chemother.* **37:**2474–2477.

Chuang, O. N., P. M. Schlievert, C. L. Wells, D. A. Manias, T. J. Tripp, and G. M. Dunny. 2009. Multiple functional domains of *Enterococcus faecalis* aggregation substance Asc10 contribute to endocarditis virulence. *Infect. Immun.* **77:**539–548.

Clewell, D. B. 2007. Properties of *Enterococcus faecalis* plasmid pAD1, a member of a widely disseminated family of pheromone-responding, conjugative, virulence elements encoding cytolysin. *Plasmid* **58:** 205–227.

Clewell, D. B., and G. Dunny. 2002. Conjugation and genetic exchange in enterococci, p. 265–300. *In* M. S. Gilmore (ed.), *The Enterococci: Pathogenesis, Molecular Biology, and Antibiotic Resistance.* ASM Press, Washington, DC.

Contreras, G. A., C. A. DiazGranados, L. Cortes, J. Reyes, S. Vanegas, D. Panesso, S. Rincon, L. Diaz, G. Prada, B. E. Murray, and C. A. Arias. 2008. Nosocomial outbreak of *Enterococcus gallinarum:* untaming of rare species of enterococci. *J. Hosp. Infect.* **70:**346–352.

DeVriese, L., M. Baele, and P. Butaye. 2006. The genus *Enterococcus*: taxonomy, p. 163–174. *In* M. Dworkin, S. Falkow, E. Rosenberg, K.-H. Schleifer, and E. Stackebrandt (ed.), *The Prokaryotes*, 3rd ed., vol. 4. Springer, New York, NY.

Domann, E., T. Hain, R. Ghai, A. Billion, C. Kuenne, K. Zimmermann, and T. Chakraborty. 2007. Comparative genomic analysis for the presence of potential enterococcal virulence factors in the probiotic *Enterococcus faecalis* strain Symbioflor 1. *Int. J. Med. Microbiol.* **297:**533–539.

Dunny, G. M. 2007. The peptide pheromone-inducible conjugation system of *Enterococcus faecalis* plasmid pCF10: cell-cell signaling, gene transfer, complexity and evolution. *Philos. Trans. R. Soc. Lond. B Biol. Sci.* **362:**1185–1193.

Engelbert, M., E. Mylonakis, F. M. Ausubel, S. B. Calderwood, and M. S. Gilmore. 2004. Contribution of gelatinase, serine protease, and *fsr* to the pathogenesis of *Enterococcus faecalis* endophthalmitis. *Infect. Immun.* **72:**3628–3633.

Flannagan, S. E., J. W. Chow, S. M. Donabedian, W. J. Brown, M. B. Perri, M. J. Zervos, Y. Ozawa, and D. B. Clewell. 2003. Plasmid content of a vancomycin-resistant *Enterococcus faecalis* isolate from a patient also colonized by *Staphylococcus aureus* with a VanA phenotype. *Antimicrob. Agents Chemother.* **47:**3954–3959.

Foulquie Moreno, M. R., P. Sarantinopoulos, E. Tsakalidou, and L. De Vuyst. 2006. The role and application of enterococci in food and health. *Int. J. Food. Microbiol.* **106:**1–24.

Freitas, A. R., C. Novais, P. Ruiz-Garbajosa, T. M. Coque, and L. Peixe. 2009a. Clonal expansion within clonal complex 2 and spread of vancomycin-resistant plasmids among different genetic lineages of *Enterococcus faecalis* from Portugal. *J. Antimicrob. Chemother.* **63:**1104–1111.

Freitas, A. R., C. Novais, P. Ruiz-Garbajosa, T. M. Coque, and L. Peixe. 2009b. Dispersion of multidrug-resistant *Enterococcus faecium* isolates belonging to major clonal complexes in different Portuguese settings. *Appl. Environ. Microbiol.* **75:**4904–4908.

Garsin, D. A., C. D. Sifri, E. Mylonakis, X. Qin, K. V. Singh, B. E. Murray, S. B. Calderwood, and F. M. Ausubel. 2001. A simple model host for identifying Gram-positive virulence factors. *Proc. Natl. Acad. Sci. USA* **98:**10892–10897.

Gilmore, M. S., and J. J. Ferretti. 2003. Microbiology. The thin line between gut commensal and pathogen. *Science* **299:**1999–2002.

Gold, O. G., H. V. Jordan, and J. van Houte. 1975. The prevalence of enterococci in the human mouth and their pathogenicity in animal models. *Arch. Oral Biol.* **20:**473–477.

Gorski, A., and B. Weber-Dabrowska. 2005. The potential role of endogenous bacteriophages in controlling invading pathogens. *Cell. Mol. Life Sci.* **62:**511–519.

Grissa, I., G. Vergnaud, and C. Pourcel. 2007. The CRISPRdb database and tools to display CRISPRs and to generate dictionaries of spacers and repeats. *BMC Bioinformatics* **8:**172.

Haft, D. H., J. Selengut, E. F. Mongodin, and K. E. Nelson. 2005. A guild of 45 CRISPR-associated (Cas) protein families and multiple CRISPR/Cas subtypes exist in prokaryotic genomes. *PLoS Comput. Biol.* **1:**e60.

Hale, C. R., P. Zhao, S. Olson, M. O. Duff, B. R. Graveley, L. Wells, R. M. Terns, and M. P. Terns. 2009. RNA-guided RNA cleavage by a CRISPR RNA-Cas protein complex. *Cell* **139:**945–956.

Hancock, L. E., and M. S. Gilmore. 2002. The capsular polysaccharide of *Enterococcus faecalis* and its relationship to other polysaccharides in the cell wall. *Proc. Natl. Acad. Sci. USA* **99:**1574–1579.

Hancock, L. E., B. D. Shepard, and M. S. Gilmore. 2003. Molecular analysis of the *Enterococcus faecalis* serotype 2 polysaccharide determinant. *J. Bacteriol.* **185:**4393–4401.

Handwerger, S., B. Raucher, D. Altarac, J. Monka, S. Marchione, K. V. Singh, B. E. Murray, J. Wolff, and B. Walters. 1993. Nosocomial outbreak due to *Enterococcus faecium* highly resistant to vancomycin, penicillin, and gentamicin. *Clin. Infect. Dis.* **16:**750–755.

Heikens, E., W. van Schaik, H. L. Leavis, M. J. Bonten, and R. J. Willems. 2008. Identification of a novel genomic island specific to hospital-acquired clonal complex 17 *Enterococcus faecium* isolates. *Appl. Environ. Microbiol.* **74:**7094–7097.

Hidron, A. I., J. R. Edwards, J. Patel, T. C. Horan, D. M. Sievert, D. A. Pollock, and S. K. Fridkin. 2008. NHSN annual update: antimicrobial-resistant pathogens associated with healthcare-associated infections: annual summary of data reported to the National Healthcare Safety Network at the Centers for Disease Control and Prevention, 2006–2007. *Infect. Control Hosp. Epidemiol.* **29:**996–1011.

Hirt, H., P. M. Schlievert, and G. M. Dunny. 2002. In vivo induction of virulence and antibiotic resistance transfer in *Enterococcus faecalis* mediated by the sex pheromone-sensing system of pCF10. *Infect. Immun.* **70:**716–723.

Horvath, P., and R. Barrangou. 2010. CRISPR/Cas, the immune system of bacteria and archaea. *Science* **327:**167–170.

Huycke, M. M., M. S. Gilmore, B. D. Jett, and J. L. Booth. 1992. Transfer of pheromone-inducible plasmids between *Enterococcus faecalis* in the Syrian hamster gastrointestinal tract. *J. Infect. Dis.* **166:**1188–1191.

Huycke, M. M., C. A. Spiegel, and M. S. Gilmore. 1991. Bacteremia caused by hemolytic, high-level gentamicin-resistant *Enterococcus faecalis*. *Antimicrob. Agents Chemother.* **35:**1626–1634.

Ike, Y., H. Hashimoto, and D. B. Clewell. 1984. Hemolysin of *Streptococcus faecalis* subspecies *zymogenes* contributes to virulence in mice. *Infect. Immun.* **45:**528–530.

Ike, Y., K. Tanimoto, H. Tomita, K. Takeuchi, and S. Fujimoto. 1998. Efficient transfer of the pheromone-independent *Enterococcus faecium* plasmid pMG1 (Gm^r) (65.1 kilobases) to *Enterococcus* strains during broth mating. *J. Bacteriol.* **180:**4886–4892.

Jakubauskas, A., E. Kriukiene, L. Trinkunaite, R. Sapranauskas, S. Jurenaite-Urbanaviciene, and A. Lubys. 2009. Bioinformatic and partial functional analysis of pEspA and pEspB, two plasmids from *Exiguobacterium arabatum* sp. nov. RFL1109. *Plasmid* **61:**52–64.

Jansen, R., J. D. Embden, W. Gaastra, and L. M. Schouls. 2002. Identification of genes that are associated with DNA repeats in prokaryotes. *Mol. Microbiol.* **43:**1565–1575.

Jett, B. D., and M. S. Gilmore. 1990. The growth-inhibitory effect of the *Enterococcus faecalis* bacteriocin encoded by pAD1 extends to the oral streptococci. *J. Dent. Res.* **69:**1640–1645.

Jett, B. D., H. G. Jensen, R. E. Nordquist, and M. S. Gilmore. 1992. Contribution of the pAD1-encoded cytolysin to the severity of experimental *Enterococcus faecalis* endophthalmitis. *Infect. Immun.* **60:**2445–2452.

Kawalec, M., M. Gniadkowski, and W. Hryniewicz. 2000. Outbreak of vancomycin-resistant enterococci in a hospital in Gdask, Poland, due to horizontal transfer of different Tn*1546*-like transposon variants and clonal spread of several strains. *J. Clin. Microbiol.* **38:**3317–3322.

Kawalec, M., Z. Pietras, E. Danilowicz, A. Jakubczak, M. Gniadkowski, W. Hryniewicz, and R. J. Willems. 2007. Clonal structure of *Enterococcus faecalis* isolated from Polish hospitals: characterization of epidemic clones. *J. Clin. Microbiol.* **45:**147–153.

Kirkpatrick, B. D., S. M. Harrington, D. Smith, D. Marcellus, C. Miller, J. Dick, L. Karanfil, and T. M. Perl. 1999. An outbreak of vancomycin-dependent *Enterococcus faecium* in a bone marrow transplant unit. *Clin. Infect. Dis.* **29:**1268–1273.

Leavis, H., J. Top, N. Shankar, K. Borgen, M. Bonten, J. van Embden, and R. J. Willems. 2004. A novel putative enterococcal pathogenicity island linked to the *esp* virulence gene of *Enterococcus faecium* and associated with epidemicity. *J. Bacteriol.* **186:**672–682.

Leavis, H. L., R. J. Willems, J. Top, and M. J. Bonten. 2006. High-level ciprofloxacin resistance from point mutations in *gyrA* and *parC* confined to global hospital-adapted clonal lineage CC17 of *Enterococcus faecium*. *J. Clin. Microbiol.* **44:**1059–1064.

Leavis, H. L., R. J. Willems, W. J. van Wamel, F. H. Schuren, M. P. Caspers, and M. J. Bonten. 2007. Insertion sequence-driven diversification creates a globally dispersed emerging multiresistant subspecies of *E. faecium*. *PLoS Pathog.* **3:**e7.

Lebreton, F., E. Riboulet-Bisson, P. Serror, M. Sanguinetti, B. Posteraro, R. Torelli, A. Hartke, Y. Auffray, and J. C. Giard. 2009. *ace*, which encodes an adhesin in *Enterococcus faecalis*, is regulated by Ers and is involved in virulence. *Infect. Immun.* **77:**2832–2839.

Leendertse, M., E. Heikens, L. M. Wijnands, M. van Luit-Asbroek, G. J. Teske, J. J. Roelofs, M. J. Bonten, T. van der Poll, and R. J. Willems. 2009. Enterococcal surface protein transiently aggravates *Enterococcus faecium*-induced urinary tract infection in mice. *J. Infect. Dis.* **200:** 1162–1165.

Lepage, E., S. Brinster, C. Caron, C. Ducroix-Crepy, L. Rigottier-Gois, G. Dunny, C. Hennequet-Antier, and P. Serror. 2006. Comparative genomic hybridization analysis of *Enterococcus faecalis*: identification of genes absent from food strains. *J. Bacteriol.* **188:**6858–6868.

Libisch, B., Z. Lepsanovic, J. Top, M. Muzslay, M. Konkoly-Thege, M. Gacs, B. Balogh, M. Fuzi, and R. J. Willems. 2008. Molecular characterization of vancomycin-resistant *Enterococcus* spp. clinical isolates from Hungary and Serbia. *Scand. J. Infect. Dis.* **40:**778–784.

Licht, T. R., D. Laugesen, L. B. Jensen, and B. L. Jacobsen. 2002. Transfer of the pheromone-inducible plasmid pCF10 among *Enterococcus faecalis* microorganisms colonizing the intestine of mini-pigs. *Appl. Environ. Microbiol.* **68:**187–193.

Luria, S. E., and M. L. Human. 1952. A nonhereditary, host-induced variation of bacterial viruses. *J. Bacteriol.* **64:**557–569.

Makarova, K. S., N. V. Grishin, S. A. Shabalina, Y. I. Wolf, and E. V. Koonin. 2006. A putative RNA-interference-based immune system in prokaryotes: computational analysis of the predicted enzymatic machinery, functional analogies with eukaryotic RNAi, and hypothetical mechanisms of action. *Biol. Direct* **1:**7.

Manson, J. M., L. Hancock, and M. S. Gilmore. 2010. Mechanism of chromosomal transfer of *Enterococcus faecalis* pathogenicity island, capsule, antimicrobial resistance and other traits. *Proc. Natl. Acad. Sci. USA.* **107:**12269–12274.

Marraffini, L. A., and E. J. Sontheimer. 2008. CRISPR interference limits horizontal gene transfer in staphylococci by targeting DNA. *Science* **322:**1843–1845.

Mazaheri Nezhad Fard, R., M. D. Barton, and M. W. Heuzenroeder. 2010. Novel Bacteriophages in *Enterococcus* spp. *Curr. Microbiol.* **60:**400–406.

McBride, S. M., V. A. Fischetti, D. J. Leblanc, R. C. Moellering, Jr., and M. S. Gilmore. 2007. Genetic diversity among *Enterococcus faecalis*. *PLoS One* **2:**e582.

Mojica, F. J., C. Diez-Villasenor, J. Garcia-Martinez, and E. Soria. 2005. Intervening sequences of regularly spaced prokaryotic repeats derive from foreign genetic elements. *J. Mol. Evol.* **60:**174–182.

Mojica, F. J., C. Diez-Villasenor, E. Soria, and G. Juez. 2000. Biological significance of a family of regularly spaced repeats in the genomes of archaea, bacteria and mitochondria. *Mol. Microbiol.* **36:**244–246.

Murray, B. E. 1990. The life and times of the *Enterococcus*. *Clin. Microbiol. Rev.* **3:**46–65.

Murray, N. E. 2002. Immigration control of DNA in bacteria: self versus non-self. *Microbiology* **148:**3–20.

Nallapareddy, S. R., K. V. Singh, R. W. Duh, G. M. Weinstock, and B. E. Murray. 2000. Diversity of *ace*, a gene encoding a microbial surface component recognizing adhesive matrix molecules, from different strains of *Enterococcus faecalis* and evidence for production of *ace* during human infections. *Infect. Immun.* **68:**5210–5217.

Nallapareddy, S. R., H. Wenxiang, G. M. Weinstock, and B. E. Murray. 2005. Molecular characterization of a widespread, pathogenic, and antibiotic resistance-receptive *Enterococcus faecalis* lineage and dissemination of its putative pathogenicity island. *J. Bacteriol.* **187:**5709–5718.

O'Driscoll, J., D. F. Heiter, G. G. Wilson, G. F. Fitzgerald, R. Roberts, and D. van Sinderen. 2006. A genetic dissection of the *Lla*JI restriction cassette reveals insights on a novel bacteriophage resistance system. *BMC Microbiol.* **6:**40.

Palmer, K. L., K. Carniol, J. M. Manson, D. Heiman, T. Shea, S. Young, Q. Zeng, D. Gevers, M. Feldgarden, B. Birren, and M. S. Gilmore. 2010. High-quality draft genome sequences of 28 *Enterococcus* sp. isolates. *J Bacteriol.* **192:**2469–2470.

Paulsen, I. T., L. Banerjei, G. S. Myers, K. E. Nelson, R. Seshadri, T. D. Read, D. E. Fouts, J. A. Eisen, S. R. Gill, J. F. Heidelberg, H. Tettelin, R. J. Dodson, L. Umayam, L. Brinkac, M. Beanan, S. Daugherty, R. T. DeBoy, S. Durkin, J. Kolonay, R. Madupu, W. Nelson, J. Vamathevan, B. Tran, J. Upton, T. Hansen, J. Shetty, H. Khouri, T. Utterback, D. Radune, K. A. Ketchum, B. A. Dougherty, and C. M. Fraser. 2003. Role of mobile DNA in the evolution of vancomycin-resistant *Enterococcus faecalis. Science* **299:**2071–2074.

Pillar, C. M., and M. S. Gilmore. 2004. Enterococcal virulence—pathogenicity island of *E. faecalis. Front. Biosci.* **9:**2335–2346.

Pourcel, C., G. Salvignol, and G. Vergnaud. 2005. CRISPR elements in *Yersinia pestis* acquire new repeats by preferential uptake of bacteriophage DNA, and provide additional tools for evolutionary studies. *Microbiology* **151:**653–663.

Pournaras, S., A. Tsakris, M. E. Kaufmann, J. Douboyas, and A. Antoniadis. 2000. Outbreak of infections in a Greek university hospital involving a single clone of high-level aminoglycoside-resistant *Enterococcus faecalis. Infect. Control Hosp. Epidemiol.* **21:**786–789.

Roberts, R. J. 1982. Restriction and modification enzymes and their recognition sequences. *Nucleic Acids Res.* **10:**r117–r144.

Roberts, R. J., T. Vincze, J. Posfai, and D. Macelis. 2010. REBASE—a database for DNA restriction and modification: enzymes, genes and genomes. *Nucleic Acids Res.* **38:**D234–D236.

Roberts, R. J., T. Vincze, J. Posfai, and D. Macelis. 2007. REBASE—enzymes and genes for DNA restriction and modification. *Nucleic Acids Res.* **35:**D269–D270.

Rogers, C. G., and W. B. Sarles. 1963. Characterization of *Enterococcus* bacteriophages from the small intestine of the rat. *J. Bacteriol.* **85:**1378–1385.

Ruiz-Garbajosa, P., M. J. Bonten, D. A. Robinson, J. Top, S. R. Nallapareddy, C. Torres, T. M. Coque, R. Canton, F. Baquero, B. E. Murray, R. del Campo, and R. J. Willems. 2006. Multilocus sequence typing scheme for *Enterococcus faecalis* reveals hospital-adapted genetic complexes in a background of high rates of recombination. *J. Clin. Microbiol.* **44:**2220–2228.

Sahm, D. F., J. Kissinger, M. S. Gilmore, P. R. Murray, R. Mulder, J. Solliday, and B. Clarke. 1989. In vitro susceptibility studies of vancomycin-resistant *Enterococcus faecalis. Antimicrob. Agents Chemother.* **33:**1588–1591.

Samuel, J., H. Coutinho, A. Galloway, C. Rennison, M. E. Kaufmann, and N. Woodford. 2008. Glycopeptide-resistant *Enterococcus raffinosus* in a haematology unit: an unusual cause of a nosocomial outbreak. *J. Hosp. Infect.* **70:**294–296.

Scott, I. U., R. H. Loo, H. W. Flynn, Jr., and D. Miller. 2003. Endophthalmitis caused by *Enterococcus faecalis*: antibiotic selection and treatment outcomes. *Ophthalmology* **110:**1573–1577.

Serfiotis-Mitsa, D., G. A. Roberts, L. P. Cooper, J. H. White, M. Nutley, A. Cooper, G. W. Blakely, and D. T. Dryden. 2008. The Orf18 gene product from conjugative transposon Tn*916* is an ArdA antirestriction protein that inhibits type I DNA restriction-modification systems. *J. Mol. Biol.* **383:**970–981.

Shankar, N., A. S. Baghdayan, and M. S. Gilmore. 2002. Modulation of virulence within a pathogenicity island in vancomycin-resistant *Enterococcus faecalis. Nature* **417:**746–750.

Shankar, N., C. V. Lockatell, A. S. Baghdayan, C. Drachenberg, M. S. Gilmore, and D. E. Johnson. 2001. Role of *Enterococcus faecalis* surface protein Esp in the pathogenesis of ascending urinary tract infection. *Infect. Immun.* **69:**4366–4372.

Shankar, V., A. S. Baghdayan, M. M. Huycke, G. Lindahl, and M. S. Gilmore. 1999. Infection-derived *Enterococcus faecalis* strains are enriched in *esp*, a gene encoding a novel surface protein. *Infect. Immun.* **67:**193–200.

Sifri, C. D., E. Mylonakis, K. V. Singh, X. Qin, D. A. Garsin, B. E. Murray, F. M. Ausubel, and S. B. Calderwood. 2002. Virulence effect of *Enterococcus faecalis* protease genes and the quorum-sensing locus *fsr* in *Caenorhabditis elegans* and mice. *Infect. Immun.* **70:**5647–5650.

Singh, K. V., S. R. Nallapareddy, J. Sillanpaa, and B. E. Murray. 2010. Importance of the collagen adhesin Ace in pathogenesis and protection against *Enterococcus faecalis* experimental endocarditis. *PLoS Pathog.* **6:**e1000716.

Singh, K. V., X. Qin, G. M. Weinstock, and B. E. Murray. 1998. Generation and testing of mutants of *Enterococcus faecalis* in a mouse peritonitis model. *J. Infect. Dis.* **178:**1416–1420.

Solheim, M., A. Aakra, L. G. Snipen, D. A. Brede, and I. F. Nes. 2009. Comparative genomics of *Enterococcus faecalis* from healthy Norwegian infants. *BMC Genomics* **10:**194.

Stein, D. C., J. S. Gunn, M. Radlinska, and A. Piekarowicz. 1995. Restriction and modification systems of *Neisseria gonorrhoeae. Gene* **157:**19–22.

Stevens, R. H., O. D. Porras, and A. L. Delisle. 2009. Bacteriophages induced from lysogenic root canal isolates of *Enterococcus faecalis. Oral Microbiol. Immunol.* **24:**278–284.

Suzuki, T., T. Wada, S. Kozai, Y. Ike, M. S. Gilmore, and Y. Ohashi. 2008. Contribution of secreted proteases to the pathogenesis of postoperative *Enterococcus faecalis* endophthalmitis. *J. Cataract Refract. Surg.* **34:**1776–1784.

Tanimoto, K., and Y. Ike. 2008. Complete nucleotide sequencing and analysis of the 65-kb highly conjugative *Enterococcus faecium* plasmid pMG1: identification of the transfer-related region and the minimum region required for replication. *FEMS Microbiol. Lett.* **288:**186–195.

Tannock, G. W., and G. Cook. 2002. Enterococci as members of the intestinal microflora of humans, p. 101–132. *In* M. S. Gilmore (ed.), *The Enterococci: Pathogenesis, Molecular Biology, and Antibiotic Resistance.* ASM Press, Washington, DC.

Tendolkar, P. M., A. S. Baghdayan, M. S. Gilmore, and N. Shankar. 2004. Enterococcal surface protein, Esp, enhances biofilm formation by *Enterococcus faecalis. Infect. Immun.* **72:**6032–6039.

Tock, M. R., and D. T. Dryden. 2005. The biology of restriction and anti-restriction. *Curr. Opin. Microbiol.* **8:**466–472.

Top, J., R. Willems, and M. Bonten. 2008. Emergence of CC17 *Enterococcus faecium*: from commensal to hospital-adapted pathogen. *FEMS Immunol. Med. Microbiol.* **52:**297–308.

Uchiyama, J., M. Rashel, Y. Maeda, I. Takemura, S. Sugihara, K. Akechi, A. Muraoka, H. Wakiguchi, and S. Matsuzaki. 2008. Isolation and characterization of a novel *Enterococcus faecalis* bacteriophage ϕEF24C as a therapeutic candidate. *FEMS Microbiol. Lett.* **278:**200–206.

Urwin, R., and M. C. Maiden. 2003. Multi-locus sequence typing: a tool for global epidemiology. *Trends Microbiol.* **11:**479–487.

Valdezate, S., C. Labayru, A. Navarro, M. A. Mantecon, M. Ortega, T. M. Coque, M. Garcia, and J. A. Saez-Nieto. 2009. Large clonal outbreak of multidrug-resistant CC17 ST17 *Enterococcus faecium* containing Tn*5382* in a Spanish hospital. *J. Antimicrob. Chemother.* **63:**17–20.

Weaver, K. E., L. B. Rice, and G. Churchward. 2002. Plasmids and transposons, p. 219–263. *In* M. S. Gilmore (ed.), *The Enterococci: Pathogenesis, Molecular Biology, and Antibiotic Resistance.* ASM Press, Washington, DC.

Weigel, L. M., D. B. Clewell, S. R. Gill, N. C. Clark, L. K. McDougal, S. E. Flannagan, J. F. Kolonay, J. Shetty, G. E. Killgore, and F. C. Tenover. 2003. Genetic analysis of a high-level vancomycin-resistant isolate of *Staphylococcus aureus. Science* **302:**1569–1571.

Willems, R. J., W. Homan, J. Top, M. van Santen-Verheuvel, D. Tribe, X. Manzioros, C. Gaillard, C. M. Vandenbroucke-Grauls, E. M. Mascini, E. van Kregten, J. D. van Embden, and M. J. Bonten. 2001. Variant *esp* gene as a marker of a distinct genetic lineage of vancomycin-resistant *Enterococcus faecium* spreading in hospitals. *Lancet* **357:**853–855.

Willems, R. J., J. Top, D. J. Smith, D. I. Roper, S. E. North, and N. Woodford. 2003. Mutations in the DNA mismatch repair proteins MutS and MutL of oxazolidinone-resistant or -susceptible *Enterococcus faecium. Antimicrob. Agents Chemother.* **47:**3061–3066.

Wu, R., C. T. King, and E. Jay. 1978. A new sequence-specific endonuclease from *Streptococcus faecalis* subsp. *zymogenes. Gene* **4:**329–336.

Xu, Q., R. D. Morgan, R. J. Roberts, and M. J. Blaser. 2000. Identification of type II restriction and modification systems in *Helicobacter pylori* reveals their substantial diversity among strains. *Proc. Natl. Acad. Sci. USA* **97:**9671–9676.

Yasmin, A., J. G. Kenny, J. Shankar, A. C. Darby, N. Hall, C. Edwards, and M. J. Horsburgh. 2010. Comparative genomics and transduction potential of *Enterococcus faecalis* temperate bacteriophages. *J. Bacteriol.* **192:**1122–1130.

Zheng, B., H. Tomita, T. Inoue, and Y. Ike. 2009. Isolation of VanB-type *Enterococcus faecalis* strains from nosocomial infections: first report of the isolation and identification of the pheromone-responsive plasmids pMG2200, encoding VanB-type vancomycin resistance and a Bac41-type bacteriocin, and pMG2201, encoding erythromycin resistance and cytolysin (Hly/Bac). *Antimicrob. Agents Chemother.* **53:**735–747.

Zhu, X., B. Zheng, S. Wang, R. J. Willems, F. Xue, X. Cao, Y. Li, S. Bo, and J. Liu. 2009. Molecular characterisation of outbreak-related strains of vancomycin-resistant *Enterococcus faecium* from an intensive care unit in Beijing, China. *J. Hosp. Infect.* **72:**147–154.

VIRAL INFECTIONS

HOST-DRIVEN PLASTICITY OF THE HUMAN IMMUNODEFICIENCY VIRUS GENOME

Stephen Norley and Reinhard Kurth

9

Reports coming from the United States in the early 1980s of an apparently infectious disease causing profound immunodeficiency in homosexual men were the first public manifestations of a tragedy of epic proportions that was already unfolding in Africa and was about to hit the rest of the planet. The AIDS pandemic has already claimed an estimated 25 million lives, and UNAIDS estimates that more than 33 million people are currently living with human immunodeficiency virus (HIV)/AIDS and that 2.7 million new infections and 2.0 million deaths occur each year (UNAIDS, 2009). The disease (being sexually transmitted) targets those members of the population most needed to care for children and to work productively. In addition to the obvious suffering of those infected with HIV, particularly in developing nations, AIDS therefore has a profound impact on both the social and economic stability of the regions most heavily afflicted. Despite intense efforts on a global scale, an effective AIDS vaccine remains elusive, and the antiviral drugs that have so effectively limited disease progression in those living in industrialized nations must be taken throughout the life of the individual, at a cost which renders them unavailable to the vast majority of those in need.

Why has HIV/AIDS proven to be such a difficult problem to solve? Certainly, the fact that the virus infects and disrupts the very cells of the body needed to mount an effective antiviral immune response is important. In addition, difficulties such as the lack of a suitable animal model, the lack of a known "correlate of protective immunity," and a general reluctance of the pharmaceutical industry to make a major commitment to AIDS vaccine development play a role. However, one of the most frequently cited reasons for HIV being a difficult nut to crack is the virus's astonishing degree of genomic plasticity.

It is probably no exaggeration to claim that HIV is one of the most rapidly evolving biological entities on this planet. Indeed, HIV evolves not only on a global scale but also dramatically within the infected individual. In this chapter we describe the scale and driving force behind the profound genomic plasticity of HIV, discuss the intense interplay between the virus and the immune system of the host, and speculate on the impact of this variability on the prospects for the development of effective vaccines and novel therapies.

Stephen Norley, Robert Koch Institute, Berlin, Germany. *Reinhard Kurth,* Ernst Schering Foundation and Robert Koch Institute, Berlin, Germany.

Genome Plasticity and Infectious Diseases,
Edited by J. Hacker, U. Dobrindt, and R. Kurth,

GENOMIC STRUCTURE AND LIFE CYCLE OF HIV

Like all retroviruses, the HIV genome has the four prototypic open reading frames *gag*, *pro*, *pol*, and *env*. The polyprotein coded for by *gag* is subsequently cleaved into structural proteins used to build the virus, *pro* codes for the protease enzyme needed to perform this cleavage, *pol* gives rise to the reverse transcriptase and integrase enzymes needed to produce the DNA copy of the RNA genome and insert it into the host's cellular DNA, and *env* codes for the outer and transmembrane glycoproteins gp120 and gp41, which are responsible for recognizing the host cell and effecting viral entry. In addition to these standard retroviral genes, HIV possesses a number of regulatory genes (*vif*, *vpr*, *tat*, *rev*, *vpu*, and *nef*) that are needed to overcome cellular inhibitory systems, accelerate virion production, or enhance infection in vivo.

HIV recognizes its target cell by interaction between the gp120 glycoprotein and the cellular CD4 molecule plus a coreceptor (usually CCR5 or CXCR4). This induces the gp41 transmembrane envelope glycoprotein to undergo conformational changes, pulling the cellular and viral membranes together and allowing their fusion, which in turn results in the viral core entering the cell. Within the cell, the reverse transcriptase enzyme makes a double-stranded copy of the viral RNA genome that is carried to the nucleus and inserted into a host cell chromosome by the integrase enzyme. This provirus can be read immediately or remain dormant for a long time until the cell is activated. Upon transcription, the mRNA is initially spliced and transported to the cytoplasm, where it is translated to yield Tat and Rev proteins, which facilitate virion production and allow transport of the full-length, unspliced RNA genome from the nucleus. Production of structural proteins then follows, the Env polypeptide is transported and cleaved via the Golgi apparatus to be expressed on the cell surface, while Gag and Gag-Pol polypeptides accumulate together with the viral RNA on the inner side of the membrane. These then bud out of the cell, and final maturation through the action of the protease enzyme results in infectious viral particles.

MECHANISMS OF GENOMIC VARIATION

HIV has a number of properties that contribute to its having an extraordinarily high degree of genomic variation (Fig. 1). First, like other retroviruses, HIV lacks a mechanism for proofreading the copies of its genome, in this case the DNA copies of the genome produced by the viral reverse transcriptase upon entry into the host cell. This lack of error correction means that the HIV genome has a mutation rate of

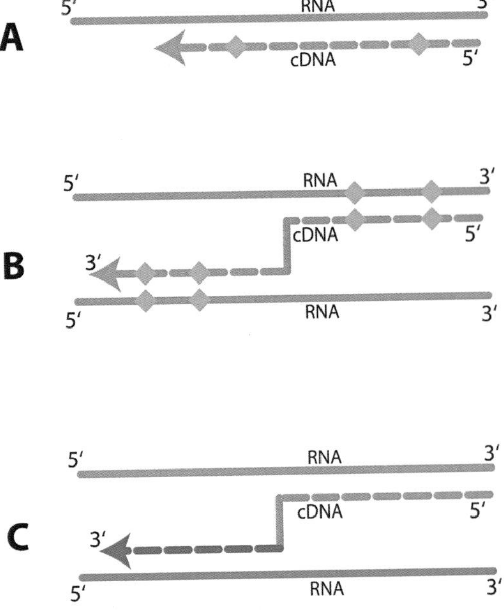

FIGURE 1 Mechanisms of genomic variation. Three main mechanisms contribute to the extensive genomic variation within the HIV genome. (A) In the absence of a proofreading function, transcription errors made by the viral reverse transcriptase enzyme during the synthesis of a DNA copy of the RNA genome result in (nearly) random mutations that accumulate if beneficial. (B) Template switching of reverse transcriptase from one RNA template to another. Distinct mutations in regions either side of the switching event can then become incorporated into a single genome. (C) Template switching between distinct viral subtypes. In the rare cases of simultaneous infection with two viral subtypes, switching can occur yielding a radically new virus with a mosaic genome. Adapted from Ramirez et al. (2008).

3×10^{-5} per nucleotide base for each cycle of replication. This, coupled with the production of between 10^8 and 10^{10} new virus particles per day (Perelson et al., 1996; Wei et al., 1995) in the infected host, means that at any given time (once infection is established), every possible genotypic variant with a single-nucleotide substitution is theoretically present. This gives natural selection a lot of material to work with. However, this is not to say that all mutations are equally likely. There is a preference for G-to-A mutations and for transitions (purine to purine or pyrimidine to pyrimidine) rather than transversions (purine to pyrimidine or vice versa) (Keulen et al., 1996). Furthermore, double mutations are very rare (Das and Berkhout, 2010).

Given that the mutated genomes arising in vivo are usually single-nucleotide substitutions and that advantageous phenotypes often require two or more mutations (e.g., the addition of a compensatory mutation to restore an escape mutant's replicative fitness), one could speculate that the formation of newly adapted strains might be an unlikely occurrence. However, the reverse transcriptase enzyme has another trick up its sleeve that partially overcomes this limitation to variation: recombination. Each viral particle carries two copies of the RNA genome that may or may not be identical. During reverse transcription of the RNA to complementary DNA (cDNA), the enzyme can switch from one template to the other; if the copies carry separate mutations at locations either side of the template switching, the resulting DNA copy now carries both. Indeed, although as discussed above, the mutation rate of HIV is very high, recombination events occur even more frequently, with at least 2.8 crossovers per genome per cycle (Zhuang et al., 2002). One important aspect of the role played by recombination in the evolution of HIV within the infected host is the fact that in the case of double infections of the cell, the mutations have already been selected for fitness in the "donor" virus. They are therefore far more likely to be of benefit to the virus than are the reverse transcription errors, which are predominantly neutral or detrimental to the virus.

As with mutations, recombination events during reverse transcription are not totally random: there are hot spots of recombination located throughout the genome. For example, a 112-bp region near the start of the *gag* gene containing a number of pause bands comprising runs of guanosine residues has been identified as a preferential site of crossing over (Shen et al., 2009). Similarly, due to both mechanistic processes of recombination and the purifying effect of selective pressure discarding nonfunctional proteins, recombination events within the *env* gene (which can obviously profoundly affect the tropism of the resulting virus) tend to cluster within six well-defined regions (Simon-Loriere et al., 2009).

Recombinations within the host originally infected with one or a small number of viruses from a single quasispecies pool enhance the apparent rate of mutation but do not drastically and immediately affect the phenotype of the resulting virus in a way that could not be achieved by mutation alone. However, in the albeit unusual situation in which an individual is coinfected with two different strains of HIV (either through an uninfected individual being infected twice from different sources within a short time or through the more rare incidences of superinfection of an infected host), then template switching can, in one fell swoop, create a mosaic virus that is entirely new. Such viruses have entire genes or gene segments derived from either progenitor and can therefore have dramatically altered characteristics with regard to tropism and fitness.

This facility for recombination was clearly demonstrated by Desrosiers and colleagues, who inoculated a rhesus macaque in one leg with an SIV attenuated by deletions in the *nef* gene and in the other leg with an SIV with deletions in *vpr* and *vpx* (Wooley et al., 1997). Within 2 weeks the animal was found to be productively infected with the full-length wild-type virus formed by recombination of the two attenuated viruses. Such an effect was also seen when macaques were infected intravaginally with the two attenuated viruses, either simultaneously or one shortly after the other (Kim et al., 2005). It is therefore clear that, provided both "donor" viruses are replicating to a degree sufficient to allow simultaneous infection of a single target cell, recombination is a likely event. If the resulting progeny virus has a selective advantage over its two parent viruses, it will rapidly dominate the viral population.

ORIGIN OF HIV

Around 40 species of African primates are currently known to be infected with (usually) their own specific strain of simian immunodeficiency virus (SIV) (Aghokeng et al., 2010) (Fig. 2). The one obvious and dramatic feature of these infections is that these "natural hosts" remain free of AIDS despite being infected with the HIV-related viruses for most of their adult lives. Molecular and epidemiological data indicate that the SIVs have been present for many thousands of years at least, and it is assumed that over this long period of coevolution the virus and host have become adapted to each other and have reached a state of peaceful coexistence. Relatively recently, however, SIV entered the unprepared human population to give rise to the HIV pandemic. Despite first becoming known in the early 1980s, the HIV pandemic had already been slowly progressing for many years. Indeed, the earliest human plasma sample definitively demonstrated to contain the virus was taken from an individual living in Kinshasa, present-day Democratic Republic of the Congo, in 1959 (Zhu et al., 1998). Phylogenetic analysis placed this virus near the ancestral node of subtypes B and D, indicating that it might be a progenitor virus that had only shortly before entered the human population. However, a second sample taken in Kinshasa only 1 year later was found to harbor a virus considerably divergent from the 1959 one (Worobey et al., 2008), being located close to the ancestral node for clade A viruses. This suggests either that the HIV epidemic had been progressing long enough for the virus to have diverged considerably or that at least two epidemics resulting from separate incursions into humans had occurred. By comparing the sequences of modern main-group (M) isolates, it was possible to estimate that the initial sustained zoonotic transmission to humans occurred in the 1920s or earlier (Korber et al., 2000; Worobey et al., 2008). The virus had therefore been spreading in Africa for 50 years before coming to the attention of Western science. Indeed, molecular evidence suggests that HIV was circulating in the United States for about 12 years before being recognized in 1981 (Gilbert et al., 2007).

As mentioned above, there are around 40 known primate species carrying their own variety of SIV (Aghokeng et al., 2010). It is now clear that, in addition to the presumed zoonotic event of 1931, SIVs have become established in humans on at least eight other occasions to give rise to the N and O groups of HIV type 1 (HIV-1) and the eight clades of HIV-2 (Hahn et al., 2000; Van Heuverswyn and Peeters, 2007). Although the origin of HIV-2 had long been known (Gao et al., 1992) to be SIVsmm, a virus endemic in African sooty mangabeys *(Cercocebus atys)*, the precise origin of HIV-1 was less clear. Specimens from wild-caught chimpanzees (or from their fecal matter) were sporadically found to contain HIV-related retroviruses (Peeters et al., 1989), and the source of HIV in humans was narrowed down to the chimpanzee subspecies *Pan troglodytes troglodytes* (Gao et al., 1999). However, it was for some time unclear whether chimpanzees represented the original, natural host of the virus or whether they were merely acting as a temporary reservoir or conduit for a virus naturally infecting another primate species. More recently, extensive analysis of new isolates of SIVcpz*Ptt* established *P. t. troglodytes* as indeed the natural host of the virus that became HIV-1 (Keele et al., 2006; Nerrienet et al., 2005). It is, however, intriguing that SIVcpz (and therefore HIV-1) appears to be a mosaic virus formed by the recombination of two viruses (SIVrcm and SIVgsn) that infect two separate species of monkey known to be hunted by chimpanzees: red-capped mangabeys *(Cercocebus torquatus)*, and greater spot-nosed monkeys *(Cercopithecus nictitans)* (Bailes et al., 2003) (Fig. 3). The SIVcpz *pol* gene clusters with that of SIVrcm whereas its *env* gene is closely related to that of SIVgsn. As well as initiating the HIV

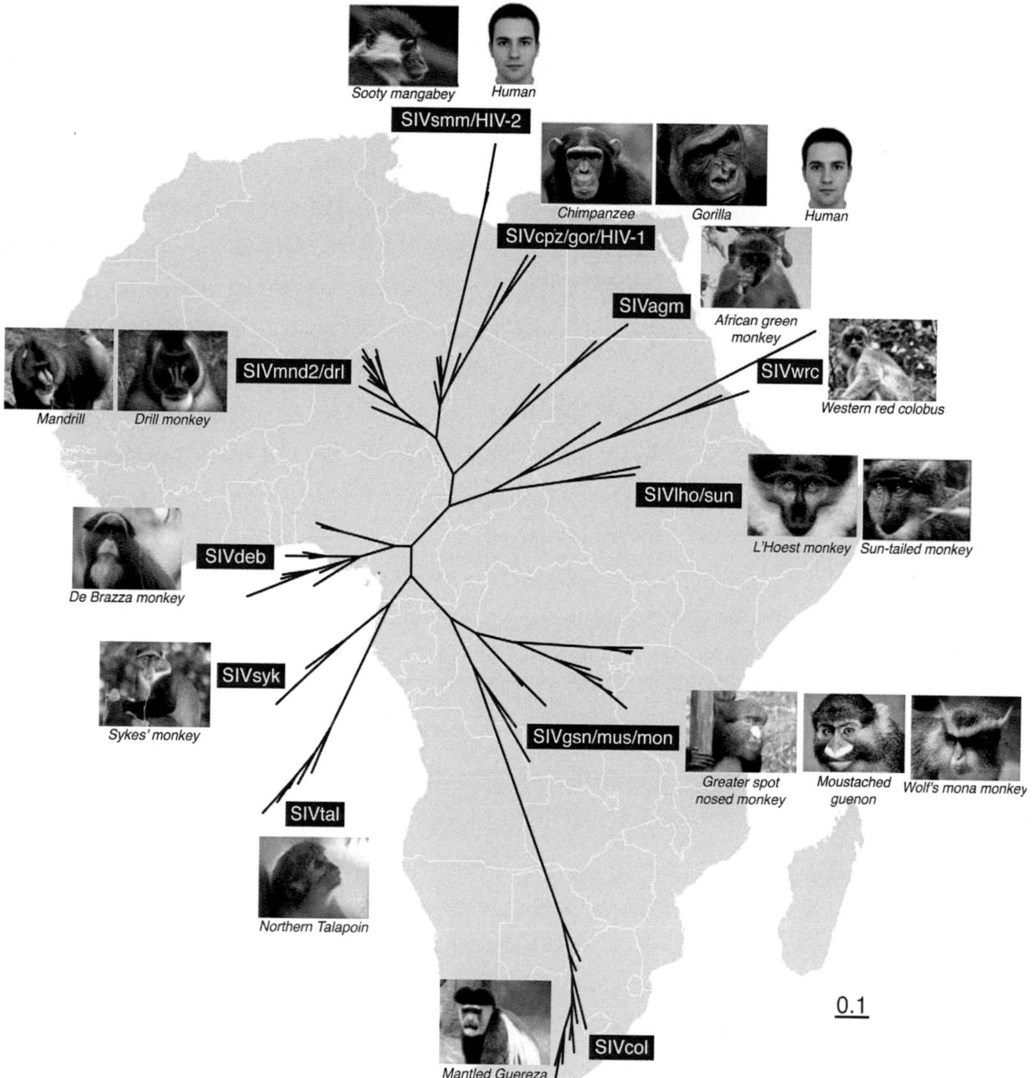

FIGURE 2 Phylogenetic relationships between strains of SIV infecting diverse species of African primates. Shown is the degree of heterogeneity within a portion of the *pol* gene, with the bar representing 0.1 replacement per site. Adapted from Aghokeng et al. (2010).

pandemic in humans, the mosaic virus SIVcpz-*Ptt* has spread to wild gorilla populations in the Cameroon to give SIVgor (Neel et al., 2010; Takehisa et al., 2009).

GLOBAL VARIABILITY

One only has to look at the most recent edition of the *HIV Sequence Compendium* (Kuiken et al., 2010) to realize how extensive the variability of HIV and SIV has become on a global scale. There are over 330,000 sequences in the HIV Sequence Database, and near-full-length sequences of over 2,500 viruses are now available, all of which are unique. Influenza virus, due to its capacity for antigenic drift and antigen shift (reassortment), is commonly regarded as one of the more capricious human pathogens, but the degree of variation of, for

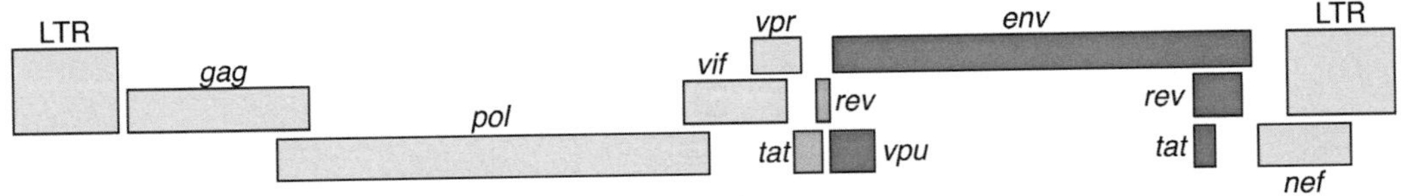

FIGURE 3 Mosaic genome of SIVcpz (and therefore HIV-1). Sequence analyses reveal that the LTRs and the *gag, pol, vif, vpr,* and *nef* genes are derived from the SIVrcm lineage whereas the *env* gene and the 3′ exons of *tat* and *rev* originate from the SIVgsn/mus/mon lineage. The origin of the 5′ exons of *tat* and *rev* is unclear. Adapted from Sharp and Hahn (2010).

example, the H3N2 hemagglutinin on a global scale is matched by that of HIV Env within a single infected individual and is dwarfed by the extensive sequence variability of HIV within just one African nation (Korber et al., 2000; Weiss, 2003) (Fig. 4).

HIV is divided into a number of groups (M, N, O, and tentatively P) representing the progeny of presumed individual zoonotic events. By far the majority of infections worldwide are with viruses belonging to the M (major) group, and this is itself divided into subtypes (or clades) A through K based on sequence homology (subtypes E and I are no longer recognized because they have been shown to consist of recombinants of other subtypes). In addition to the accepted subtypes, a number of circulating recombinant forms (CRFs) have been identified (in addition to the previous subtypes E and I), and indeed such viruses are predominant in some areas. CRF02_AG, for example, accounts for 28% of infections in West Africa (Hemelaar et al., 2006). However, tracing the ancestry of HIV subtypes is complicated, and there is strong evidence to suggest that CRF02_AG is actually an original founding subtype which gave rise to a CRF now erroneously classified as subtype G (Abecasis et al., 2007).

Arising as they did in Africa, infections with all subtypes can be found throughout that continent. However, presumably due primarily to founder effect and subsequent local epidemics, infections in different regions of the rest of the world tend to be dominated by one or a few subtypes. In the United States and Europe subtype B is predominant, whereas in India and other parts of Asia subtype C is most common. This extreme variability further compounds the

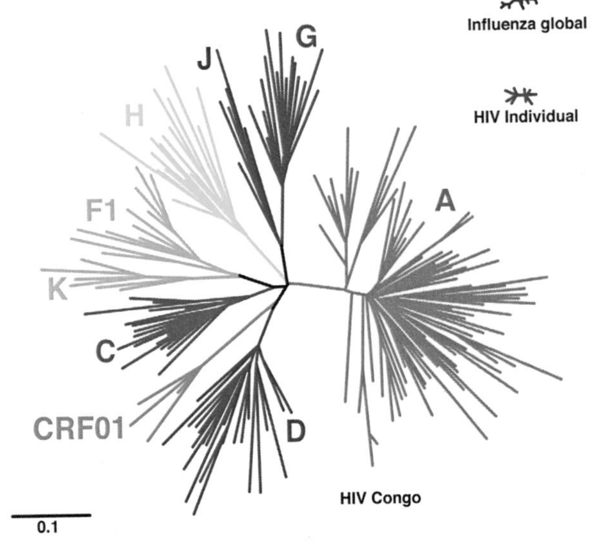

FIGURE 4 Comparison of genomic variability. The degree of variation within the HIV envelope glycoprotein in a long-term singly infected individual is comparable to the global variation of the influenza A H3 hemagglutinin protein in 1 year. Variation of the envelope gene within one African nation (Democratic Republic of Congo) is dramatically higher. Adapted from Weiss (2003).

already significant problems facing the development of an AIDS vaccine.

EVOLUTION IN THE SINGLE INDIVIDUAL

The evolution of HIV is, as with all organisms, driven predominantly by Darwinian natural selection that comprises two fully independent but essential components. The first is the production of random mutations that form a pool of organisms differing slightly in phenotype. This provides the material with which the second component, nonrandom survival of variants, can work. Certainly, genetic drift in the absence of overt selective pressure can accumulate and result in changes in the consensus genotype and phenotype of a population, but, as discussed later in more detail, it is selective pressure that drives the rapid and spectacular evolution of HIV.

Most individuals are infected by a single virus, and the majority of the rest receive a small number of closely related viruses (Keele et al., 2008) which means that with each new infection, the HIV quasispecies present in the "donor" experiences a dramatic bottleneck, giving intrapatient evolution initially very little to work with. However, due to the mechanisms of mutation and recombination, the population of viruses in the newly infected host rapidly expands and diversifies. One study showed the almost complete replacement of the infecting virus with variant populations by 2 months after infection, and by 12 to 20 months a quasispecies of variants with mutations at 17 to 34 discrete locations had developed (Salazar-Gonzalez et al., 2009). Indeed, if the selective pressure is high enough, the entire body's viral population can be replaced with mutants within a matter of days (Wei et al., 1995).

FORCES DRIVING HIV EVOLUTION

The combination of high mutation rate, high recombination rate, and high rate of viral replication provides a wealth of material upon which natural selection can operate. However, aside from the stochastic and unpredictable mechanisms of genetic drift and founder effect, such variability would do little to produce new viral populations without some form of purifying selection; i.e., the newly created variants must have some form of advantage if they are to replace the original viruses. These driving forces include adaptation to the new host or to a new target cell and, more recently, escape from the inhibitory effects of antiviral drugs. However, by far the most potent selective pressure exerted on the virus comes from the host immune response. Although they are by no means mutually exclusive, these forces deserve to be addressed individually.

Adaptation to the Host

Infection by HIV starts with a single virus (or a very limited number of related viruses), and this bottleneck by itself constitutes a selective pressure, because the transmitted virus must be one suited (in most cases) to infect and propagate in the mucosal tissues at the point of entry. Once through this "filter" and into the host's lymphoid tissue, however, the virus that comes to predominate during this early phase will be one best suited to take advantage of the ready-to-use pool of target cells in the body. Determining the primary target for HIV during acute infection of humans is difficult because (i) the time of infection is usually unknown and patients first notice symptoms some weeks following the event and (ii) tissue biopsies of internal organs are generally not possible. However, such studies can and have been done using the SIVmac/rhesus macaque model for AIDS, and the results clearly demonstrate that the $CD4^+$ T cells of the gut-associated lymphoid tissue are massively infected during the acute phase of infection (Chase et al., 2007; Lay et al., 2009). These cells, being predominantly activated, serve as ideal targets for HIV, and this huge reservoir is severely depleted within weeks of infection. It is also significant that these cells usually express the CCR5 coreceptor. It has been known for some time that the viruses isolated from patients during the initial years of infection (non-syncytium inducing and macrophage tropic) use the CCR5 coreceptor to recognize and infect their target cells and that often these viruses later mutate and switch to using the CXCR4 receptor (syncytium inducing and T-cell tropic) (Cheng-Mayer et al., 1988; Fenyo et al., 1988; Tersmette et al., 1988). However, even if a person is infected by contact with a "donor" having predominantly CXCR4-tropic viruses, the initial isolates are almost exclusively CCR5 tropic (van't Wout et al., 1994). The existence of this large pool of highly susceptible $CD4^+$, $CCR5^+$ activated T cells in the gut-associated lymphoid tissue explains the rapid selection of CCR5-tropic variants, since such viruses would have an enormous advantage over CXCR4-tropic viruses during this initial phase of infection. Years later, when activated $CCR5^+$ T cells are a limiting resource for the virus, a mutant able to infect via the CXCR4 receptor might once again have a selective advantage and come to dominate the personal quasispecies of the host.

It is of interest that this "requirement" for CCR5 tropism in the infecting virus renders a particular subset of humans practically resistant to HIV infection. Approximately 10 to 20% of Caucasians carry a 32-bp deletion in one copy of their *CCR5* gene, a mutation that prevents expression of the receptor at the cell surface. Due, presumably, to this lower density of CCR5 expression, such individuals have a slower progression to disease than those with two functional copies of the gene (Liu et al., 1996). Furthermore, the approximately 1% of the population who are homozygous for the CCR5-Δ32 mutation, and who therefore express no CCR5 on the surface of their T cells, are virtually resistant to infection through sexual contact (Dean et al., 1996), although occasional infections with CXCR4-tropic viruses have been reported (Sheppard et al., 2002). Unfortunately, this "protective" mutation is virtually absent in Africa (Martinson et al., 1997).

In addition to the generalized competition to dominate, HIV can adapt to different environments within the individual body. For example, variants of HIV may arise that can replicate within the brain of the host and propagate within this niche (Monken et al., 1995). Indeed, separate regions of the brain can contain compartmentalized quasispecies, each with its own evolutionary history (Morris et al., 1999; Wong et al., 1997). Such compartmentalization can also occur in the spleen, with individual white pulps harboring their own variants of HIV (Cheynier et al., 1995; Delassus et al., 1992) and acting as powerhouses of recombination and genetic variation (Jung et al., 2002).

During the first week or so of massive, exponential expansion of the virus throughout the body, there is no significant pressure from the immune system and selection is limited to competition for resources (i.e., target cells) and possible adaptation to the new host. However, as the body becomes flooded with viral antigen and virus-infected cells, the immune system becomes dramatically activated and responds by producing virus-specific antibodies and T cells. The resulting interplay between virus and immune system is complex, and the fact the virus is not cleared from the body by the host's immunity but, rather, continues its high-level replication for years means that this battle continues for an unusually long time. Such conditions are naturally ideal for the development of escape mutants.

Escape from Immune Control: Neutralizing Antibodies

The body responds to infection by producing antibodies specific for the various virus proteins. A subset of those antibodies specific for the outer and transmembrane envelope glycoproteins interfere with the recognition of (or entry into) the target cell and effectively neutralizes the virion's infectivity. In other lentiviruses such as equine infectious anemia virus, the interplay between the neutralizing-antibody response of the infected horse and the development of neutralizing antibodies is clear (Montelaro et al., 1984; Salinovich et al., 1986). The horse becomes infected and experiences high viral loads before developing neutralizing antibodies that suppress the virus. This is followed by the almost inevitable appearance of an escape mutant not recognized by the circulating neutralizing antibodies, and this allows another burst of high virus load before the immune system can again respond with antibodies specific for the new virus. This interaction continues until the virus exhausts its options for viable escape mutations (or, presumably, the horse exhausts its repertoire of B cells). Such obvious boom-and-bust cycles do not occur with HIV, and the role played by HIV-specific neutralizing antibodies during natural infection remained controversial for some time. Certainly, cultivating HIV in the presence of suboptimal levels of neutralizing antibodies results in the outgrowth of escape mutants (McKeating et al., 1989; Nakowitsch et al., 2005; Shibata et al., 2007; Watkins et al., 1996) and the emergence of neutralizing escape mutants has been documented in vivo, both during acute infection (Richman et al., 2003) and in so-called long-term nonprogressors (LTNPs), i.e., therapy-naive individuals who have been infected for a long time (usually 10 years or more) without developing signs of disease (Bradney et al., 1999).

Although broadly specific neutralizing antibodies appear only after many months or years of infection, type-specific neutralizing antibodies generally appear quickly in the infected host. Nevertheless, HIV continues to replicate, and it is therefore clear that the virus must have some means of avoiding the effects of such antibodies. A neutralizing escape mutant is usually thought to be a virus that has mutated its envelope glycoprotein so that the corresponding epitope is no longer recognized by the antibody, either directly or through conformational change. Indeed, such direct escape mutations have been observed (Frost et al., 2005), and viruses that resist neutralizing-antibody recognition via allosteric changes in the envelope glycoproteins by mutations in the intracytoplasmic tail of the transmembrane glycoprotein have also been generated (Kalia et al., 2005). However, in the case of HIV, neutralizing escape mutants that rapidly replaced the original infecting virus were often found to have mutations that did not map to known epitopes but instead involved changes in glycosylation patterns (Wei et al., 2003). This implies that HIV can modify its glycan shield to prevent access by neutralizing antibodies without actually altering the target epitopes that are usually needed for target cell recognition and entry.

Although HIV-infected humans do not experience the obvious cycles of immune response and viral escape seen with equine infectious anemia virus infection, many groups have shown a pattern of later virus isolates being resistant to neutralization by antibodies generated earlier; i.e., the neutralizing-antibody response continually lags behind the emergence of new escape mutants (Bradney et al., 1999; Bunnik et al., 2008; Mahalanabis et al., 2009). It appears that early during infection, the neutralizing antibodies produced are relatively type specific and targeted to one or two regions of the envelope glycoprotein that are relatively free to mutate without the virus taking a significant fitness hit (Moore et al., 2009; Rong et al., 2009).

Despite the sometimes contradictory nature of the observations, it seems clear that the neutralizing-antibody response to HIV does limit, at least to some degree, the replication of the virus. This is inferred by the emergence of escape mutants, because such viruses would not have an advantage over the wild-type viruses if no selective pressure existed. Whether or not neutralizing antibodies contribute significantly to prevention of disease progression is still unclear, however. Certainly, early analyses of the immune responses in LTNPs appeared to indicate that such individuals were more likely to possess broadly reactive neutralizing antibodies (Cao et al., 1995; Carotenuto et al., 1998; Cecilia et al., 1999; Pilgrim et al., 1997), the logical conclusion being that such antibodies can control the circulating population of HIV and any variants that might arise. It is therefore surprising that the viral population in antiviral drug-naive "elite controllers" (individuals who maintain undetectable virus loads for over 1 year without therapy) and "viremic controllers" (those maintaining virus loads under 2,000 RNA copies/ml [Walker, 2007]) is predominantly neutralization resistant (Mahalanabis et al., 2009) and that the development of broadly neutralizing antibodies in LTNPs is associated with higher viral loads and greater sequence diversity in the *env* gene (Braibant et al., 2008). This suggests that the continuous interplay between immune system and virus, with new variants forming and new antibodies being produced in response, is the reason for LTNPs having broadly specific neutralizing-antibody responses rather than such antibodies being responsible for their prolonged survival.

Escape from Immune Control: Cytotoxic T Lymphocytes

With the onset of the AIDS pandemic, it soon became clear that the course of disease differed significantly between individuals, with some progressing rapidly to AIDS and others falling under the heading of "long-term nonprogressors" or even "elite controllers." Analysis of patient major histocompatibility complex (MHC) haplotypes revealed a strong association between positivity for certain alleles (HLA-B27, HLA-B57, and HLA-B51 in European patients; B5703, B5801, and B8101 in African patients) and protection from disease progression (Frater et al., 2007; Kiepiela et al., 2004; O'Brien et al., 2001). As MHC molecules are involved in presentation of viral protein fragments to specific cytotoxic T lymphocytes (CTLs), a potential role for antiviral CTLs in virus control appeared obvious.

If the CTL response in infected humans exerts a powerful inhibitory effect on viral replication, one would expect the rapid appearance of HIV escape mutants able to circumvent this control. And indeed, this is exactly what has been observed. A series of papers in the early and mid-1990s demonstrated the outgrowth of CTL escape mutants in infected individuals (Borrow et al., 1997; Phillips et al., 1991; Rowland-Jones et al., 1992; Wolinsky et al., 1996). Furthermore, in a cohort of HLA-B27-positive patients who had remained healthy for up to 14 years, rapid progression to disease (loss of $CD4^+$ T cells, rise in plasma viral load) was observed in two patients whose viruses mutated a B27-restricted CTL epitope in Gag, rendering them invisible to the (presumably) controlling CTLs (Goulder et al., 1997).

Analysis of the interplay between host cellular immune response and virus variability in HIV-infected humans is confounded by a number of factors including a lack of knowledge concerning the nature of the infecting virus, heterogeneity in the MHC background of the infected patients, and (generally) a lack of virus and T-cell samples from the acute phase of infection. These problems can be largely overcome by using the SIV/macaque animal model in which animals with common MHC alleles can be infected with a known, clonal virus and samples can be taken at regular intervals thereafter. One of the first such studies examining variation over time in 10 distinct CTL epitopes within the Env and Nef proteins of SIVmac from a family of infected macaques found that all 10 epitopes accumulated nonsynonomous mutations through positive selection, with many of the mutations reducing or even eliminating CTL recognition or MHC binding (Evans et al., 1999). A similar study of animals with the Mamu-A*01 MHC haplotype found that mutations accumulated in epitopes within the Tat protein recognized by the corresponding CTL (Allen et al., 2000), and a further study involving 21 macaques found CTL escape during acute infection in 19 animals (O'Connor et al., 2002).

Due to the techniques used, studies looking at the variation occurring in vivo after infection are limited to a description of the dominant viral variants in circulation at the time of sampling. Recent advances in sequencing technologies have allowed the viral quasispecies to be subjected to ultradeep pyrosequencing (Bimber et al., 2009). This has revealed that, in addition to the one or two dominant variants detected by classical Sanger sequencing, by 17 days postinfection the quasispecies contained lower frequencies of viral variants representing mutations at most amino acid positions of the major CTL epitope (Fig. 5). Such rapid and profound variation within a target for CTLs clearly demonstrates both the extreme plasticity of the HIV/SIV genome and the intense selective pressure exerted on the virus during the acute phase of infection.

Mechanisms of CTL Escape

The options open to the virus for escaping CTL recognition are numerous (Fig. 6). First, it may alter one of the amino acids in the epitope

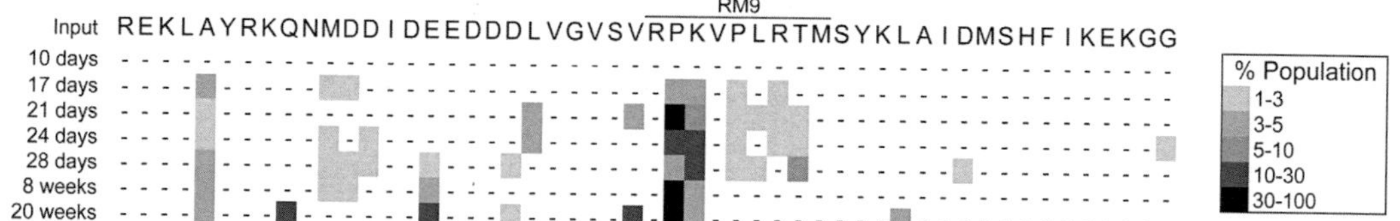

FIGURE 5 Rapid and extensive variation within a CTL epitope. Ultradeep pyrosequencing of the SIVmac *nef* gene after infection of cynomolgus macaques reveals the appearance of variants within only 17 days. Such variants, particularly those with mutations within the RM9 CTL epitope, come to dominate the viral population during the ensuing weeks. Adapted from Bimber et al. (2009).

necessary for recognition by the corresponding CTL T-cell receptor (within the context of the presenting MHC-I molecule). Such a change would probably be only a temporary respite because a new population of CTLs specific for the new epitope could soon appear. If, however, a mutation occurred within the epitope at one of the anchor residues responsible for holding the protein fragment within the MHC-I molecule cleft, it is possible that the new sequence would not be presented by the MHC molecule at all, leaving the immune response unable to respond anew.

Some regions of viral proteins are essential for virion viability, and any alteration results in a dramatic reduction in fitness. CTL epitopes within such conserved regions are therefore resistant to escape. However, it is possible that mutations in the residues flanking the epitope will interfere with the correct processing and presentation of the protein fragment, rendering the virus invisible to the effects of CTLs without exacting the corresponding fitness hit. Finally, if an effective CTL response to an epitope within an essential, conserved region is effectively preventing viral replication, an escape mutant may still have an advantage over the wild-type predecessors, albeit with a vastly reduced fitness, and may therefore come to dominate the viral population. Under such conditions it is possible for a second, compensatory mutation at a distant location to restore the protein to full functionality, leading to a rebound in viral load. Such events have been observed in real time in vivo (Peyerl et al., 2003), and analysis of sequence databases suggests that such tandem mutations occur frequently.

EVOLUTION OF HIV WITHIN THE HUMAN POPULATION

So far, we have discussed the profound influence that the powerful immune response to HIV has on its evolution within the individual infected host. The pattern of epitopes recognized by CTLs varies from person to person depending on the particular mix of MHC-I molecules expressed on the surface of their cells. Upon entering a new host, these epitopes come under extreme selective pressure to mutate and escape. What, then, occurs when such escape mutants, viruses that may have taken a significant fitness hit to circumvent immune control, are transferred to a new host with a different repertoire of MHC-I molecules?

As one would expect, in most cases a virus bearing escape mutations in CTL epitopes that render the protein in question less efficient would suddenly find itself free of the selective pressure (at least with regards to those epitopes) and a mutation that restores the "wild-type" sequence would impart an enormous replicative advantage. Such reversions upon transfer to MHC-mismatched hosts have been documented in humans (Duda et al., 2009; Leslie et al., 2004; Novitsky et al., 2010) and underscore both the efficacy of immune control by CTL and the fitness costs paid by the virus in escaping this control. As usual, it is often easier to monitor such events using the SIV/macaque animal model because one can infect animals of selected MHC background with a standardized virus isolate. One such study (Friedrich et al., 2004), in which virus engineered to contain three "escaped" CTL epitopes was used to infect MHC-matched and -mismatched

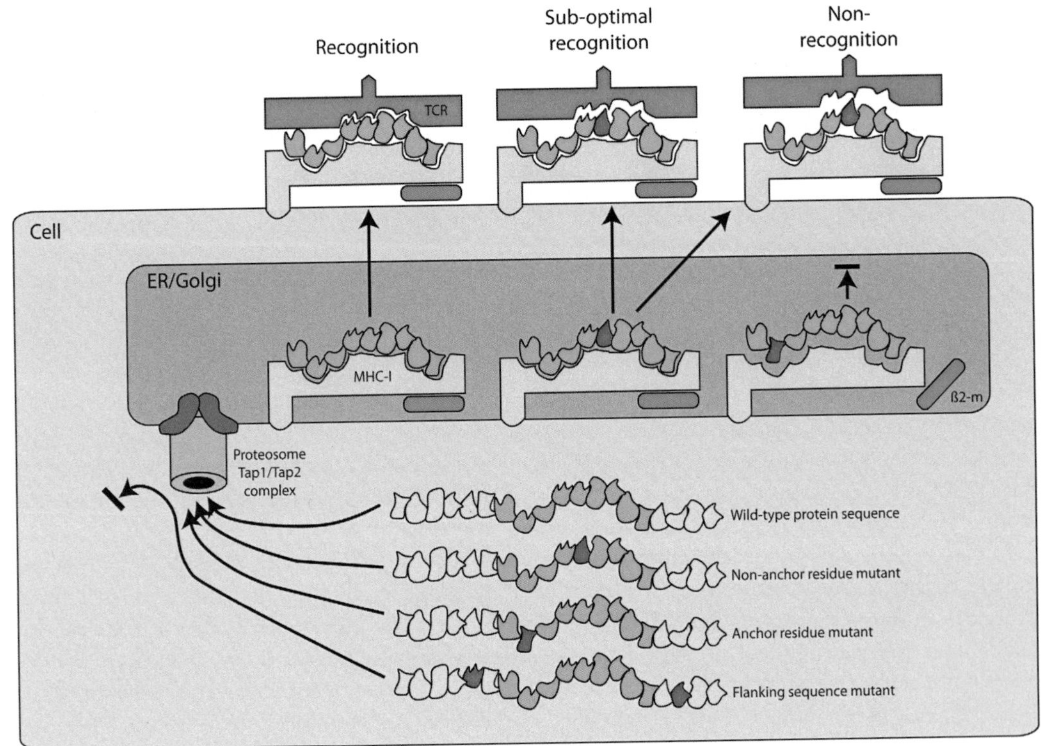

FIGURE 6 Escape from virus-specific CTL recognition. A CTL epitope (blue) within a viral protein is normally processed, bound to an MHC-I molecule, and presented via the endoplasmic reticulum (ER)/Golgi complex on the surface of the cell to be recognized by the corresponding T-cell receptor (TCR) expressed by a CTL. Mutations resulting in the substitution (red) of an amino acid normally recognized by the TCR may result in suboptimal or even no recognition. Mutations resulting in changes of an "anchor" residue can inhibit formation of the MHC-I/β2-microglobulin/epitope complex, preventing expression at the cell surface. Finally, changes in amino acids flanking the epitope may prevent even the wild-type sequence from being processed and expressed. Adapted from Koup (1994).

macaques, found preservation of the escaped versions in animals possessing MHC haplotypes matching those in which the escape is known to occur, but rapid reversion in animals lacking such haplotypes and therefore unable to respond to the wild-type reversion. Another study (Fernandez et al., 2005) showed reversion of a CTL escape mutant within 2 weeks after transfer to MHC-mismatched animals.

Superficially, one might expect that the net result of transmissions from host to host would be zero, i.e., that sequences corresponding to individual CTL epitopes would switch back and forth between "escape/low fitness" and "wild type/high fitness" depending on the MHC environment in which virus finds itself. Although, as mentioned above, this is partially true, it is not the whole story. First, certain MHC-I alleles are very common among particular human populations (HLA-A*0201, for example, is present in over 50% of some groups), which means that CTL escape mutations restricted to such alleles are often still under selective pressure upon transmission and tend to become fixed. Indeed, such "ready-made" escape mutants are already resistant to immune control during the acute phase. This can be a particular problem with mother-to-child transmission because of the high likelihood of the child sharing the MHC allele in question (Goulder et al., 2001). On the other hand, if the escape mutation has an attenuating effect on viral fitness, this virus is maintained in the MHC-matched recipient and, in the absence of an immune response to an otherwise immunodominant epitope, faciliates control by CTLs specific for subdominant epitopes (Schneidewind et al., 2009b).

The second scenario in which reversion to the wild type may not occur is when the escape mutation has little or no effect on viral fitness. Under such conditions, release from immune control by transmission to an MHC-mismatched host lacking the ability to mount a CTL response to the "escaped" epitope does not exert significant selective pressure to revert to wild type. For example, transmission of two distinct escape mutants within one immunodominant CTL epitope to MHC-mismatched recipients (Leslie et al., 2004) resulted in the rapid reversion of one (due to a fitness cost of escape) but maintenance of the other (no fitness cost). Indeed, in populations where a particular MHC allele is common, footprints of CTL escape can commonly be found in infected individuals lacking this allele (Leslie et al., 2004; Matthews et al., 2009).

The third mechanism by which CTL escape mutants can accumulate at the population level is when the loss of fitness caused by the escape mutation is compensated for by a second mutation elsewhere. In this way, even variants carrying potentially attenuating escape mutations can "pass through" individuals lacking the relevant MHC and become fixed at the population level (Schneidewind et al., 2009a, 2009b).

When these data are taken together, it is clear that the population of HIV variants circulating within the human population is evolving and will continue to evolve within an environment that, from the virus's point of view, involves drastic shifts in selective pressure as it moves from one host to another. On the one hand, an escape mutation that renders a virus less fit will tend to persist if the corresponding MHC allele is common within the target population. Although potentially leading to an attenuation of the virus over time, evolution in this direction would also gradually lead to the disappearance of immunodominant epitopes susceptible to immunologic control, a situation that could cause significant problems for vaccine development (Kawashima et al., 2009).

ESCAPE FROM ANTIVIRAL DRUGS

In addition to the extreme selection pressure exerted on HIV by the immune system, there is an additional "artificial" pressure driving HIV evolution, particularly in industrialized countries. Most HIV-infected individuals in such nations have access to highly active antiretroviral therapy (HAART), a cocktail of anti-HIV drugs targeting different aspects of the viral replication cycle. Given the high variability of HIV in vivo, it is no surprise that if suppressed by a single drug, HIV soon responds with an escape mutant. Such mutations quickly negated the benefits of the first antiretroviral, AZT, used to combat HIV (Larder et al., 1989; Larder and Kemp, 1989), and the speed with which HIV can escape control by a single drug first became clear with the advent of protease inhibitors in the mid-1990s (Perelson et al., 1996; Wei et al., 1995). However, by administering a combination of antiviral drugs targeting different viral proteins in different ways, it is possible to suppress the rate of virus replication to a very low level. This greatly diminishes the pool of available variants and makes it very unlikely that a multiple mutant resistant to all drugs being taken will arise. There is now a plethora of antiretrovirals available, some inhibiting the viral reverse transcriptase by a variety of mechanisms and others targeting the viral protease enzyme, the viral integrase, or the transmembrane glycoprotein (Menendez-Arias, 2010). Unfortunately, similar to the situation with antibiotics, poor compliance by patients receiving HAART and other factors can result in the emergence of resistant mutants of HIV. Patients are therefore usually monitored for the appearance of such variants and can be switched to alternative drugs when it becomes necessary.

One worrying aspect of drug resistance is the circulation of escape mutants in the general population, even in those as yet therapy naive (Jakobsen et al., 2010; Recordon-Pinson et al., 2009; Vercauteren et al., 2009; Wensing et al., 2005). Similar to the situation with CTL escape variants, if the mutations leading to drug resistance have no significant effect on viral fitness (or if the effects are nullified by compensatory mutations elsewhere), one can expect such resistance mutations to accumulate in the general population. This has obvious and alarming implications for the future of AIDS therapeutics.

CONCLUSIONS

HIV is almost certainly the most rapidly evolving biological entity on the planet at present. The combination of high error rate during replication, the tendency for separate genomes to recombine with one another through template switching of the viral reverse transcriptase enzyme, and the establishment of what is essentially an acute infection lasting for years provides an almost unlimited pool of viral variants for natural selection to work on. Although the founder effect caused by the bottleneck of transmission and the pressures of adaptation to different tissues and target cells within the new host will drive evolution to some degree, by far the greatest selection force exerted on the virus comes from the host immune response, particularly the virus-specific cytotoxic T-cell response. Although the host CTL response to HIV infection is intense and effective at dramatically reducing virus replication, escape mutants almost inevitably arise. The resulting interplay between virus variation, fitness, and immune response continues for years and is extremely complex, indeed almost chaotic, in nature. Since its introduction from African monkeys to humans via chimpanzees approximately 80 years ago, HIV has diversified and evolved at an alarming rate and continues to evolve today. The challenges posed by the extraordinary plasticity of the HIV genome with regard to vaccine development and therapy are enormous, but it is only by understanding the mechanisms, extent, and limitations of this plasticity that these challenges will hopefully one day be overcome.

REFERENCES

Abecasis, A. B., P. Lemey, N. Vidal, T. de Oliveira, M. Peeters, R. Camacho, B. Shapiro, A. Rambaut, and A. M. Vandamme. 2007. Recombination confounds the early evolutionary history of human immunodeficiency virus type 1: subtype G is a circulating recombinant form. *J. Virol.* **81:**8543–8551.

Aghokeng, A. F., A. Ayouba, E. Mpoudi-Ngole, S. Loul, F. Liegeois, E. Delaporte, and M. Peeters. 2010. Extensive survey on the prevalence and genetic diversity of SIVs in primate bushmeat provides insights into risks for potential new cross-species transmissions. *Infect. Genet. Evol.* **10:**386–396.

Allen, T. M., D. H. O'Connor, P. Jing, J. L. Dzuris, B. R. Mothe, T. U. Vogel, E. Dunphy, M. E. Liebl, C. Emerson, N. Wilson, K. J. Kunstman, X. Wang, D. B. Allison, A. L. Hughes, R. C. Desrosiers, J. D. Altman, S. M. Wolinsky, A. Sette, and D. I. Watkins. 2000. Tat-specific cytotoxic T lymphocytes select for SIV escape variants during resolution of primary viraemia. *Nature* **407:**386–390.

Bailes, E., F. Gao, F. Bibollet-Ruche, V. Courgnaud, M. Peeters, P. A. Marx, B. H. Hahn, and P. M. Sharp. 2003. Hybrid origin of SIV in chimpanzees. *Science* **300:**1713.

Bimber, B. N., B. J. Burwitz, S. O'Connor, A. Detmer, E. Gostick, S. M. Lank, D. A. Price, A. Hughes, and D. O'Connor. 2009. Ultradeep pyrosequencing detects complex patterns of $CD8^+$ T-lymphocyte escape in simian immunodeficiency virus-infected macaques. *J. Virol.* **83:**8247–8253.

Borrow, P., H. Lewicki, X. Wei, M. S. Horwitz, N. Peffer, H. Meyers, J. A. Nelson, J. E. Gairin, B. H. Hahn, M. B. Oldstone, and G. M. Shaw. 1997. Antiviral pressure exerted by HIV-1-specific cytotoxic T lymphocytes (CTLs) during primary infection demonstrated by rapid selection of CTL escape virus. *Nat. Med.* **3:**205–211.

Bradney, A. P., S. Scheer, J. M. Crawford, S. P. Buchbinder, and D. C. Montefiori. 1999. Neutralization escape in human immunodeficiency virus type 1-infected long-term nonprogressors. *J. Infect. Dis.* **179:**1264–1267.

Braibant, M., H. Agut, C. Rouzioux, D. Costagliola, B. Autran, and F. Barin. 2008. Characteristics of the env genes of HIV type 1 quasispecies in long-term nonprogressors with broadly neutralizing antibodies. *J. Acquir. Immune Defic. Syndr.* **47:**274–284.

Bunnik, E. M., L. Pisas, A. C. van Nuenen, and H. Schuitemaker. 2008. Autologous neutralizing humoral immunity and evolution of the viral envelope in the course of subtype B human immunodeficiency virus type 1 infection. *J. Virol.* **82:**7932–7941.

Cao, Y., L. Qin, L. Zhang, J. Safrit, and D. D. Ho. 1995. Virologic and immunologic characterization of long-term survivors of human immunodeficiency virus type 1 infection. *N. Engl. J. Med.* **332:**201–208.

Carotenuto, P., D. Looij, L. Keldermans, F. de Wolf, and J. Goudsmit. 1998. Neutralizing antibodies are positively associated with CD4$^+$ T-cell counts and T-cell function in long-term AIDS-free infection. *AIDS* **12:**1591–1600.

Cecilia, D., C. Kleeberger, A. Munoz, J. V. Giorgi, and S. Zolla-Pazner. 1999. A longitudinal study of neutralizing antibodies and disease progression in HIV-1-infected subjects. *J. Infect. Dis.* **179:**1365–1374.

Chase, A. J., A. R. Sedaghat, J. R. German, L. Gama, M. C. Zink, J. E. Clements, and R. F. Siliciano. 2007. Severe depletion of CD4$^+$ CD25$^+$ regulatory T cells from the intestinal lamina propria but not peripheral blood or lymph nodes during acute simian immunodeficiency virus infection. *J. Virol.* **81:**12748–12757.

Cheng-Mayer, C., D. Seto, M. Tateno, and J. A. Levy. 1988. Biologic features of HIV-1 that correlate with virulence in the host. *Science* **240:**80–82.

Cheynier, R., S. Henrichwark, F. Hadida, E. Pelletier, E. Oksenhendler, B. Autran, and S. Wain-Hobson. 1995. Clonal expansion of T cells and HIV genotypes in microdissected splenic white pulps indicates viral replication in situ and infiltration of HIV-specific cytotoxic T lymphocytes. *Adv. Exp. Med. Biol.* **374:**173–182.

Das, A. T., and B. Berkhout. 2010. HIV-1 evolution: frustrating therapies, but disclosing molecular mechanisms. *Philos. Trans. R. Soc. Lond. B* **365:** 1965–1973.

Dean, M., M. Carrington, C. Winkler, G. A. Huttley, M. W. Smith, R. Allikmets, J. J. Goedert, S. P. Buchbinder, E. Vittinghoff, E. Gomperts, S. Donfield, D. Vlahov, R. Kaslow, A. Saah, C. Rinaldo, R. Detels, and S. J. O'Brien. 1996. Genetic restriction of HIV-1 infection and progression to AIDS by a deletion allele of the CKR5 structural gene. Hemophilia Growth and Development Study, Multicenter AIDS Cohort Study, Multicenter Hemophilia Cohort Study, San Francisco City Cohort, ALIVE Study. *Science* **273:**1856–1862.

Delassus, S., R. Cheynier, and S. Wain-Hobson. 1992. Nonhomogeneous distribution of human immunodeficiency virus type 1 proviruses in the spleen. *J. Virol.* **66:**5642–5645.

Duda, A., L. Lee-Turner, J. Fox, N. Robinson, S. Dustan, S. Kaye, H. Fryer, M. Carrington, M. McClure, A. R. McLean, S. Fidler, J. Weber, R. E. Phillips, and A. J. Frater. 2009. HLA-associated clinical progression correlates with epitope reversion rates in early human immunodeficiency virus infection. *J. Virol.* **83:**1228–1239.

Evans, D. T., D. H. O'Connor, P. Jing, J. L. Dzuris, J. Sidney, J. da Silva, T. M. Allen, H. Horton, J. E. Venham, R. A. Rudersdorf, T. Vogel, C. D. Pauza, R. E. Bontrop, R. DeMars, A. Sette, A. L. Hughes, and D. I. Watkins. 1999. Virus-specific cytotoxic T-lymphocyte responses select for amino-acid variation in simian immunodeficiency virus Env and Nef. *Nat. Med.* **5:**1270–1276.

Fenyo, E. M., L. Morfeldt-Manson, F. Chiodi, B. Lind, A. von Gegerfelt, J. Albert, E. Olausson, and B. Asjo. 1988. Distinct replicative and cytopathic characteristics of human immunodeficiency virus isolates. *J. Virol.* **62:**4414–4419.

Fernandez, C. S., I. Stratov, R. De Rose, K. Walsh, C. J. Dale, M. Z. Smith, M. B. Agy, S. L. Hu, K. Krebs, D. I. Watkins, D. H. O'Connor, M. P. Davenport, and S. J. Kent. 2005. Rapid viral escape at an immunodominant simian-human immunodeficiency virus cytotoxic T-lymphocyte epitope exacts a dramatic fitness cost. *J. Virol.* **79:**5721–5731.

Frater, A. J., H. Brown, A. Oxenius, H. F. Gunthard, B. Hirschel, N. Robinson, A. J. Leslie, R. Payne, H. Crawford, A. Prendergast, C. Brander, P. Kiepiela, B. D. Walker, P. J. Goulder, A. McLean, and R. E. Phillips. 2007. Effective T-cell responses select human immunodeficiency virus mutants and slow disease progression. *J. Virol.* **81:**6742–6751.

Friedrich, T. C., E. J. Dodds, L. J. Yant, L. Vojnov, R. Rudersdorf, C. Cullen, D. T. Evans, R. C. Desrosiers, B. R. Mothe, J. Sidney, A. Sette, K. Kunstman, S. Wolinsky, M. Piatak, J. Lifson, A. L. Hughes, N. Wilson, D. H. O'Connor, and D. I. Watkins. 2004. Reversion of CTL escape-variant immunodeficiency viruses in vivo. *Nat. Med.* **10:**275–281.

Frost, S. D., T. Wrin, D. M. Smith, S. L. Kosakovsky Pond, Y. Liu, E. Paxinos, C. Chappey, J. Galovich, J. Beauchaine, C. J. Petropoulos, S. J. Little, and D. D. Richman. 2005. Neutralizing antibody responses drive the evolution of human immunodeficiency virus type 1 envelope during recent HIV infection. *Proc. Natl. Acad. Sci. USA* **102:**18514–18519.

Gao, F., E. Bailes, D. L. Robertson, Y. Chen, C. M. Rodenburg, S. F. Michael, L. B. Cummins, L. O. Arthur, M. Peeters, G. M. Shaw, P. M. Sharp, and B. H. Hahn. 1999. Origin of HIV-1 in the chimpanzee *Pan troglodytes troglodytes*. *Nature* **397:**436–441.

Gao, F., L. Yue, A. T. White, P. G. Pappas, J. Barchue, A. P. Hanson, B. M. Greene, P. M. Sharp, G. M. Shaw, and B. H. Hahn. 1992. Human infection by genetically diverse SIVSM-related HIV-2 in west Africa. *Nature* **358:**495–499.

Gilbert, M. T., A. Rambaut, G. Wlasiuk, T. J. Spira, A. E. Pitchenik, and M. Worobey. 2007. The emergence of HIV/AIDS in the Americas and beyond. *Proc. Natl. Acad. Sci. USA* **104:**18566–18570.

Goulder, P. J., C. Brander, Y. Tang, C. Tremblay, R. A. Colbert, M. M. Addo, E. S. Rosenberg, T. Nguyen, R. Allen, A. Trocha, M. Altfeld, S. He, M. Bunce, R. Funkhouser, S. I. Pelton, S. K. Burchett, K. McIntosh, B. T. Korber, and B. D. Walker. 2001. Evolution and transmission of stable CTL escape mutations in HIV infection. *Nature* **412:**334–338.

Goulder, P. J., R. E. Phillips, R. A. Colbert, S. McAdam, G. Ogg, M. A. Nowak, P. Giangrande, G. Luzzi, B. Morgan, A. Edwards, A. J. McMichael, and S. Rowland-Jones. 1997. Late escape from an immunodominant cytotoxic T-lymphocyte response associated with progression to AIDS. *Nat. Med.* **3:**212–217.

Hahn, B. H., G. M. Shaw, K. M. De Cock, and P. M. Sharp. 2000. AIDS as a zoonosis: scientific and public health implications. *Science* **287:**607–614.

Hemelaar, J., E. Gouws, P. D. Ghys, and S. Osmanov. 2006. Global and regional distribution of HIV-1 genetic subtypes and recombinants in 2004. *AIDS* **20:**W13–W23.

Jakobsen, M. R., M. Tolstrup, O. S. Sogaard, L. B. Jorgensen, P. R. Gorry, A. Laursen, and L. Ostergaard. 2010. Transmission of HIV-1 drug-resistant variants: prevalence and effect on treatment outcome. *Clin. Infect. Dis.* **50:**566–573.

Jung, A., R. Maier, J. P. Vartanian, G. Bocharov, V. Jung, U. Fischer, E. Meese, S. Wain-Hobson, and A. Meyerhans. 2002. Recombination: multiply infected spleen cells in HIV patients. *Nature* **418:**144.

Kalia, V., S. Sarkar, P. Gupta, and R. C. Montelaro. 2005. Antibody neutralization escape mediated by point mutations in the intracytoplasmic tail of human immunodeficiency virus type 1 gp41. *J. Virol.* **79:**2097–2107.

Kawashima, Y., K. Pfafferott, J. Frater, P. Matthews, R. Payne, M. Addo, H. Gatanaga, M. Fujiwara, A. Hachiya, H. Koizumi, N. Kuse, S. Oka, A. Duda, A. Prendergast, H. Crawford, A. Leslie, Z. Brumme, C. Brumme, T. Allen, C. Brander, R. Kaslow, J. Tang, E. Hunter, S. Allen, J. Mulenga, S. Branch, T. Roach, M. John, S. Mallal, A. Ogwu, R. Shapiro, J. G. Prado, S. Fidler, J. Weber, O. G. Pybus, P. Klenerman, T. Ndung'u, R. Phillips, D. Heckerman, P. R. Harrigan, B. D. Walker, M. Takiguchi, and P. Goulder. 2009. Adaptation of HIV-1 to human leukocyte antigen class I. *Nature* **458:**641–645.

Keele, B. F., E. E. Giorgi, J. F. Salazar-Gonzalez, J. M. Decker, K. T. Pham, M. G. Salazar, C. Sun, T. Grayson, S. Wang, H. Li, X. Wei, C. Jiang, J. L. Kirchherr, F. Gao, J. A. Anderson, L. H. Ping, R. Swanstrom, G. D. Tomaras, W. A. Blattner, P. A. Goepfert, J. M. Kilby, M. S. Saag, E. L. Delwart, M. P. Busch, M. S. Cohen, D. C. Montefiori, B. F. Haynes, B. Gaschen, G. S. Athreya, H. Y. Lee, N. Wood, C. Seoighe, A. S. Perelson, T. Bhattacharya, B. T. Korber, B. H. Hahn, and G. M. Shaw. 2008. Identification and characterization of transmitted and early founder virus envelopes in primary HIV-1 infection. *Proc. Natl. Acad. Sci. USA* **105:**7552–7557.

Keele, B. F., F. Van Heuverswyn, Y. Li, E. Bailes, J. Takehisa, M. L. Santiago, F. Bibollet-Ruche, Y. Chen, L. V. Wain, F. Liegeois, S. Loul, E. M. Ngole, Y. Bienvenue, E. Delaporte, J. F. Brookfield, P. M. Sharp, G. M. Shaw, M. Peeters, and B. H. Hahn. 2006. Chimpanzee reservoirs of pandemic and nonpandemic HIV-1. *Science* **313:**523–526.

Keulen, W., C. Boucher, and B. Berkhout. 1996. Nucleotide substitution patterns can predict the requirements for drug-resistance of HIV-1 proteins. *Antiviral Res.* **31:**45–57.

Kiepiela, P., A. J. Leslie, I. Honeyborne, D. Ramduth, C. Thobakgale, S. Chetty, P. Rathnavalu, C. Moore, K. J. Pfafferott, L. Hilton, P. Zimbwa, S. Moore, T. Allen, C. Brander, M. M. Addo, M. Altfeld, I. James, S. Mallal, M. Bunce, L. D. Barber, J. Szinger, C. Day, P. Klenerman, J. Mullins, B. Korber, H. M. Coovadia, B. D. Walker, and P. J. Goulder. 2004. Dominant influence of HLA-B in mediating the potential co-evolution of HIV and HLA. *Nature* **432:**769–775.

Kim, E.-Y., M. Busch, K. Abel, L. Fritts, P. Bustamante, J. Stanton, D. Lu, S. Wu, J. Glowczwskie, T. Rourke, D. Bogdan, M. Piatak, Jr., J. D. Lifson, R. C. Desrosiers, S. Wolinsky, and C. J. Miller. 2005. Retroviral recombination in vivo: viral replication patterns and genetic structure of simian immunodeficiency virus (SIV) populations in rhesus macaques after simultaneous or sequential intravaginal inoculation with SIVmac239Δ*vpx*/Δ*vpr* and SIVmac239Δ*nef*. *J. Virol.* **79:**4886–4895.

Korber, B., M. Muldoon, J. Theiler, F. Gao, R. Gupta, A. Lapedes, B. H. Hahn, S. Wolinsky, and T. Bhattacharya. 2000. Timing the ancestor of the HIV-1 pandemic strains. *Science* **288:**1789–1796.

Koup, R. A. 1994. Virus escape from CTL recognition. *J. Exp. Med.* **180:**779–782.

Kuiken, C., B. Foley, T. Leitner, C. Apetrei, B. Hahn, I. Mizrachi, J. Mullins, A. Rambaut, S. Wolinsky, and B. Korber (ed.). 2010. *HIV Sequence Compendium 2010.* Los Alamos National Laboratory, Los Alamos, NM.

Larder, B. A., G. Darby, and D. D. Richman. 1989. HIV with reduced sensitivity to zidovudine (AZT) isolated during prolonged therapy. *Science* **243:**1731–1734.

Larder, B. A., and S. D. Kemp. 1989. Multiple mutations in HIV-1 reverse transcriptase confer high-level resistance to zidovudine (AZT). *Science* **246:**1155–1158.

Lay, M. D., J. Petravic, S. N. Gordon, J. Engram, G. Silvestri, and M. P. Davenport. 2009. Is the gut the major source of virus in early simian immunodeficiency virus infection? *J. Virol.* **83:**7517–7523.

Leslie, A. J., K. J. Pfafferott, P. Chetty, R. Draenert, M. M. Addo, M. Feeney, Y. Tang, E. C. Holmes, T. Allen, J. G. Prado, M. Altfeld, C. Brander, C. Dixon, D. Ramduth, P. Jeena, S. A. Thomas, A. St John, T. A. Roach, B. Kupfer, G. Luzzi, A. Edwards, G. Taylor, H. Lyall, G. Tudor-Williams, V. Novelli, J. Martinez-Picado, P. Kiepiela, B. D. Walker, and P. J. Goulder. 2004. HIV evolution: CTL escape mutation and reversion after transmission. *Nat. Med.* **10:**282–289.

Liu, R., W. A. Paxton, S. Choe, D. Ceradini, S. R. Martin, R. Horuk, M. E. MacDonald, H. Stuhlmann, R. A. Koup, and N. R. Landau. 1996. Homozygous defect in HIV-1 coreceptor accounts for resistance of some multiply-exposed individuals to HIV-1 infection. *Cell* **86:**367–377.

Mahalanabis, M., P. Jayaraman, T. Miura, F. Pereyra, E. M. Chester, B. Richardson, B. Walker, and N. L. Haigwood. 2009. Continuous viral escape and selection by autologous neutralizing antibodies in drug-naive human immunodeficiency virus controllers. *J. Virol.* **83:**662–672.

Martinson, J. J., N. H. Chapman, D. C. Rees, Y. T. Liu, and J. B. Clegg. 1997. Global distribution of the CCR5 gene 32-basepair deletion. *Nat. Genet.* **16:**100–103.

Matthews, P. C., A. J. Leslie, A. Katzourakis, H. Crawford, R. Payne, A. Prendergast, K. Power, A. D. Kelleher, P. Klenerman, J. Carlson, D. Heckerman, T. Ndung'u, B. D. Walker, T. M. Allen, O. G. Pybus, and P. J. Goulder. 2009. HLA footprints on human immunodeficiency virus type 1 are associated with interclade polymorphisms and intraclade phylogenetic clustering. *J. Virol.* **83:**4605–4615.

McKeating, J. A., J. Gow, J. Goudsmit, L. H. Pearl, C. Mulder, and R. A. Weiss. 1989. Characterization of HIV-1 neutralization escape mutants. *AIDS* **3:**777–784.

Menendez-Arias, L. 2010. Molecular basis of human immunodeficiency virus drug resistance: an update. *Antiviral Res.* **85:**210–231.

Monken, C. E., B. Wu, and A. Srinivasan. 1995. High resolution analysis of HIV-1 quasispecies in the brain. *AIDS* **9:**345–349.

Montelaro, R. C., B. Parekh, A. Orrego, and C. J. Issel. 1984. Antigenic variation during persistent infection by equine infectious anemia virus, a retrovirus. *J Biol Chem.* **259:**10539–10544.

Moore, P. L., N. Ranchobe, B. E. Lambson, E. S. Gray, E. Cave, M. R. Abrahams, G. Bandawe, K. Mlisana, S. S. Abdool Karim, C. Williamson, and L. Morris. 2009. Limited neutralizing antibody specificities drive neutralization escape in early HIV-1 subtype C infection. *PLoS Pathog.* **5:**e1000598.

Morris, A., M. Marsden, K. Halcrow, E. S. Hughes, R. P. Brettle, J. E. Bell, and P. Simmonds. 1999. Mosaic structure of the human immunodeficiency virus type 1 genome infecting lymphoid cells and the brain: evidence for frequent in vivo recombination events in the evolution of regional populations. *J. Virol.* **73:**8720–8731.

Nakowitsch, S., H. Quendler, H. Fekete, R. Kunert, H. Katinger, and G. Stiegler. 2005. HIV-1 mutants escaping neutralization by the human antibodies 2F5, 2G12, and 4E10: in vitro experiments versus clinical studies. *AIDS* **19:**1957–1966.

Neel, C., L. Etienne, Y. Li, J. Takehisa, R. S. Rudicell, I. N. Bass, J. Moudindo, A. Mebenga, A. Esteban, F. Van Heuverswyn, F. Liegeois, P. J. Kranzusch, P. D. Walsh, C. M. Sanz, D. B. Morgan, J. B. Ndjango, J. C. Plantier, S. Locatelli, M. K. Gonder, F. H. Leendertz, C. Boesch, A. Todd, E. Delaporte, E. Mpoudi-Ngole, B. H. Hahn, and M. Peeters. 2010. Molecular epidemiology of simian immunodeficiency virus infection in wild-living gorillas. *J. Virol.* **84:**1464–1476.

Nerrienet, E., M. L. Santiago, Y. Foupouapouognigni, E. Bailes, N. I. Mundy, B. Njinku, A. Kfutwah, M. C. Muller-Trutwin, F. Barre-Sinoussi, G. M. Shaw, P. M. Sharp, B. H. Hahn, and A. Ayouba. 2005. Simian immunodeficiency virus infection in wild-caught chimpanzees from Cameroon. *J. Virol.* **79:**1312–1319.

Novitsky, V., R. Wang, L. Margolin, J. Baca, S. Moyo, R. Musonda, and M. Essex. 2010. Dynamics and timing of in vivo mutations at Gag residue 242 during primary HIV-1 subtype C infection. *Virology* **403:**37–46.

O'Brien, S. J., X. Gao, and M. Carrington. 2001. HLA and AIDS: a cautionary tale. *Trends Mol. Med.* **7:**379–381.

O'Connor, D. H., T. M. Allen, T. U. Vogel, P. Jing, I. P. DeSouza, E. Dodds, E. J. Dunphy, C. Melsaether, B. Mothe, H. Yamamoto, H. Horton, N. Wilson, A. L. Hughes, and D. I. Watkins. 2002. Acute phase cytotoxic T lymphocyte escape is a hallmark of simian immunodeficiency virus infection. *Nat. Med.* **8:**493–499.

Peeters, M., C. Honore, T. Huet, L. Bedjabaga, S. Ossari, P. Bussi, R. W. Cooper, and E. Delaporte. 1989. Isolation and partial characterization of an HIV-related virus occurring naturally in chimpanzees in Gabon. *AIDS* **3:**625–630.

Perelson, A. S., A. U. Neumann, M. Markowitz, J. M. Leonard, and D. D. Ho. 1996. HIV-1 dynamics in vivo: virion clearance rate, infected cell life-span, and viral generation time. *Science* **271:**1582–1586.

Peyerl, F. W., D. H. Barouch, W. W. Yeh, H. S. Bazick, J. Kunstman, K. J. Kunstman, S. M. Wolinsky, and N. L. Letvin. 2003. Simian-human immunodeficiency virus escape from cytotoxic T-lymphocyte recognition at a structurally constrained epitope. *J. Virol.* **77:**12572–12578.

Phillips, R. E., S. Rowland-Jones, D. F. Nixon, F. M. Gotch, J. P. Edwards, A. O. Ogunlesi, J. G. Elvin, J. A. Rothbard, C. R. Bangham, C. R. Rizza, et al. 1991. Human immunodeficiency virus genetic variation that can escape cytotoxic T cell recognition. *Nature* **354:**453–459.

Pilgrim, A. K., G. Pantaleo, O. J. Cohen, L. M. Fink, J. Y. Zhou, J. T. Zhou, D. P. Bolognesi, A. S. Fauci, and D. C. Montefiori. 1997. Neutralizing antibody responses to human immunodeficiency virus type 1 in primary infection and long-term-nonprogressive infection. *J. Infect. Dis.* **176:**924–932.

Ramirez, B. C., E. Simon-Loriere, R. Galetto, and M. Negroni. 2008. Implications of recombination for HIV diversity. *Virus Res.* **134:**64–73.

Recordon-Pinson, P., G. Anies, M. Bruyand, D. Neau, P. Morlat, J. L. Pellegrin, A. Groppi, R. Thiebaut, F. Dabis, H. Fleury, and B. Masquelier. 2009. HIV type-1 transmission dynamics in recent seroconverters: relationship with transmission of drug resistance and viral diversity. *Antivir. Ther.* **14:**551–556.

Richman, D. D., T. Wrin, S. J. Little, and C. J. Petropoulos. 2003. Rapid evolution of the neutralizing antibody response to HIV type 1 infection. *Proc. Natl. Acad. Sci. USA* **100:**4144–4149.

Rong, R., B. Li, R. M. Lynch, R. E. Haaland, M. K. Murphy, J. Mulenga, S. A. Allen, A. Pinter, G. M. Shaw, E. Hunter, J. E. Robinson, S. Gnanakaran, and C. A. Derdeyn. 2009. Escape from autologous neutralizing antibodies in acute/early subtype C HIV-1 infection requires multiple pathways. *PLoS Pathog.* **5:**e1000594.

Rowland-Jones, S. L., R. E. Phillips, D. F. Nixon, F. M. Gotch, J. P. Edwards, A. O. Ogunlesi, J. G. Elvin, J. A. Rothbard, C. R. Bangham, C. R. Rizza, and A. McMichael. 1992. Human immunodeficiency virus variants that escape cytotoxic T-cell recognition. *AIDS Res. Hum. Retroviruses* **8:**1353–1354.

Salazar-Gonzalez, J. F., M. G. Salazar, B. F. Keele, G. H. Learn, E. E. Giorgi, H. Li, J. M. Decker, S. Wang, J. Baalwa, M. H. Kraus, N. F. Parrish, K. S. Shaw, M. B. Guffey, K. J. Bar, K. L. Davis, C. Ochsenbauer-Jambor, J. C. Kappes, M. S. Saag, M. S. Cohen, J. Mulenga, C. A. Derdeyn, S. Allen, E. Hunter, M. Markowitz, P. Hraber, A. S. Perelson, T. Bhattacharya, B. F. Haynes, B. T. Korber, B. H. Hahn, and G. M. Shaw. 2009. Genetic identity, biological phenotype, and evolutionary pathways of transmitted/founder viruses in acute and early HIV-1 infection. *J. Exp. Med.* **206:**1273–1289.

Salinovich, O., S. L. Payne, R. C. Montelaro, K. A. Hussain, C. J. Issel, and K. L. Schnorr. 1986. Rapid emergence of novel antigenic and genetic variants of equine infectious anemia virus during persistent infection. *J. Virol.* **57:**71–80.

Schneidewind, A., Z. L. Brumme, C. J. Brumme, K. A. Power, L. L. Reyor, K. O'Sullivan, A. Gladden, U. Hempel, T. Kuntzen, Y. E. Wang, C. Oniangue-Ndza, H. Jessen, M. Markowitz, E. S. Rosenberg, R. P. Sekaly, A. D. Kelleher, B. D. Walker, and T. M. Allen. 2009a. Transmission and long-term stability of compensated CD8 escape mutations. *J. Virol.* **83:**3993–3997.

Schneidewind, A., Y. Tang, M. A. Brockman, E. G. Ryland, J. Dunkley-Thompson, J. C. Steel-Duncan, M. A. St John, J. A. Conrad, S. A. Kalams, F. Noel, T. M. Allen, C. D. Christie, and M. E. Feeney. 2009b. Maternal transmission of human immunodeficiency virus escape mutations subverts HLA-B57 immunodominance but facilitates viral control in the haploidentical infant. *J. Virol.* **83:**8616–8627.

Sharp, P. M., and B. H. Hahn. 2010. The evolution of HIV-1 and the origin of AIDS. *Philos. Trans. R. Soc. Lond. B* **365:**2487–2494.

Shen, W., L. Gao, M. Balakrishnan, and R. A. Bambara. 2009. A recombination hot spot in HIV-1 contains guanosine runs that can form a G-quartet structure and promote strand transfer in vitro. *J. Biol. Chem.* **284:**33883–33893.

Sheppard, H. W., C. Celum, N. L. Michael, S. O'Brien, M. Dean, M. Carrington, D. Dondero, and S. P. Buchbinder. 2002. HIV-1 infection in individuals with the CCR5-Delta32/Delta32 genotype: acquisition of syncytium-inducing virus at seroconversion. *J. Acquir. Immune Defic. Syndr.* **29:**307–313.

Shibata, J., K. Yoshimura, A. Honda, A. Koito, T. Murakami, and S. Matsushita. 2007. Impact of V2 mutations on escape from a potent neutralizing anti-V3 monoclonal antibody during in vitro selection of a primary human immunodeficiency virus type 1 isolate. *J. Virol.* **81:**3757–3768.

Simon-Loriere, E., R. Galetto, M. Hamoudi, J. Archer, P. Lefeuvre, D. P. Martin, D. L. Robertson, and M. Negroni. 2009. Molecular mechanisms of recombination restriction in the envelope gene of the human immunodeficiency virus. *PLoS Pathog.* **5:**e1000418.

Takehisa, J., M. H. Kraus, A. Ayouba, E. Bailes, F. Van Heuverswyn, J. M. Decker, Y. Li, R. S.

Rudicell, G. H. Learn, C. Neel, E. M. Ngole, G. M. Shaw, M. Peeters, P. M. Sharp, and B. H. Hahn. 2009. Origin and biology of simian immunodeficiency virus in wild-living western gorillas. *J. Virol.* **83:**1635–1648.

Tersmette, M., R. E. de Goede, B. J. Al, I. N. Winkel, R. A. Gruters, H. T. Cuypers, H. G. Huisman, and F. Miedema. 1988. Differential syncytium-inducing capacity of human immunodeficiency virus isolates: frequent detection of syncytium-inducing isolates in patients with acquired immunodeficiency syndrome (AIDS) and AIDS-related complex. *J. Virol.* **62:**2026–2032.

UNAIDS. 2009. *AIDS Epidemic Update 2009.* UNAIDS. Geneva, Switzerland. http://www.unaids.org/en/KnowledgeCentre/HIVData/EpiUpdate/EpiUpdArchive/2009/default.asp.

Van Heuverswyn, F., and M. Peeters. 2007. The origins of HIV and implications for the global epidemic. *Curr. Infect. Dis. Rep.* **9:**338–346.

van't Wout, A. B., N. A. Kootstra, G. A. Mulder-Kampinga, N. Albrecht-van Lent, H. J. Scherpbier, J. Veenstra, K. Boer, R. A. Coutinho, F. Miedema, and H. Schuitemaker. 1994. Macrophage-tropic variants initiate human immunodeficiency virus type 1 infection after sexual, parenteral, and vertical transmission. *J. Clin. Investig.* **94:**2060–2067.

Vercauteren, J., A. M. Wensing, D. A. van de Vijver, J. Albert, C. Balotta, O. Hamouda, C. Kucherer, D. Struck, J. C. Schmit, B. Asjo, M. Bruckova, R. J. Camacho, B. Clotet, S. Coughlan, Z. Grossman, A. Horban, K. Korn, L. Kostrikis, C. Nielsen, D. Paraskevis, M. Poljak, E. Puchhammer-Stockl, C. Riva, L. Ruiz, M. Salminen, R. Schuurman, A. Sonnerborg, D. Stanekova, M. Stanojevic, A. M. Vandamme, and C. A. Boucher. 2009. Transmission of drug-resistant HIV-1 is stabilizing in Europe. *J. Infect. Dis.* **200:**1503–1508.

Walker, B. D. 2007. Elite control of HIV Infection: implications for vaccines and treatment. *Top. HIV Med.* **15:**134–136.

Watkins, B. A., S. Buge, K. Aldrich, A. E. Davis, J. Robinson, M. S. Reitz, Jr., and M. Robert-Guroff. 1996. Resistance of human immunodeficiency virus type 1 to neutralization by natural antisera occurs through single amino acid substitutions that cause changes in antibody binding at multiple sites. *J. Virol.* **70:**8431–8437.

Wei, X., J. M. Decker, S. Wang, H. Hui, J. C. Kappes, X. Wu, J. F. Salazar-Gonzalez, M. G. Salazar, J. M. Kilby, M. S. Saag, N. L. Komarova, M. A. Nowak, B. H. Hahn, P. D. Kwong, and G. M. Shaw. 2003. Antibody neutralization and escape by HIV-1. *Nature* **422:**307–312.

Wei, X., S. K. Ghosh, M. E. Taylor, V. A. Johnson, E. A. Emini, P. Deutsch, J. D. Lifson, S. Bonhoeffer, M. A. Nowak, B. H. Hahn, M. S. Saag, and G. Shaw. 1995. Viral dynamics in human immunodeficiency virus type 1 infection. *Nature* **373:**117–122.

Weiss, R. A. 2003. HIV and AIDS in relation to other pandemics. *EMBO Rep.* **4**(Spec. No.)**:**S10–S14.

Wensing, A. M., D. A. van de Vijver, G. Angarano, B. Asjo, C. Balotta, E. Boeri, R. Camacho, M. L. Chaix, D. Costagliola, A. De Luca, I. Derdelinckx, Z. Grossman, O. Hamouda, A. Hatzakis, R. Hemmer, A. Hoepelman, A. Horban, K. Korn, C. Kucherer, T. Leitner, C. Loveday, E. MacRae, I. Maljkovic, C. de Mendoza, L. Meyer, C. Nielsen, E. L. Op de Coul, V. Ormaasen, D. Paraskevis, L. Perrin, E. Puchhammer-Stockl, L. Ruiz, M. Salminen, J. C. Schmit, F. Schneider, R. Schuurman, V. Soriano, G. Stanczak, M. Stanojevic, A. M. Vandamme, K. Van Laethem, M. Violin, K. Wilbe, S. Yerly, M. Zazzi, and C. A. Boucher. 2005. Prevalence of drug-resistant HIV-1 variants in untreated individuals in Europe: implications for clinical management. *J. Infect. Dis.* **192:**958–966.

Wolinsky, S. M., B. T. Korber, A. U. Neumann, M. Daniels, K. J. Kunstman, A. J. Whetsell, M. R. Furtado, Y. Cao, D. D. Ho, and J. T. Safrit. 1996. Adaptive evolution of human immunodeficiency virus-type 1 during the natural course of infection. *Science* **272:**537–542.

Wong, J. K., C. C. Ignacio, F. Torriani, D. Havlir, N. J. Fitch, and D. D. Richman. 1997. In vivo compartmentalization of human immunodeficiency virus: evidence from the examination of pol sequences from autopsy tissues. *J. Virol.* **71:**2059–2071.

Wooley, D. P., R. A. Smith, S. Czajak, and R. C. Desrosiers. 1997. Direct demonstration of retroviral recombination in a rhesus monkey. *J. Virol.* **71:**9650–9653.

Worobey, M., M. Gemmel, D. E. Teuwen, T. Haselkorn, K. Kunstman, M. Bunce, J. J. Muyembe, J. M. Kabongo, R. M. Kalengayi, E. Van Marck, M. T. Gilbert, and S. M. Wolinsky. 2008. Direct evidence of extensive diversity of HIV-1 in Kinshasa by 1960. *Nature* **455:**661–664.

Zhu, T., B. T. Korber, A. J. Nahmias, E. Hooper, P. M. Sharp, and D. D. Ho. 1998. An African HIV-1 sequence from 1959 and implications for the origin of the epidemic. *Nature* **391:**594–597.

Zhuang, J., A. E. Jetzt, G. Sun, H. Yu, G. Klarmann, Y. Ron, B. D. Preston, and J. P. Dougherty. 2002. Human immunodeficiency virus type 1 recombination: rate, fidelity, and putative hot spots. *J. Virol.* **76:**11273–11282.

GENOME PLASTICITY OF INFLUENZA VIRUSES

Silke Stertz and Peter Palese

10

Influenza viruses have caused devastating pandemics and epidemics in the past, and they continue to be a major health problem causing a huge economic burden worldwide. Thus, it is important to understand the characteristics of influenza viruses and to elucidate the extensive interplay between virus and host.

Influenza viruses belong to the family *Orthomyxoviridae*, which includes the genera *Influenzavirus A, B,* and *C, Thogotovirus*, and *Isavirus* (Palese and Shaw, 2007). Members of the family are characterized by a segmented, single-stranded negative-sense RNA genome which consists of eight segments in influenza A and B viruses and seven segments in influenza C virus. Influenza A viruses are further classified into different subtypes according to their surface glycoproteins, the hemagglutinin (HA) and the neuraminidase (NA). To date, 16 different types of HA and 9 types of NA have been isolated, and multiple subtypes with various combinations of HA and NA can be found in different animal species, including aquatic birds. However, in humans only three subtypes have been circulating: H1N1, H2N2, and H3N2. Different subtypes have not been described for influenza B and C viruses. The nomenclature for influenza viruses includes the genus, the species from which the virus was isolated (except for humans), the location, the isolate number, and the year of virus isolation (Palese and Shaw, 2007). As an example, the virus strain A/Brisbane/59/2007 is an influenza A virus which was the 59th isolate from humans in Brisbane, Australia, in 2007.

Influenza A viruses display a pleomorphic structure: spherical particles of about 100 nm in diameter have been described as well as filamentous particles which can be more than 300 nm in length. The virions consist of a lipid bilayer which is derived from the plasma membrane of the host cell and harbors the viral glycoproteins HA and NA and the ion channel M2, a layer of matrix protein M1 underneath the lipid bilayer, and the ribonucleoprotein (RNP) complexes in the lumen of the virion (Fig. 1A and B). Each RNP consists of an RNA segment encapsidated by the viral nucleoprotein (NP) and the viral polymerase complex containing PB1, PB2, and PA bound to the ends of the RNA. Besides the eight structural proteins, influenza A virus encodes the three nonstructural proteins NS1, NEP, and PB1-F2 (Palese and Shaw, 2007).

Silke Stertz and Peter Palese, Department of Microbiology, Mount Sinai School of Medicine, 1 Gustave Levy Pl., New York, NY 10029-6574.

Genome Plasticity and Infectious Diseases,
Edited by J. Hacker, U. Dobrindt, and R. Kurth,

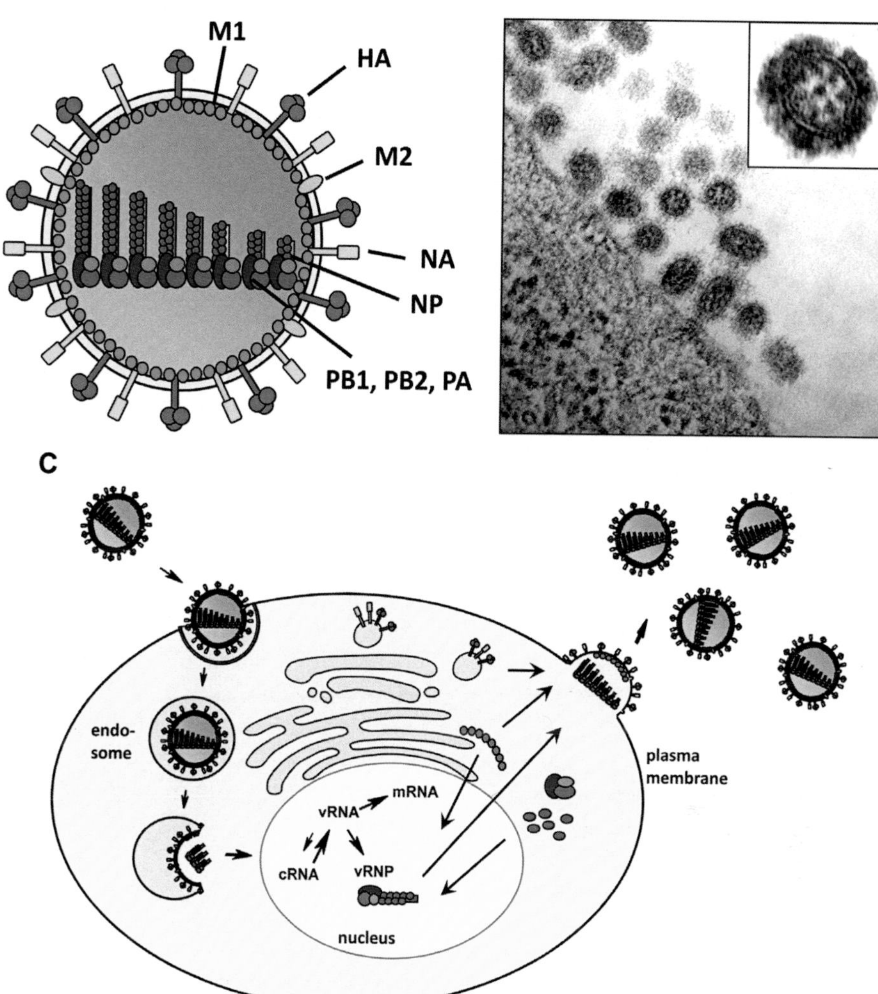

FIGURE 1 (A) Schematic representation of the influenza A virus particle. The virion possesses a membrane which is derived from the host cell plasma membrane and harbors the viral glycoproteins hemagglutinin (HA) and neuraminidase (NA) as well as the ion channel M2. The inner side of the membrane is lined with the matrix protein M1. The viral ribonucleoprotein complexes (RNPs) consist of viral RNA which is encapsidated with the nucleoprotein NP and associated with the polymerase complex, which consists of the three subunits PB1, PB2, and PA. (B) Electron micrographs of influenza A virus particles. MDCK cells were infected with influenza A virus strain A/WSN/33 at a high multiplicity of infection. At 20 h postinfection, samples were fixed (2.5% glutaraldehyde in 0.1 M cacodylate buffer, followed by 2% osmium tetraoxide) and en bloc staining was performed (2% uranyl acetate). Samples were dehydrated and embedded in Epon 812 resin mixture. Ultrathin sections were stained with 2% uranyl acetate in 70% ethanol followed by Reynolds lead. Sections were examined with an H-7650 electron microscope (Hitachi) operated at 80 kV. A section of an MDCK cell from which progeny virions are budding is shown. The inset shows a higher magnification of one of the virions. In this cross section the eight RNP segments are visible as dot-like structures within the particle. These pictures were kindly provided by Yi-ying Chou, Mount Sinai School of Medicine, New York, NY. (C) Schematic representation of the influenza A virus replication cycle. Virions are taken up by endocytosis after binding of HA to sialic acid on surface proteins of the host cell plasma membrane. Upon acidification of the endosome, HA mediates fusion of the viral membrane with the endosomal membrane and the viral RNPs are released into the cytosol. The RNPs are transported to the nucleus, where transcription and replication occur. The late stages of the replication cycle take place at the budding sites at the plasma membrane, where the structural components of the virus form progeny virions.

The viral glycoprotein HA is responsible for binding to the receptor sialic acid on the host cell and thereby facilitates endocytic uptake of the virus (Fig. 1C). Upon acidification of the endosome, HA undergoes major conformational changes which lead to fusion of the viral membrane with the endosomal membrane. The ion channel M2 ensures that the lumen of the virion gets acidified in the endosome, which enables the RNPs to detach from the matrix protein M1 (Matlin et al., 1981) and to be released into the cytosol of the host cell after fusion of the viral membrane with the endosomal membrane. Next, the RNPs are imported into the nucleus of the host cell (Martin and Helenius, 1991), where the viral polymerase facilitates transcription and replication of the viral genome. Late in the replication cycle, the newly synthesized glycoproteins are transported to the budding site at the plasma membrane via vesicular transport pathways. Progeny viral genomic RNA which is encapsidated by NP and bound to the polymerase complex is then exported from the nucleus by the viral nuclear export protein NEP and the matrix protein M1 (Palese and Shaw, 2007). It is unclear to date how these complexes are transported to the budding site after exiting the nucleus. The assembly process takes place at the plasma membrane, and HA is thought to be the driving force of budding (Leser and Lamb, 2005). However, the molecular mechanism of budding is not well understood. The viral NA is crucial for the last step of the replication cycle, the release of virions: by cleaving off sialic acids, NA prevents virions from being bound to the host cell and enables the release of progeny virions (Fig. 1C) (Palese and Shaw, 2007).

While influenza B and C viruses circulate only in humans, influenza A viruses infect a wide range of animals. The natural reservoir of all influenza A virus subtypes is aquatic birds, but some subtypes are maintained in humans, domestic poultry, pigs, dogs, horses, and other species (Wright et al., 2007). In humans, influenza A, B, and C viruses can cause disease. However, infection by influenza C virus usually leads to very mild symptoms whereas influenza A and influenza B viruses can cause more severe disease. The symptoms of influenza include fever, headache, dry cough, sore throat, runny or stuffy nose, muscle aches, and, in some cases, especially in young children, gastrointestinal symptoms. Striking predominantly in the winter months, influenza is a severe problem, with millions of people getting infected every year. In the United States, for example, 5 to 20% of the population is infected each year, which causes more than 200,000 hospitalizations and approximately 36,000 deaths in most years (www.cdc.gov/flu/about/disease/index.htm). It is important to note that there are both direct costs due to medical treatment for patients and indirect costs due to sick leave, for example.

In addition to the problems caused by seasonal influenza, there is the threat of an emerging influenza pandemic, as occurred in 1918, 1957, 1968, and 2009. Pandemics are the result of an introduction into the human population of an influenza A virus to which no or very little preexisting immunity is present. This happened in 1918, when the so-called Spanish flu killed more than 50 million people (Johnson and Mueller, 2002) and in 1957 when an H2N2 virus caused the Asian flu pandemic. In recent years there was the threat of a pandemic caused by H5N1 viruses. From 1997 to 2010, the H5N1 viruses caused close to 300 lethal infections in humans. However, these viruses have not yet gained the ability to spread efficiently from human to human. In spring 2009, the focus shifted to a novel virus of the H1N1 subtype which spread around the globe within a few months. In this outbreak (which was declared a pandemic by the World Health Organization), in contrast to the other pandemics, there was no change of subtype. Taken together, influenza viruses pose a major problem for human health and thereby cause a substantial economic burden. It is crucial to determine which viral features are associated with increased virulence and also which factors on the host side contribute to severe outcomes of influenza virus infections. In recent years, great progress in characterizing genetic virulence factors of the virus has been made; however, much less is known about genetic susceptibility factors on the host side, especially in humans. In this chapter we discuss the current knowledge of these factors.

VIRAL FACTORS

To be successful, an influenza virus must replicate and produce progeny virions in a given host. The advanced understanding of viral features which contribute to efficient virus replication is summarized below.

The Viral Glycoproteins HA and NA

The influenza pandemics which occurred in the past century share the fact that new subtypes of influenza A viruses were introduced into the human population. This phenomenon is based on reassortment of RNA segments between different virus strains. Within a host cell that is infected by two different viruses, progeny with different combinations of segments can be produced. Most combinations are less fit in a given host than the parental strains which have adapted to the host. However, in some instances a virus strain which is more efficient in replication or transmission might evolve and therefore propagate efficiently. In 1968, reassortment of two viruses resulted in a new pandemic virus which had six segments from the seasonal virus circulating around that time plus two new segments encoding a novel type of hemagglutinin (H3) and a different PB1 subunit of the polymerase complex (Kawaoka et al., 1989). The exchange of HA enabled the virus to replicate and spread efficiently since there was no or little preexisting immunity in the population. The contribution of PB1 is less well understood, but it is possible that it led to an improved function of the polymerase complex. Alternatively, the presence of PB1-F2, which is encoded in an alternative open reading frame on the PB1 segment, could have resulted in increased fitness of the virus. The introduction of a new subtype is called antigenic shift and is considered a hallmark of influenza A virus evolution. Besides antigenic shift, a process called antigenic drift is the main mechanism by which the virus evades preexisting immunity. It consists of the gradual accumulation of point mutations in the glycoproteins HA and NA due to positive selection of mutants by neutralizing antibodies (Fig. 2). As a consequence of this constant change of the antigenicity of the virus, the vaccine for seasonal influenza has to be updated frequently.

HA is a key factor for virulence. Besides its ability to constantly change antigenically, it contributes to virulence by defining receptor specificity as well as the range of target tissues. The HA protein is produced as a precursor (HA0) which is posttranslationally cleaved into HA1 and HA2. The site for proteolytic cleavage is an important determinant of virulence. In highly pathogenic avian influenza viruses the proteolytic cleavage site contains multiple basic amino acids (Kawaoka and Webster, 1988), enabling cleavage by ubiquitously expressed subtilisin-related proteases like furin (Wright et al., 2007). Viruses with multibasic cleavage sites can cause systemic infections, whereas viruses with a single arginine at the cleavage site rely on specific proteases which are expressed only in the respiratory tract in mammals or the gastrointestinal tract in birds. Tryptase Clara, for example, is expressed in cells of the respiratory tract of mice and rats and can mediate cleavage of HA (Kido et al., 1992).

Tissue tropism of a virus is further determined by its receptor specificity. HA binds sialic acid (SA) as a receptor on the host cell surface to initiate infection. Specifically, HA recognizes terminal sialic acids linked to galactose by either an α2,3 linkage (SAα2,3Gal) or an α2,6 linkage (SAα2,6Gal). Avian viruses preferentially bind SAα2,3Gal, whereas human viruses prefer to bind to SAα2,6Gal (Connor et al., 1994). This roughly matches the distribution of SA in the respiratory tract of humans, where SAα2,6Gal is predominant on epithelial cells of the upper respiratory tract, and the gastrointestinal tract of birds, where SAα2,3Gal is most prevalent (Couceiro et al., 1993; Ito et al., 1998). In viruses of the H2 and H3 subtypes, receptor specificity is determined by amino acids 226 and 228: glutamine at position 226 and glycine 228 result in a preference for SAα2,3Gal binding in avian viruses, whereas leucine 226 and serine 228 are

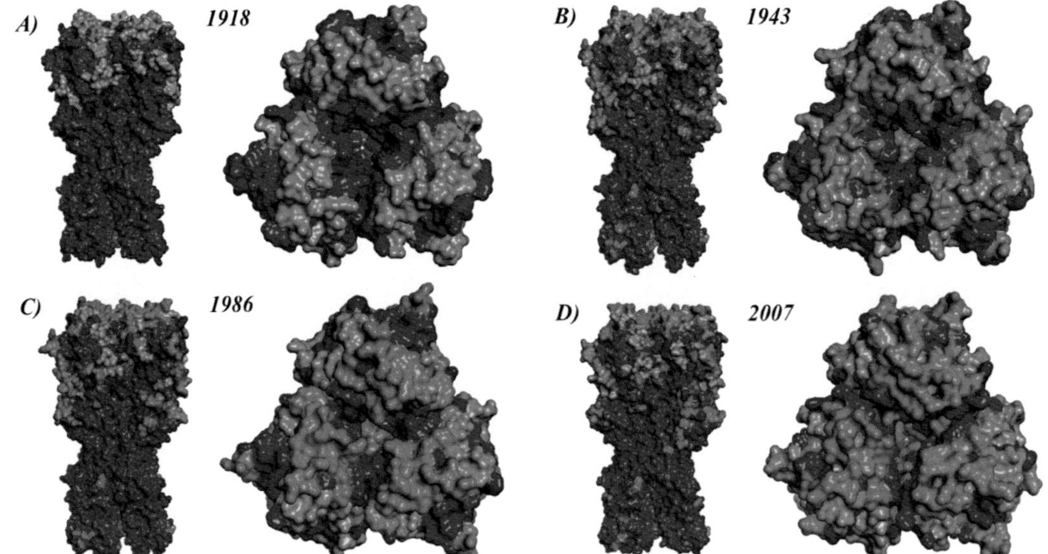

FIGURE 2 Antigenic drift of H1N1 viruses from 1918, 1943, 1986, and 2007. The HA trimeric complex is shown for virus strains A/Brevig Mission/1/1918, A/Weiss/43, A/Taiwan/1/1986, and A/Brisbane/59/2007 to illustrate the gradual accumulation of amino acid changes in the antigenic sites over the years. The structure of 1918 HA was obtained from the PDB server (ID: 2WRG), and the modeling for the other HA proteins was performed using the Swiss Model software. The left side shows the trimer from the side; the right side displays a zenithal view of the trimer. Blue corresponds to conserved amino acids, and red represents amino acids that differ from the 1918 HA. The antigenic sites are colored in light blue. Most neutralizing antibodies bind to the antigenic sites on the upper part of the trimeric complex. Thus, most amino acid changes occur at these sites. The structure modeling was kindly provided by Estanislao Nistal-Villan (Manicassamy et al., 2010).

found in human viruses and mediate binding to SAα2,6Gal (Neumann and Kawaoka, 2006). In viruses of the H1 subtype, amino acid 190 seems to be most critical for receptor specificity (Glaser et al., 2005). Glutamate at position 190 is found in avian viruses, whereas aspartate is dominant in human isolates. Additional contributions to specificity have been reported for positions 136, 195, and 225 in the H1 subtype (van Riel et al., 2006; Wright et al., 2007).

For many years, the dogma was that avian viruses cannot infect humans because of this difference in receptor specificity. However, in 1997, when H5N1 viruses infected humans and even led to fatal outcomes, it became clear that in some instances avian viruses can infect humans. This can be explained by recent findings that SAα2,3Gal is present on certain cell types in the lower human respiratory tract and that this might enable infections with avian viruses (van Riel et al., 2006). It should be noted, though, that infections of humans with avian viruses are a rare event. Furthermore, mutations in HA might also affect the replication efficiency of the virus. As an example, amino acid substitutions at positions 119 and 186 in the HA of the live-attenuated vaccine virus for the pandemic H1N1 virus of 2009 resulted in increased replication efficiency (Chen et al., 2010). Directly linked to the receptor specificity of the virus is the activity of its NA. As mentioned above, NA cleaves off sialic acids on the host cell and thereby allows for efficient release of progeny virions. To this aim, receptor binding affinity and receptor-destroying activity need to be balanced well. When the N2 type of NA was introduced into humans, its cleavage activity for SAα2,6Gal increased, most probably as a consequence of the increased affinity of HA to SAα2,6Gal (Baum and Paulson, 1991; Kobasa et al., 1999). This example illustrates that evolution selects for viruses with correlating HA and NA activities. In summary, the glycoproteins HA and NA determine the antigenicity, receptor binding, and tissue tropism of a virus and thus are important determinants of virulence.

The Viral Polymerase Complex

In addition to the glycoproteins, the polymerase complex is a major determinant of virulence and host adaptation. The polymerase complex consists of three subunits: PB1, PB2, and PA. Furthermore, the viral nucleoprotein NP is needed for efficient transcription and replication of the viral genome. The polymerase activity occurs in the nucleus of a host cell and relies on numerous host cell processes, e.g., the cellular import machinery for nuclear proteins. It is evident that a successful virus needs a polymerase which can use the host cell machinery efficiently and produce viral transcripts and genomes at a high rate. Indeed, many studies have shown that more pathogenic viruses possess higher polymerase activities than less pathogenic viruses (Gabriel et al., 2005; Salomon et al., 2006; Grimm et al., 2007), confirming that replication efficiency is crucial for virulence. In recent years, several amino acids critical for efficient replication have been identified in the polymerase complex. The most prominent is residue 627 in PB2. Avian viruses usually carry a glutamic acid (E) at this position; most human viruses have replaced the glutamic acid with a lysine (K). Initially, the E627K mutation was described as a determinant of host range in vitro (Subbarao et al., 1993). In 2001, an in vivo study showed that the presence of lysine at position 627 determined whether a virus of the H5N1 subtype was lethal in mice (Hatta et al., 2001). Furthermore, an H7N7 virus isolated from a human with a fatal case of influenza in The Netherlands had a lysine at position 627 of PB2 whereas all the viruses isolated from patients with nonfatal cases and from chickens had a glutamic acid (Munster et al., 2007). Subsequent in vitro studies revealed that polymerase complexes with the 627K substitution replicate better in mammalian cells. This difference was most obvious at 37°C (the body temperature of humans), while there was no significant difference at 41°C, the body temperature of birds (Massin et al., 2001). While many studies have confirmed that E627K can mediate adaptation to mammalian cells, it also became clear that it is not an absolute prerequisite. Several virus isolates from patients with severe H5N1 infections were shown to have a glutamic acid at position 627, suggesting that other residues can mediate adaptation to mammalian cells. Indeed, it could be demonstrated in an H5N1 model as well as in a study using H7N7 viruses that D701N in PB2 can also lead to enhanced polymerase activity in mammalian cells (Gabriel et al., 2005; Li et al., 2005; Steel et al., 2009).

The novel H1N1 virus of the 2009 pandemic has developed yet another strategy. It possesses the avian signature amino acids at positions 627 and 701 but has two unique amino acids which lead to increased polymerase activity in mammalian cells: serine at 590 and arginine at 591 (Mehle and Doudna, 2009). Interestingly, structural modeling predicts the juxtaposition of arginine at 591 to lysine at 627, suggesting that the mechanism by which 627K and 591R mediate enhancement of polymerase function might be the same. However, the molecular mechanism has not been elucidated yet. At least two different modes of action are possible. (i) The adaptive mutations could help overcome a cellular restriction factor which inhibits avian viruses in mammalian cells. (ii) Alternatively, interaction of the polymerase with a required host cell factor could be improved and thereby polymerase function could be more efficient. Overall, PB2 seems to play a crucial role in adaptation to mammalian cells, but it is unclear to date how this works. Furthermore, PB1 and PA can also contribute to replication efficiency. Several amino acids in PB1 and PA have been identified in different model systems, but in contrast to PB2, no dominant amino acid change has been described so far.

The Viral Nonstructural Protein PB1-F2

In 2001 it was found that the PB1 segment encodes an additional protein, PB1-F2, which is transcribed from an alternative +1 reading frame

(Chen et al., 2001). Not all influenza A virus strains encode a functional PB1-F2 protein; it is an accessory protein which has been implicated in virulence by several studies. PB1-F2 has been shown to increase virulence by promoting secondary bacterial infections, increasing cell infiltration and cytokine release, and delaying viral clearance in the lungs (Zamarin et al., 2006; Conenello et al., 2007; McAuley et al., 2007), but the mechanism behind these findings is unclear. In vitro studies revealed a proapoptotic function of PB1-F2 (Gibbs et al., 2003; Zamarin et al., 2005), but this has not been confirmed in vivo yet. In support of its role as a virulence factor, PB1-F2 was found to be encoded by the pandemic viruses of 1918, 1957, and 1968 as well as by H5N1 viruses. Closer analysis revealed that amino acid 66 of PB1-F2 is of particular interest (Conenello et al., 2007). H5N1 viruses which displayed a highly pathogenic phenotype in mice, as well as the highly virulent virus of the 1918 pandemic, have a serine (S) at position 66, whereas less pathogenic viruses possess an asparagine (N) at this position. Mutation of S66 to N drastically reduced pathogenicity in both the H5N1 and the 1918 background, and so PB1-F2 with S66 can be defined as a virulence factor (Conenello et al., 2007).

The Viral Nonstructural Protein NS1

Segment 8 of influenza A virus encodes two proteins: nonstructural protein 1 (NS1) and the nuclear export protein (NEP). The unspliced mRNA transcribed from segment 8 is translated into NS1, and a spliced transcript derived from the same mRNA encodes NEP. Despite its small size of approximately 26 kDa, NS1 has multiple functions and activities. It has been implicated in regulating viral RNA synthesis, viral mRNA translation, splicing of mRNAs, and several cellular signaling pathways (Hale et al., 2008). Its main function is to antagonize the innate immune response of the host by blocking the induction of alpha/beta interferon (IFN-α /β) (Garcia-Sastre et al., 1998). These cytokines are the key regulators of the host's innate immune response to virus infections (Haller et al., 2006). They work in an autocrine and paracrine manner and lead to the upregulation of more than 300 IFN-stimulated genes. The gene products can then induce an antiviral state in the IFN-exposed cells, and virus spread can thus be limited. Since the adaptive immune response relies on an efficient innate response, inhibition of the IFN system also causes a delay of the adaptive response (Goodbourn et al., 2000). Influenza viruses with an NS1 deletion are severely attenuated in IFN-competent hosts (Egorov et al., 1998; Garcia-Sastre et al., 1998).

The mechanism of IFN suppression is to some extent strain specific, but two main modes of action can be described. First, NS1 limits the induction of the IFN response by blocking the activation of a crucial sensor of viral infections, RIG-I (Pichlmair et al., 2006; Mibayashi et al., 2007; Gack et al., 2009). Second, NS1 interferes with cellular mRNA processing (Nemeroff et al., 1992; Qiu and Krug, 1994; Noah et al., 2003). The fact that at least two independent mechanisms for suppression of the IFN system have evolved shows that this function is critical for the virus. This was confirmed by multiple experimental studies which showed that impairment of the ability to suppress the induction of IFN attenuates the virus (Garcia-Sastre et al., 1998; Talon et al., 2000; Kochs et al., 2007). In 2002, an additional level of counteracting the IFN system was described for the NS1 proteins of highly pathogenic H5N1 viruses: they were shown to confer resistance to IFN treatment, and glutamic acid at position 92 was found to be required for the observed resistance (Seo et al., 2002). Since H5N1 infections induce high levels of proinflammatory cytokines, it is obvious that the ability to replicate in the presence of IFN is a big advantage for the virus. It is still unclear, though, if the excessive cytokine levels found upon H5N1 infections are the cause or the consequence of the high pathogenicity of these viruses. It should also be noted that H5N1 viruses with glutamic acid at position 92 in NS1 can no longer be isolated and this mutation has not been found in viruses of a subtype other than H5N1. Recent studies suggest that the C terminus of NS1 can also contribute to virulence.

Sequence analysis revealed that avian influenza virus isolates have the consensus sequence of a PDZ domain ligand (ESEV or EPEV) in amino acids 227 to 230 (Obenauer et al. 2006). This motif was never found in human or any other nonavian virus isolates. Furthermore, it was shown that avian NS1 proteins as well as NS1 from the 1918 pandemic virus were able to bind to PDZ domain-containing proteins whereas NS1 proteins from human viruses isolated after 1918 did not. The introduction of such a binding motif into NS1 of the mouse-adapted strain A/WSN/33 increased the virulence of the virus (Jackson et al., 2008). The current hypothesis is that avian NS1 proteins can interact with PDZ domain-containing proteins in human cells and thereby interfere with signaling pathways, leading to increased virulence.

Resistance to Antiviral Drugs

There are two classes of US Food and Drug Administration-approved drugs against influenza: inhibitors of the ion channel M2 and NA inhibitors. The first group comprises the adamantanes, rimantadine and amantadine, which both act by inhibiting the viral ion channel M2 and thereby block the step of uncoating during virus entry. These inhibitors are effective against influenza A viruses but do not inhibit influenza B viruses. Oseltamivir, zanamivir, and peramivir are the members of the second group, and they are active against influenza A and B viruses. They bind to NA and inhibit its enzymatic function. This prevents the release of progeny virions from infected cells and thus limits the spread of the virus. Unfortunately, resistance to M2 inhibitors can occur spontaneously or emerge rapidly during treatment with the drug (Belshe et al., 1988). Resistance can be conferred by an amino acid change at position 26, 27, 30, 31, or 34 in M2 (Bright et al., 2005), and it was shown that resistance can occur without compromising virus replication (Sweet et al., 1991).

In recent years, almost 100% of the seasonal H3N2 viruses circulating in humans were found to be resistant to the adamantanes. Also, the pandemic virus of 2009 is resistant to this class of drugs. Luckily, both the seasonal H3N2 viruses as well as the pandemic virus of 2009 are still sensitive to the NA inhibitors. However, resistance to oseltamivir has become an increasing problem. Before 2008, oseltamivir-resistant viruses were only rarely detected, but then resistant seasonal H1N1 viruses appeared and became the dominant virus type. For NAs of the N1 subtype, resistance is conferred by an amino acid change at position 274: Whereas viruses with a histidine at this position are sensitive, viruses with a tyrosine are relatively resistant to oseltamivir treatment. As mentioned above, viruses of the H3N2 subtype are usually sensitive to oseltamivir, but two mutations in NA which both can confer resistance have been described: E119V and R292K (Wright et al., 2007; Bouvier et al., 2008). It becomes clear that circulating influenza viruses need to be closely monitored for resistance to the available drugs. Furthermore, the development of new influenza virus drugs is crucial.

Compatibility of Segments

The examples above show that in many studies single amino acid substitutions had a huge impact on virulence. However, it is also true that virulence is often a multigenic trait and a combination of different segments is needed to recapitulate full virulence. This can be explained by the fact that different functions like polymerase activity and receptor binding need to be efficient for successful virus replication. Furthermore, it became clear early on that only certain segments are compatible with each other whereas other combinations of segments do not work well together. This compatibility of genes might even differ between different host systems, making predictions about the virulence of reassortant viruses extremely difficult. Segment incompatibility can be illustrated in the example of the NS gene of the 1918 pandemic virus. When the NS1 gene from the 1918 virus was introduced into strain A/WSN/33, the resulting virus replicated well in tissue culture but was attenuated in mice (Basler et al., 2001). This was somehow unexpected since the NS1 protein of the 1918 virus was very efficient at blocking the IFN response

(Basler et al.. 2001). Clearly, the NS1 protein of the 1918 virus is not optimal in the background of the mouse-adapted strain A/WSN/33. This might be because interactions with mouse cellular factors are impaired or the interaction of NS1 with the other viral gene products is not optimal. It can be concluded that multiple functions of the virus contribute to virulence and that these functions need to play together and be optimized in a given host system.

The prominent markers of virulence which have been identified to date are summarized in Table 1.

HOST FACTORS

In general, influenza viruses are associated with a low mortality rate in humans. Even the deadly pandemic virus of 1918 had a mortality rate of only about 2% (Johnson and Mueller, 2002). Still, thousands of people die each year from influenza because of the great number of infected individuals each year. Which factors make some individuals more susceptible to infection and disease than others? In contrast to the viral factors which contribute to a severe outcome of infection, not much is known about the host factors. The information available at present is summarized below.

Host Proteins Required for Influenza Virus Replication

Viruses are strictly dependent on host cells for their propagation, since they use the host cell machinery for each step of their replication cycle. Thus, an influenza virus which has established a lineage in a host species has evolved to interact with the host proteins of this species. However, it is possible that within the same host species genetic polymorphisms may occur and influence the ability of the virus to use the host proteins. One example that could be envisioned is the abundance of the receptor SAα2,6Gal on human cells, which could vary among individuals. Indeed, one study evaluated the binding of influenza virus to erythrocytes from 100 individuals and found differences of up to 40-fold (Rumyantsev, 2006). However, so far no genetic polymorphism has been described and linked to increased or decreased susceptibility to influenza in humans. Recently, several studies identified sets of host proteins which are required for efficient influenza virus replication in human cells (Brass et al., 2009; Shapira et al., 2009; Karlas et al., 2010; Konig et al., 2010). As an example, the influenza virus-host protein interaction network identified in one of the studies is displayed in Fig. 3 (Konig et al., 2010). These data could provide a basis for future studies of genetic polymorphisms in humans.

Health and Immunity Status of Individuals

Age and health status are major determinants of the outcome of influenza. Infants, elderly people, individuals with underlying chronic diseases, and transplant patients are at high risk for complications. Their immune system may be impaired, which can result in delayed clearance of the virus and high susceptibility to secondary bacterial

TABLE 1 Summary of virulence markers

Marker of virulence	Property	Increasing virulence	Decreasing virulence
HA	Cleavage site between HA1 and HA2	Multibasic	Monobasic
	Receptor specificity	SAα2,6Gal	SAα2,3Gal
	Immunity in population	No	Partial
Polymerase complex	Replication efficiency	High	Low
	Amino acid 627 in PB2	Lysine	Glutamic acid
	Amino acid 701 in PB2	Aspartate	Asparagine
PB1-F2	Presence	Yes	No
	Amino acid 66	Serine	Asparagine
NS1	Inhibition of IFN induction	Yes	No
	Inhibition of IFN signaling	Yes	No

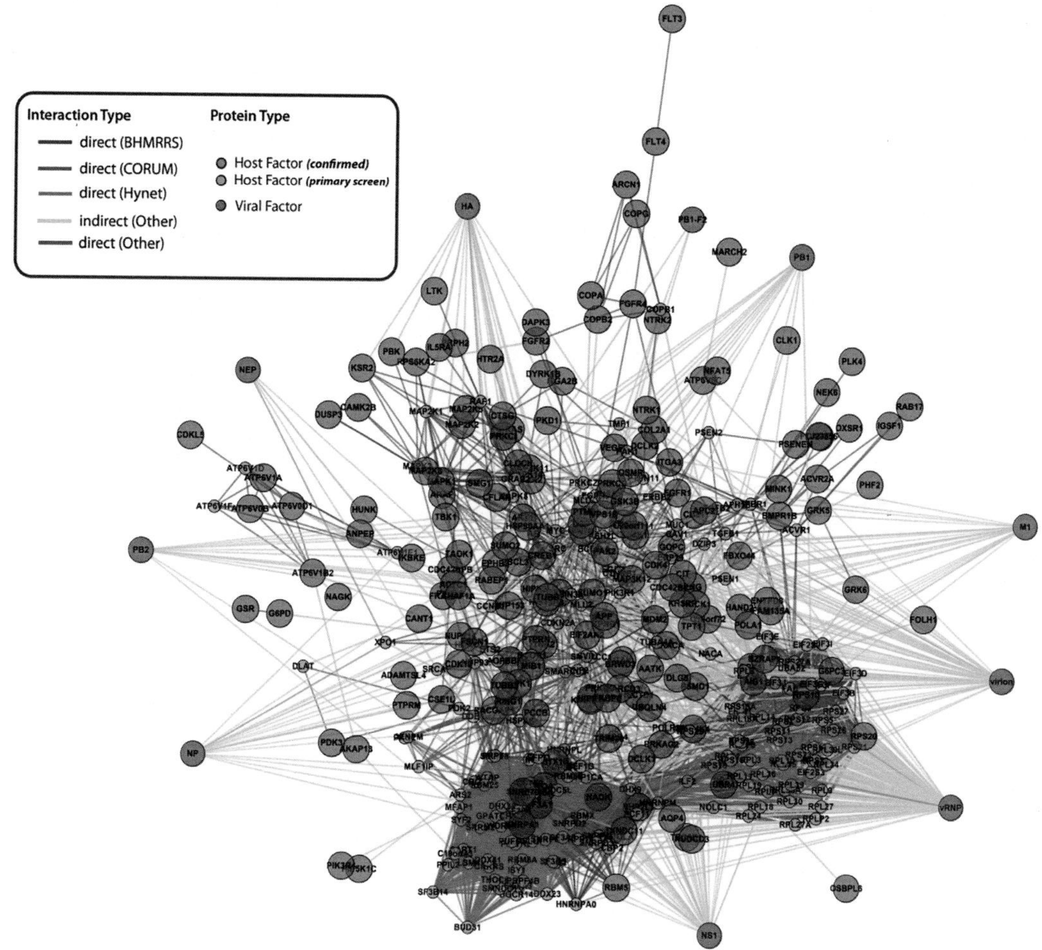

FIGURE 3 Influenza host-pathogen interaction map. Analysis of protein-protein interaction data for the host cell factors which were found to be required for influenza virus replication resulted in a highly significant ($P < 0.001$, permutation test) host-pathogen interaction map containing 4,266 interactions between 181 confirmed influenza virus-host cellular factors (green circles), 10 influenza virus-encoded proteins or complexes (red circles), and a further 184 cellular proteins (orange circles). Interaction data were elucidated based on binary protein interaction data derived from publicly available databases including BIND, HPRD, MINT, Reactome, Rual et al., and Stelzl et al. (Rual et al., 2005; Stelzl et al., 2005) (BHMRRS; blue connections), curated protein complex data (CORUM; pink connections), the Hynet yeast two-hybrid database (aqua connections), and published viral-protein interaction data (yellow and green connections). Red circles indicate influenza nodes, green circles represent confirmed factors, and orange circles indicate unconfirmed influenza host proteins identified in the primary RNAi screen. Viral nodes are abbreviated as follows: HA, hemagglutinin; NS1, NS1 protein; M1, M1 matrix protein; NEP, NEP/NS2 protein; NP, NP protein; PB1 and PB2, the polymerase subunits PB1 and PB2; PB1-F2, PB1-F2 protein; vRNP, influenza virus ribonucleoprotein complex; virion, proteins incorporated into virions. Adapted from Konig et al. (2010).

infections. The high mortality rate in very young children and elderly people during the 1918 pandemic is illustrated in Fig. 4. Both ends of the curve show an increased death rate, which is observed for most influenza viruses. Interestingly, there are two age groups which have relatively low mortality rates. Children 4 to 15 years of age seem to be protected against severe outcomes. This phenomenon has also been observed for infections with other viruses, like Epstein-Barr

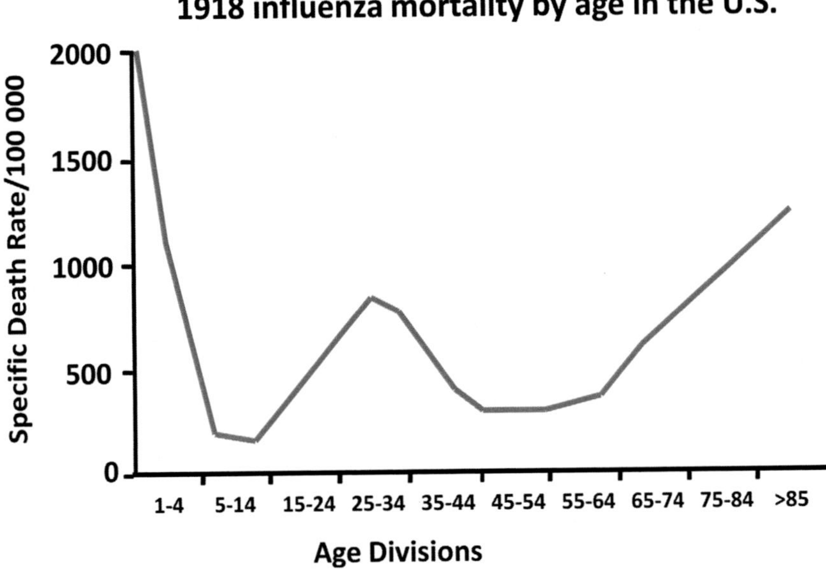

FIGURE 4 1918 influenza mortality by age in the United States. The death rate during the 1918 influenza pandemic per 100,000 individuals is shown for different age groups. The resulting curve has a characteristic W shape, with the highest mortality in infants followed by elderly people. Children 5 to 14 years of age as well as adults 45 to 60 years of age displayed partial protection. Adapted from Palese (2004).

virus, measles virus, and mumps virus. For reasons which are not yet fully understood, children of this age can deal much better with lytic virus infections than can adults. The second age group which displayed some protection comprised individuals between 45 and 65 years of age. The hypothesis to date is that people aged 45 years or older were exposed to a similar virus in the 1870s or 1880s. Cross-reactive antibodies from this exposure could explain the protection seen in this group. The older population (>65 years) was also in contact with the earlier virus, but the weakened immune system probably outweighed any advantage. Thus, besides age and health status, preexisting immunity due to previous infections or vaccinations affects the outcome of an influenza virus infection.

Genetic Polymorphisms Affecting the Immune Response to Influenza Virus

As mentioned above, no genetic polymorphism has been clearly linked to susceptibility to influenza in humans. However, a few studies have addressed the role of the genetic background for the generation of an efficacious antibody response to influenza vaccination. One of them found that certain human leukocyte antigen (HLA) class II alleles are overrepresented in people with low titers of neutralizing antibodies after vaccination whereas other alleles are overrepresented in groups with particularly high antibody titers (Gelder et al., 2002). While it is plausible that HLA class II alleles affect the immune response to influenza vaccination, it should be noted that some people who have the allele that is associated with low responses did mount a good antibody response. This indicates that it is more likely that a gene linked to HLA class II is responsible rather than HLA class II itself. Another study evaluated the frequencies of single-nucleotide polymorphisms (SNPs) in the mannose-binding lectin (MBL)-2 gene and in the tumor necrosis factor alpha (TNF-α) and interleukin-10 (IL-10) promoter regions in an influenza vaccine trial (Tang et al., 2007). The authors identified a SNP in codon 54 of the

MBL-2 gene which was independently associated with poor and adverse responses to the vaccine. They did not find any significant correlation for the SNPs in the TNF-α promoter region, but they identified a SNP in the IL-10 promoter region which was associated with reduced risk for adverse events. While these results are certainly interesting, they need to be confirmed in different study groups.

Since it is difficult to identify genetic polymorphisms associated with severe outcome in humans, the focus has been on the identification of such factors in mice. Inbred mouse strains have defined genetics and can be tested in controlled experimental setups. Once such factors have been identified in mice, databases with human sequences could be searched for polymorphisms in these genes. This would guide the way for future studies of genetic risk factors in humans. Indeed, comparison of different inbred mouse strains and their response to influenza virus infection has shown that there can be drastic differences in the severity of disease between different mouse strains (Trammell and Toth, 2008; Boon et al., 2009). These studies have identified a number of genes for which differential expression in susceptible versus nonsusceptible strains was found. Most of these genes are involved in the innate or adaptive immune response to infection. However, for most of these genes it has not yet been shown that the observed differences in expression are the cause of the different outcomes of infection. One of the few examples where a gene has been clearly linked to susceptibility to influenza virus infection is the murine Mx1 gene. It has been demonstrated that Mx1 confers protection against influenza virus (Horisberger et al., 1983; Grimm et al., 2007; Tumpey et al., 2007); even the highly pathogenic virus of the 1918 pandemic is greatly attenuated in Mx1-positive mice (Tumpey et al., 2007). It was found that most laboratory mouse strains have a deletion or a premature stop codon in their Mx1 gene so that they do not encode a functional version of the Mx1 protein (Staeheli et al., 1988). In contrast, a few mouse strains like SL/NiA or A2G do encode functional Mx1 and are much more resistant to influenza virus. It was shown that Mx1 is located in the nucleus and that it inhibits primary transcription of the viral RNA (Dreiding et al., 1985; Pavlovic et al,, 1992). Humans also encode Mx proteins: MxA and MxB. For MxA, antiviral activity against a variety of viruses like influenza virus, bunyaviruses, and measles virus could be demonstrated; no antiviral activity has been found for MxB so far (Haller et al., 2009). While genetic polymorphisms in the Mx gene have been identified in chicken and in swine (Ko et al., 2002; Palm et al., 2007), it is unclear to date if there are genetic polymorphisms in the human MxA gene which affect the outcome of influenza virus infection.

For influenza viruses to survive, they need to be transmitted from host to host. If replication is efficient and high viral loads are achieved, transmission is most probably easier. However, transmission efficiency is not simply a function of replication efficiency; other factors also contribute. While transmission in humans remains a complex area of study, successful animal models using ferrets and guinea pigs have been developed and have led to a better understanding of the transmission process (Herlocher et al., 2001, 2004; Lowen et al., 2006). In particular, environmental factors which influence transmission have been identified: low temperature and low humidity work in favor of the virus, which at least partially explains the seasonality of influenza (Lowen et al., 2007).

PERSPECTIVES

In recent years much progress has been made in the influenza virus field. The development of reverse genetics techniques has greatly advanced our understanding of the virus and its replication cycle. We have learned much about the different viral proteins and how they contribute to virulence. Furthermore, we have begun to elucidate how influenza virus interacts with its host and how these interactions contribute to the outcome of an influenza virus infection. However, there are still many open questions to be addressed in the future. We still have only a limited understanding of the transmission of influenza viruses within the same species or between different species. Furthermore, the evolution of influenza viruses, for example the frequency of gene reassortment, is poorly understood. Especially for humans, very little is known about genetic factors of the host which contribute to the outcome of infection. The challenges for future research will be to unravel the multiple interactions of virus and host at a molecular level and to use this knowledge to design improved anti-influenza drugs and vaccines.

REFERENCES

Basler, C. F., A. H. Reid, J. K. Dybing, T. A. Janczewski, T. G. Fanning, H. Zheng, M. Salvatore, M. L. Perdue, D. E. Swayne, A. Garcia-Sastre, P. Palese, and J. K. Taubenberger. 2001. Sequence of the 1918 pandemic influenza virus nonstructural gene (NS) segment and characterization of recombinant viruses bearing the 1918 NS genes. *Proc. Natl. Acad. Sci. USA* **98:**2746–2751.

Baum, L. G., and J. C. Paulson. 1991. The N2 neuraminidase of human influenza virus has acquired a substrate specificity complementary to the hemagglutinin receptor specificity. *Virology* **180:**10–15.

Belshe, R. B., M. H. Smith, C. B. Hall, R. Betts, and A. J. Hay. 1988. Genetic basis of resistance to rimantadine emerging during treatment of influenza virus infection. *J. Virol.* **62:**1508–1512.

Boon, A. C., J. deBeauchamp, A. Hollmann, J. Luke, M. Kotb, S. Rowe, D. Finkelstein, G. Neale, L. Lu, R. W. Williams, and R. J. Webby. 2009. Host genetic variation affects resistance to infection with a highly pathogenic H5N1 influenza A virus in mice. *J. Virol.* **83:**10417–10426.

Bouvier, N. M., A. C. Lowen, and P. Palese. 2008. Oseltamivir-resistant influenza A viruses are transmitted efficiently among guinea pigs by direct contact but not by aerosol. *J. Virol.* **82:**10052–10058.

Brass, A. L., I. C. Huang, Y. Benita, S. P. John, M. N. Krishnan, E. M. Feeley, B. J. Ryan, J. L. Weyer, L. van der Weyden, E. Fikrig, D. J. Adams, R. J. Xavier, M. Farzan, and S. J. Elledge. 2009. The IFITM proteins mediate cellular resistance to influenza A H1N1 virus, West Nile virus, and dengue virus. *Cell* **139:**1243–1254.

Bright, R. A., M. J. Medina, X. Xu, G. Perez-Oronoz, T. R. Wallis, X. M. Davis, L. Povinelli, N. J. Cox, and A. I. Klimov. 2005. Incidence of adamantane resistance among influenza A (H3N2) viruses isolated worldwide from 1994 to 2005: a cause for concern. *Lancet* **366:**1175–1181.

Chen, W., P. A. Calvo, D. Malide, J. Gibbs, U. Schubert, I. Bacik, S. Basta, R. O'Neill, J. Schickli, P. Palese, P. Henklein, J. R. Bennink, and J. W. Yewdell. 2001. A novel influenza A virus mitochondrial protein that induces cell death. *Nat. Med.* **7:**1306–1312.

Chen, Z., W. Wang, H. Zhou, A. L. Suguitan, Jr., C. Shambaugh, L. Kim, J. Zhao, G. Kemble, and H. Jin. 2010. Generation of live attenuated novel influenza virus A/California/7/09 (H1N1) vaccines with high yield in embryonated chicken eggs. *J. Virol.* **84:**44–51.

Conenello, G. M., D. Zamarin, L. A. Perrone, T. Tumpey, and P. Palese. 2007. A single mutation in the PB1-F2 of H5N1 (HK/97) and 1918 influenza A viruses contributes to increased virulence. *PLoS Pathog.* **3:**1414–1421.

Connor, R. J., Y. Kawaoka, R. G. Webster, and J. C. Paulson. 1994. Receptor specificity in human, avian, and equine H2 and H3 influenza virus isolates. *Virology* **205:**17–23.

Couceiro, J. N., J. C. Paulson, and L. G. Baum. 1993. Influenza virus strains selectively recognize sialyloligosaccharides on human respiratory epithelium; the role of the host cell in selection of hemagglutinin receptor specificity. *Virus Res.* **29:**155–165.

Dreiding, P., P. Staeheli, and O. Haller. 1985. Interferon-induced protein Mx accumulates in nuclei of mouse cells expressing resistance to influenza viruses. *Virology* **140:**192–196.

Egorov, A., S. Brandt, S. Sereining, J. Ramonova, B. Ferko, D. Katinger, A. Grassauer, G. Alexandrova, H. Katinger, and T. Muster. 1998. Transfectant influenza A viruses with long deletions in the NS1 protein grow efficiently in Vero cells. *J. Virol.* **72:**6437–6441.

Gabriel, G., B. Dauber, T. Wolff, O. Planz, H. D. Klenk, and J. Stech. 2005. The viral polymerase mediates adaptation of an avian influenza virus to a mammalian host. *Proc. Natl. Acad. Sci. USA* **102:**18590–18595.

Gack, M. U., R. A. Albrecht, T. Urano, K. S. Inn, I. C. Huang, E. Carnero, M. Farzan, S. Inoue, J. U. Jung, and A. Garcia-Sastre. 2009. Influenza A virus NS1 targets the ubiquitin ligase TRIM25 to evade recognition by the host viral RNA sensor RIG-I. *Cell Host Microbe* **5:**439–449.

Garcia-Sastre, A., A. Egorov, D. Matassov, S. Brandt, D. E. Levy, J. E. Durbin, P. Palese, and T. Muster. 1998. Influenza A virus lacking the NS1 gene replicates in interferon-deficient systems. *Virology* **252:**324–330.

Gelder, C. M., R. Lambkin, K. W. Hart, D. Fleming, O. M. Williams, M. Bunce, K. I. Welsh, S. E. Marshall, and J. Oxford. 2002. Associations between human leukocyte antigens and nonresponsiveness to influenza vaccine. *J. Infect. Dis.* **185:**114–117.

Gibbs, J. S., D. Malide, F. Hornung, J. R. Bennink, and J. W. Yewdell. 2003. The influenza A virus PB1-F2 protein targets the inner mitochondrial membrane via a predicted basic amphipathic helix that disrupts mitochondrial function. *J. Virol.* **77:**7214–7224.

Glaser, L., J. Stevens, D. Zamarin, I. A. Wilson, A. Garcia-Sastre, T. M. Tumpey, C. F. Basler, J. K. Taubenberger, and P. Palese. 2005. A single amino acid substitution in 1918 influenza virus hemagglutinin changes receptor binding specificity. *J. Virol.* **79:**11533–11536.

Goodbourn, S., L. Didcock, and R. E. Randall. 2000. Interferons: cell signalling, immune modulation, antiviral responses and virus countermeasures. *J. Gen. Virol.* **81:**2341–2364.

Grimm, D., P. Staeheli, M. Hufbauer, I. Koerner, L. Martinez-Sobrido, A. Solorzano, A. Garcia-Sastre, O. Haller, and G. Kochs. 2007. Replication fitness determines high virulence of influenza A virus in mice carrying functional Mx1 resistance gene. *Proc. Natl. Acad. Sci. USA* **104:**6806–6811.

Hale, B. G., R. E. Randall, J. Ortin, and D. Jackson. 2008. The multifunctional NS1 protein of influenza A viruses. *J. Gen. Virol.* **89:**2359–2376.

Haller, O., G. Kochs, and F. Weber. 2006. The interferon response circuit: induction and suppression by pathogenic viruses. *Virology* **344:**119–130.

Haller, O., P. Staeheli, and G. Kochs. 2009. Protective role of interferon-induced Mx GTPases against influenza viruses. *Rev. Sci. Tech.* **28:**219–231.

Hatta, M., P. Gao, P. Halfmann, and Y. Kawaoka. 2001. Molecular basis for high virulence of Hong Kong H5N1 influenza A viruses. *Science* **293:**1840–1842.

Herlocher, M. L., S. Elias, R. Truscon, S. Harrison, D. Mindell, C. Simon, and A. S. Monto. 2001. Ferrets as a transmission model for influenza: sequence changes in HA1 of type A (H3N2) virus. *J. Infect. Dis.* **184:**542–546.

Herlocher, M. L., R. Truscon, S. Elias, H. L. Yen, N. A. Roberts, S. E. Ohmit, and A. S. Monto. 2004. Influenza viruses resistant to the antiviral drug oseltamivir: transmission studies in ferrets. *J. Infect. Dis.* **190:**1627–1630.

Horisberger, M. A., P. Staeheli, and O. Haller. 1983. Interferon induces a unique protein in mouse cells bearing a gene for resistance to influenza virus. *Proc. Natl. Acad. Sci. USA* **80:**1910–1914.

Ito, T., J. N. Couceiro, S. Kelm, L. G. Baum, S. Krauss, M. R. Castrucci, I. Donatelli, H. Kida, J. C. Paulson, R. G. Webster, and Y. Kawaoka. 1998. Molecular basis for the generation in pigs of influenza A viruses with pandemic potential. *J. Virol.* **72:**7367–7373.

Jackson, D., M. J. Hossain, D. Hickman, D. R. Perez, and R. A. Lamb. 2008. A new influenza virus virulence determinant: the NS1 protein four C-terminal residues modulate pathogenicity. *Proc. Natl. Acad. Sci. USA* **105:**4381–4386.

Johnson, N. P., and J. Mueller. 2002. Updating the accounts: global mortality of the 1918–1920 "Spanish" influenza pandemic. *Bull. Hist. Med.* **76:**105–115.

Karlas, A., N. Machuy, Y. Shin, K. P. Pleissner, A. Artarini, D. Heuer, D. Becker, H. Khalil, L. A. Ogilvie, S. Hess, A. P. Maurer, E. Muller, T. Wolff, T. Rudel, and T. F. Meyer. 2010. Genome-wide RNAi screen identifies human host factors crucial for influenza virus replication. *Nature* **463:**818–822.

Kawaoka, Y., S. Krauss, and R. G. Webster. 1989. Avian-to-human transmission of the PB1 gene of influenza A viruses in the 1957 and 1968 pandemics. *J. Virol.* **63:**4603–4608.

Kawaoka, Y., and R. G. Webster. 1988. Sequence requirements for cleavage activation of influenza virus hemagglutinin expressed in mammalian cells. *Proc. Natl. Acad. Sci. USA* **85:**324–328.

Kido, H., Y. Yokogoshi, K. Sakai, M. Tashiro, Y. Kishino, A. Fukutomi, and N. Katunuma. 1992. Isolation and characterization of a novel trypsin-like protease found in rat bronchiolar epithelial Clara cells—a possible activator of the viral fusion glycoprotein. *J. Biol. Chem.* **267:**13573–13579.

Ko, J. H., H. K. Jin, A. Asano, A. Takada, A. Ninomiya, H. Kida, H. Hokiyama, M. Ohara, M. Tsuzuki, M. Nishibori, M. Mizutani, and T. Watanabe. 2002. Polymorphisms and the differential antiviral activity of the chicken Mx gene. *Genome Res.* **12:**595–601.

Kobasa, D., S. Kodihalli, M. Luo, M. R. Castrucci, I. Donatelli, Y. Suzuki, T. Suzuki, and Y. Kawaoka. 1999. Amino acid residues contributing to the substrate specificity of the influenza A virus neuraminidase. *J. Virol.* **73:**6743–6751.

Kochs, G., I. Koerner, L. Thiel, S. Kothlow, B. Kaspers, N. Ruggli, A. Summerfield, J. Pavlovic, J. Stech, and P. Staeheli. 2007. Properties of H7N7 influenza A virus strain SC35M lacking interferon antagonist NS1 in mice and chickens. *J. Gen. Virol.* **88:**1403–1409.

Konig, R., S. Stertz, Y. Zhou, A. Inoue, H. H. Hoffmann, S. Bhattacharyya, J. G. Alamares, D. M. Tscherne, M. B. Ortigoza, Y. Liang, Q. Gao, S. E. Andrews, S. Bandyopadhyay, P. De Jesus, B. P. Tu, L. Pache, C. Shih, A. Orth, G. Bonamy, L. Miraglia, T. Ideker, A. Garcia-Sastre, J. A. Young, P. Palese, M. L. Shaw, and S. K. Chanda. 2010. Human host factors required for influenza virus replication. *Nature* **463:**813–817.

Leser, G. P., and R. A. Lamb. 2005. Influenza virus assembly and budding in raft-derived microdomains: a quantitative analysis of the surface distribution of HA, NA and M2 proteins. *Virology* **342:** 215–227.

Li, Z., H. Chen, P. Jiao, G. Deng, G. Tian, Y. Li, E. Hoffmann, R. G. Webster, Y. Matsuoka, and K. Yu. 2005. Molecular basis of replication of duck H5N1 influenza viruses in a mammalian mouse model. *J. Virol.* **79:**12058–12064.

Lowen, A. C., S. Mubareka, J. Steel, and P. Palese. 2007. Influenza virus transmission is dependent on relative humidity and temperature. *PLoS Pathog.* **3:**1470–1476.

Lowen, A. C., S. Mubareka, T. M. Tumpey, A. Garcia-Sastre, and P. Palese. 2006. The guinea pig as a transmission model for human influenza viruses. *Proc. Natl. Acad. Sci. USA* **103:**9988–9992.

Manicassamy, B., R. A. Medina, R. Hai, T. Tsibane, S. Stertz, E. Nistal-Villan, P. Palese, C. F. Basler, and A. Garcia-Sastre. 2010. Protection of mice against lethal challenge with 2009 H1N1 influenza A virus by 1918-like and classical swine H1N1 based vaccines. *PLoS Pathog.* **6:**e1000745.

Martin, K., and A. Helenius. 1991. Transport of incoming influenza virus nucleocapsids into the nucleus. *J. Virol.* **65:**232–244.

Massin, P., S. van der Werf, and N. Naffakh. 2001. Residue 627 of PB2 is a determinant of cold sensitivity in RNA replication of avian influenza viruses. *J. Virol.* **75:**5398–5404.

Matlin, K. S., H. Reggio, A. Helenius, and K. Simons. 1981. Infectious entry pathway of influenza virus in a canine kidney cell line. *J. Cell. Biol.* **91:**601–613.

McAuley, J. L., F. Hornung, K. L. Boyd, A. M. Smith, R. McKeon, J. Bennink, J. W. Yewdell, and J. A. McCullers. 2007. Expression of the 1918 influenza A virus PB1-F2 enhances the pathogenesis of viral and secondary bacterial pneumonia. *Cell Host Microbe* **2:**240–249.

Mehle, A., and J. A. Doudna. 2009. Adaptive strategies of the influenza virus polymerase for replication in humans. *Proc. Natl. Acad. Sci. USA* **106:**21312–21316.

Mibayashi, M., L. Martinez-Sobrido, Y. M. Loo, W. B. Cardenas, M. Gale, Jr., and A. Garcia-Sastre. 2007. Inhibition of retinoic acid-inducible gene I-mediated induction of beta interferon by the NS1 protein of influenza A virus. *J. Virol.* **81:**514–524.

Munster, V. J., E. de Wit, D. van Riel, W. E. Beyer, G. F. Rimmelzwaan, A. D. Osterhaus, T. Kuiken, and R. A. Fouchier. 2007. The molecular basis of the pathogenicity of the Dutch highly pathogenic human influenza A H7N7 viruses. *J. Infect. Dis.* **196:**258–265.

Nemeroff, M. E., U. Utans, A. Kramer, and R. M. Krug. 1992. Identification of *cis*-acting intron and exon regions in influenza virus NS1 messenger RNA that inhibit splicing and cause the formation of aberrantly sedimenting presplicing complexes. *Mol. Cell. Biol.* **12:**962–970.

Neumann, G., and Y. Kawaoka. 2006. Host range restriction and pathogenicity in the context of influenza pandemic. *Emerg. Infect. Dis.* **12:**881–886.

Noah, D. L., K. Y. Twu, and R. M. Krug. 2003. Cellular antiviral responses against influenza A virus are countered at the posttranscriptional level by the viral NS1A protein via its binding to a cellular protein required for the 3' end processing of cellular pre-mRNAS. *Virology* **307:**386–395.

Obenauer, J. C., J. Denson, P. K. Mehta, X. Su, S. Mukatira, D. B. Finkelstein, X. Xu, J. Wang, J. Ma, Y. Fan, K. M. Rakestraw, R. G. Webster, E. Hoffmann, S. Krauss, J. Zheng, Z. Zhang, and C. W. Naeve. 2006. Large-scale sequence analysis of avian influenza isolates. *Science* **311:**1576–1580.

Palese, P. 2004. Influenza: old and new threats. *Nat. Med.* **10**(12 Suppl.):S82–S87.

Palese, P., and M. L. Shaw. 2007. Orthomyxoviridae: the viruses and their replication, p. 1647–1689. *In* D. M. Knipe and P. M. Howley (ed.), *Fields Virology*, 5th ed., vol. 2. Lippincott Williams & Wilkins, Philadelphia. PA.

Palm, M., M. Leroy, A. Thomas, A. Linden, and D. Desmecht. 2007. Differential anti-influenza activity among allelic variants at the Sus scrofa Mx1 locus. *J. Interferon Cytokine Res.* **27:**147–155.

Pavlovic, J., O. Haller, and P. Staeheli. 1992. Human and mouse Mx proteins inhibit different steps of the influenza virus multiplication cycle. *J. Virol.* **66:**2564–2569.

Pichlmair, A., O. Schulz, C. P. Tan, T. I. Naslund, P. Liljestrom, F. Weber, and C. Reis e Sousa. 2006. RIG-I-mediated antiviral responses to single-stranded RNA bearing 5′-phosphates. *Science* **314:**997–1001.

Qiu, Y., and R. M. Krug. 1994. The influenza virus NS1 protein is a poly(A)-binding protein that inhibits nuclear export of mRNAs containing poly(A). *J. Virol.* **68:**2425–2432.

Rual, J. F., K. Venkatesan, T. Hao, T. Hirozane-Kishikawa, A. Dricot, N. Li, G. F. Berriz, F. D. Gibbons, M. Dreze, N. Ayivi-Guedehoussou, N. Klitgord, C. Simon, M. Boxem, S. Milstein, J. Rosenberg, D. S. Goldberg, L. V. Zhang, S. L. Wong, G. Franklin, S. Li, J. S. Albala, J. Lim, C. Fraughton, E. Llamosas, S. Cevik, C. Bex, P. Lamesch, R. S. Sikorski, J. Vandenhaute, H. Y. Zoghbi, A. Smolyar, S. Bosak, R. Sequerra, L. Doucette-Stamm, M. E. Cusick, D. E. Hill, F. P. Roth. and M. Vidal. 2005. Towards a proteome-scale map of the human protein-protein interaction network. *Nature* **437:**1173–1178.

Rumyantsev, S. N. 2006. Genetic immunity and influenza pandemics. *FEMS Immunol. Med. Microbiol.* **48:**1–10.

Salomon, R., J. Franks, E. A. Govorkova, N. A. Ilyushina, H. L. Yen, D. J. Hulse-Post, J. Humberd, M. Trichet, J. E. Rehg, R. J. Webby, R. G. Webster, and E. Hoffmann. 2006. The polymerase complex genes contribute to the high virulence of the human H5N1 influenza virus isolate A/Vietnam/1203/04. *J. Exp. Med.* **203**:689–697.

Seo, S. H., E. Hoffmann, and R. G. Webster. 2002. Lethal H5N1 influenza viruses escape host antiviral cytokine respones. *Nat. Med.* **8:**950–954.

Shapira, S. D., I. Gat-Viks, B. O. Shum, A. Dricot, M. M. de Grace, L. Wu, P. B. Gupta, T. Hao, S. J. Silver, D. E. Root, D. E. Hill, A. Regev, and N. Hacohen. 2009. A physical and regulatory map of host-influenza interactions reveals pathways in H1N1 infection. *Cell* **139:**1255–1267.

Staeheli, P., R. Grob, E. Meier, J. G. Sutcliffe, and O. Haller. 1988. Influenza virus-susceptible mice carry Mx genes with a large deletion or a nonsense mutation. *Mol. Cell. Biol.* **8:**4518–4523.

Steel, J., A. C. Lowen, S. Mubareka, and P. Palese. 2009. Transmission of influenza virus in a mammalian host is increased by PB2 amino acids 627K or 627E/701N. *PLoS Pathog.* **5:**e1000252.

Stelzl, U., U. Worm, M. Lalowski, C. Haenig, F. H. Brembeck, H. Goehler, M. Stroedicke, M. Zenkner, A. Schoenherr, S. Koeppen, J. Timm, S. Mintzlaff, C. Abraham, N. Bock, S. Kietzmann, A. Goedde, E. Toksoz, A. Droege, S. Krobitsch, B. Korn, W. Birchmeier, H. Lehrach, and E. E. Wanker. 2005. A human protein-protein interaction network: a resource for annotating the proteome. *Cell* **122:**957–968.

Subbarao, E. K., W. London, and B. R. Murphy. 1993. A single amino acid in the PB2 gene of influenza A virus is a determinant of host range. *J. Virol.* **67:**1761–1764.

Sweet, C., F. G. Hayden, K. J. Jakeman, S. Grambas, and A. J. Hay. 1991. Virulence of rimantadine-resistant human influenza A (H3N2) viruses in ferrets. *J. Infect. Dis.* **164:**969–972.

Talon, J., M. Salvatore, R. E. O'Neill, Y. Nakaya, H. Zheng, T. Muster, A. Garcia-Sastre, and P. Palese. 2000. Influenza A and B viruses expressing altered NS1 proteins: a vaccine approach. *Proc. Natl. Acad. Sci. USA* **97:**4309–4314.

Tang, Y. W., H. Li, H. Wu, Y. Shyr, and K. M. Edwards. 2007. Host single-nucleotide polymorphisms and altered responses to inactivated influenza vaccine. *J. Infect. Dis.* **196:**1021–1025.

Trammell, R. A., and L. A. Toth. 2008. Genetic susceptibility and resistance to influenza infection and disease in humans and mice. *Expert Rev. Mol. Diagn.* **8:**515–529.

Tumpey, T. M., K. J. Szretter, N. Van Hoeven, J. M. Katz, G. Kochs, O. Haller, A. Garcia-Sastre, and P. Staeheli. 2007. The Mx1 gene protects mice against the pandemic 1918 and highly lethal human H5N1 influenza viruses. *J. Virol.* **81:**10818–10821.

van Riel, D., V. J. Munster, E. de Wit, G. F. Rimmelzwaan, R. A. Fouchier, A. D. Osterhaus, and T. Kuiken. 2006. H5N1 virus attachment to lower respiratory tract. *Science* **312:**399.

Wright, P. F., G. Neumann, and Y. Kawaoka. 2007. Orthomyxoviruses, p. 1691–1740. *In* D. M. Knipe and P. M. Howley (ed.), *Fields Virology*, 5th ed., vol. 2. Lippincott Williams & Wilkins, Philadelphia, PA.

Zamarin, D., A. Garcia-Sastre, X. Xiao, R. Wang, and P. Palese. 2005. Influenza virus PB1-F2 protein induces cell death through mitochondrial ANT3 and VDAC1. *PLoS Pathog.* **1:**e4.

Zamarin, D., M. B. Ortigoza, and P. Palese. 2006. Influenza A virus PB1-F2 protein contributes to viral pathogenesis in mice. *J. Virol.* **80:**7976–7983.

PLASTICITY OF THE HEPATITIS C VIRUS GENOME

Joerg Timm and Michael Roggendorf

11

With approximately 3% of the world's population (~130 million people) infected with hepatitis C virus (HCV), the World Health Organization has declared HCV a global health problem (World Health Organization, 1999). Upon acute infection, up to 80% of subjects develop chronic hepatitis with viral persistence and are at risk of developing liver cirrhosis and hepatocellular carcinoma. One characteristic of HCV is its enormous sequence diversity, which represents a significant hurdle to the development of both effective vaccines and novel therapeutic interventions.

GENETIC DIVERSITY OF HCV: GENOTYPES AND SUBTYPES

Phylogenetic analysis of HCV genomes revealed that sequences fall into different clusters. This observation led to a classification of HCV into different genotypes, and a standardized nomenclature was proposed in a consensus paper in 1994 (Simmonds et al., 1994). The global distribution of HCV genotypes is regionally specific. The predominant genotype in most areas is genotype 1; however, some areas are infected almost exclusively with other genotypes. For example, the predominant genotype in Egypt is genotype 4, and the HCV epidemic in this country could be linked to parenteral treatment of schistosomiasis in the 1950s (Ray et al., 2000a). In some regions in Africa, genotype 2 is more frequent. In some areas of Asia, however, genotypes 3 and 6 are predominant. Despite substantial sequence variation, all genotypes share the same genome structure with genes of nearly identical size. The genotype-specific variation of the different genes is remarkably consistent and has enabled many of the currently recognized variants of HCV to be provisionally classified based on partial sequences from subgenomic regions such as core/E1 and NS5B. The original nomenclature was recently updated further, with the nomenclature of existing variants standardized (Simmonds et al., 2005). Based on phylogenetic analysis, a classification into seven major genotypes was proposed and criteria for the designation of new HCV variants were formulated. These proposals provide an HCV nomenclature scheme for the three major public HCV sequence databases (Combet et al., 2007; Kuiken et al., 2005) and eliminate inconsistencies of the current classification procedures. HCV genotypes differ from each other by 31 to

Joerg Timm and Michael Roggendorf, Institute of Virology, University of Duisburg-Essen, Virchowstr. 179, 45147 Essen, Germany.

Genome Plasticity and Infectious Diseases,
Edited by J. Hacker, U. Dobrindt, and R. Kurth,

33% at the nucleotide level (Simmonds, 2004). The genotypes are further divided into multiple epidemiologically distinct subtypes differing by 20 to 25% from one another (Simmonds, 2004). A phylogenetic tree depicting all published complete HCV genomes is shown in Fig. 1. For many of the HCV subtypes, particularly the less common ones, complete genome sequences are not available.

ORGANIZATION OF THE HCV GENOME AND REPLICATION

The HCV genome is an RNA molecule of approximately 9,600 nucleotides structured in a coding region that contains one large open reading frame and is flanked by nontranslated regions at the 5′ and 3′ ends (Fig. 2, top). The polyprotein is cleaved into structural (core, envelope 1, and envelope 2) and nonstructural (NS2, NS3, NS4A, NS4B, NS5A, and NS5B) proteins, with one additional small protein at the junction between the structural and nonstructural elements (p7 protein [Fig. 2, bottom]) (Lindenbach and Rice, 2005). The 5′ nontranslated region forms a highly structured RNA element that contains an internal ribosomal entry site (IRES) that allows interaction with the 40S ribosomal subunit and initiation of cap-independent translation of the viral RNA. A single large reading frame is translated into one polyprotein, which is subsequently cleaved by host cellular proteases and virally encoded proteases into the individual proteins. The structural proteins core, envelope 1, and envelope 2 are cleaved by host cellular proteases. Processing of these proteins is thought to take place in a membrane-associated complex at the endoplasmatic reticulum by signal peptidases. The core protein forms the viral capsid, binds the RNA, and interacts with envelope proteins to form viral particles. Different receptors have been suggested for the interaction of viral particles with the hepatocytes that mediate HCV

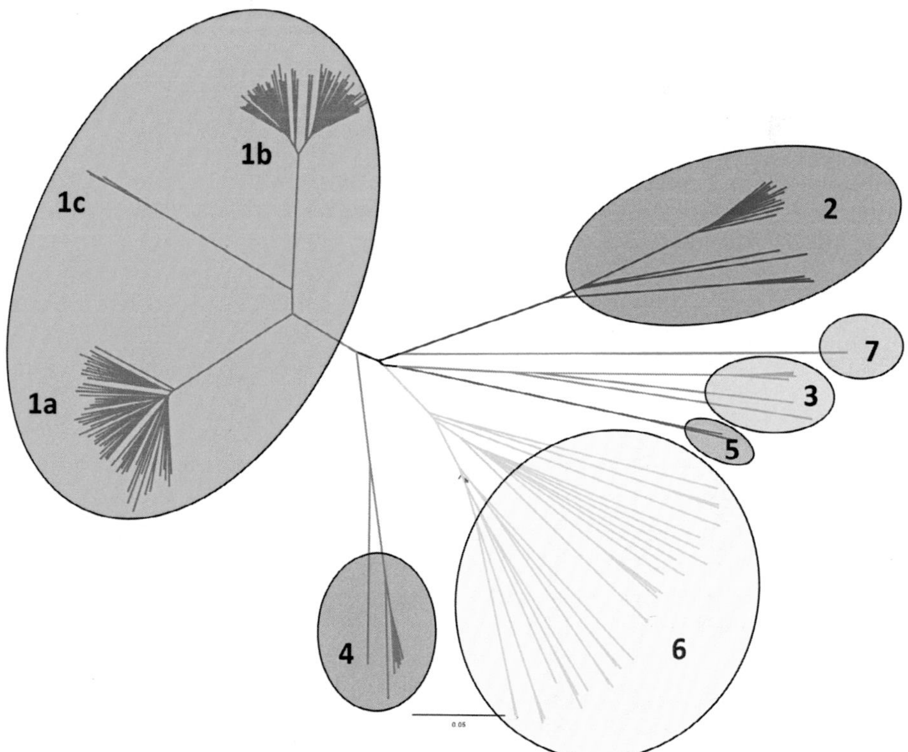

FIGURE 1 Phylogenetic tree depicting HCV sequences retrieved from the HCV sequence database. HCV sequences fall into seven different clusters (genotypes 1 through 7) and are further classified into subtypes.

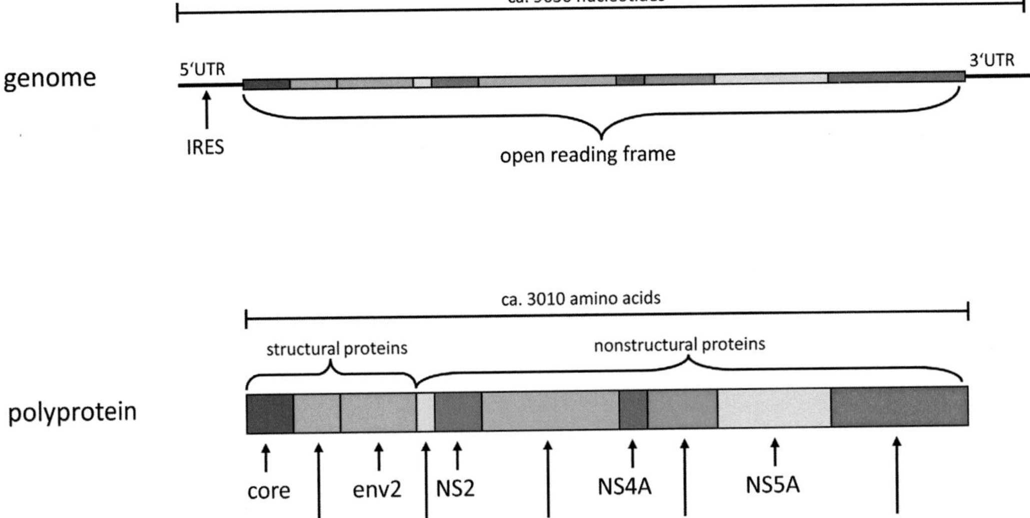

FIGURE 2 Organization of the HCV genome and polyprotein. The HCV genome is an RNA molecule of approximately 9,600 nucleotides structured in a coding region that contains one large open reading frame and is flanked by nontranslated regions at the 5′ and 3′ ends. The polyprotein is cleaved into structural (core, envelope 1, and envelope 2) and nonstructural (NS2, NS3, NS4A, NS4B, NS5A, and NS5B) proteins with one additional small protein at the junction between the structural and nonstructural elements (p7 protein).

entry. These receptors include CD81, scavenger receptor class B type I (SR-BI), claudin-1, and occluding.

These structural components of HCV are flanked by the nonstructural proteins NS2 to NS5B. The function of one additional protein (p7) between these elements remains to be elucidated. It has been suggested that p7 forms an ion channel in planar lipid bilayers. NS2 contains an autoprotease, which cleaves the junction between NS2 and NS3. NS3 is a multifunctional protein with an N-terminal protease domain and a C-terminal RNA helicase/NTPase domain. The NS3 protease cleaves the remaining nonstructural proteins with NS4A as a cofactor for this activity. The NS3 RNA helicase/NTPase unwinds RNA and DNA; however, its role during viral replication is unclear. The integral membrane protein NS4B is sufficient to induce membranous web formation and has been proposed to serve as a scaffold for replication complex assembly. The role of NS5A is again unclear. Numerous protein-protein interactions have been suggested, including a role in silencing the host's innate immune response and determining responsiveness to interferon alpha (Tellinghuisen and Rice, 2002). NS5B encodes the viral RNA-dependent RNA polymerase. In the viral replication cycle the plus-strand RNA genome serves as a template to make a minus-strand intermediate, which then serves as a template to produce multiple copies of plus-strand RNA genomes. One additional protein resulting from frameshifted translation of the core protein has been identified (alternative reading frame protein ARFP). However, the function of this protein is unknown.

MODEL SYSTEMS FOR HCV REPLICATION

Until the development of subgenomic replicons in 1999, no cell culture system was available for studies of HCV replication. The first in vitro replication system for HCV was a bicistronic RNA molecule with the IRES of HCV initiating translation of a resistance gene for subsequent selection and the IRES of the encephalomyocarditis virus followed by the nonstructural HCV proteins NS3 to NS5B that are needed for replication of the RNA (Lohmann et al., 1999). Numerous more advanced variants of these original subgenomic replicons have been developed since then (Bartenschlager, 2006). This includes replicons of different HCV genotypes, replicons with reporter genes such as luciferase or green fluorescent protein that can be used in transient-replication assays, and replicons with improved replication capacity. Improvement of replication was an important step for many applications. This was achieved by replication-enhancing mutations (REMs) in the nonstructural genes that were selected after continuous replication in vitro. Interestingly, although some of these REMs increased viral titers about 100-fold in vitro, they were not beneficial for virus replication in vivo in the chimpanzee model. Despite these shortcomings, subgenomic replicons continue to be a powerful tool for studies of HCV replication and, more importantly, for the development of inhibitors that can be used as therapeutic agents.

Another advancement of this in vitro replication system was the development of genomic replicons that contained all components of HCV including the structural and nonstructural protein-coding genes. Although the structural elements of the virus were included, the first systems were unable to produce virus particles. The reasons for this lack of particle production are still not fully clarified. In 2005 a subgenomic replicon was found in a genotype 2a background that yielded high RNA titers in vitro even without any additional REMs. This isolate was derived from a Japanese patient with fulminant hepatitis C and was therefore called JFH1. Different groups used this isolate and eventually succeeded in developing a cell culture system for HCV that has a full replication cycle including production of virus particles and entry of uninfected cells (Bartenschlager, 2006).

THE QUASISPECIES NATURE OF HCV

As a member of the *Flaviviridae*, HCV has a virally encoded RNA polymerase that lacks a proofreading function. Replication of this plus-strand RNA genome is therefore characterized by ongoing error rates between 1 in 10,000 and 1 in 100,000 bp copied, which are typically found for RNA polymerases. Together with a high turnover rate in vivo of an estimated 10^{12} virions per day (Neumann et al., 1998), this means that, theoretically, every possible mutation in every single position of the genome will be generated in one infected host every day. This high error rate is reflected in the generation of a heterogeneous but closely related swarm of viruses within the same host, referred to as quasispecies in vivo. Although the cell culture systems for HCV have been substantially improved over the past few years, this important characteristic is not reflected by all available in vitro systems. The quasispecies nature of HCV can be best illustrated by sequence analysis of a short but highly polymorphic region in envelope 2 designated hypervariable region 1 (HVR1). Analysis of clonal sequences reveals that sequences of the viral population from the same subject are highly variable but still phylogenetically closely related. In public databases, the consensus sequence of the quasispecies is normally presented as the most predominant residue at any given position.

THE TRANSMISSION EVENT

The quasispecies nature of HCV may have important consequences during a transmission event. Depending on the transmission route, the number of transmitted viral RNA copies can be limited and may not represent the true complexity of the sequence diversity of the donor. This bottleneck phenomenon has been described for sexual transmission of HCV (Quer et al., 2005) and in the chimpanzee model (Nainan et al., 2006). However, the bottleneck could also be interpreted as selection of the optimal strain in the new host during the earliest infection events. With more advanced sequencing technologies now becoming available, the bottleneck phenomenon upon transmission is being readdressed. These studies indicate that indeed the complexity of the quasispecies population is very limited early after infection and that the quasispecies may expand from only a few or even a single molecular clone upon infection of a new host

(Wang et al., 2010). These data are supported by similar observations upon liver transplantation in patients with chronic hepatitis C. Virtually all patients undergo reinfection of the donor organ. This reinfection is associated with a dramatic shift in the complexity of the quasispecies population, suggesting that only a limited number of viral variants establish reinfection (Feliu et al., 2004).

SEQUENCE DIFFERENCES BETWEEN HCV ISOLATES OF THE SAME SUBTYPE

Beyond the sequence differences in the quasispecies population within a single individual, there are more substantial sequence differences between HCV isolates from different individuals. The existence of different genotypes and subtypes has already been discussed; however, even between isolates of the same subtype there are substantial sequence differences. Longitudinal analysis of isolates from subjects with chronic HCV infection calculated a mutation rate on the order of 1.5×10^{-3} to 2.0×10^{-3} nucleotide substitutions per site per genome per year (Rispeter et al., 2000). Figure 3 shows sequences from a large HCV genotype 1b outbreak. The red sequences are clonal sequences from the infection source and represent members of the quasispecies population of the inoculum. The black sequences are bulk sequences derived from different patients 30 years after infection from this common source. Importantly, the sequences from the infection source are located close to the center of the tree whereas the viruses from different patients continuously evolve away from the center. In the model of neutral evolution, mutations are selectively neutral. The spread of these neutral mutations is influenced mainly by stochastic factors and is called genetic drift. As a consequence of this stochastic process, even disadvantageous mutations can reach fixation when the virus circulates through a sufficiently small population. In turn, advantageous mutations are also affected by genetic drift when they are rare and are occasionally lost from the population. On the amino acid level it seems that the majority of mutations in the HCV polyprotein are not selectively neutral. These differences on the protein level are mainly the result of virus-host interactions that are continuously at work and that are an important driving force for viral evolution.

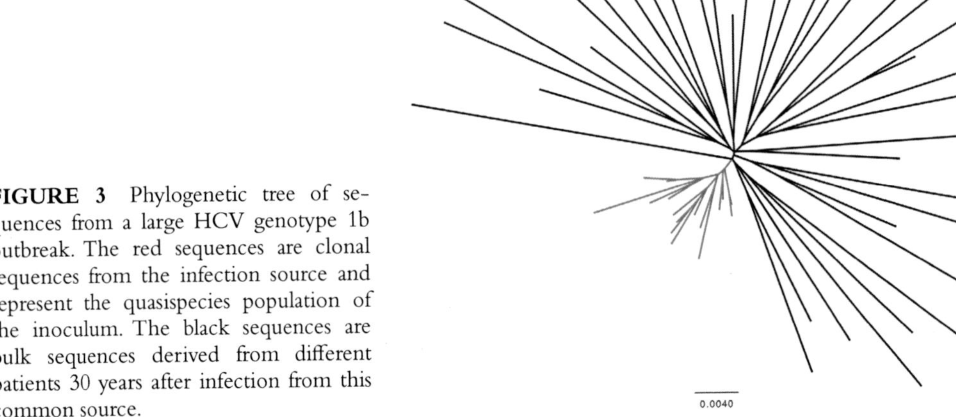

FIGURE 3 Phylogenetic tree of sequences from a large HCV genotype 1b outbreak. The red sequences are clonal sequences from the infection source and represent the quasispecies population of the inoculum. The black sequences are bulk sequences derived from different patients 30 years after infection from this common source.

Positive Selection Pressure by the Humoral Immune Response

Similar to other highly variable pathogens, a complex process of continuous selection has been proposed for HCV (Grenfell et al., 2004). Theoretically, infections with persistent viruses such as HCV have time to evolve within the same host before being transmitted to the next host and may adapt to the specific environment in an individual. The evolution of HCV may therefore be substantially influenced by host factors mediating selection pressure on the virus. Even though the consensus sequence may be close to the maximum of viral replication capacity at any one time, the existence of a large and diverse viral population allows rapid, adaptive changes in response to changes in the replication environment. Many variants that are beneficial in a new environment may already be present at a low frequency in the quasispecies population and subsequently outcompete the existing dominant sequence. The impact of the quasispecies complexity on the clinical outcome can be profound. Farci et al. (2000) analyzed sequences covering HVR1 obtained during the acute phase of infection in subjects who spontaneously resolved viremia and subjects who continued to chronic infection. Spontaneous resolution of viremia was predicted by a decrease in quasispecies complexity during the first weeks of infection. In turn, patients with viral persistence harbored viruses with increasing diversity, suggesting a fast adaptation process to the new environment.

As mentioned above, the most variable region in the HCV genome is a short fragment spanning 27 amino acids of envelope 2 and is therefore designated hypervariable region 1 (HVR1). There is strong evidence that the profound sequence diversity in this region is the result of immune pressure by virus-specific antibodies. Importantly, there is a close association between the observed sequence diversity in this region and the appearance of HCV-specific antibodies in the sera of subjects with acute infection (Kato et al., 1994; Weiner et al., 1992). Patients suffering from common variable immune deficiency (CVID) who present with hypogammaglobulinemia are not able to produce high titers of HCV-specific antibodies and therefore are not able to mount humoral immune selection pressure. Analysis of sequences of HVR1 revealed that patients with hypogammaglobulinemia had significantly fewer amino acid substitutions in this region over time than controls had (Booth et al., 1998). In a similar analysis, the rates of nonsynonymous and synonymous mutations in the core and envelope in patients with and without CVID were compared (Christie et al., 1999). The rates of synonymous or silent mutations were similar in the core and envelope proteins. In patients without CVID, as expected, the rate of nonsynonymous mutations was much higher in the envelope than in the core, a protein that is known to be highly conserved. However, this high rate of nonsynonymous mutations in the envelope was not observed in patients with CVID, suggesting that evolution is triggered by the presence of anti-HCV antibodies. It was demonstrated in the chimpanzee model that a high turnover rate is not sufficient to explain HVR1 sequence diversity. Only minor sequence variation was observed in this region upon serial infection with passage of an infectious HCV clone in eight different animals (Ray et al., 2000b). It is noteworthy that samples for the subsequent infection of the next animal were taken during the acute phase before antibodies became detectable. Again, this study indicates that this region in the envelope remains stable in the absence of antibodies despite high-level viremia that was present in all animals during the acute phase of infection. Taken together, all these studies suggest that without immune selection pressure, only minor sequence changes occur in HVR1.

The lack of an in vitro culture system has hampered direct evaluation of these putative escape mechanisms in the envelope protein. Recently, more elegant tools for this type of analysis became available by pseudotyping retroviral particles with HCV glycoproteins. Von Hahn et al. (2007) used this technique to demonstrate the impact of neutralizing antibodies on the evolution of HVR1. In this study, longitudinal samples were obtained over a period of 26 years from patient H, who was infected in 1977 with genotype 1a. Sera were analyzed for the presence of neutralizing antibodies against the autologous isolate present at the time of sampling. A neutralizing antibody response to the inoculum strain could be detected as early as 8 weeks after infection. Interestingly, the antibodies present in a given sample continuously failed to neutralize HCV pseudoparticles bearing the autologous sequence from the same time point. Longitudinal analysis demonstrated continuous escape from emerging antibodies over the time of infection, indicating that humoral immune pressure is the major driving force for the observed sequence diversity in HVR1.

Positive Selection Pressure by the Cellular Immune Response

Mutational escape from CD8 T cells targeting viral proteins has been well documented for highly variable pathogens such as HCV. Selection of mutations in CD8 epitopes that inhibit recognition by specific T cells has been found in the chimpanzee model of HCV infection (Weiner et al., 1995). In a follow-up analysis, the majority of targeted CD8 epitopes in chimpanzees infected with HCV evolved over time, and an important role for mutational escape as a contributor for viral persistence has been suggested (Erickson et al., 2001). More recently, several longitudinal studies of patients with acute HCV infection provided compelling evidence for CD8 escape in humans as well (Cox et al., 2005; Guglietta et al., 2005; Tester et al., 2005; Timm et al., 2004). Probably the most comprehensive analysis was done by Cox et al. (2005). They prospectively monitored subjects with ongoing intravenous drug use and high-risk behavior for evidence of acute HCV infection. Using this approach, they were able to identify eight patients with acute HCV infection. Samples from these patients were obtained during acute infection (at the time of diagnosis) and after 6 months. Utilizing comprehensive techniques with overlapping peptides spanning the entire HCV polyprotein, they determined the breadth of the immune response. At the same time, they analyzed sequence evolution between the first sample and the one obtained 6 months later. Of 25 targeted epitopes, 17 evolved over time, consistent with selection of escape mutations. Of note, the single subject without selection of escape mutations cleared viremia spontaneously. In turn, 50% of the observed sequence changes outside envelope were associated with a detectable CD8 response. In line with these findings, Ray et al. (2005) analyzed sequences from a single-source outbreak with HCV genotype 1b and observed reproducible selection of mutations in previously described CD8 epitopes in subjects expressing the restricting HLA allele.

The observation of widespread escape in individuals during acute HCV infection prompted efforts to determine whether adaptation to HLA class I-restricted selection pressure also occurs at the population level. Indeed, analysis of circulating HCV isolates in various populations revealed accumulation of viral sequence polymorphisms at different sites of the protein in patients with the same HLA allele. Many of these sequence polymorphisms were located inside previously described CD8 epitopes that are restricted by the associated HLA class I allele. An example of an HLA class I-associated sequence polymorphism is illustrated in Fig. 4. Viral sequences from a large HCV genotype 1b outbreak are aligned with a prototype genotype 1b sequence in a previously described HLA B35-restricted CD8 epitope. Differences from the prototype sequence are significantly more frequent in HLA-B35-positive subjects than in HLA B35-negative subjects, indicating that there is reproducible selection pressure on this region in HLA B35-positive subjects. Collectively, these studies suggest that selection pressure by CD8 T cells contributes to the evolution of HCV.

Positive Selection Pressure by Antiviral Drugs

The current standard treatment regimen for patients with chronic hepatitis C is a combination of pegylated alpha interferon with ribavirin (Fried et al., 2002; Manns et al., 2001). Interestingly, the response rate to this treatment

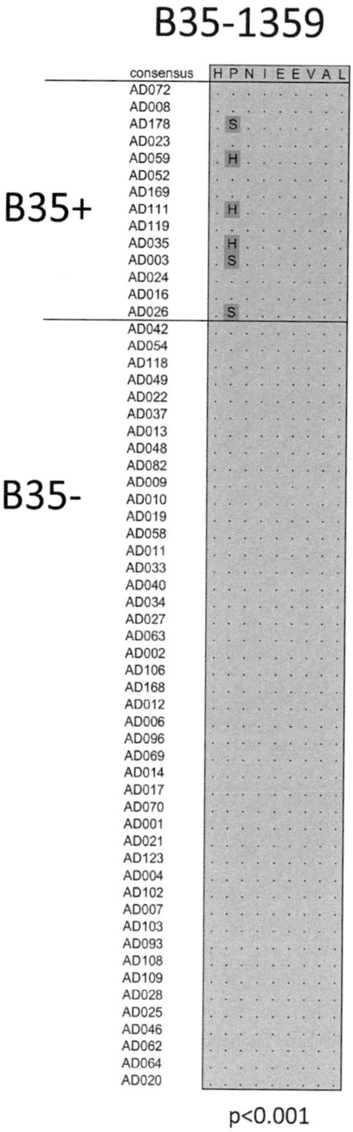

FIGURE 4 HLA class I-associated evolution in an HLA-B35-restricted CD8 epitope in a large HCV genotype 1b outbreak. Viral sequences are aligned with a consensus sequence and sorted into sequences derived from HLA-B35-positive and HLA-B35-negative subjects. Differences from the consensus sequence are significantly more frequent in HLA-B35-positive subjects ($P < 0.001$).

regimen is dependent on the infecting genotype, suggesting that sequence differences between genotypes influence the susceptibility to these drugs. Patients infected with genotype 2 or 3 usually show a much faster decline in viral load after initiation of therapy associated with higher sustained response rates. The determinants of this differential responsiveness of different genotypes are poorly understood. Alpha interferon predominantly modulates the innate immune system (Feld and Hoofnagle, 2005). Engagement of its specific receptor turns on a cascade of interferon-stimulated genes resulting in a non-pathogen-specific antiviral state. Different HCV sequences seem to have different capabilities to interfere with this antiviral strategy. The rates of response to treatment dramatically differ not only between different genotypes but also between isolates of the same subtype. Comparison of sequences of successfully treated isolates with sequences of isolates that did not respond has put a 40-amino-acid stretch of the HCV NS5A protein into the spotlight (Chayama et al., 1997). The degree of sequence variation in this region has been associated with treatment outcome and has therefore been designated the interferon sensitivity-determining region (ISDR). Subsequently, conflicting results have been published in similar studies; however, a meta-analysis supported the impact of this region on treatment outcome (Pascu et al., 2004). A correlate of this observation may be the reported inhibitory action of HCV NS5A on protein kinase R (Gale et al., 1998). For this interaction, the ISDR and an additional C-terminal 26-amino-acid stretch of NS5A are crucial. Therefore, selection of viral variants during treatment that successfully enhance this interaction seems reasonable. However, selection of mutations was not observed in the presence of this antiviral drug in vitro (aus dem Siepen et al., 2007), and selection of variants during treatment in longitudinal studies has not formally been shown. It therefore remains unclear how alpha interferon contributes to evolution.

The exact antiviral mechanisms of ribavirin are even less well established. Several mechanisms have been suggested, including inhibition of the HCV polymerase and early chain termination during the replication process. Higher mutation rates in the presence of ribavirin have been reported, potentially resulting in an "error catastrophe." Two recent studies analyzed the mutation rate in the presence and absence of ribavirin in patients receiving treatment. Hofmann et al. (2007) analyzed the NS3 and NS5B genes in 14 subjects receiving either ribavirin monotherapy or in combination with alpha interferon. Based on a comparison of clonal sequences in the quasispecies population before and after initiation of therapy, they concluded that the mutation rate of HCV is higher in the presence of ribavirin. These results were reproducible in cell culture with HCV replicon-bearing hepatoma cell lines. Even though the overall effect was weak, a dose dependency could be demonstrated, and the inactive L-enantiomer did not show the same effect. In a similar analysis by Lutchman et al. (2007), the mutation rate for NS5B was calculated based on analysis of bulk and clonal sequences of the NS5B gene in 18 subjects receiving ribavirin and 13 subjects receiving placebo. A significant increase of the mutation rate in the presence of ribavirin was observed after 4 weeks of treatment; however, there was no significant difference between the mutation rates after 24 weeks in the drug recipients and the placebo group. The authors of this latter study conclude that ribavirin is unlikely to act through an increase of the mutational error rate, resulting in an error catastrophe. One study demonstrated selection of a Phe-to-Tyr mutation at position 415 of the HCV NS5B protein in the presence of ribavirin (Young et al., 2003). This mutation was associated with a less susceptible phenotype for this drug when tested in the replicon model in vitro. This mutation was also observed in 5 of 16 subjects infected with genotype 1a in the study by Lutchman et al. However, it was not reproducible in HCV genotype 1b. Whether specific mutations are selected in the presence of ribavirin is therefore still unclear.

Future treatment strategies will include small molecules as inhibitors of virus-specific protein functions. Drugs such as protease and polymerase inhibitors have proven to be extremely powerful in early clinical trials for the treatment of HCV infection. In recent years, many compounds have been tested as inhibitors of the HCV protease and polymerase. Some are now in phase III clinical trials and are expected to be available soon. The first specific HCV inhibitor that was tested in humans was the protease inhibitor ciluprevir. In patients infected with genotype 1, the viral load was dramatically decreased after only 2 days of treatment (Hinrichsen, 2004). However, the drug was designed to inhibit the HCV protease from a genotype 1 isolate with high affinity. As expected, the efficacy was therefore much lower in subjects infected with HCV genotype 2 or 3 (Reiser et al., 2005). Due to observed toxic effects of this drug at high dosage in animal models, further clinical trials were stopped. Other protease inhibitors (telaprevir and boceprevir) have meanwhile been tested in phase III clinical trials and are now available. Along with their proof of excellent efficacy in vitro and in vivo, several reports have been published describing resistance mutations. Sarrazin et al. (2007) analyzed clonal sequences from subjects treated with the protease inhibitor telaprevir in a clinical trial; they found that mutations associated with phenotypic resistance were rapidly selected during treatment and the number of resistant clones in each patient correlated well with the virologic response to the drug. The mutations were reproducibly located in only a few positions in the HCV protease gene. Interestingly, the number of resistant clones decreased after cessation of therapy, indicating that some mutations are associated with fitness costs and revert to wild type in the absence of the drug. Future studies will show if combinations of different drugs such as polymerase and protease inhibitors are beneficial for decreasing the risk of resistance mutations, similar to the situation with human immunodeficiency virus.

LIMITATIONS TO HCV EVOLUTION: NEGATIVE SELECTION PRESSURE

Analysis of available HCV full-genome sequences from public databases shows that the degree of sequence variation varies both between different proteins and between regions of the same protein (Fig. 5). Some regions are highly conserved even across different HCV genotypes. Many of these highly conserved regions represent functionally important motifs in the viral

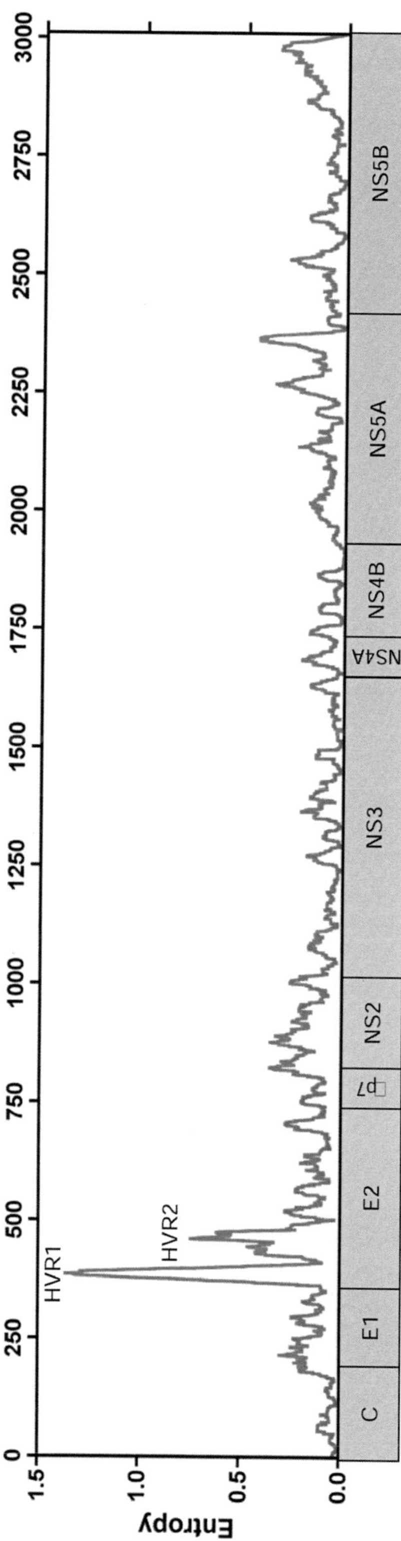

FIGURE 5 Entropy across the HCV polyprotein. All HCV genotype 1b sequences were retrieved from the Los Alamos National Laboratory HCV Sequence Database. The entropy score was calculated for all windows of 20 residues.

protein in which substantial sequence variation is not tolerated. Viral evolution is clearly limited by structural constraints forcing the virus into a state in which it is able to functionally exist. Many mutations that occur during the replication process are deleterious or disadvantageous to the fitness of the virus and are therefore negatively selected. In contrast, forces such as immune or drug selection pressure drive the virus away from the consensus sequence in the individual. Selection of variants is therefore a trade-off between host pressure and functional needs. Purifying selection describes the driving force toward a sequence with optimal replication capacity in the absence of outside pressure on the virus. Reversion in HCV was first described for an escape mutation that has been selected by virus-specific cytotoxic T lymphocytes (Timm et al., 2004). In this study, a virus harboring an escape mutation in an HLA-B8 restricted epitope in NS3 was transmitted to a host who was HLA-B8 negative and therefore was not able to mount the same T-cell response. In the new host, the virus continued to evolve back to the prototype sequence and the variant disappeared. Similarly to the reversion of cytotoxic T-lymphocyte escape mutations, Sarrazin et al. (2007) described, in their study on drug resistance to the protease inhibitor telaprevir, reversion to the wild-type sequence after treatment was discontinued. These studies illustrate the main selecting forces of HCV evolution. On one side there is positive selection pressure, mainly by the immune system but also in the presence of antiviral drugs. These selection forces are not constant and vary in different hosts and different environments, largely depending on the host's genetic background. On the other side there is negative selection pressure, which forces the virus into a state of optimal replication capacity. This force is more or less constant but depends largely on the preexisting sequence configuration such as the genotype or presence of compensatory mutations.

REFERENCES

aus dem Siepen, M., C. Oniangue-Ndza, M. Wiese, S. Ross, M. Roggendorf, and S. Viazov. 2007. Interferon-alpha and ribavirin resistance of Huh7 cells transfected with HCV subgenomic replicon. *Virus Res.* **125:**109–113.

Bartenschlager, R. 2006. Hepatitis C virus molecular clones: from cDNA to infectious virus particles in cell culture. *Curr. Opin. Microbiol.* **9:**416–422.

Booth, J. C., U. Kumar, D. Webster, J. Monjardino, and H. C. Thomas. 1998. Comparison of the rate of sequence variation in the hypervariable region of E2/NS1 region of hepatitis C virus in normal and hypogammaglobulinemic patients. *Hepatology* **27:**223–227.

Chayama, K., A. Tsubota, M. Kobayashi, K. Okamoto, M. Hashimoto, Y. Miyano, H. Koike, M. Kobayashi, I. Koida, Y. Arase, S. Saitoh, Y. Suzuki, N. Murashima, K. Ikeda, and H. Kumada. 1997. Pretreatment virus load and multiple amino acid substitutions in the interferon sensitivity-determining region predict the outcome of interferon treatment in patients with chronic genotype 1b hepatitis C virus infection. *Hepatology* **25:**745–749.

Christie, J. M., H. Chapel, R. W. Chapman, and W. M. Rosenberg. 1999. Immune selection and genetic sequence variation in core and envelope regions of hepatitis C virus. *Hepatology* **30:**1037–1044.

Combet, C., N. Garnier, C. Charavay, D. Grando, D. Crisan, J. Lopez, A. Dehne-Garcia, C. Geourjon, E. Bettler, C. Hulo, P. Le Mercier, R. Bartenschlager, H. Diepolder, D. Moradpour, J. M. Pawlotsky, C. M. Rice, C. Trepo, F. Penin, and G. Deleage. 2007. euHCVdb: the European hepatitis C virus database. *Nucleic Acids Res.* **35:**D363–D366.

Cox, A. L., T. Mosbruger, Q. Mao, Z. Liu, X. H. Wang, H. C. Yang, J. Sidney, A. Sette, D. Pardoll, D. L. Thomas, and S. C. Ray. 2005. Cellular immune selection with hepatitis C virus persistence in humans. *J. Exp. Med.* **201:**1741–1752.

Erickson, A. L., Y. Kimura, S. Igarashi, J. Eichelberger, M. Houghton, J. Sidney, D. McKinney, A. Sette, A. L. Hughes, and C. M. Walker. 2001. The outcome of hepatitis C virus infection is predicted by escape mutations in epitopes targeted by cytotoxic T lymphocytes. *Immunity* **15:**883–895.

Farci, P., A. Shimoda, A. Coiana, G. Diaz, G. Peddis, J. C. Melpolder, A. Strazzera, D. Y. Chien, S. J. Munoz, A. Balestrieri, R. H. Purcell, and H. J. Alter. 2000. The outcome of acute hepatitis C predicted by the evolution of the viral quasispecies. *Science* **288:**339–344.

Feld, J. J., and J. H. Hoofnagle. 2005. Mechanism of action of interferon and ribavirin in treatment of hepatitis C. *Nature* **436:**967–972.

Feliu, A., E. Gay, M. Garcia-Retortillo, J. C. Saiz, and X. Forns. 2004. Evolution of hepatitis C virus quasispecies immediately following liver transplantation. *Liver Transpl.* **10:**1131–1139.

Fried, M. W., M. L. Shiffman, K. R. Reddy, C. Smith, G. Marinos, F. L. Goncales, Jr., D. Haussinger, M. Diago, G. Carosi, D. Dhumeaux, A. Craxi, A. Lin, J. Hoffman, and J. Yu. 2002. Peginterferon alfa-2a plus ribavirin for chronic hepatitis C virus infection. *N. Engl. J. Med.* **347:**975–982.

Gale, M., Jr., C. M. Blakely, B. Kwieciszewski, S. L. Tan, M. Dossett, N. M. Tang, M. J. Korth, S. J. Polyak, D. R. Gretch, and M. G. Katze. 1998. Control of PKR protein kinase by hepatitis C virus nonstructural 5A protein: molecular mechanisms of kinase regulation. *Mol. Cell. Biol.* **18:**5208–5218.

Grenfell, B. T., O. G. Pybus, J. R. Gog, J. L. Wood, J. M. Daly, J. A. Mumford, and E. C. Holmes. 2004. Unifying the epidemiological and evolutionary dynamics of pathogens. *Science* **303:**327–332.

Guglietta, S., A. R. Garbuglia, V. Pacciani, C. Scotta, M. P. Perrone, L. Laurenti, E. Spada, A. Mele, M. R. Capobianchi, G. Taliani, A. Folgori, A. Vitelli, L. Ruggeri, A. Nicosia, E. Piccolella, and P. Del Porto. 2005. Positive selection of cytotoxic T lymphocyte escape variants during acute hepatitis C virus infection. *Eur. J. Immunol.* **35:**2627–2637.

Hinrichsen, H., Y. Benhamou, H. Wedemeyer, M. Reiser, R. E. Sentjens, J. L. Calleja, X. Forns, A. Erhardt, J. Cronlein, R. L. Chaves, C. L. Yong, G. Nehmiz, and G. G. Steinmann. 2004. Short-term antiviral efficacy of BILN 2061, a hepatitis C virus serine protease inhibitor, in hepatitis C genotype 1 patients. *Gastroenterology* **127:**1347–1355.

Hofmann, W. P., A. Polta, E. Herrmann, U. Mihm, B. Kronenberger, T. Sonntag, V. Lohmann, B. Schonberger, S. Zeuzem, and C. Sarrazin. 2007. Mutagenic effect of ribavirin on hepatitis C nonstructural 5B quasispecies in vitro and during antiviral therapy. *Gastroenterology* **132:**921–930.

Kato, N., Y. Ootsuyama, H. Sekiya, S. Ohkoshi, T. Nakazawa, M. Hijikata, and K. Shimotohno. 1994. Genetic drift in hypervariable region 1 of the viral genome in persistent hepatitis C virus infection. *J. Virol.* **68:**4776–4784.

Kuiken, C., K. Yusim, L. Boykin, and R. Richardson. 2005. The Los Alamos hepatitis C sequence database. *Bioinformatics* **21:**379–384.

Lindenbach, B. D., and C. M. Rice. 2005. Unravelling hepatitis C virus replication from genome to function. *Nature* **436:**933–938.

Lohmann, V., F. Korner, J. Koch, U. Herian, L. Theilmann, and R. Bartenschlager. 1999. Replication of subgenomic hepatitis C virus RNAs in a hepatoma cell line. *Science* **285:**110–113.

Lutchman, G., S. Danehower, B. C. Song, T. J. Liang, J. H. Hoofnagle, M. Thomson, and M. G. Ghany. 2007. Mutation rate of the hepatitis C virus NS5B in patients undergoing treatment with ribavirin monotherapy. *Gastroenterology* **132:**1757–1766.

Manns, M. P., J. G. McHutchison, S. C. Gordon, V. K. Rustgi, M. Shiffman, R. Reindollar, Z. D. Goodman, K. Koury, M. Ling, and J. K. Albrecht. 2001. Peginterferon alfa-2b plus ribavirin compared with interferon alfa-2b plus ribavirin for initial treatment of chronic hepatitis C: a randomised trial. *Lancet* **358:**958–965.

Nainan, O. V., L. Lu, F. X. Gao, E. Meeks, B. H. Robertson, and H. S. Margolis. 2006. Selective transmission of hepatitis C virus genotypes and quasispecies in humans and experimentally infected chimpanzees. *J. Gen. Virol.* **87:**83–91.

Neumann, A. U., N. P. Lam, H. Dahari, D. R. Gretch, T. E. Wiley, T. J. Layden, and A. S. Perelson. 1998. Hepatitis C viral dynamics in vivo and the antiviral efficacy of interferon-alpha therapy. *Science* **282:**103–107.

Pascu, M., P. Martus, M. Hohne, B. Wiedenmann, U. Hopf, E. Schreier, and T. Berg. 2004. Sustained virological response in hepatitis C virus type 1b infected patients is predicted by the number of mutations within the NS5A-ISDR: a meta-analysis focused on geographical differences. *Gut* **53:**1345–1351.

Quer, J., J. I. Esteban, J. Cos, S. Sauleda, L. Ocana, M. Martell, T. Otero, M. Cubero, E. Palou, P. Murillo, R. Esteban, and J. Guardia. 2005. Effect of bottlenecking on evolution of the nonstructural protein 3 gene of hepatitis C virus during sexually transmitted acute resolving infection. *J. Virol.* **79:**15131–15141.

Ray, S. C., R. R. Arthur, A. Carella, J. Bukh, and D. L. Thomas. 2000a. Genetic epidemiology of hepatitis C virus throughout Egypt. *J. Infect. Dis.* **182:**698–707.

Ray, S. C., L. Fanning, X. H. Wang, D. M. Netski, E. Kenny-Walsh, and D. L. Thomas. 2005. Divergent and convergent evolution after a common-source outbreak of hepatitis C virus. *J. Exp. Med.* **201:**1753–1759.

Ray, S. C., Q. Mao, R. E. Lanford, S. Bassett, O. Laeyendecker, Y. M. Wang, and D. L. Thomas. 2000b. Hypervariable region 1 sequence stability during hepatitis C virus replication in chimpanzees. *J. Virol.* **74:**3058–3066.

Reiser, M., H. Hinrichsen, Y. Benhamou, H. W. Reesink, H. Wedemeyer, C. Avendano, N. Riba, C. L. Yong, G. Nehmiz, and G. G.

Steinmann. 2005. Antiviral efficacy of NS3-serine protease inhibitor BILN-2061 in patients with chronic genotype 2 and 3 hepatitis C. *Hepatology* **41:**832–835.

Rispeter, K., M. Lu, S. E. Behrens, C. Fumiko, T. Yoshida, and M. Roggendorf. 2000. Hepatitis C virus variability: sequence analysis of an isolate after 10 years of chronic infection. *Virus Genes* **21:**179–188.

Sarrazin, C., T. L. Kieffer, D. Bartels, B. Hanzelka, U. Muh, M. Welker, D. Wincheringer, Y. Zhou, H. M. Chu, C. Lin, C. Weegink, H. Reesink, S. Zeuzem, and A. D. Kwong. 2007. Dynamic hepatitis C virus genotypic and phenotypic changes in patients treated with the protease inhibitor telaprevir. *Gastroenterology* **132:**1767–1777.

Simmonds, P. 2004. Genetic diversity and evolution of hepatitis C virus—15 years on. *J. Gen. Virol.* **85:**3173–3188.

Simmonds, P., A. Alberti, H. J. Alter, F. Bonino, D. W. Bradley, C. Brechot, J. T. Brouwer, S. W. Chan, K. Chayama, and D. S. Chen. 1994. A proposed system for the nomenclature of hepatitis C viral genotypes. *Hepatology* **19:**1321–1324.

Simmonds, P., J. Bukh, C. Combet, G. Deleage, N. Enomoto, S. Feinstone, P. Halfon, G. Inchauspe, C. Kuiken, G. Maertens, M. Mizokami, D. G. Murphy, H. Okamoto, J. M. Pawlotsky, F. Penin, E. Sablon, I. T. Shin, L. J. Stuyver, H. J. Thiel, S. Viazov, A. J. Weiner, and A. Widell. 2005. Consensus proposals for a unified system of nomenclature of hepatitis C virus genotypes. *Hepatology* **42:**962–973.

Tellinghuisen, T. L., and C. M. Rice. 2002. Interaction between hepatitis C virus proteins and host cell factors. *Curr. Opin. Microbiol.* **5:**419–427.

Tester, I., S. Smyk-Pearson, P. Wang, A. Wertheimer, E. Yao, D. M. Lewinsohn, J. E. Tavis, and H. R. Rosen. 2005. Immune evasion versus recovery after acute hepatitis C virus infection from a shared source. *J. Exp. Med.* **201:**1725–1731.

Timm, J., G. M. Lauer, D. G. Kavanagh, I. Sheridan, A. Y. Kim, M. Lucas, T. Pillay, K. Ouchi, L. L. Reyor, J. Schulze zur Wiesch, R. T. Gandhi, R. T. Chung, N. Bhardwaj, P. Klenerman, B. D. Walker, and T. M. Allen. 2004. CD8 epitope escape and reversion in acute HCV infection. J. Exp. Med. **200:**1593–1604.

von Hahn, T., J. C. Yoon, H. Alter, C. M. Rice, B. Rehermann, P. Balfe, and J. A. McKeating. 2007. Hepatitis C virus continuously escapes from neutralizing antibody and T-cell responses during chronic infection in vivo. *Gastroenterology* **132:**667–678.

Wang, G. P., S. A. Sherrill-Mix, K. M. Chang, C. Quince, and F. D. Bushman. 2010. Hepatitis C virus transmission bottlenecks analyzed by deep sequencing. *J. Virol.* **84:**6218–6228.

Weiner, A., A. L. Erickson, J. Kansopon, K. Crawford, E. Muchmore, A. L. Hughes, M. Houghton, and C. M. Walker. 1995. Persistent hepatitis C virus infection in a chimpanzee is associated with emergence of a cytotoxic T lymphocyte escape variant. *Proc. Natl. Acad. Sci. USA* **92:**2755–2759.

Weiner, A. J., H. M. Geysen, C. Christopherson, J. E. Hall, T. J. Mason, G. Saracco, F. Bonino, K. Crawford, C. D. Marion, and K. A. Crawford. 1992. Evidence for immune selection of hepatitis C virus (HCV) putative envelope glycoprotein variants: potential role in chronic HCV infections. *Proc. Natl. Acad. Sci. USA* **89:**3468–3472.

World Health Organization. 1999. Hepatitis C—global prevalence (update). *Wkly. Epidemiol. Rec.* **74:**425.

Young, K. C., K. L. Lindsay, K. J. Lee, W. C. Liu, J. W. He, S. L. Milstein, and M. M. Lai. 2003. Identification of a ribavirin-resistant NS5B mutation of hepatitis C virus during ribavirin monotherapy. *Hepatology* **38:**869–878.

GENOME DIVERSITY AND HOST INTERACTION OF NOROVIRUSES

Eckart Schreier

12

The epidemic and sporadic forms of gastroenteritis are common causes of morbidity in developed countries and of morbidity and mortality in developing countries. Although the current review focuses on viral causes of acute gastroenteritis, it can also be caused by bacteria or parasites. Recent studies employing molecular and antigenic methods for detection of enteric viruses showed that the majority of acute viral gastroenteritis cases worldwide are caused by noroviruses (NVs). NVs form a genus of the virus family *Caliciviridae*, which also includes the genera *Sapovirus*, *Vesivirus*, and *Lagovirus*. Recently, a fifth genus, provisionally named *Becovirus (Nabovirus)*, and a sixth genus named *Recovirus* were proposed because certain viruses show significant differences from the other four *Caliciviridae* genera (Oliver et al., 2006; Farkas et al., 2008) (Table 1).

NVs and sapoviruses, the only *Caliciviridae* that infect humans, are the major agents of acute gastroenteritis in nonbacterial outbreaks, and may account for more than 90% of such outbreaks. According to the Centers for Disease Control and Prevention, NVs are responsible for at least 23 million gastroenteritis infections annually in the United States (Mead et al., 1999). Viral gastroenteritis is a serious and debilitating illness that affects people of all ages. It is characterized by a rapid onset of nausea, vomiting, and/or diarrhea. NVs are classified by the National Institute of Allergy and Infectious Diseases as class B bioterrorism agents because they are highly contagious, extremely stable in the environment, and infectious at low doses (<10 viral particles) (Teunis et al., 2008) and they have an extended period of viral shedding. Viral transmission occurs via fecal-oral spread through contaminated water, via containers or food, or even via airborne transfer during emesis by infected individuals. Outbreaks occur most frequently in nursing homes, retirement communities, hospitals, day care centers, cruise and military ships, and military barracks. The spread during an outbreak occurs predominantly via direct person-to-person transmission. The incubation period is generally 12 to 48 hours, with symptoms typically lasting for 12 to 72 hours. However, the virus can also persist asymptomatically for several weeks postinfection. Although these viruses are usually self-limiting in an immunocompetent host, the exposure in immunocompromised patients can last for several years.

Eckart Schreier, Department of Infectious Diseases, Robert Koch Institute, Nordufer 20, 13353 Berlin, Germany.

Genome Plasticity and Infectious Diseases,
Edited by J. Hacker, U. Dobrindt, and R. Kurth,

TABLE 1 Taxonomic structure of the *Caliciviridae*

Genus	Type species	GenBank accession no. of representative virus strain
Norovirus	Norwalk virus	M87661
	Murine norovirus	AY228235
	Bovine norovirus	AJ011099
Sapovirus	Sapporo virus	U65427
Vesivirus	Vesicular exanthema of swine virus	U76874
	Feline calicivirus	M86379
Lagovirus	Rabbit hemorrhagic disease virus	M67473
	European brown hare syndrome virus	Z69620
Becovirus (Nabovirus)[a]	Bovine enteric calicivirus Nebraska (BEC-NB)	AY082891
	Bovine enteric calicivirus Newbury agent 1	DQ13304
Recovirus[a]	Rhesus monkey calicivirus (Tulane virus)	EU391643

[a]*Becovirus* and *Recovirus* are tentative genera not yet accepted by the International Commitee on Taxonomy of Viruses.

Diagnosis of NV infection is generally based on clinical features, with confirmation by molecular analysis using polymerase chain reaction (PCR) and enzyme immunoassay.

Evidence for protective immunity—i.e., the prevention of NV infection due to prior exposure—is controversial. Published reports suggest that NV antibodies provide short-term immunity, but conflicting reports claim that they provide no immunity (Rockx et al., 2005a). If NVs induce only a short immunity, even against homologous antigenic virus variants, the development of effective vaccines will be difficult. Although scientists' understanding of NV immunity is still incomplete, the rapid clearance of NV infection in immunocompetent patients suggests that the innate immune system can be a powerful weapon. However, despite much effort over the last few years, human NVs generally fail to replicate in tissue culture, and this has seriously restricted scientists' understanding of the pathogenesis and immunology of NV disease.

Two recently developed models for NV replication have potential to improve our understanding of NV pathogenesis and immunity and may aid in the development of antiviral agents: the gnotobiotic pig model for understanding the mechanisms of NV replication (Cheetham et al., 2006), and the murine norovirus (MNV) for in vivo or in vitro modeling of NV replication in human macrophages and dendritic cells (Karst et al., 2003; Wobus et al., 2004). However, additional research is required to make these tools relevant and useful for investigation of human NVs.

The molecular cloning of the Norwalk virus RNA in 1990 and the subsequent cloning of many other NV strains were important steps in the understanding of its pathogenesis, molecular epidemiology, and immunology and for the development of diagnostic assays. Different expression systems that promote the self-assembly of recombinant major proteins (capsid proteins) of different NV strains into virus-like particles (VLPs) with antigenic activity against the original viruses provided important tools for study of host-virus interaction, immune responses, and development of NV vaccines. However, because the VLPs do not always undergo the same assembly and maturation process as native virions, the particular expression system may influence capsid protein expression. Overall, the preparation of recombinant VLPs (Jiang et al., 1992; Prasad et al., 1996) was an important milestone in NV research.

GENOMIC ORGANIZATION OF NOROVIRUSES

NVs were first described in 1972 by Albert Kapikian (Kapikian et al., 1972), who used immunoelectron microscopy to visualize the virus (then called the "Norwalk-like virus") in passed stool filtrate from an outbreak in Norwalk, OH. But a detailed understanding of the genomic structure of NVs was not revealed until the early 1990s when the first cDNA clones of NV were obtained (Xi et al., 1990) and the sequence of the entire NV genome was reported (Lambden et al., 1993; Jiang et al., 1993).

The molecular cloning and genomic characterization of other viral strains has greatly facilitated our understanding of the genetic structure and classification of NVs. Additionally, the molecular cloning of NVs associated with infections in animals has shown that this group of viruses has a broad range of host organisms.

NVs are small round viruses, approximately 38 nm in diameter, with icosohedral symmetry, and possessing a single-stranded, positive-sense RNA genome of ~7.5 kb (Fig. 1). The 5′ untranslated region is covalently linked to a viral nonstructural protein (VPg) (Daughenbaugh et al., 2003). In vitro, this VPg interacts with components of the translation machinery and may play a role in initiating translation of NV RNA (Daughenbaugh et al., 2003). Thus, NVs possess neither the ribosomal entry sites nor cap structures typical of eukaryotic mRNA. The 5′ end sequence is repeated internally in the genome and may be relevant during recombination events. The 3′ end bears a short untranslated region followed by a poly(A) tail of variable length. In conclusion, the 5′ and 3′ untranslated regions of NV genome contains RNA elements that bind to cellular proteins.

The RNA genome is organized into three open reading frames (ORFs) (Fig. 2). ORF1 encodes an ~200-kDa polyprotein that is cleaved by the virus-encoded 3C-like protease into six nonstructural proteins and their precursors, including the RNA-dependent RNA polymerase (RdRp) with the motif GDD (Gly-Asp-Asp). Polymerases with this motif are found in many

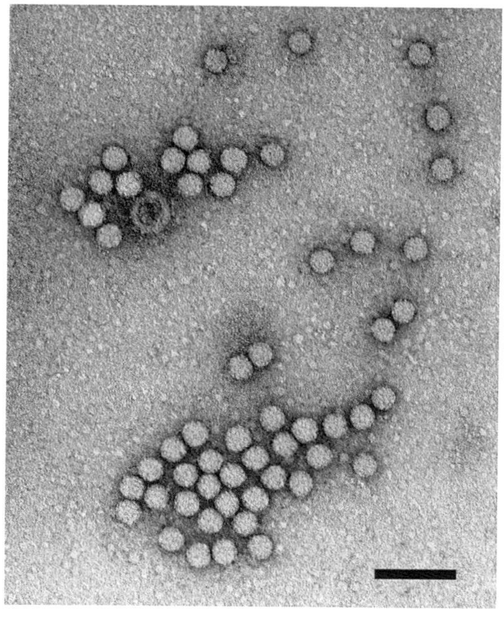

FIGURE 1 NV particles from a stool filtrate of a patient with acute gastroenteritis. The particles were negatively stained with uranyl acetate and visualized by electron microscopy. They are about 35 nm in diameter. Bar, 100 nm. Courtesy of the Robert Koch Institute, Berlin, Germany.

plus-strand RNA viruses. ORF1 and ORF2 encode the major (VP1) and minor (VP2) capsid proteins, respectively. The VP1 protein forms two principal domains: the conserved shell (S) and the more variable P (protruding) domains, the latter of which is subdivided into P1-1, P1-2, and P2. The P domains bear antigenic determinants that affect the immunological and host specificity (Fig. 3). Expression of the P domain in bacteria results in the formation of dimers or higher-order structures, the P particles. In the assembled viral particle, the P domain also participates in dimeric interactions that are thought to stabilize the capsid.

The VP1 protein may be processed proteolytically into a soluble protein which differs from the P domain only in the absence of a 4- to 7-residue arginine-rich sequence at the C terminus (referred to as P polypeptide). This P polypeptide could play a role in the replication, pathogenesis, and host immune response

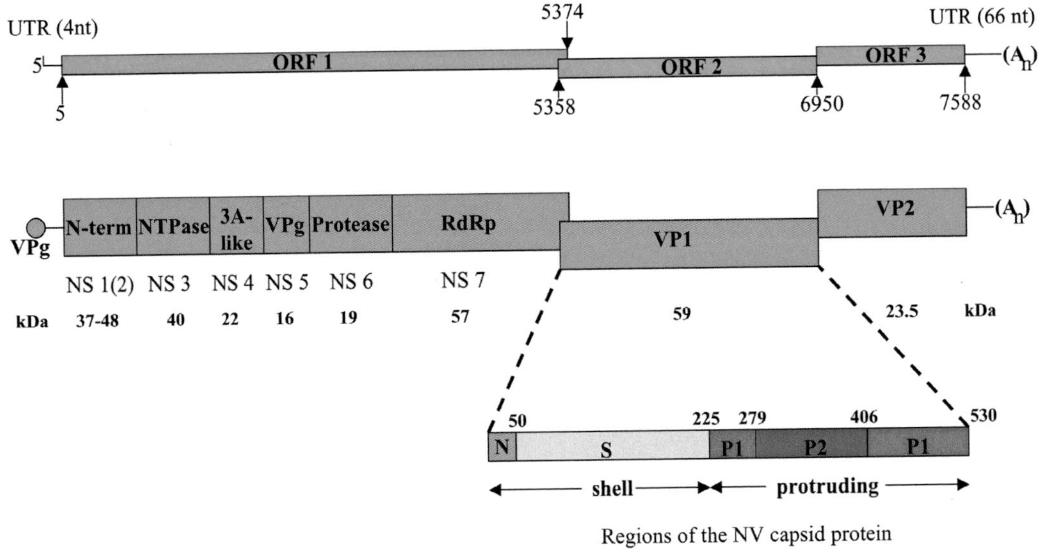

FIGURE 2 Schematic diagram showing the organization of the NV genome and putative cleavage products of the ORF1 polyprotein. Values represent the molecular mass of the predicted protein products (in kilodaltons). The nucleotide position (GenBank accession number M87661) is indicated along the top.

of NV RNA (Tan et al., 2006). The function of the protein encoded by ORF3 is not clear, although it was suggested that it upregulates VP1 or acts as a histone-like protein to stabilize the capsid RNA complex (Glass et al., 2000; Bertolotti-Ciarlet et al., 2003).

GENETIC DIVERSITY AND CLASSIFICATION OF NOROVIRUSES

There is huge genetic diversity among the human NVs because the viruses change during each NV outbreak and even between each outbreak period. Activity at the RdRp region of ORF1, combined with recombination events, leads to an extraordinarily high frequency of mutations. This high degree of variation is caused by a lack of genetic proofreading, which allows the expression of mutations. The most recently proposed classification of NV variants was based on sequence comparison from different regions of the viral genome (i.e., genotyping). Unfortunately, direct serotyping based on neutralization assays is not possible as long as NVs cannot be grown in culture.

Until recently, NV classifications were based exclusively on the RdRp region of ORF1. However, novel studies showed that comparison of the nucleotide sequences of the capsid region ORF2 enabled superior differentiation. The identification of naturally occurring recombinant NVs (Hardy et al., 1997; Jiang et al., 1999; Schreier et al., 2000) showed that recombination can affect the classification of NVs, so recombinants could be missed if only the ORF1 region is sequenced. A dual typing method using phylogenetic analysis of two different genome regions (ORF1 and ORF3) was already developed in 1999 (Schreier et al., 2000).

The International Committee on Taxonomy of Viruses has no guidelines for the classification of viruses below the species level, so no clear consensus criteria are used for NV classification. For NVs, the reverse transcription-polymerase chain reaction (RT-PCR) in combination with genomic sequencing in the ORF1 and ORF2 region is currently the primary method used for classification and characterization of different strains. For rapid detection of NV by multiplex real-time RT-PCR, recently developed assays are faster than conventional RT-PCR. However, these systems appear to amplify the short, conserved sequences that are common in the

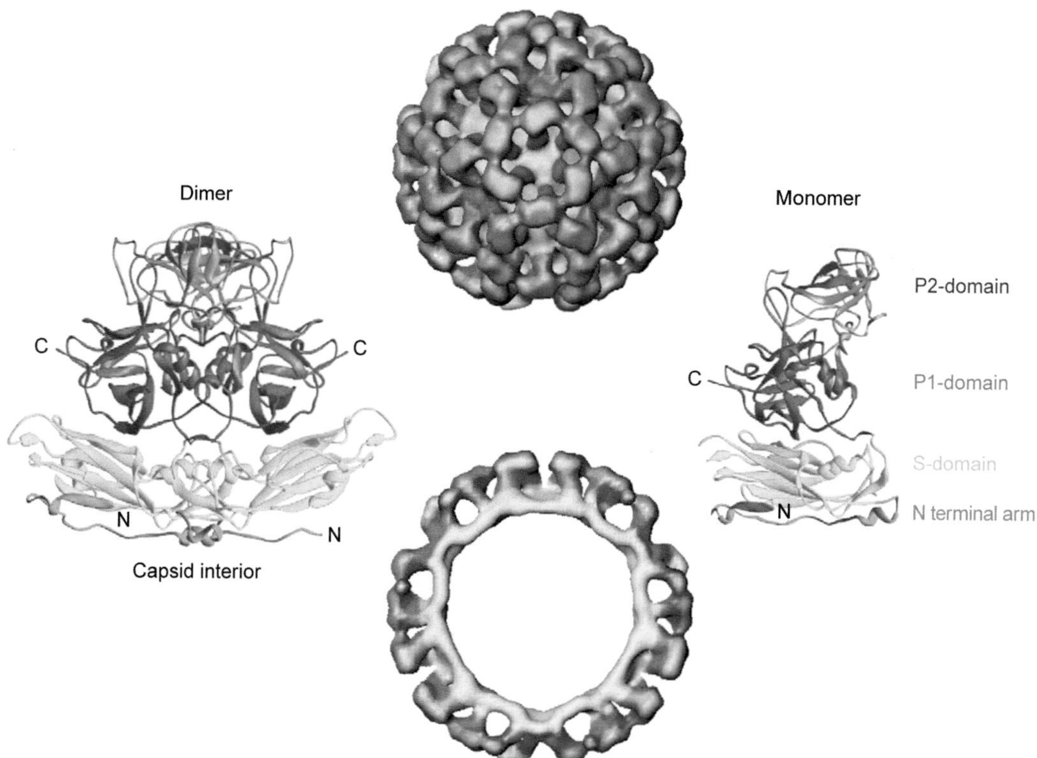

FIGURE 3 Capsid structure of the NV VLP solved by cryoelectron microscopic reconstruction (top, surface representation; bottom, cross section) and by X-ray crystallography. The VLP contains 90 dimers of capsid protein assembled in T=3 icosahedral symmetry (left, ribbon diagram). Each monomeric capsid protein (right, ribbon diagram) is divided into an N-terminal arm region (green) facing the interior of the VLP, a shell (S) domain (yellow) that forms the continuous surface of the VLP, and a protruding (P) domain that constitutes the arch at the surface of the VLP. The P domain is further divided into subdomains P1 and P2 (red and blue, respectively). The P2 subdomain is implicated in virus-host interactions. Reprinted from Hutson et al. (2004) with permission.

ORF1-ORF2 junction region and are usually not suitable for genotyping.

Up to now, five distinct genogroups have been identified and have been tentatively classified by phylogenetic analysis of RdRp sequences or complete capsid gene sequences (Fig. 4). Infections in humans have been described for three genogroups, GI, GII, and GIV, whereas the GIII and GV strains have so far been found only in cattle and mice, respectively. Within genogroups, NVs are subdivided further into more than 40 genotypes. Based on partial capsid N/S domain region and RdRp sequences, 14 genotypes in GI and 17 genotypes in GII have been reported (Kageyama et al., 2004). Using the entire capsid sequence of human NV, GI can be subdivided into eight genotypes (GI.1 to GI.8) and GII can be subdivided into at least 16 genotypes (GII.1 to GII.10 and GII.12 to GII.17) (Zheng et al., 2006), or even 19 genotypes if porcine NVs are included (Wang et al., 2007). Based on phylogenetic analysis, GII porcine NVs have been classified into three genotypes (GII.11, GII.18, and GII.19). Two genotypes in GIII (GIII.1 and GIII.2) are recognized as bovine NV. Phylogenetic analysis of full-length genomes of 26 murine NV (MNV) isolates revealed a single genotype in GV, and genogroup GIV contains only a single human genotype (GIV.1). Genogroup GIV NVs (classified as genotype GIV.2) have been detected in a dead lion cub (Martella

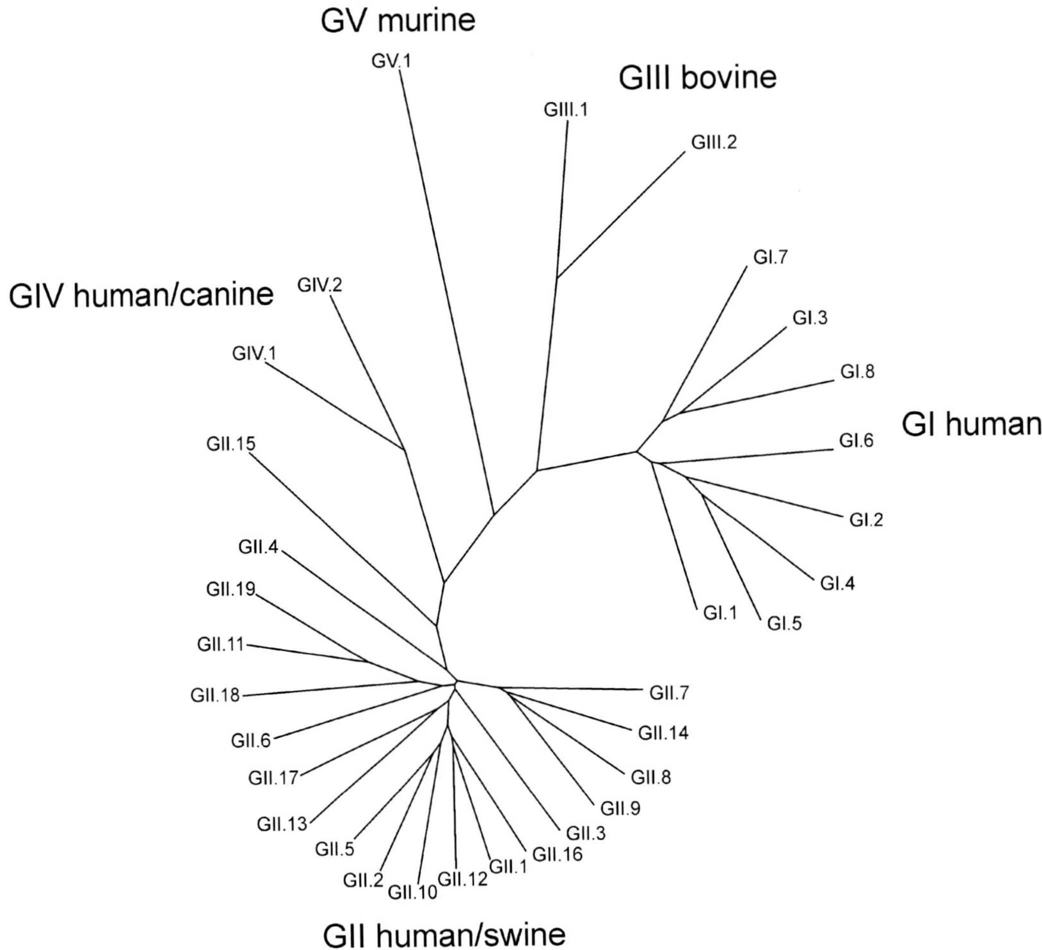

FIGURE 4 Phylogenetic relationships within the genus *Norovirus.* Full-length capsid nucleotide sequences were used for the phylogenetic analysis and included a representative strain from each genotype of genogroups GI to GV. Phylogenetic analysis (neighbor-joining method) was performed with BioEdit (version 7.09, copyright T. A. Hall), which includes the Phylogeny Interference Package (PHYLIP) from J. Felsenstein. Evolutionary distances were calculated by the Kimura two-parameter method (Kimura, 1980). The scale bar represents the phylogenetic distances expressed as units of expected nucleotide substitutions per site. GenBank accession numbers for the genotypes in the analysis were as follows: GI.1 (M87661), GI.2 (L07418), GI.3 (U04469), GI.4 (AB042808), GI.5 (AJ277614), GI.6 (AF093797), GI.7 (AJ277609), GI.8 (AF538679), GII.1 (U07611), GII.2 (AY134748), GII.3 (U22498), GII.4 (X86557), GII.5 (AJ277607), GII.6 (AJ277620), GII.7 (AJ277608), GII.8 (AF195848), GII.9 (AY038599),GII.10 (AF427118), GII.11 (AB074893), GII.12 (AJ277618), GII.13 (AY113106), GII.14 (AY130761), GII.15 (AY130762), GII.16 (AY502010), GII.17 (AY502009), GII.18 (AY823304), GII.19 (AY823306), GIII.1 (AJ011099), GIII.2 (AF320625), GIV.1 (AF195847), GIV.2 (EF450827), and GV (AY228235).

et al., 2007) and in a canine (Martella et al., 2008) (Table 2).

The fact that some human NV strains are closely related to strains infecting animals, particularly porcines, strengthens the hypothesis that human infections may result via zoonotic transmission from a nonhuman reservoir. At present, there is no evidence that the same strains circulate in both the human and nonhuman species. However, the recent detection of human GII.4 sequences in retail swine meat and cattle stool samples in Canada (Mattison et al., 2007) has increased discussion regarding a possible interspecies transmission. Previous studies indicated that some nonhuman caliciviruses are capable of crossing species barriers and potentially using humans as their hosts (Smith et al., 1998a, 1998b). Moreover, experimental infections of gnotobiotic calves and pigs with a human GII.4 strain (Cheetham et al., 2006; Souza et al., 2008) showed that NV replication is not restricted to a specific host. Evidence of recombination events in human or nonhuman NVs with a resulting emergence of recombinant virus strains would be extremely important. However, NV recombinant events detected up to now were exclusively between human NVs, and no recombinant events between human and nonhuman NVs have been reported.

Not surprisingly, additional NV classification schemes have been recommended.

TABLE 2 Distribution of norovirus genogroups and genotypes across the various human and animal species

Host	Genotype(s) of genogroup:				
	GI	GII	GIII	GIV	GV
Human	GI.1–GI.8	GII.1–GII.10, GII.12–GII.17		GIV.1	
Pig		GII.11, GII.18, GII.19			
Cattle			GIII.1, GIII.2		
Mouse					GV.1
Lion, dog				GIV.2	

Multiple short amino acid motifs located at the N terminus, S domain, P1 domain, P2 domain, and C terminus of capsid genes have been used to define seven phylogenetic NV genogroups (Phan et al., 2007). GI, GIV, GVI, and GVII were found exclusively in humans. GIII and GV infected only bovines and murines, respectively. Genogroup GII comprised human and porcine NV strains. GI was subdivided into 16 genotypes with 32 subgenotypes, and GII was subdivided into 23 genotypes with 34 subgenotypes. Inconsistent classification can result from use of partial sequences and may depend on the genome region selected. At present, molecular classification of NV strains is based on the scheme published by Zheng et al. (2006). However, a proposal was drafted for a new NV nomenclature in compliance with the classification published in *Fields Virology*, 5th ed. (Green, 2007). Currently, a publicly available NV genotyping system is available at www.rivm.nl/mpf/norovirus/typingtool.

The genetic diversity among NVs is generally much higher than that of other single-stranded RNA viruses, such as hepatitis C virus or enteroviruses. Comparison of full-length genomic sequences or full-length capsid sequences of NV strains showed that strains within a genogroup differ by up to 30% while strains belonging to different genogroups can differ by up to about 60% (Zheng et al., 2006).

RECOMBINATION

In addition to the accumulation of point mutations (antigenic drift), inter- or intratypic recombination events (antigenic shift) are major driving forces in RNA virus evolution. Recombination is also a major determinant of viral virulence and is implicated in the generation of new virus strains with increased biological fitness and increased pathogenicity. The recombinant strains are derived from two parental strains with quasichimeric character. NV genotyping based solely on the ORF1, ORF2, or ORF3 sequences may not be sufficient for detection of recombinants. The first evidence for recombination events in German strains of NV was obtained in 1999 and 2000. Two German

NV isolates were obtained from outbreaks in 1998, and sequencing of the ORF1 and ORF3 regions did not show phylogenetic equivalence (Schreier et al., 2000).

The first indication of a naturally occurring recombinant with a potential recombination site at ORF1/ORF2 was found in stool specimens from children hospitalized with diarrhea in Mendoza, Argentina. This recombinant bears ORFs belonging to the genetic clusters GII.4 (ORF1/RdRp region) and GII.3 (ORF2/capsid region) (Jiang et al., 1999) Recently, an NV recombinant with a breakpoint outside the ORF1/ORF2 junction region, i.e., a double recombination event, was identified. Recombination within the capsid gene has also been detected (for a review, see Bull et al. [2007]).

At present there is no perfect classification system for recombinant NVs. A recent worldwide study identified 20 NV recombinant strains in current circulation (Bull et al., 2007). NV recombinants and their recombination sites were identified by phylogenetic analysis, SimPlot analysis, and the maximum x method. NV strains were defined as recombinant types only if the recombination breakpoint met the criteria for all three methods. All 20 defined recombinants (1 in genogroup GI, 17 in GII, and 2 in GIII) were intergenotypic recombinants. Not surprisingly, most of the recombinants came from GII; this is the most prevalent NV genogroup worldwide, and a large number of GII sequences have been deposited in GenBank. Of the 17 NV GII recombinants identified, GII.4 and GII.b polymerases predominate, regardless of their corresponding capsid genotypes. GIIb polymerase variants were initially detected in France in 2000 and have been associated with outbreaks worldwide (Bon et al., 2005), but this polymerase variant does not correspond to any known genotype. Evidence of intragenomic recombination events in the capsid gene, i.e., recombination between NV strains from the same genotype, has been published (Rohayem et al., 2005; Phan et al., 2006). However, this result was not confirmed in a more recent study (Bull et al., 2007).

The recent detection in India of an intergenogroup recombination between genotype GI.3 and GII.4 indicates an additional step in the evolution of NVs (Nayak et al., 2008). The site of recombination in all recombinants was reported to be mainly at the junction point of ORF1 and ORF2 (Jiang et al., 1999; Bull et al., 2005, 2007; Nayak et al., 2008). This result is not surprising because sequence alignment of NV strains of different genogroups or genotypes showed that the junction region of ORF1 and ORF2 is highly conserved. The presence of such a conserved nucleotide motif at the overlapping site of ORF1/ORF2, in connection with the presence of stem-loop (hairpin) structure in this part of the RNA genome, can lead to switching of the viral RdRp complex during replication from one RNA template to another. NV recombinants with a crossover site outside the ORF1-ORF2 junction region (Waters et al., 2007) or with double breakpoints known for other infections (e.g., polioviruses) are very rare (Bull et al., 2007).

Although recombination between human and animal NVs has never been reported, such events are entirely possible. Intertypic recombination between genotypes of bovine NV and between genotypes of MNVs was demonstrated via a comparison of complete genome sequences and incongruent clustering of subgenomic sequence fragments from different regions (Han et al., 2004; Mueller et al., 2007). We described MNV recombinants in which the putative crossover point is located within 100 nucleotides of the ORF1/ORF2 region. Because this junction region is highly conserved in MNV strains, this recombination may be driven by homologous RNA interactions comparable to polioviruses and murine coronaviruses (Makino et al., 1986, 1987; Kirkegaard and Baltimore, 1986. The occurrence of subgenomic RNA during replication of MNV supports this model (Karst et al., 2003). Recently, we also showed that MNV recombination events are possible in vitro after propagation of two different MNV strains in RAW 264.7 cells (Mueller, 2009). Intertypic recombination events were also detected in sapoviruses (Chanit et al., 2009; Hansman et al., 2005).

In summary, published data from sources throughout the world suggest that recombination events are not a rare phenomenon among NVs and indicate that these events contribute to the genetic diversity of these viruses.

PREVALENCE OF NV GENOTYPE GII.4 VARIANTS

Numerous molecular epidemiological studies from around the world showed that most recent outbreaks involved genotypes of genogroups GI and, especially, GII. Genotype GII.4 occurs much more frequently than other GII genotypes; its potential for pandemic spread was first recognized in the mid-1990s. However, it was recently reported that almost half of the strains involved in gastroenteritis outbreaks in Argentina belong to genogroup GIV (Gomes et al., 2007).

Since the initiation of molecular genetic surveillance of NV strains by sequence analysis in the early 1990s, it was recognized that antigenic drift variants of GII.4 are responsible for many NV gastroenteritis outbreaks worldwide. Between 2000 and 2004, two new GII.4 variants replaced an old GII.4 strain (strain US95/96) in the United States. The old strain was highly prevalent in the United States and The Netherlands in 1995 and 1996. At around the same time, in the winter of 2002–2003, an increased incidence of NV outbreaks was reported in Europe and a new GII.4 variant (formerly denoted GII.4b) was identified (Lopman et al., 2004). An unexpectedly large number of outbreaks in the spring and summer of 2006 coincided with the emergence of two new GII.4 variants (named GII.4 2006a and b) and was followed by a larger number of outbreaks than usual in the winter of 2006–2007 (Verhoef et al., 2008; Kroneman et al., 2006). Thus, distinct GII.4 lineages emerged in 1995–1996, 2002–2003, 2004–2005, and 2006–2007.

Up to now, five (or six) GII.4 lineages have been identified. In Europe these epidemic antigenic drift variants of genotype GII.4 are usually named after their year of detection: 1996, 2002, 2004, 2006a, and 2006b (and possibly 2008) (Siebenga et al., 2007b, 2009). National surveillance data in Germany showed that between 2001 and 2006, the emergence of significant new variants of GII.4 strains was correlated with higher NV activity. During the interepidemic phases (2001–2002, 2003–2004, and

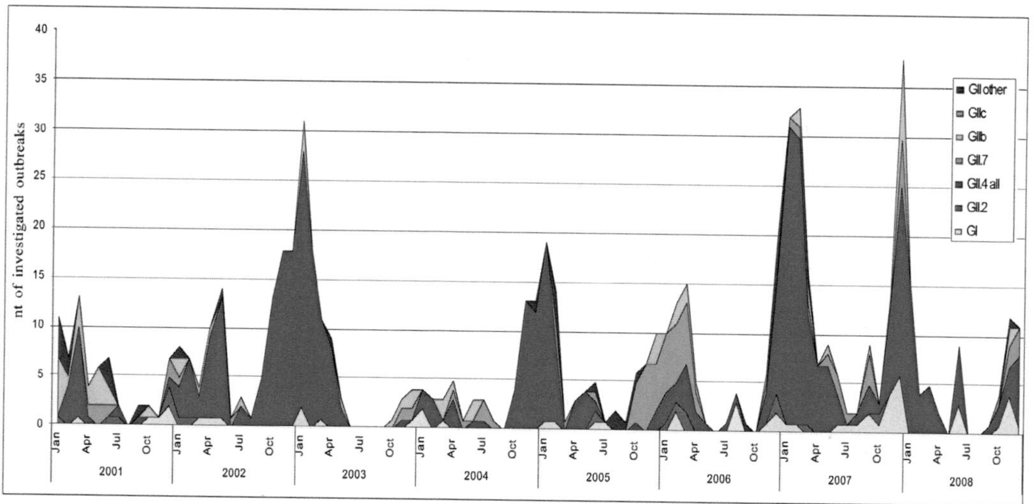

FIGURE 5 Distribution of major NV genotypes in Germany between January 2001 and December 2008. Genotyping was done based on partial RdRp sequence data (M. Hoehne and E. Schreier, Robert Koch Institute, Berlin, Germany, unpublished data). The numbers of reported NV cases in Germany are as follows: 9,292 (2001), 51,619 (2002), 41,755 (2003), 64,794 (2004), 62,773 (2005), 75,865 (2006), 201,227 (2007), and 212,692 (2008) (see http://www3.rki.de/SurvStat).

2005–2006) there was more cocirculation of different genotypes of GI and GII (Fig. 5). Since the 2006–2007 season, the number of reported cases in Germany has been constantly large and the GII.4 2006a and 2006b strains have predominated. These two new variants have been detected worldwide and are responsible for simultaneous outbreaks. In the 2008–2009 season, a new GII.4 drift variant (tentatively denoted GII.4 2008) was detected in several countries; it will be interesting to see if this drift variant continues in future outbreaks.

There are many possible explanations for the high prevalence of GII.4 variants: increased stability of the virus in the environment, superior transmission compared to other genotypes, changes in the P2 subdomain-host receptor interaction, or low population immunity to the emerging variant. Recent reports suggested that GII.4 strains are more transmissible than other genotypes in health care settings, where close contact favors person-to-person transmission (Siebenga et al., 2007a; Buesa et al., 2008). A recent Swedish study of the genetic diversity of NV infections in food-related and water-related outbreaks showed that water-related outbreaks of NV GI were by far the most common (Lysen et al., 2009). A higher prevalence of GI NVs in water-related outbreaks was also observed in Finland (Maunula and Von Bonsdorff, 2005).

Several studies were undertaken in recent years to improve understanding of the mechanisms and biological advantages of GII.4 epidemic strains. In The Netherlands, epidemic GII.4 strains collected between 1995 and 2006 were sequenced in the capsid gene and the genetic changes in the capsid protein were analyzed (Siebenga et al., 2007b). This study showed that GII.4 NVs evolve stepwise by highly significant preferential accumulation and fixation of nucleotide and amino acid mutations in the protruding part of the capsid protein. Interestingly, strains belonging to GII.4 2006b variants are grouped closer to the 2002 variant than to the 2006a variant, which constitutes a subgroup of variant 2004. This indicates the existence of two different clusters: the 2002-2006b and the 2004-2006a variants. This observation has also been confirmed by phylogenetic analyses based on partial sequences of the RdRp (Buesa et al., 2008).

An evolutionary analysis investigated the extent of amino acid diversity in the capsid region for the clusters of GII.4 viruses, using representative strains collected in the United States from 1987 to 2005. Diversity was approximately 2% overall and approximately 10% between the earliest cluster and the extant clusters (Lindesmith et al., 2008). The fact that most amino acid replacements occurred within the protruding P2 subdomain of the capsid protein is not surprising since amino acid residues are surface exposed in the virion. Overall, previous phylogenetic and evolutionary analyses of the P2 domain suggest that the GII.4 viruses have evolved fairly linearly over the years in terms of antigenic drift. This suggests that the P2 subdomain evolves by immune escape in response to preexisting human herd immunity to altered antigenicity. However, no long-term immunity to NV infection has been reported so far. The hypothesis that herd immunity is a driving force for GII.4 evolution is supported by results from a surrogate neutralization assay, which measured the blockade of histo-blood group antigen (HBGA) binding by using a panel of GII.4 VLPs representing strains isolated in 1987, 1997, 2002, and 2006 from acute- and convalescent-phase sera collected during outbreaks. The blockade of GII.4 VLP-HBGA binding was greater with convalescent-phase sera collected near the time of origin of the VLP (Cannon et al., 2009). HBGA expression on the gut mucosa correlates with susceptibility to infection with the prototype Norwalk virus (Hutson et al., 2002; Lindesmith et al., 2003).

The diversity of GII.4 NV can account for its persistence among humans (Lindesmith et al., 2008; Siebenga et al., 2007b), and studies with VLPs from the GII.4 genocluster support this concept (Donaldson et al., 2008). In this context it is very interesting that a single amino acid substitution in the P2 domain of the capsid protein of MNV is sufficient for escape from antibody neutralization (Lochridge and Hardy, 2007).

In a Spanish study, partial sequencing of the RdRp gene enabled the identification of five genetic variants of GII.4 associated with outbreaks during 2001 and 2006 (Buesa et al., 2008). The 1996 variant was still detected in 2001 and even in 2003 but was largely displaced in 2002 by the variant GII.4 2002. The fact that old variants can still be detected at low levels has also been reported by other researchers (Gallimore et al., 2007). A huge increase in the incidence of NV outbreaks was observed in the winter of 2006 with the occurrence of the new variants 2006a and 2006b. This replacement of a viral species by a new emerging species happened within a 4-month period in the late winter to early spring.

The fact that minor nucleotide changes in the NV RdRp gene are related to the incidence of GII.4-associated gastroenteritis outbreaks had already been shown for European outbreak strains from the epidemic years 2002 and 2004 (Lopman et al., 2004). Analysis of the RdRp region characterized a hexanucleotide sequence AACTTG in the predominant variant of 2001, which changed to AATCTG in the epidemic year 2002. That this specific 6-nucleotide motif could act as a marker of major GII.4 epidemics was also shown in studies of gastroenteritis outbreaks in Australia from 2001 to 2005 (Bruggink and Marshall, 2008). In each epidemic year the predominant hexamer sequence changed relative to the previous year. It should be noted that the six-nucleotide variants in the RdRp are in frame to code for the amino acids asparagine and leucine. Therefore, the generalization that GII.4 epidemics correlate with the appearance of such new hexamer variants is not yet confirmed. However, it is known that the exchange of a single nucleotide can change the fitness of viruses. New emerging species of NV strains belonging to the GII.4 genotype were a predominant cause of nosocomial outbreaks of viral gastroenteritis in Sweden in 1997 to 2005 (Johansen et al., 2008). During the 2002–2003 winter season the incidence of NV infections in major Swedish hospitals was almost fourfold that of *Clostridium difficile* diarrhea.

It is impossible to predict which of the currently active GII.4 variants will cause gastroenteritis epidemics in coming years. Investigation of NV RNA evolution among individuals with prolonged NV excretion is important in this regard. Swedish researchers analyzed the evolution of polymerase and the capsid gene in an immunosuppressed individual with chronic diarrhea (lasting >2 years) and prolonged NV shedding (Nilsson et al., 2003). Nucleotide sequencing of the RdRp gene revealed only sporadic and scattered nucleotide changes, with only one substitution over a 1-year period. Comparative sequence analysis of the entire capsid gene revealed a total of 32 amino acid changes within the protruding hypervariable P2 domain of the capsid protein during the 1-year period. The accumulated amino acid changes in the P2 domain resulted in predictable structural changes which could potentially induce a new NV phenotype. However, mutations in the RdRp gene result more often from a lack of proofreading of the viral RdRp than from amino acid substitutions. Changes in the P2 domain are probably driven by immune mechanisms.

Three other cases of prolonged NV shedding in patients with immune dysfunction or in immunocompetent individuals have been reported. In a child with cartilage hair hypoplasia (T-cell deficiency), no amino acid mutations were found in a partial capsid sequence of 277 nucleotides in the 5′ region of ORF2 (GII.3 strain/ARG 320/1999/US like) over a 6-month period (Gallimore et al., 2004).

Recently, single-nucleotide and amino acid substitutions in the NV capsid region were detected in two immunocompetent individuals in Japan during viral shedding that lasted for up to 2 months. However, these substitutions were not restricted to a distinct region.

A hospital in The Netherlands reported significantly prolonged periods of NV-related gastroenteritis combined with shedding over long durations in patients infected with GII.4 or the recombinant GIIb-GII.3 strains (Siebenga et al., 2008). This study showed that the NV capsid protein accumulates mutations more rapidly in healthy immunocompetent individuals than in immunocompromised individuals. The rate of mutation accumulation was lowest among individuals who had the most severe immune dysfunction.

Two potentially immunologically significant epitopes (termed A and B) in the highly variable P2 domain of the capsid protein of GII.4 variants were recently characterized, and these may provide important insights into the fitness of NV strains (Allen et al., 2008). Amino acid substitutions, especially in surface-exposed antigenic regions of the NV P2 domain, can change not only the immunogenicity of virus epitopes but also the properties of virus binding to putative cell receptors and may be responsible for the emergence of novel NV strains. This can also lead to strains with altered host tropism. In this study, 66 P2 sequences from viruses isolated during outbreaks occurring between 1997 and 2006 in the United Kingdom showed diversity of up to 20%. Detailed analysis identified numerous mutation hot spots. Analysis of mutations at these hot spots and their mapping onto the three-dimensional crystal structure of a specific NV GII.4 strain (Cao et al., 2007) revealed two sites, both 3 amino acid residues in length, one located near the N terminus and one near the C terminus of the P2 domain. Both sites were located in exposed loops of the P2 domain of the capsid protein, and changes in both sites were strongly associated with the emergence of epidemiologically significant virus strains, which—possibly due to lack of herd immunity—resulted in gastroenteritis epidemics. Mutations at both of these sites resulted in conformational changes that altered the antigenic properties of the virus. In connection with recently published crystal structure data for the GII.4 strain (Cao et al., 2007), it is assumed that these two sites together act as variant-specific epitopes.

In addition to these putative variant-specific amino acid changes, a seventh surface-exposed position is notable. This amino acid position is part of a putative RGD (arginyl-glycyl-aspartic) motif which is positioned in a loop of the P2 domain. Although the biological relevance of this position is unknown, the amino acid change generated an integrin-binding RGD motif in GII.4 strains in the 2002–2003 epidemic (Allen et al., 2008; Siebenga et al., 2008). The RGD motif is sterically close to both the binding pocket and the HBGA binding site (Tan et al., 2003; Cao et al., 2007) and may be involved in immune evasion. The association of amino acid substitutions in the capsid protein with the emergence of new epidemic NV strains was also shown in a study in The Netherlands (Siebenga et al., 2007b). However, these authors also showed that individual amino acid changes in regions other than the P2 domain have been associated with European epidemics.

In conclusion, the association of sequence changes at the nucleotide and amino acid level with the emergence of new epidemic strains of NV genotype GII.4 is an important part of molecular epidemiological investigations. Less is known about the genetic evolution of other NV genotypes that are less prevalent in the population and cause only sporadic outbreaks in limited geographic regions. Recently, Iritani and coworkers compared more than 30 complete capsid gene sequences of NV genotype GII.2 strains, obtained from outbreaks or sporadic cases in The Netherlands and Japan between 1994 and 2005 (Iritani et al., 2008). Some strains were characterized as recombinants. Molecular analysis of the GII.2 capsids showed differences between recombinant and nonrecombinant genomes with regard to antigenic drift. Fixation of amino acid substitutions over time could be used as an indicator for genetic drift only if recombinants were excluded from the sequence alignment.

The finding that various NV recombinant strains behave differently during NV infections demonstrates the importance of molecular epidemiological and evolution studies. Not surprisingly, the P2 domain in GII.2 strains showed a significantly higher rate of substitutions than did the P1 and S regions, although the rate of change was clearly lower than in genogroup GII.4 strains. The fact that NVs belonging to this rarer genotype also evolved by accumulation of mutations in the surface-exposed region of the major capsid protein suggests that these changes were induced by the immune response.

For many RNA viruses, high mutation rates may facilitate the development of a quasispecies population in an infected patient (Domingo et al., 1998; Domingo, 1997; Domingo and Holland, 1997; Eigen, 1993, 1996). Within this heterogeneous cloud of genetically related virus variants, mutants with an increased capacity to adapt to various environments may be generated (Domingo et al., 1998; Forns et al., 1999). This quasispecies nature of RNA viruses plays an important role in their persistence. Recent data concerning quasispecies dynamics and molecular evolution of the NV capsid protein P region during chronic infection are very interesting in this regard. Carlsson et al. (2009b) sequenced the P1-1 and P2 regions from an individual infected for 3 years with NV genotype GII.3 and used an evolutionary trace algorithm to identify conserved amino acid residues and to correlate these with quasispecies behavior. The results showed that more amino acid residues were conserved in the P1-1 region than in the P2 region. This result is not surprising, as the P2 domain has far more surface exposure than the P1-1 domain. More interesting was the finding that most amino acid positions of the putative carbohydrate-binding pocket within the hypervariable P2 domain remained absolutely conserved during chronic infection, presumably because there was no selective advantage to alter the HBGA receptor-binding specificity. Previously, crystal structure studies of a GII.4 NV suggested that these amino acid residues in the P2 domain are involved in carbohydrate binding (Cao et al., 2007; Chakravarty et al., 2005). Mutational analyses of receptor-binding specificity have also shown that such amino acid residues are important in the binding of NV particles to putative carbohydrate receptor molecules (Bu et al., 2008). Although the receptors or coreceptors for human NV and MNV are different, it is interesting that a single amino acid substitution in the P2 domain of the VP1 protein of MNV leads to escape from antibody neutralization (Lochridge and Hardy, 2007). These data, which were obtained in studies of a native virus, suggest that the NV particle domains which are important for functional interactions may be similar to those of MNV, even though the cell tropism for the two viruses is quite different.

NOROVIRUS-HOST INTERACTIONS

Due to the difficulty of culturing these viruses, the relationship between NV genotypes and their phenotypes or antigenic profiles is poorly understood. Therefore, it is doubtful whether the MNV can be helpful in this context.

The recent discovery of an association between specific HBGAs and clinical NV infections, along with published evidence that NVs recognize HBGAs as receptors in a strain-specific manner, were breakthroughs in the understanding of the NV-host interaction (Marionneau et al., 2002; Lindesmith et al., 2003; Huang et al., 2003, 2005; Hutson et al., 2003; Harrington et al., 2002, 2004). HBGAs are a highly heterogeneous group of carbohydrates, normally found on the surface of red blood cells, expressed on mucosal surfaces and respiratory epithelia, and frequently present as free antigens in body fluids such as saliva and intestinal contents. Many viruses and other microorganisms use HBGAs to attach to the surface of the host cell. Humans of different blood types may have increased or decreased susceptibility to particular diseases, and even natural factors such as the decoy receptors in milk may interfere or compete with pathogens for specific receptors and thus may influence the NV infection or the outcome of infection. Breast-fed infants seem to be less susceptible to NV diarrhea, although this depends on the maternal HBGA type and elements (e.g., decoy receptors), which can block binding of NV to HBGAs (Jiang et al., 2004).

HBGA expression is regulated by several genes that determine which of the three biosynthetic pathways is followed, and this variation leads to polymorphic blood groups (ABO), Lewis, and secretor phenotypes. The *FUT3* gene encodes an α1,3 or α1,4 fucosyltransferase, which is responsible for the synthesis of the Lewis A (Le^a) phenotype (also known as the nonsecretor phenotype). The gene responsible for the secretor phenotype, FUT2, encodes an α1,2-fucosyltranferase that generates the H type 1 and the H type 3 antigens. ABO, Lewis, and secretor phenotypes and enzymatic pathways have been described in detail (Hutson et al., 2004; Green et al., 1988; Clausen and Hakomori, 1989). Eight carbohydrate-binding patterns involved in NV recognition belong to either the ABO, or the Lewis or secretor families (Huang et al., 2003; Tan and Jiang, 2005, 2007). These binding patterns interact with specific NV structures—mostly VLPs—via saliva from individuals with different phenotypes, via blood type-specific hemagglutination assays, or through binding of histo-blood group antigens on gastroduodenal epithelia cells of secretor individuals (Harrington et al., 2002; Huang et al., 2003; Hutson et al., 2002, 2003; Marionneau et al., 2002). Challenge studies showed that secretor-negative individuals (i.e., nonsecretors, or individuals with a defect in the FUT2 α1,2-fucosyltranferase gene) are less susceptible or even resistant to infection with the prototype strain, the Norwalk virus (Lindesmith et al., 2003; Hutson et al., 2005). Approximately 20% of northern Europeans and Caucasian Americans are secretor negative.

Recent studies of GII.3 and GII.4 NV outbreaks revealed an association between HBGA phenotypes and viral infection (Tan et al., 2008; Kindberg et al., 2007). The combination of the variable expression of the putative HBGA receptors and the strain-specific binding may explain differences in susceptibility to NV infections. However, no structural explanations have clarified the difference between ligand recognition of NVs from different genogroups. Although the prototype GI.1 virus (the Norwalk virus) specifically recognizes A- and H-type HBGAs, it does not bind type B antigen when challenged with a GII.4 NV that recognized A, B, and H antigens of human HBGAs (Cao et al., 2007). Individuals with HBGA type B infection may thus be protected against infection with GI infection but are not protected against GII NVs (Rockx et al., 2005a).

There is no evidence for an association between HBGA type and susceptibility to clinical infections with GII NVs (Halperin et al., 2008). NV strains belonging to the GII.4 NV cluster can infect all HBGA secretors, regardless of their blood type.

Interestingly, crystal structure data of GI (GI.1 genotype) and GII (GII.4 genotype) NV P domains, either alone or with HBGA type A carbohydrate antigen, provided evidence of different receptor-binding modes. Results showed that although the P domain of both strain variants bound the same A antigens, the binding mode and the amino acids involved in the interaction with the HBGAs were quite different (Bu et al., 2008). However, the binding region for both strains was located in the same region of the hypervariable P2 domain. These data support the genetic classification of NV but also indicate that the two strains are not from the same evolutionary lineage in terms of selection by the human HBGAs. A recent study showed that some NV GII strains (GII.3 and GII.4VLPs) but not the GI.1 prototype strain (Norwalk virus) have at least two binding specificities: one secretor gene dependent which is related to α1,2-fucosylated carbohydrates, and another related to α2,3-sialylated carbohydrates (Rydell et al., 2009a, 2009b). This sialic-acid-dependent binding also applies to other GII strains, but it is not clear whether it applies to human NVs of GI. Recent data indicated that MNV can use terminal sialic acid as an attachment receptor during binding to murine macrophages (Taube et al., 2009). Many viruses, including the feline calicivirus, use sialic acid as a receptor for infection (Stuart and Brown, 2007).

The fact that individuals who are NV antibody positive may be secretor negative, though often with significantly lower titers, suggests that secretor-independent infections can occur with some NV strains (Harrington et al., 2002; Huang et al., 2005). NV infections in nonsecretors have been reported (Rockx et al., 2005c; Lindesmith et al., 2005). In a recent GII.4 outbreak, one symptomatic patient infected with the GII.4 strain was a nonsecretor (Carlsson et al., 2009a). Surprisingly, however, previous data suggesting that a homozygous nonsense mutation in the human secretor FUT2 gene (G428A) provides complete resistance to symptomatic

GII NV infections (Kindberg et al., 2007; Thorven et al., 2005) were not confirmed. In the GII.4 outbreak reported by Carlsson et al., the Lewis status (Lewis positive or Lewis negative) was not identified as a susceptibility marker for symptomatic GII.4 NV infection. Early in vitro binding studies suggested that the Lewis status could affect susceptibility to NV (Huang et al., 2005). Other studies showed that individuals of blood type O were more susceptible to NV infection than were individuals of other blood types (Hutson et al., 2002). However, a more recent study with a GII.2 NV showed that blood type and secretor status did not correlate with susceptibility to NV infection (Lindesmith et al., 2005). In summary, despite the diverse binding profiles of NV genogroups GI and GII, the polymorphic nature of putative NV receptors appears to ensure that nearly all individuals are susceptible to NV infection.

Molecules other than HBGAs may participate in the NV-host cell interaction. For example, a cellular 105-kDa membrane protein and heparin sulfate bind specifically to NV-like particles (VLPs) (Tamura et al., 2000, 2004). Thus, many questions about NV-host interaction remain unanswered; for example, are HBGAs the natural receptor, or are they cofactors in the NV infection? Much of our understanding of the interactions between NVs and their host cells was obtained through study of recombinant NV capsid proteins, which spontaneously form copious amounts of VLPs in *Baculovirus* expression systems (Jiang et al., 1992) (Fig. 6). VLPs were also generated with the human endothelial kidney cell line 293T (Taube et al., 2005) and the Venezuelan equine encephalitis (VEE) replicon system, in which the NV capsid gene is inserted in place of the viral VEE structure genes. The VEE replicon particles are capable of infecting cells and generating VLPs (Baric et al., 2002).

The X-ray crystal structure of VLP shows that the capsid has a T=3 icosahedral symmetry organized into 90 dimers of the capsid protein (Prasad et al., 1999), in which each monomer forms two distinct domains—the shell (S) and the protruding P domain – that are linked by a flexible hinge. The S domain is involved in the formation of the icosahedral shell, whereas the P domain, which is divided into subdomains P1 and P2, is extensively involved in the dimeric contacts. The P1 subdomain connects the S domain and the P2 subdomain. Interestingly, despite noticeable structural differences among the different genera of the *Caliciviridae* family, the unique modular S-P1-P2 domain organization of the capsid protein is duplicated in all genera of this family (Chen et al., 2004). Based on the X-ray structure of the recombinant NV capsid, it is hypothesized that the S domain functions to provide a scaffold for icosahedral assembly, the P2 subdomain functions as a quasi replaceable module to confer host specificity and strain diversity, and the P1 subdomain provides additional fine-tuning to position the P2 domain. As mentioned earlier, the P2 subdomain is the most surface-exposed region of the capsid protein, contains the most variable sequences, and may play an essential role in interactions with HBGA carbohydrates.

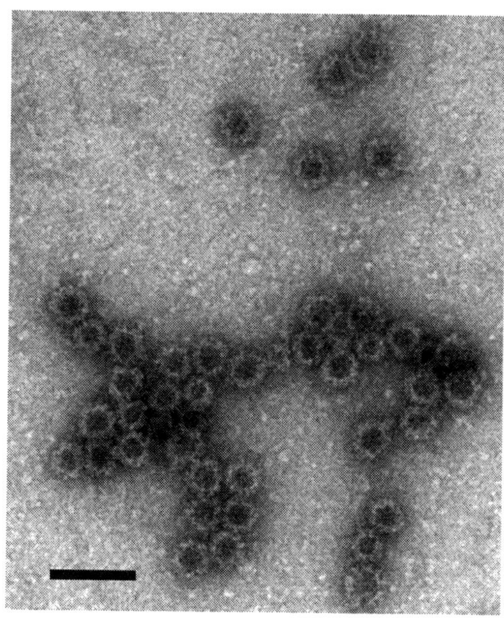

FIGURE 6 Electron micrograph of baculovirus-expressed NV capsid protein (VLPs) negatively stained with uranyl acetate. Bar, 100 nm. (M. Hoehne, M. Laue, and E. Schreier, Robert Koch Institute, Berlin, Germany, unpublished data.)

The involvement of the P2 domain in receptor binding is supported by studies with synthetic carbohydrates and monoclonal antibodies and by reverse genetic experiments involving mutational analysis of the GI and GII NV structures (Hutson et al., 2003; Harrington et al., 2004; Lochridge et al., 2005). Experiments with chimeric capsids, in which the S and P domains were imported from parent strains with different receptor-binding patterns, provided evidence for the importance of the P2 domain in interactions with putative receptor molecules.

The high variability and plasticity of the NV capsid protein P2 domain can alter or even completely block the binding of various NV strains to HBGAs. Thus, the evolution of NVs is influenced not only by the host immune response but also by the polymorphism of the HBGA system, which enables selection of new NV variants for different host susceptibilities. However, it is not clear why the GII.4 NV genoclusters have evolved to produce pandemic strains over the past 20 years while other NV genotypes have not produced such potent strains. Comparison of the VP1 monomer structure of the NV GI.1 or GII.3 P domains to the GII.4 P domain showed that these three proteins are structurally different in the hypervariable P2 subdomain. Such differences in proximal regions, as well as differences in the S or P1 domain of the NV capsid protein, can drastically change the interaction of the capsid protein with the cellular receptor responsible for viral attachment and entry. Recent X-ray crystallographic analysis of the P-domain dimer, both alone and in a complex with A- and H- type HBGAs, described the interactions responsible for binding specificity and provided a molecular explanation for why the HBGA-binding pattern of GI NVs is more restricted than that of GII NVs. The alignment of representative GI NV sequences around the HBGA-binding site showed conservation of the amino acid residues involved in carbohydrate binding. None of these residues are conserved in the GII NVs—this binding epitope in the P domain is highly conserved only in the GI NVs (Choi et al., 2008). The HBGA-binding site in GII.4 variants is thus distinct from that in the GI NV strains. This difference in the HBGA-binding site of GI and GII NVs and the fact that GII.4 NVs recognize a broad spectrum of HBGAs compared to other GII and GI genotypes may explain why GII.4 variants are more prevalent in human populations. However, the HBGA-binding site among GII.4 strains appears to be well conserved, indicating that HBGA-binding specificity is not a major contributing factor in the epochal evolution of GII.4 strains (Prasad, 2010).

Recent results of qualitative and quantitative studies of the binding of pre- and post-2002 GII.4 NV variants onto synthetic HBGAs showed a increased affinity of post-2002 GII.4 variants for HBGAs (de Rougemont et al., 2011). This matches with the increased incidence of NV outbreaks since 2002–2003 (Lopman et al., 2004). The use of distinctly different epitopes for binding of GI and GII NVs to HBGAs supports the hypothesis that the evolution of NVs in human populations is related to blood type distribution (Le Pendu et al., 2006). Even if currently active GII.4 NV variants persist by altering their HBGA carbohydrate-binding targets, it should be emphasized that other structures such as receptors, coreceptors, or enzymes may be necessary for NV persistence, attachment, or cellular internalization (Guix et al., 2007) and may thereby influence NV evolution. Transfection of NV RNA isolated from human stool samples into human hepatoma Huh-7 cells leads to viral replication, with expression of viral antigens, RNA replication, and release of viral particles into the medium. However, no viral spread from NV-transfected cells to naive cells occurred (Guix et al., 2007). Further high-resolution structural studies are necessary to determine the role of the P2 subdomain in host interactions and to understand its possible role in NV strain diversity.

The unique modular organization of the human NV capsid protein and the published phylogenetic data indicating that GII.4 viruses evolved in response to pandemic outbreaks (Siebenga et al., 2007b; Lindesmith et al.,

2008) marked the beginning of a new epoch in the understanding of NVs. The term "epochal evolution" is used to describe a rapid burst of change (e.g., the emergence of new phenotypes) following a period of stasis (van Nimwegen, 2006). For GII.4 NVs, the emergence of the predominant epidemic GII.4 cluster in 2002 and 2003 marked the beginning of a new epoch and also marked the beginning of a fascinating story.

A recent study showed that the GII.4 genotype evolves in response to herd immunity (Lindesmith et al., 2008). Each new GII.4 antigenic drift variant acquires unique immunologic properties. The functional effects of these variants on single structural proteins are surprisingly broad; they can affect assembly, receptor recognition, host specificity, or immune evasion. However, an important caveat should be mentioned for all published studies reporting interactions of NV capsid protein regions with putative receptor molecules such as the HBGAs: the synthetic HBGAs used (synthetic trisaccharides) probably do not represent biologically relevant HBGAs. Due to the huge variability of NVs, many questions about NV-receptor interactions in vivo remain unanswered. The gnotobiotic pig model described earlier is currently being used to study host genetic susceptibility to individual NV variants via binding to specific HBGAs (Cheetham et al., 2007). In addition, the sensitivity of receptor-binding activity to certain host factors may influence the in vitro cultivation of NV. For example, addition of stool extracts produced a significant increase in binding of some NV strains to human saliva.

Despite the ongoing difficulty in cultivating the rapidly changing human NVs, significant advances have been made in understanding virus-host interactions. Continuous molecular surveillance of NVs is essential if we are to understand its evolution. The two major NV genogroups GI and GII represent an evolutionary lineage with distinct genetic traits. Divergent and convergent evolution, as well as changes in human HBGAs, have likely contributed to NV diversity. Monitoring of the variability of circulating NVs, along with precise understanding of virus-host interactions during viral attachment and cell entry, will aid in the development of effective vaccines or antiviral agents.

CONCLUSIONS AND PROSPECTS

Despite much effort over the last 40 years, our understanding of noroviruses and NV-induced disease is limited. For example, little is known about morphological and functional changes in the human intestinal mucosa. NV pathogenesis in gnotobiotic pig and calf models showed a rapid and self-limiting diarrheal disease (Cheetham et al., 2006; Souza et al., 2008), which is similar to the human response. In pigs infected with a human GII.4 strain, NV was detected in enterocytes of villi in the proximal small intestine. Interestingly, similar morphological and functional changes were reported for intestinal samples from humans with acute NV infection, and it was concluded that human NV infection leads to both epithelial transport dysfunction and barrier dysfunction (Troeger et al., 2009). Interestingly, the lack of routine in vitro cell culture assays for NVs appears to have produced new and valuable systems for investigation. For example, the recent generation of NV replicon-bearing BHK21 (baby hamster kidney) and Huh 7 (human hepatoma) cells (Chang et al., 2006) may provide important tools for basic research on NV.

Complex systems such as the gnotobiotic pig or calf models, or the commonly used MNV model, may help to elucidate the mechanisms of infection, replication, or immune response in NV-induced gastroenteritis. How far into the future these findings will remain relevant is an entirely different question. Experimental NV infections in nonhuman species, including primates, may be relevant. Chimpanzees inoculated intravenously with human NV did not show clinical signs of gastroenteritis, but the onset and duration of NV shedding in stool and serum antibody responses were similar to those observed in humans (Bok et al., 2011). Rhesus macaques are also susceptible to NV infection, but have a longer latency until the development of NV-specific immunoglobulin M and G responses (Rockx et al., 2005b). More recent models such as the gnotobiotic pig NV or MNV have already yielded many insights, including an understanding of the relative roles of innate and adaptive immunity in the response to NV infection. Two reverse genetic systems for recovery of genetically defined infectious MNV in tissue culture were recently described (Chaudhry et al., 2007; Ward et al., 2007) and may provide a powerful tool for investigation of the molecular determinants of NV virulence and for analysis of pathogenic variations. A reverse genetic system applied in vivo recently demonstrated that a single amino acid substitution in the MNV capsid protein is sufficient to attenuate symptoms (Bailey et al., 2008). Finally, different methods used to predict the secondary structure of caliciviruses are becoming increasingly important due to the growing availability of nucleotide sequences in the *Caliciviridae* virus family; these have provided valuable evidence about the evolutionary development of RNA structural elements.

In summary, the immense genetic diversity of human NVs circulating throughout the world's population and the high mutability (metamorphosis) of this genus have proved to be a catastrophe for individual humans but simultaneously a gift for researchers who seek to understand NVs or to understand the behavior of viruses in general.

REFERENCES

Allen, D. J., J. J. Gray, C. I. Gallimore, J. Xerry, and M. Iturriza-Gomara. 2008. Analysis of amino acid variation in the P2 domain of the GII-4 norovirus VP1 protein reveals putative variant-specific epitopes. *PLoS One* **3:**e1485.

Bailey, D., L. B. Thackray, and I. G. Goodfellow. 2008. A single amino acid substitution in the murine norovirus capsid protein is sufficient for attenuation in vivo. *J. Virol.* **82:**7725–7728.

Baric, R. S., B. Yount, L. Lindesmith, P. R. Harrington, S. R. Greene, F. C. Tseng, N. Davis, R. E. Johnston, D. G. Klapper, and C. L. Moe. 2002. Expression and self-assembly of Norwalk virus capsid protein from Venezuelan equine encephalitis virus replicons. *J. Virol.* **76:** 3023–3030.

Bertolotti-Ciarlet, A., S. E. Crawford, A. M. Hutson, and M. K. Estes. 2003. The 3′ end of Norwalk virus mRNA contains determinants that regulate the expression and stability of the viral capsid protein VP1: a novel function for the VP2 protein. *J. Virol.* **77:**11603 –11615.

Bok, K., G. I. Parra, T. Mitra, E. Abente, C. K. Shaver, D. Boon, R. Engle, C. Yu, A. Z. Kapikian, S. V. Sosnovtsev, R. H. Purcell, and K. Y. Green. 2011. Chimpanzees as an animal model for human norovirus infection and vaccine development. *Proc. Natl. Acad. Sci. USA* **108:**325–330.

Bon, F., K. Ambert-Balay, H. Giraudon, J. Kaplon, S. Le Guyader, M. Pommepuy, A. Gallay, V. Vaillant, H. de Valk, R. Chikhi-Brachet, A. Flahaut, P. Pothier, and E. Kohli. 2005. Molecular epidemiology of caliciviruses detected in sporadic and outbreak cases of gastroenteritis in France from December 1998 to February 2004. *J. Clin. Microbiol.* **43:**4659–4664.

Bruggink, L., and J. Marshall. 2008. Molecular changes in the norovirus polymerase gene and their association with incidence of GII.4 norovirus-associated gastroenteritis outbreaks in Victoria, Australia, 2001–2005. *Arch. Virol.* **153:**729–732.

Bu, W., A. Mamedova, M. Tan, M. Xia, X. Jiang, and R. S. Hegde. 2008. Structural basis for the receptor binding specificity of Norwalk virus. *J. Virol.* **82:**5340–5347.

Buesa, J., R. Montava, R Abu-Mallouh, M. Fos, J. M. Ribes, R. Bartolome, H. Vanaclocha, N. Torner, and A. Dominguez. 2008. Sequential evolution of genotype GII.4 norovirus variants causing gastroenteritis outbreaks from 2001 to 2006 in Eastern Spain. *J. Med. Virol.* **80:**1288–1295.

Bull, R. A., G. S. Hansman, L. E. Clancy, M. M. Tanaka, W. D. Rawlinson, and P. A. White. 2005. Norovirus recombination in ORF1/ORF2 overlap. *Emerg. Infect. Dis.* **11:**1079–1085.

Bull, R. A., M. M. Tanaka, and P. A. White. 2007. Norovirus recombination. *J. Gen. Virol.* **88:**3347–3359.

Cannon, J. L., L. C. Lindesmith, E. F. Donaldson, L. Saxe, R. S. Baric, and J. Vinje. 2009. Herd immunity to GII.4 noroviruses is supported by outbreak patient sera. *J. Virol.* **83:**5363–5374.

Cao, S., Z. Lou, M. Tan, Y. Chen, Y. Liu, Z. Zhang, X. C. Zhang, X. Jiang, X. Li, and Z. Rao. 2007. Structural basis for the recognition of blood group trisaccharides by norovirus. *J. Virol.* **81:** 5949–5957.

Carlsson, B., E. Kindberg, J. Buesa, G. E. Rydell, M. F. Lidon, R. Montava, R. Abu Mallouh, A. Grahn, J. Rodriguez-Diaz, J. Bellido, A. Arnedo, G. Larsson, and L. Svensson. 2009a. The G428A nonsense mutation in FUT2 provides strong but not absolute protection against symptomatic GII.4 norovirus infection. *PLoS One* **4:**e5593.

Carlsson, B., A. M. Lindberg, J. Rodriguez-Diaz, K. O. Hedlund, B. Persson, and L. Svensson. 2009b. Quasispecies dynamics and molecular evolution of human norovirus capsid P region during chronic infection. *J. Gen. Virol.* **90:**432–441.

Chakravarty, S., A. M. Hutson, M. K. Estes, and B. V. Prasad. 2005. Evolutionary trace residues in noroviruses: importance in receptor binding, antigenicity, virion assembly, and strain diversity. *J. Virol.* **79:**554–568.

Chang, K. O., S. V. Sosnovtsev, G. Belliot, A. D. King, and K. Y. Green. 2006. Stable expression of a Norwalk virus RNA replicon in a human hepatoma cell line. *Virology* **353:**463–473.

Chanit, W., A. Thongprachum, P. Khamrin, S. Okitsu, M. Mizuguchi, and H. Ushijima. 2009. Intergenogroup recombinant sapovirus in Japan, 2007–2008. *Emerg. Infect. Dis.* **15:**1084–1087.

Chaudhry, Y., M. A. Skinner, and I. G. Goodfellow. 2007. Recovery of genetically defined murine norovirus in tissue culture by using a fowlpox virus expressing T7 RNA polymerase. *J. Gen. Virol.* **88:**2091–2100.

Cheetham, S., M. Souza, R. McGregor, T. Meulia, Q. Wang, and L. J. Saif. 2007. Binding patterns of human norovirus-like particles to buccal and intestinal tissues of gnotobiotic pigs in relation to A/H histo-blood group antigen expression. *J. Virol.* **81:**3535–3544.

Cheetham, S., M. Souza, T. Meulia, S. Grimes, M. G. Han, and L. J. Saif. 2006. Pathogenesis of a genogroup II human norovirus in gnotobiotic pigs. *J. Virol.* **80:**10372–10381.

Chen, R., J. D. Neill, J. S. Noel, A. M. Hutson, R. I. Glass, M. K. Estes, and B. V. Prasad. 2004. Inter- and intragenus structural variations in caliciviruses and their functional implications. *J. Virol.* **78:**6469–6479.

Choi, J. M., A. M. Hutson, M. K. Estes, and B. V. Prasad. 2008. Atomic resolution structural characterization of recognition of histo-blood group antigens by Norwalk virus. *Proc. Natl. Acad. Sci. USA* **105:**9175–9180.

Clausen, H., and S. Hakomori. 1989. ABH and related histo-blood group antigens; immunochemical differences in carrier isotypes and their distribution. *Vox Sang.* **56:**1–20.

Daughenbaugh, K. F., C. S. Fraser, J. W. Hershey, and M. E. Hardy. 2003. The genome-linked protein VPg of the Norwalk virus binds eIF3, suggesting its role in translation initiation complex recruitment. *EMBO J.* **22:**2852–2859.

de Rougemont, A., N. Ruvoen-Clouet, B. Simon, M. Estienney, C. Elie-Caille, S. Aho, P. Pothier, J. Le Pendu, W. Boireau, and G. Belliot. 2011. Qualitative and quantitative analysis of the binding of GII.4 norovirus variants onto human blood group antigens. *J. Virol.* **85:**4057–4070.

Domingo, E. 1997. RNA virus evolution, population dynamics, and nutritional status. *Biol. Trace Elem. Res.* **56:**23–30.

Domingo, E., C. Escarmis, N. Sevilla and E. Baranowski. 1998. Population dynamics in the evolution of RNA viruses. *Adv. Exp. Med. Biol.* **440:**721–727.

Domingo, E., and J. J. Holland. 1997. RNA virus mutations and fitness for survival. *Annu. Rev. Microbiol.* **51:**151–178.

Donaldson, E. F., L. C. Lindesmith, A. D. Lobue, and R. S. Baric. 2008. Norovirus pathogenesis: mechanisms of persistence and immune evasion in human populations. *Immunol. Rev.* **225:**190–211.

Eigen, M. 1993. The origin of genetic information: viruses as models. *Gene* **135:**37–47.

Eigen, M. 1996. On the nature of virus quasispecies. *Trends Microbiol.* **4:**216–218.

Farkas, T., K. Sestak, C. Wei, and X. Jiang. 2008. Characterization of a rhesus monkey calicivirus representing a new genus of *Caliciviridae*. *J. Virol.* **82:**5408–5416.

Forns, X., R. H. Purcell, and J. Bukh. 1999. Quasispecies in viral persistence and pathogenesis of hepatitis C virus. *Trends Microbiol.* **7:**402–410.

Gallimore, C. I., M. Iturriza-Gomara, J. Xerry, J. Adigwe, and J. J. Gray. 2007. Inter-seasonal diversity of norovirus genotypes: emergence and selection of virus variants. *Arch. Virol.* **152:**1295–1303.

Gallimore, C. I., D. Lewis, C. Taylor, A. Cant, A. Gennery, and J. J. Gray. 2004. Chronic excretion of a norovirus in a child with cartilage hair hypoplasia (CHH). *J. Clin. Virol.* **30:**196–204.

Glass, P. J., L. J. White, J. M. Ball, I. Leparc-Goffart, M. E. Hardy, and M. K. Estes. 2000. Norwalk virus open reading frame 3 encodes a minor structural protein. *J. Virol.* **74:**6581–6591.

Gomes, K. A., J. A. Stupka, J. Gomez, and G. I. Parra. 2007. Molecular characterization of calicivirus strains detected in outbreaks of gastroenteritis in Argentina. *J. Med. Virol.* **79:**1703–1709.

Green, F. R., P. Greenwell, L. Dickson, B. Griffiths, J. Noades, and D. M. Swallow. 1988. Expression of the ABH, Lewis, and related antigens on the glycoproteins of the human jejunal brush border. *Subcell. Biochem.* **12:**119–153.

Green, K. Y. 2007. *Caliciviridae:* the noroviruses, p. 949–978. *In* D. M. Knipe and P. M. Howley (ed.), *Fields Virology*, 5th ed., vol. 1. Lippincott Williams & Wilkins, Philadelphia, PA.

Guix, S., M. Asanaka, K. Katayama, S. E. Crawford, F. H. Neill, R. L. Atmar, and M. K. Estes.

2007. Norwalk virus RNA is infectious in mammalian cells. *J. Virol.* **81:**12238–12248.

Halperin, T., H. Vennema, M. Koopmans, G. Kahila Bar-Gal, R. Kayouf, T. Sela, R. Ambar, and E. Klement. 2008. No association between histo-blood group antigens and susceptibility to clinical infections with genogroup II norovirus. *J. Infect. Dis.* **197:**63–65.

Han, M. G., J. R. Smiley, C. Thomas, and L. J. Saif. 2004. Genetic recombination between two genotypes of genogroup III bovine noroviruses (BoNVs) and capsid sequence diversity among BoNVs and Nebraska-like bovine enteric caliciviruses. *J. Clin. Microbiol.* **42:**5214–5224.

Hansman, G. S., N. Takeda, T. Oka, M. Oseto, K. O. Hedlund, and K. Katayama. 2005. Intergenogroup recombination in sapoviruses. *Emerg. Infect. Dis.* **11:**1916–1920.

Hardy, M. E., S. F. Kramer, J. J. Treanor, and M. K. Estes. 1997. Human calicivirus genogroup II capsid sequence diversity revealed by analyses of the prototype Snow Mountain agent. *Arch. Virol.* **142:**1469–1479.

Harrington, P. R., L. Lindesmith, B. Yount, C. L. Moe, and R. S. Baric. 2002. Binding of Norwalk virus-like particles to ABH histo-blood group antigens is blocked by antisera from infected human volunteers or experimentally vaccinated mice. *J. Virol.* **76:**12335–12343.

Harrington, P. R., J. Vinje, C. L. Moe, and R. S. Baric. 2004. Norovirus capture with histo-blood group antigens reveals novel virus-ligand interactions. *J. Virol.* **78:**3035–3045.

Huang, P., T. Farkas, S. Marionneau, W. Zhong, N. Ruvoen-Clouet, A. L. Morrow, M. Altaye, L. K. Pickering, D. S. Newburg, J. LePendu, and X. Jiang. 2003. Noroviruses bind to human ABO, Lewis, and secretor histo-blood group antigens: identification of 4 distinct strain-specific patterns. *J. Infect. Dis.* **188:**19–31.

Huang, P., T. Farkas, W. Zhong, M. Tan, S. Thornton, A. L. Morrow, and X. Jiang. 2005. Norovirus and histo-blood group antigens: demonstration of a wide spectrum of strain specificities and classification of two major binding groups among multiple binding patterns. *J. Virol.* **79:**6714–6722.

Hutson, A. M., F. Airaud, J. LePendu, M. K. Estes, and R. L. Atmar. 2005. Norwalk virus infection associates with secretor status genotyped from sera. *J. Med. Virol.* **77:**116–120.

Hutson, A. M., R. L. Atmar, and M. K. Estes. 2004. Norovirus disease: changing epidemiology and host susceptibility factors. *Trends Microbiol.* **12:**279–287.

Hutson, A. M., R. L. Atmar, D. Y. Graham, and M. K. Estes. 2002. Norwalk virus infection and disease is associated with ABO histo-blood group type. *J. Infect. Dis.* **185:**1335–1337.

Hutson, A. M., R. L. Atmar, D. M. Marcus, and M. K. Estes. 2003. Norwalk virus-like particle hemagglutination by binding to h histo-blood group antigens. *J. Virol.* **77:**405–415.

Iritani, N., H. Vennema, J. J. Siebenga, R. J. Siezen, B. Renckens, Y. Seto, A. Kaida, and M. Koopmans. 2008. Genetic analysis of the capsid gene of genotype GII.2 noroviruses. *J. Virol.* **82:**7336–7345.

Jiang, X., C. Espul, W. M. Zhong, H. Cuello, and D. O. Matson. 1999. Characterization of a novel human calicivirus that may be a naturally occurring recombinant. *Arch. Virol.* **144:**2377–2387.

Jiang, X., P. Huang, W. Zhong, M. Tan, T. Farkas, A. L. Morrow, D. S. Newburg, G. M. Ruiz-Palacios, and L. K. Pickering. 2004. Human milk contains elements that block binding of noroviruses to human histo-blood group antigens in saliva. *J. Infect. Dis.* **190:**1850–1859.

Jiang, X., M. Wang, D. Y. Graham, and M. K. Estes. 1992. Expression, self-assembly, and antigenicity of the Norwalk virus capsid protein. *J. Virol.* **66:**6527–6532.

Jiang, X., M. Wang, K. Wang, and M. K. Estes. 1993. Sequence and genomic organization of Norwalk virus. *Virology* **195:**51–61.

Johansen, K., K. Mannerqvist, A. Allard, Y. Andersson, L. G. Burman, L. Dillner, K. O. Hedlund, K. Jonsson, U. Kumlin, T. Leitner, et al. 2008. Norovirus strains belonging to the GII.4 genotype dominate as a cause of nosocomial outbreaks of viral gastroenteritis in Sweden 1997–2005. Arrival of new variants is associated with large nationwide epidemics. *J. Clin. Virol.* **42:**129–134.

Kageyama, T., M. Shinohara, K. Uchida, S. Fukushi, F. B. Hoshino, S. Kojima, R. Takai, T. Oka, N. Takeda, and K. Katayama. 2004. Coexistence of multiple genotypes, including newly identified genotypes, in outbreaks of gastroenteritis due to norovirus in Japan. *J. Clin. Microbiol.* **42:**2988–2995.

Kapikian, A . Z., R. G. Wyatt, R. Dolin, T. S. Thornhill, A. R. Kalica, and R. M. Chanock. 1972. Visualization by immune electron microscopy of a 27-nm particle associated with acute infectious nonbacterial gastroenteritis. *J. Virol.* **10:**1075–1081.

Karst, S. M., C. E. Wobus, M. Lay, J. Davidson, and H. W. Virgin. 2003. STAT1-dependent innate immunity to a Norwalk-like virus. *Science* **299:**1575–1578.

Kimura, M. 1980. A simple method for estimating evolutionary rate of base substitutions through comparative studies of nucleotide sequences. *J. Mol. Evol.* **16:**111–120.

Kindberg, E., B. Akerlind, C. Johnsen, J. D. Knudsen, O. Heltberg, G. Larson, B. Bottiger, and

L. Svensson. 2007. Host genetic resistance to symptomatic norovirus (GGII.4) infections in Denmark. *J. Clin. Microbiol.* **45:**2720–2722.

Kirkegaard, K., and D. Baltimore. 1986. The mechanism of RNA recombination in poliovirus. *Cell* **47:**433–443.

Kroneman, A., H. Vennema, J. Harris, G. Reuter, C. H. von Bonsdorff, K. O. Hedlund, K. Vainio, V. Jackson, P. Pothier, J. Koch, et al. 2006. Increase in norovirus activity reported in Europe. *Euro Surveill.* **11:**E061214.1.

Lambden, P. R., E. O. Caul, C. R. Ashley, and I. N. Clarke. 1993. Sequence and genome organization of a human small round-structured (Norwalk-like) virus. *Science* **259:**516–519.

Le Pendu, J., N. Ruvoen-Clouet, E. Kindberg, and L. Svensson. 2006. Mendelian resistance to human norovirus infections. *Semin. Immunol.* **18:**375–386.

LePendu, J., and R. Baric. 2003. Human susceptibility and resistance to Norwalk virus infection. *Nat. Med.* **9:**548–553.

Lindesmith, L., C. Moe, J. Lependu, J. A. Frelinger, J. Treanor, and R. S. Baric. 2005. Cellular and humoral immunity following Snow Mountain virus challenge. *J. Virol.* **79:**2900–2909.

Lindesmith, L., C. Moe, S. Marionneau, N. Ruvoen, X. Jiang, L. Lindblad, P. Stewart, J. LePendu, and R. Baric. 2003. Human susceptibility and resistance to Norwalk virus infection. *Nat. Med.* **9:**548–553.

Lindesmith, L. C., E. F. Donaldson, A. D. Lobue, J. L. Cannon, D. P. Zheng, J. Vinje, and R. S. Baric. 2008. Mechanisms of GII.4 norovirus persistence in human populations. *PLoS Med.* **5:**e31.

Lochridge, V. P., and M. E. Hardy. 2007. A single-amino-acid substitution in the P2 domain of VP1 of murine norovirus is sufficient for escape from antibody neutralization. *J. Virol.* **81:**12316–12322.

Lochridge, V. P., K. L. Jutila, J. W. Graff, and M. E. Hardy. 2005. Epitopes in the P2 domain of norovirus VP1 recognized by monoclonal antibodies that block cell interactions. *J. Gen. Virol.* **86:**2799–2806.

Lopman, B., H. Vennema, E. Kohli, P. Pothier, A. Sanchez, A. Negredo, J. Buesa, E. Schreier, M. Reacher, D. Brown, et al. 2004. Increase in viral gastroenteritis outbreaks in Europe and epidemic spread of new norovirus variant. *Lancet* **363:**682–688.

Lysen, M., M. Thorhagen, M. Brytting, M. Hjertqvist, Y. Andersson, and K. O. Hedlund. 2009. Genetic diversity among food-borne and waterborne norovirus strains causing outbreaks in Sweden. *J. Clin. Microbiol.* **47:**2411–2418.

Makino, S., J. O. Fleming, J. G. Keck, S. A. Stohlman, and M. M. Lai. 1987. RNA recombination of coronaviruses: localization of neutralizing epitopes and neuropathogenic determinants on the carboxyl terminus of peplomers. *Proc. Natl. Acad. Sci. USA* **84:**6567–6571.

Makino, S., J. G. Keck, S. A. Stohlman, and M. M. Lai. 1986. High-frequency RNA recombination of murine coronaviruses. *J. Virol.* **57:**729–737.

Marionneau, S., N. Ruvoën, B. Le Moullac-Vaidye, M. Clement, A. Cailleau-Thomas, G. Ruiz-Palacios, P. Huang, X. Jiang, and J. Le Pendu. 2002. Norwalk virus binds to histo-blood group antigens present on gastroduodenal epithelial cells of secretor individuals. *Gastroenterology* **122:**1967–1977.

Martella, V., M. Campolo, E. Lorusso, P. Cavicchio, M. Camero, A. L. Bellacicco, N. Decaro, G. Elia, G. Greco, M. Corrente, et al. 2007. Norovirus in captive lion cub *(Panthera leo)*. *Emerg. Infect. Dis.* **13:**1071–1073.

Martella, V., E. Lorusso, N. Decaro, G. Elia, A. Radogna, M. D'Abramo, C. Desario, A. Cavalli, M. Corrente, M. Camero, et al. 2008. Detection and molecular characterization of a canine norovirus. *Emerg. Infect. Dis.* **14:** 1306–1308.

Mattison, K., A. Shukla, A. Cook, F. Pollari, R. Friendship, D. Kelton, S. Bidawid, and J. M. Farber. 2007. Human noroviruses in swine and cattle. *Emerg. Infect. Dis.* **13:**1184–1188.

Maunula, L., and C.-H. Von Bonsdorff. 2005. Norovirus genotypes causing gastroenteritis outbreaks in Finland 1998–2002. *J. Clin. Virol.* **34:**186–194.

Mead, P. S., L. Slutsker, V. Dietz, L. F. McCaig, J. S. Bresee, C. Shapiro, P. M. Griffin, and R. V. Tauxe. 1999. Food-related illness and death in the United States. *Emerg. Infect. Dis.* **5:**607–625.

Mueller, B., U. Klemm, A. Mas Marques, and E. Schreier. 2007. Genetic diversity and recombination of murine noroviruses in immunocompromised mice. *Arch. Virol.* **152:**1709–1719.

Mueller, B. 2009. *Molekulare Charakterisierung muriner Noroviren—phylogenetische und antigene Eigenschaften.* Dissertation. Humboldt-Universität zu Berlin, Berlin, Germany.

Nayak, M. K., G. Balasubramanian, G. C. Sahoo, R. Bhattacharya, J. Vinje, N. Kobayashi, M. C. Sarkar, M. K. Bhattacharya, and T. Krishnan. 2008. Detection of a novel intergenogroup recombinant Norovirus from Kolkata, India. *Virology* **377:**117–123.

Nilsson, M., K. O. Hedlund, M. Thorhagen, G. Larson, K. Johansen, A. Ekspong, and L. Svensson. 2003. Evolution of human calicivirus RNA in vivo: accumulation of mutations in the protruding P2 domain of the capsid leads to structural changes and possibly a new phenotype. *J. Virol.* **77:**13117–13124.

Oliver, S. L., E. Asobayire, A. M. Dastjerdi, and J. C. Bridger. 2006. Genomic characterization of the unclassified bovine enteric virus Newbury agent-1 (Newbury1) endorses a new genus in the family *Caliciviridae*. *Virology* **350:**240–250.

Phan, T. G., K. Kaneshi, Y. Ueda, S. Nakaya, S. Nishimura, A. Yamamoto, K. Sugita, S. Takanashi, S. Okitsu, and H. Ushijima. 2007. Genetic heterogeneity, evolution, and recombination in noroviruses. *J. Med. Virol.* **79:**1388–1400.

Phan, T. G., T. Kuroiwa, K. Kaneshi, Y. Ueda, S. Nakaya, S. Nishimura, A. Yamamoto, K. Sugita, T. Nishimura, F. Yagyu, et al. 2006. Changing distribution of norovirus genotypes and genetic analysis of recombinant GIIb among infants and children with diarrhea in Japan. *J. Med. Virol.* **78:**971–978.

Prasad, B. V. 2010. Structural biology of calicivirus capsids (state-of-the-art), p. 14. *Fourth Int. Conf. Caliciviruses*, Santa Cruz, Chile, 16 to 19 October 2010.

Prasad, B. V., M. E. Hardy, T. Dokland, J. Bella, M. G. Rossmann, and M. K. Estes. 1999. X-ray crystallographic structure of the Norwalk virus capsid. *Science* **286:**287–290.

Prasad, B. V., M. E. Hardy, X. Jiang, and M. K. Estes. 1996. Structure of Norwalk virus. *Arch. Virol. Suppl.* **12:**237–242.

Rockx, B., R. S. Baric, I. de Grijs, E. Duizer, and M. P. Koopmans. 2005a. Characterization of the homo- and heterotypic immune responses after natural norovirus infection. *J. Med. Virol.* **77:**439–446.

Rockx, B. H., W. M. Bogers, J. L. Heeney, G. van Amerongen, and M. P. Koopmans. 2005b. Experimental norovirus infections in non-human primates. *J. Med. Virol.* **75:**313–320.

Rockx, B. H., H. Vennema, C. J. Hoebe, E. Duizer, and M. P. Koopmans. 2005c. Association of histo-blood group antigens and susceptibility to norovirus infections. *J. Infect. Dis.* **191:**749–754.

Rohayem, J., J. Munch, and A. Rethwilm. 2005. Evidence of recombination in the norovirus capsid gene. *J. Virol.* **79:**4977–4990.

Rydell, G. E., A. B. Dahlin, F. Hook, and G. Larson. 2009a. QCM-D studies of human norovirus VLPs binding to glycosphingolipids in supported lipid bilayers reveal strain specific characteristics. *Glycobiology* **19:**1176–1184.

Rydell, G. E., J. Nilsson, J. Rodriguez-Diaz, N. Ruvoen-Clouet, L. Svensson, J. Le Pendu, and G. Larson. 2009b. Human noroviruses recognize sialyl Lewis x neoglycoprotein. *Glycobiology* **19:**309–320.

Schreier, E., F. Doring, and U. Kunkel. 2000. Molecular epidemiology of outbreaks of gastroenteritis associated with small round structured viruses in Germany in 1997/98. *Arch. Virol.* **145:**443–453.

Siebenga, J. J., M. F. Beersma, H. Vennema, P. van Biezen, N. J. Hartwig, and M. Koopmans. 2008. High prevalence of prolonged norovirus shedding and illness among hospitalized patients: a model for in vivo molecular evolution. *J. Infect. Dis.* **198:**994–1001.

Siebenga, J. J., H. Vennema, E. Duizer, and M. P. Koopmans. 2007a. Gastroenteritis caused by norovirus GGII.4, The Netherlands, 1994–2005. *Emerg. Infect. Dis.* **13:**144–146.

Siebenga, J. J., H. Vennema, B. Renckens, E. de Bruin, B. van der Veer, R. J. Siezen, and M. Koopmans. 2007b. Epochal evolution of GGII.4 norovirus capsid proteins from 1995 to 2006. *J. Virol.* **81:**9932–9941.

Siebenga, J. J., H. Vennema, D. P. Zheng, J. Vinje, B. E. Lee, X. L. Pang, E. C. Ho, W. Lim, A. Choudekar, S. Broor, T. Halperin, N. B. Rasool, J. Hewitt, G. E. Greening, M. Jin, Z. J. Duan, Y. Lucero, M. O'Ryan, M. Hoehne, E. Schreier, R. M. Ratcliff, P. A. White, N. Iritani, G. Reuter, and M. Koopmans. 2009. Norovirus illness is a global problem: emergence and spread of Norovirus GII.4 variants, 2001–2007. *J. Infect. Dis.* **200:**802–812.

Smith, A. W., E. S. Berry, D. E. Skilling, J. E. Barlough, S. E. Poet, T. Berke, J. Mead, and D. O. Matson. 1998a. In vitro isolation and characterization of a calicivirus causing a vesicular disease of the hands and feet. *Clin. Infect. Dis.* **26:**434–439.

Smith, A. W., D. E. Skilling, N. Cherry, J. H. Mead, and D. O. Matson. 1998b. Calicivirus emergence from ocean reservoirs: zoonotic and interspecies movements. *Emerg. Infect. Dis.* **4:**13–20.

Souza, M., M. S. Azevedo, K. Jung, S. Cheetham, and L. J. Saif. 2008. Pathogenesis and immune responses in gnotobiotic calves after infection with the genogroup II.4-HS66 strain of human norovirus. *J. Virol.* **82:**1777–1786.

Stuart, A. D., and T. D. Brown. 2007. Alpha2,6-linked sialic acid acts as a receptor for feline calicivirus. *J. Gen. Virol.* **88:**177–186.

Tamura, M., K. Natori, M. Kobayashi, T. Miyamura, and N. Takeda. 2000. Interaction of recombinant Norwalk virus particles with the 105-kilodalton cellular binding protein, a candidate receptor molecule for virus attachment. *J. Virol.* **74:**11589–11597.

Tamura, M., K. Natori, M. Kobayashi, T. Miyamura, and N. Takeda. 2004. Genogroup II noroviruses efficiently bind to heparan sulfate proteoglycan associated with the cellular membrane. *J. Virol.* **78:**3817–3826.

Tan, M., P. Huang, J. Meller, W. Zhong, T. Farkas, and X. Jiang. 2003. Mutations within the P2 domain of norovirus capsid affect binding to human histo-blood group antigens: evidence for a binding pocket. *J. Virol.* **77:**12562–12571.

Tan, M., and X. Jiang. 2005. Norovirus and its histo-blood group antigen receptors: an answer to a historical puzzle. *Trends Microbiol.* **13:**285–293.

Tan, M., and X. Jiang. 2007. Norovirus-host interaction: implications for disease control and prevention. *Expert Rev. Mol. Med.* **9:**1–22.

Tan, M., M. Jin, H. Xie, Z. Duan, X. Jiang, and Z. Fang. 2008. Outbreak studies of a GII-3 and a GII-4 norovirus revealed an association between HBGA phenotypes and viral infection. *J. Med. Virol.* **80:**1296–1301.

Tan, M., J. Meller, and X. Jiang. 2006. C-terminal arginine cluster is essential for receptor binding of norovirus capsid protein. *J. Virol.* **80:**7322–7331.

Taube, S., A. Kurth, and E. Schreier. 2005. Generation of recombinant norovirus-like particles (VLP) in the human endothelial kidney cell line 293T. *Arch. Virol.* **150:**1425–1431.

Taube, S., J. W. Perry, K. Yetming, S. P. Patel, H. Auble, L. Shu, H. F. Nawar, C. H. Lee, T. D. Connell, J. A. Shayman, and C. E. Wobus. 2009. Ganglioside-linked terminal sialic acid moieties on murine macrophages function as attachment receptors for murine noroviruses. *J. Virol.* **83:**4092–4101.

Teunis, P. F., C. L. Moe, P. Liu, S. E. Miller, L. Lindesmith, R. S. Baric, J. Le Pendu, and R. L. Calderon. 2008. Norwalk virus: how infectious is it? *J. Med. Virol.* **80:**1468–1476.

Thorven, M., A. Grahn, K. O. Hedlund, H. Johansson, C. Wahlfrid, G. Larson, and L. Svensson. 2005. A homozygous nonsense mutation (428G→A) in the human secretor (FUT2) gene provides resistance to symptomatic norovirus (GGII) infections. *J. Virol.* **79:**15351–15355.

Troeger, H., C. Loddenkemper, T. Schneider, E. Schreier, H. J. Epple, M. Zeitz, M. Fromm, and J. D. Schulzke. 2009. Structural and functional changes of the duodenum in human norovirus infection. *Gut* **58:**1070–1077.

van Nimwegen, E. 2006. Epidemiology. Influenza escapes immunity along neutral networks. *Science* **314:**1884–1886.

Verhoef, L., E. Depoortere, I. Boxman, E. Duizer, Y. van Duynhoven, J. Harris, C. Johnsen, A. Kroneman, S. Le Guyader, W. Lim, L. Maunula, H. Meldal, R. Ratcliff, G. Reuter, E. Schreier, G. Siebenga, K. Vainio, C. Varela, H. Vennema, and M. Koopmans. 2008. Emergence of new norovirus variants on spring cruise ships and prediction of winter epidemics. *Emerg. Infect. Dis.* **14:**238–243.

Wang, Q. H., V. Costantini, and L. J. Saif. 2007. Porcine enteric caliciviruses: genetic and antigenic relatedness to human caliciviruses, diagnosis and epidemiology. *Vaccine* **25:**545–5466.

Ward, V. K., C. J. McCormick, I. N. Clarke, O. Salim, C. E. Wobus, L. B. Thackray, H. W. Virgin IV, and P. R. Lambden. 2007. Recovery of infectious murine norovirus using pol II-driven expression of full-length cDNA. *Proc. Natl. Acad. Sci. USA* **104:**11050–11055.

Waters, A., S. Coughlan, and W. W. Hall. 2007. Characterisation of a novel recombination event in the norovirus polymerase gene. *Virology* **363:**11–14.

Wobus, C. E., S. M. Karst, L. B. Thackray, K. O. Chang, S. V. Sosnovtsev, G. Belliot, A. Krug, J. M. Mackenzie, K. Y. Green, and H. W. Virgin. 2004. Replication of norovirus in cell culture reveals a tropism for dendritic cells and macrophages. *PLoS Biol.* **2:**e432.

Xi, J. N., D. Y. Graham, K. N. Wang, and M. K. Estes. 1990. Norwalk virus genome cloning and characterization. *Science* **250:**1580–1583.

Zheng, D. P., T. Ando, R. L. Fankhauser, R. S. Beard, R. I. Glass, and S. S. Monroe. 2006. Norovirus classification and proposed strain nomenclature. *Virology* **346:**312–323.

GENOME DIVERSITY AND EVOLUTION OF ROTAVIRUSES

Jelle Matthijnssens and Ulrich Desselberger

13

Rotaviruses (RVs) are a major cause of acute gastroenteritis (AGE) in infants and young children worldwide, and in the young of a large variety of animals (mammals and birds). RV disease is associated with over 600,000 deaths of infants and young children per annum, mainly in developing countries (Parashar et al., 2006). Since 2006, two live attenuated RV vaccines, Rotarix and RotaTeq, have been licensed in many countries around the world after they were shown to be efficacious and safe in very large phase III clinical trials (Block et al., 2007; Linhares et al., 2008; Ruiz-Palacios et al., 2006; Vesikari et al., 2006). Both vaccines are now widely applied, also in universal mass vaccination (UMV) campaigns. The World Health Organization has issued a recommendation to use these vaccines worldwide (SAGE, 2009; O'Ryan et al., 2009). However, their broad effectiveness remains to be determined during the next 2 or 3 years.

A considerable body of basic research has been devoted to RVs (for a review, see Estes and Kapikian [2007]), and efforts to explore the molecular biology of these viruses continue. One of the main characteristics of RVs is the extensive genomic and antigenic diversity, even among cocirculating strains, and the very high fluctuations in the distribution of cocirculating genotypes from region to region, from season to season, and even within a season. In this review, the basic facts of genome diversity of RVs are described and several mechanisms driving their evolution are discussed. An attempt is made to judge how the diversity of cocirculating wild-type (wt) RVs may be influenced by the ongoing vaccination programs.

GENOME, GENE PROTEIN ASSIGNMENTS, AND VIRUS PARTICLE STRUCTURE

RVs possess a genome consisting of 11 segments of double-stranded RNA (dsRNA) ranging from 3,302 bp (segment 1) to 664 bp (segment 11), yielding a total genome size of approximately 18,500 bp. All genome segments of RVs of a particular group (see below) have short but highly conserved 5′ and 3′ ends (Table 1). Full gene-protein assignments have been carried out for several strains as shown in Table 2, where the known functions of individual RV proteins

Jelle Matthijnssens, Laboratory of Clinical and Epidemiological Virology, Department of Microbiology and Immunology, Rega Institute for Medical Research, University of Leuven, Leuven, Belgium. *Ulrich Desselberger,* Department of Medicine, University of Cambridge and Addenbrooke's Hospital, Cambridge, United Kingdom.

Genome Plasticity and Infectious Diseases,
Edited by J. Hacker, U. Dobrindt, and R. Kurth,

TABLE 1 5′- and 3′-terminal nucleotide sequences of the RNAs of group A-D rotaviruses

RV group	Host species	Terminal nucleotide sequences	
		5′ end	3′ end
A	Mammalian	GGCUUUAAA... UUU	...AUAUGACC U U G
A	Avian	GGCAAUAAA... UU U	...AUAUGACC U U G
B	Mammalian	GGCANAAAA... UU UUUU	...AAAAACCC U G
C	Mammalian	GCCAAAAAA... UUUUUU	...UGUGGCU
D	Avian	GGCAUUUAA... U	...AUAUGACC U U G

are also recorded. All the genome segments are monocistronic except segment 11, which encodes two proteins.

RV particles consist of three layers (diagrammatically shown in Fig. 1). The inner layer ("core") is formed from 120 molecules of viral protein 2 (VP2) and encloses the genome and 12 molecules each of two minor proteins, VP1 (the viral RNA-dependent RNA polymerase [RdRp]) and VP3 (the multifunctional viral "capping enzyme"). The middle layer consists of 260 trimers of VP6 (arranged in icosahedral symmetry) which form the outside of double-layered particles (DLPs). The DLPs in turn are wrapped into an outer layer, consisting of 260 trimers of VP7 and 60 trimers of the spike-like structures of VP4 (Fig. 1). The triple-layered particles (TLPs) are recognized as the infectious virions. The TLP layers are interrupted by 132 channels of three different classes of symmetry and different functions. Using the procedures of X-ray crystallography, single-particle cryo-electron microscopy, and combinations thereof, the atomic structures of many RV proteins (in isolation or as part of viral particles) have been described in recent years, which has improved our understanding of protein functions (for details, see Aoki et al. [2009], Charpilienne et al. [2002], Chen et al. [2009], Estes and Kapikian [2007], Lawton et al. [1997, 1999], Lepault et al. [2001], Li et al. [2009], Lu et al. [2008], Mathieu et al. [2001], McClain et al. [2010], Pesavento et al. [2003], Prasad et al. [1996], Yoder and Dormitzer [2006], Yoder et al. [2009], and Zhang et al. [2008]).

REPLICATION

Viral replication occurs in the mature epithelial cells of the small intestine. Replication in vitro has been studied in some detail (for a review, see Estes and Kapikian [2007]). It takes place exclusively in the cytoplasm. RV TLPs attach to the host cell and enter it by receptor-mediated endocytosis or direct penetration. There are several cellular receptors for RVs, some of which have not been fully characterized, but viral uptake follows a sequence of interactions with primary and secondary receptors (Lopez and Arias, 2004). After enzymatic removal of the outer capsid of TLPs in the cytoplasm, DLPs which are transcriptionally active emerge, producing large numbers of 11 different single-stranded RNA molecules of positive polarity, which exit the DLPs via 12 aqueous "class I" channels. The new RNA molecules either act as mRNAs, with their translation products accumulating in the cytoplasm, or are replicated in intracytoplasmic inclusion bodies termed viroplasms. Two nonstructural RV proteins, NSP2 and NSP5, are major components of viroplasms which are essential for early viral morphogenesis and RNA replication. The viroplasms also contain VP1, VP2, VP3, VP6, NSP4, and, initially, mRNAs of all genomic segments, which are later replicated to dsRNAs in nascent RV particles. NSP4 was discovered as the first viral enterotoxin (Ball et al., 1996) and found to be intimately involved in the regulation of intracellular Ca^{2+} concentrations (Berkova et al., 2006). Recently, close structural and functional association of viroplasms with the cellular organelles lipid droplets (recruited during RV replication) has been described (Cheung et al., 2010). NSP5 interacts with both VP2 and VP1. The exact order of events during early morphogenesis and the control mechanisms by which packaging

TABLE 2 Gene-protein assignments and protein functions of group A RVs[a]

RNA segment		Protein product					
No.	Size (bp)[b]	Description	Deduced mol mass (kDa)	Location (oligomeric state)	No. of molecules/virion	Posttranslational modification	Functions
1	3,302–3,305	VP1	125.0	Inner core	12		RNA-dependent RNA polymerase; single-stranded-RNA binding; complex with VP3; interaction with NSP5
2	2,684–2,753	VP2	94.0	Core	120	Myristylation	RNA binding; required for replicase activity of VP1; core scaffolding protein
3	2,582–2,592	VP3	88.0	Inner core	12		Guanylyltransferase; methyltransferase; single-stranded-RNA binding; complex with VP1
4	2,349–2,368	VP4	86.8	Outer capsid (trimer)	120	Proteolytic Cleavage to VP5* and VP8*	Hemagglutinin; cell attachment protein; neutralization antigen (antibody protective); fusogenic; protease-enhanced infectivity; virulence (mice, piglets)
5	1,564–2,122	NSP1 (VP5)	58.7	Nonstructural	NA[c]		RNA binding; virulence (mice); interacting with and degrading IRF-3 and IRF-7; nonessential for replication of some strains; involved in host specificity
6	1,347–1,362	VP6	44.8	Inner capsid (trimer)	780	Myristylation	Group- and subgroup-specific antigen; antibody partially protective (by intracellular neutralization?); required for transcription
7[d]	1,064–1,105	NSP3 (VP9)	34.6	Nonstructural (dimer)	NA		RNA binding (3′ end); competing with cellular PABP for interaction with EIF4G1 (translation); inhibiting host cell translation
8[d]	1,042–1,059	NSP2 (VP8)	36.7	Nonstructural (octamer)	NA		RNA binding; NTPase; helicase; plus-strand RNA packaging; forms viroplasms with NSP5; virulence (mice)
9[d]	1,051-1,067	VP7	37.4[e]	Outer capsid (trimer)	780	Cleavage of signal sequence; glycosylation	Neutralization antigen (antibody protective); Ca^{2+} binding
10	727–753	NSP4 (VP12)	20.3	Nonstructural	NA	Glycosylation (→VP10, NS28); trimming	Intracellular receptor for DLPs; role in morphogenesis; interacting with viroplasms; modulating transcription; viral enterotoxin (secreted cleavage product); virulence (mice, piglets); interaction with cellular integrins as receptors
11	663–820	NSP5 (VP11)	21.7	Nonstructural (dimer)	NA	O glycosylation, phosphorylation	RNA binding; protein kinase; forming viroplasms with NSP2; interacting with VP1 and NSP6
		NSP6	12.0	Nonstructural	NA		Interacting with NSP5

[a]Modified from Estes and Kapikian (2007).
[b]Gene sequences with duplications were not included.
[c]NA, not applicable.
[d]This gene-protein assignment is of the SA11 rotavirus strain.
[e]Second in-frame initiation codon located 30 codons downstream (deduced molecular mass 33.9 kDa).

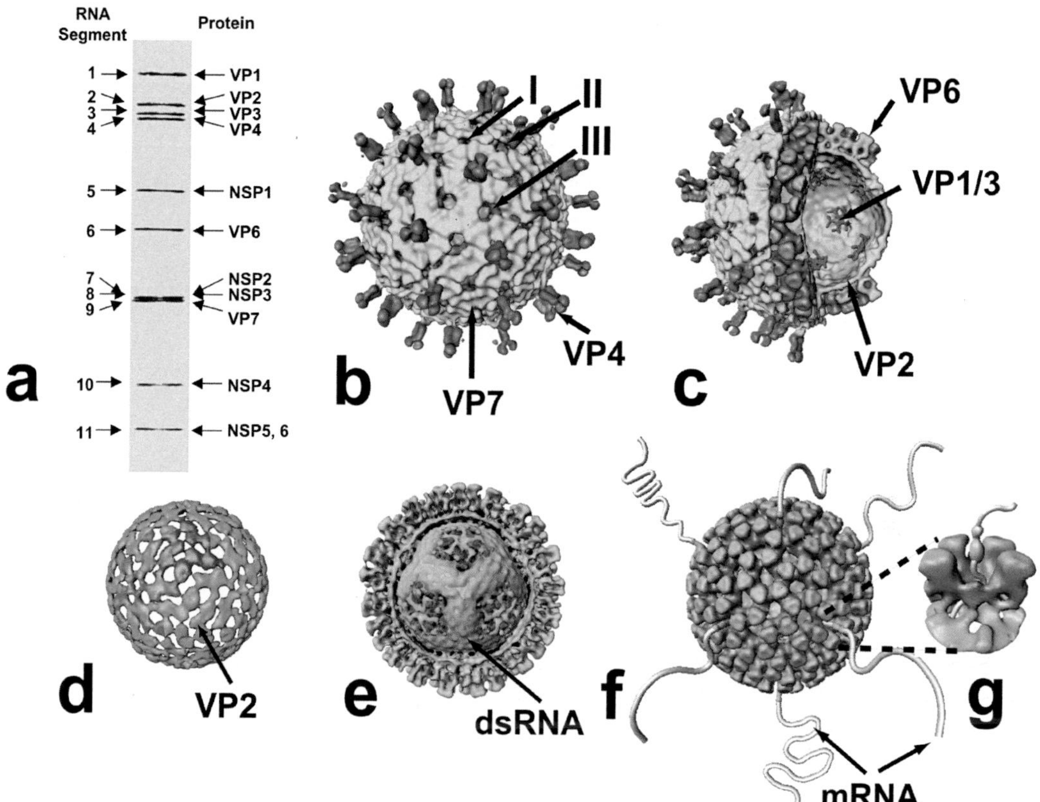

FIGURE 1 Structural organization of RVs. (a) RNA gel showing RV RNA segments and encoded products. (b) Surface representation of the RV structure: besides the VP4 spikes (red) and the VP7 outer layer (yellow), three types of channels are indicated (I, II, and III). (c) Cutaway diagram of the RV structure showing the middle VP6 (blue) and internal VP2 (green) layers. The flower-shaped VP1-VP3 complex on the inside of VP2 is shown in red. (d) Structural organization of the VP2 layer. Some of the 60 dimers forming this layer are shown in red and purple. (e) Genomic RNA in the RV structure. The VP6 and VP2 layers are half cut away to show the genomic organization. (f) Structure of the actively transcribing DLPs, with exit pathway for the single-stranded positive-sense RNAs through the class I channels at the fivefold vertex. (g) Close-up cutaway view depicting the exit pathway in one of the channels. The transcripts are shown as gray strands in panels f and g. From Pesavento et al. (2003) with kind permission from B.V.V. Prasad, Baylor College of Medicine, Houston, TX.

and reassortment of RNA segments into cores occur are at present unknown. NSP5 may have a central role in the recruitment of viroplasmic RV proteins (Contin et al., 2010). DLPs, formed in the viroplasms, contain one of each of the 11 RNA segments in the ds form. The DLPs traffic through the rough endoplasmic reticulum with NSP4 acting as an intracellular receptor for VP6. In the rough endoplasmic reticulum, VP7 and VP4 are incorporated. Triple-layer infectious virions are released by lysis of nonpolarized cells (e.g., MA104) or by budding from polarized cells (e.g., Caco-2 cells) before a cytopathic effect becomes obvious.

In cells coinfected by two different RV strains, the two genomes are transcribed in parallel and RNA segments from both parents are packaged (reassorted) into progeny virus particles. As the viral genome consists of 11 RNA segments, theoretically $2^{11} - 2$, or 2,046, different reassortants could emerge. However, reassortment appears to be highly nonrandom, and the relative frequencies of individual reassortants depend on the cell line in which reassortment has taken place (Graham et al., 1987) and probably also on the replication kinetics of coinfecting parental strains.

REVERSE GENETICS

Rescue of point mutations (engineered into a cDNA) into viable RNA viruses requires a reverse-genetics system. For RVs, this has been established for RNA segment 4 (encoding VP4), which can be rescued into a helper virus under strong immune selection pressure against the VP4 of the helper virus (Komoto et al., 2006, 2008). A modification of the system using rearranged gene segments has been described which does not require the use of selection by antibody, as rearranged genome segments appear to have a packaging advantage (Troupin et al., 2010). A dual-selection system using RV temperature-sensitive mutants and segment-specific small interfering RNAs has succeeded in obtaining RV monoreassortants by reverse-genetics manipulation of a nonstructural protein gene (Trask et al., 2010). However, a plasmid-only system like that developed for *Orthoreovirus* (Kobayashi et al., 2007) and *Orbivirus* (Boyce et al., 2008; Boyce and Roy, 2007; Matsuo et al., 2010) regrettably does not yet exist for RVs.

CLASSIFICATION

RVs are subdivided into different groups based on differences in antigenic properties of VP6, of which groups A through E are well distinguished. Groups F and G have been assigned to RVs of bird origin and are much less well characterized. Within group A RVs, several subgroups (I, II, I+II, and non-I, non-II) were characterized by the reactivity of various isolates with two VP6-specific monoclonal antibodies, 631/9 and 255/60 (Greenberg et al., 1983). More recently, molecular techniques (in particular, reverse transcription [RT]-PCR)have been used to define RV subgroups genomically (Iturriza-Gómara et al., 2002a, 2002b).

RNA-RNA hybridization of different RV genomes has been applied in the past in an attempt to classify RVs and to define reassortment events (Nakagomi and Nakagomi, 1991; Nakagomi et al., 1989; Ward et al., 1990). The procedure has been used to define genogroups. For human RV strains, three genogroups have been differentiated, represented by the reference strains Wa, DS-1, and AU-1 (Nakagomi et al., 1989; Nakagomi and Nakagomi, 1989). However, this method has been completely superseded by whole-genome sequencing (see below), which has revealed much more complex evolutionary events. The concept of genogroups has not been formally recognized as a classification category.

Serologic reactivity and the composition of genes encoding both outer layer proteins (VP7 and VP4) have been extensively used to differentiate RV types, either by cross-reactivity with type-specific monoclonal antibodies or monospecific polyclonal antibodies (serotype) or by phylogenetic analysis of gene sequences (genotype). VP7 is the determinant of G types (VP7 is a glycosylated protein), and VP4 is the determinant of P types (VP4 is cleaved by trypsin-like enzymes, i.e., is protease sensitive). For most G types, the serotype designation and the genotype designation are identical. P types are identified mainly as genotypes, due to a scarcity of type-specific antisera. Thus, P serotypes are designated by Arabic numbers and genotypes are designated by Arabic numbers in square brackets. Accordingly, the human Wa strain is classified as G1P1A[8], the human DS-1 strain as G2P1B[4], the ovine strain Lp14 as G10P[15], etc. (Estes and Kapikian, 2007).

As VP4 and VP7 are encoded by different RNA segments (segment 4 and 7, 8, or 9 [depending on the strain], respectively), various G-P combinations can occur as the consequence of ancient or recent reassortment events. Logically, the other nine RNA segments are also involved in reassortment events, and, indeed, reassortments of various genes (besides those encoding VP7 and VP4) have been discovered in cocirculating human RV strains (Maunula and Von Bonsdorff, 2002; Rahman et al., 2007b). These findings have recently led to a comprehensive classification system encompassing all 11 RNA segments (Matthijnssens et al., 2008a), in which different numbers of genotypes of every genome segment are distinguished after appropriate cut-off points had been identified (Table 3, which was constructed after over 3,000 segmental nucleotide sequences had been compared). Cutoff values are based on amino acid percent identities between RVs of different serotypes and on typical peaks of pairwise identity frequency diagrams based on nucleotide sequences (Matthijnssens et al., 2008a). RV strains are designated according to the formula VP7(G)-VP4(P)-VP6(I)-VP1(R)-VP2(C)-VP3(M)-NSP1(A)-NSP2(N)-NSP3(T)-NSP4(E)-NSP5(H); e.g., for the human RV strain Wa, the designation is G1-P1A[8]-I1-R1-C1-M1-A1-N2-T1-E1-H1. This system has been very productive in deducing the evolution of RVs (see below). In 2008, a Rotavirus Classification Working Group (RCWG) was established to support the identification of novel genotypes for all genes and avoid duplications and possible errors (Matthijnssens et al., 2008b). Between 2008 and October 2010, over 40 new genotypes for different genes were identified, and it is likely that more will be discovered in the years to come as full genome sequencing is increasingly applied to RVs. To facilitate RV classification further, an online genotyping tool, RotaC, has recently been developed (http://rotac.regatools.be). This tool is updated regularly for new genotypes of any of the 11 RNA segments (Maes et al., 2009). Up till now (October 2010), 25 G types and 34 P types of RVs have been discovered, and the search is ongoing (Abe et al., 2009; Collins et al., 2010; Esona et al., 2010a; Matthijnssens et al., 2008a; Solberg et al., 2009; Trojnar et al., 2009; Ursu et al., 2009; unpublished data on a bovine RV carrying G24P[33]). Of those, 12 G types and 12 P types have so far been found in human RV isolates.

EPIDEMIOLOGY OF RVS

RVs spread mainly via the fecal-oral route. Water, vomitus, and food may act as vehicles, but person-to-person spread is most prominent. RV particles are very resistant to environmental conditions in temperate climates. The large

TABLE 3 Nucleotide percentage similarity cutoff values defining genotypes of the 11 RV genome segments

Gene product	% Similarity cutoff value[a]	No.[b]	Genotype designation (derivation)	No. of sequences evaluated[b]
VP7	80	25 G	Glycosylated protein	>1,100
VP4	80	34 P	Protease-sensitive protein	>310
VP6	85	16 I	Inner capsid protein (middle layer)	>330
VP1	83	8 R	RNA-dependent RNA polymerase	>90
VP2	84	8 C	Core protein	>90
VP3	81	8 M	Methyltransferase (capping enzyme)	>90
NSP1	79	16 A	Antagonist of interferon	>130
NSP2	85	8 N	NTPase	>100
NSP3	85	11 T	Translation enhancer protein	>120
NSP4	85	13 E	Enterotoxin	>530
NSP5[c]	91	10 H	Phosphoprotein	>150

[a]Updated from Matthijnssens et al. (2008a).
[b]As of October 2010.
[c] NSP6, which is also encoded by RNA 11, has not been included as not all RV strains have an ORF for NSP6 and as it is not essential for replication.

number of particles in the feces of children with acute RV disease (up to 10^{11} particles/ml of feces) and the very low 50% diarrhea-causing dose (1 DD_{50} = 10 PFU [Ward et al., 1986]) lead to wide and efficient spread to any susceptible host. Prominent seasonal peaks (winter and spring) of RV outbreaks are observed in countries with temperate climates, while in tropical regions RV infections and disease occur throughout the year (Bishop, 1996; Brandt et al., 1983; Desselberger et al., 2001). Most human infections are caused by group A RVs.

The epidemiology of group A RV infections is complex, since RVs of different G types cocirculate within a geographical region at any one time and change very rapidly over time (from one season to the next or even within a season) in the same location (Desselberger et al., 2001; Gentsch et al., 1996; Iturriza-Gómara et al., 2004a; Rahman et al., 2005b; Ramachandran et al., 1998; Santos and Hoshino, 2005). In most regions with a temperate climate, over 90% of cocirculating strains are types G1 to G4 and G9, typically G1P1A[8], G2P1B[4], G3P1A[8], G4P1A[8], and G9P1A[8] (Santos and Hoshino, 2005), although G12P1A[8] RVs are also increasingly being detected worldwide (Iturriza-Gómara et al., 2011; Matthijnssens et al., 2008c, 2009a; Rahman et al., 2007b). It is currently unknown where the G12 genotype emerged and where it originated, as only one report described a porcine G12P[7] RV strain isolated in India, and its G12 gene was found to cluster in a different lineage from the G12 genes of the human RV isolates (Ghosh et al., 2006). Other genotypes may be prevalent at high frequencies in tropical countries: G5P[8] in Brazil (Araujo et al., 2007; Gouvea et al., 1994), G10P[11] in India (Iturriza-Gómara et al., 2004b), and G8P[4] and G8P[6] in Malawi (Cunliffe et al., 2000) and diverse countries in Africa (Armah et al., 2010; Mwenda et al., 2010; Page et al., 2010). Detailed reviews of the occurrence of unusual G-genotype RVs in humans have recently been published (Esona et al., 2010b; Matthijnssens et al., 2008c). Increasingly, RV infections are recognized as the cause of a significant proportion of nosocomial infections and diarrheal disease (Gleizes et al., 2006). Group B RVs have caused outbreaks of diarrhea in children and adults in China (Tao, 1988) and have been isolated from sporadic cases of AGE in Calcutta, India (Kobayashi et al., 2001; Krishnan et al., 1999), and Bangladesh (Rahman et al., 2007a; Sanekata et al., 2003). Kuga et al. (2009) recorded a significant genomic diversity of the VP7 genes of human, bovine, murine, and mainly porcine group B RVs, leading to the differentiation of at least five different G types when cutoff values similar to those of group A RVs (Matthijnssens et al., 2008a) were applied. An additional novel VP4 genotype of a bovine group B RV was recently identified (Ghosh et al., 2010). Full-genome sequencing of four human group B RVs revealed a very high level of genetic conservation. However, a high degree of overall genetic diversity was observed between group B RV from different host species, which may require a classification of genotypes of all 11 segments in the future (Yamamoto et al., 2010). Group C RVs are associated with small outbreaks of AGE in humans, sometimes in families (Caul et al., 1990; Jiang et al., 1995; Rahman et al., 2005a). In contrast to group A RVs, and similar to group B RVs, full-genome sequencing of group C RVs from different countries in southeast Asia revealed that they most likely belong to a single genotype cluster except for the VP3 gene (Yamamoto et al., 2011). Group D and E RVs were isolated from pheasants and pigs, respectively, but remain relatively poorly characterized (Devitt and Reynolds, 1993; Haynes et al., 1994; Pedley et al., 1986). The single full-genome sequence of a group D RV (strain 05V0049), isolated from a diseased chicken, showed conserved, group A-like termini of the genome segments but a very low overall degree of amino acid identity of encoded proteins to their cogent counterparts of group A, B, or C RVs (Trojnar et al., 2010). An exception was the relatively close relationships between the NSP1 gene of group D RV strain 05V0049 and avian group A RV NSP1 genes (Trojnar et al., 2010). This observation leads to the provocative idea that in a distant past a reassortment event might have happened between avian group A and group D RVs, resulting in a group A RV with an NSP1 gene segment of group D RV origin, or vice versa.

GENETIC MECHANISMS OF RV EVOLUTION

For the evolution of human RVs, the following genetic mechanisms have been found to be operative (Iturriza-Gómara et al., 2003):

1. accumulation of point mutations
2. genome reassortment
3. genome rearrangements (recombination)
4. zoonotic transmission
5. combinations of the above factors

Accumulation of Point Mutations

Due to the relatively high inborn error rate of replication by viral RdRps (Hanada et al., 2004; Jenkins et al., 2002), RNA viruses, including RVs, evolve rapidly. The error rate of the RV RdRp was found to be 5×10^{-5} in vitro, i.e., one mutation per genome per replication (Blackhall et al., 1996), but may be higher (Jenkins et al., 2002). The overall VP7 evolutionary rate (nucleotide substitutions/site/year) was recently estimated to be 1.87×10^{-3} (1.45×10^{-3} to 2.27×10^{-3}) for G9 and 1.66×10^{-3} (1.13×10^{-3} to 2.32×10^{-3}) for G12 RVs, respectively (Matthijnssens et al., 2010a). Point mutations may or may not occur sequentially and accumulate. There is evidence for this phenomenon in human RV isolates of several collections (Iturriza-Gómara et al., 2000; Martella et al., 2004; Simmonds et al., 2008). Iturriza-Gómara et al. (2000) reported failure to genotype with a P[8]-specific primer in a multiplex RT-PCR. This turned out to be due to mismatches in the primer binding region as a result of multiple nucleotide point mutations having occurred, even among strains of a geographically defined area over a short period. In Fig. 2, the mismatches between the primer 1T-1 and RV strains circulating in the United Kingdom are shown, together with the sequence of a new adapted and degenerate primer 1T-1D, which allowed typing of all previously untypeable strains as P[8]. Similar observations have been reported by others (Adah et al.,1997; Santos et al., 2003; Rahman et al., 2005c).

Genome Reassortment

Reassortment of RV genomes can be easily reproduced in vitro (Garbarg-Chenon et al., 1986) and in vivo (Gombold and Ramig, 1986) and has also been found to occur among cocirculating human wt RV strains (Iturriza-Gómara et al., 2001; Matthijnssens et al., 2006c; Maunula and Von Bonsdorff, 2002; McDonald et al., 2009; Rahman et al., 2007b), leading to a large number of different G-P combinations. The phylogenetic analyses of the VP4 and VP7 genes of two human RV strains (DRC88: G8P[8] and DRC86: G8P[6]), isolated in the Democratic Republic of Congo, are shown in Fig. 3 (Matthijnssens et al., 2006c). Complete genome analyses of these two strains had demonstrated that 10 of the 11 RNA segments were nearly identical, as is demonstrated for the VP7 genes in Fig. 3A. Only the VP4-encoding RNA segments belonged to different genotypes (P[8] and P[6] [Fig. 3B]). This is a clear example of a single-gene (mono-) reassortment between a commonly circulating G8P[6] strain with a local P[8]-carrying RV strain (Matthijnssens et al., 2006c). Reassortment events in nature depend on the frequency of RV coinfections, which is often high in tropical countries (Ahmed et al., 1991; Unicomb et al., 1999), resulting in a greater RV genome diversity. In addition, numerous reassortment events have been discovered between human and animal RV strains (see "Zoonotic Transmission" below).

Genome Rearrangements

In immunodeficient hosts and under certain experimental conditions, but also during natural evolution, RVs undergo genome rearrangements (Desselberger, 1996; Schnepf et al., 2008). These are intrasegmental recombination events leading to partial duplications of genome segments (for a review, see Desselberger [1996]). In most cases the partial duplication starts after the termination codon and reiterates sequences

Primers Con3 1T-1 1T-1D Con2

Nt 1 11 32 339 356 868 887 2359

Gene segment 4 (VP4) 5′ 3′

Consensus	(Nt 337) 5′ C C G C A C G T C A A T C C A G T A G A T A G A C A (Nt 362) 5′	
Rev. compl 1T-1D-primer	- C A **N** G T **Y** A **A** **Y** C **C** A G T A G	
Rev. compl 1T-1-primer	G C A C G T T A T C C A A G T A G	
616-96*	C C . . . . . . C G **A** T . **C** . . . . . . T A G A C A	I
202-96*	C C . . . . . . C G **A** T . **C** . . . . . C T A G A C A	I
211-96*	C C . . . A . . C . **A** T . **C** . . . . . . T A G A C A	I
117-96*	C C . . . A . . C . **A** T . **C** . . . . . . T A G A C A	I
199-96*	C C . . . A . . C . **A** T . **C** . . . . . . T A G A C A	I
564-96*	C C . . . T . . . . **A** . . **C** . . . . C . T A G A C A	I
618-96*	C C . . . T . . . . **A** . . **C** . . . . . . T A G A C A	I
591-96*	C C . . . T . . . . **A** . . **C** . . . . . . T A G A C A	I
622-96*	C C . . . T . . . . **A** . . **C** . . . . . . T A G A C A	I
630-96*	C C . . . T . . . . **A** . . **C** . . . . . . T A G A C A	I
549-96*	C C A . . . . . . G **A** T . **C** . . . . . . T A G A C A	I
626-96*	C C . . . . . . C . **A** T . **C** . . . . . . T A G A C A	II
62496*	C C . . . . . . C . **A** . . **C** . . . . . . T A G A C A	II
597-96*	C C . . . . . . C . **A** . . **C** . . . . . . T A G A C A	II
607-96*	C C . . . . . . C . **A** . . **C** . . . . . . T A G A C A	II
594-96*	C C . . . . . . C . **A** . . **C** . . . . . . T A G A C A	II
611-96*	C C . . . . **G** T . **C** . . . . . . T A G A C A	II
623-96*	C C . . . . . . C . **A** . . **C** . . . . . . T A G A C A	II
629-96*	C C . . . . . . C . **A** . . **C** . . . . . . T A G A C A	II
656-96*	C C . . . . . . C . **A** . . **C** . . . . . . T A G A C A	II
676-96*	C C . . . . . . C . **A** . . **C** . . . . . . T A G A C A	II
0.2-98*	C C . . . . . . C . **A** T . **C** . . . . . . T A G A C A	II
0.3-98*	C C . . . . . . C . **A** T . **C** . . . . . . T A G A C A	II
884-97*	C C . . . . . . C G **A** T . **C** . . . . . . T A G A C A	III
892-97*	C C . . . . . . C G **A** T . **C** . . . . . . T A G A C A	III
480-97*	C C . . . . . . C R **A** T . **C** . . . . . . T A G A C A	III
1226-97*	C C . . . T . . . . **A** . T **C** . . . . . . T A G A C A	III
1221-97*	C C . . . . . . C G **A** T . **C** . . . . . . T A G A C A	III
1207-97*	C C . . . . . . C G **A** T . **C** . . . . . . T A G A C A	III
221-97*	C C . . . . . . C G **A** T . **C** . . . . . . T A G A C A	III
429-97*	C C A . . . . . . G **A** T . **C** . . . . . . T A G A C A	III
431-97*	C C A . . . . . . G **A** T . **C** . . . . . . T A G A C A	III
873-97*	C C . . . . . . C G **A** T . **C** . . . . . . T A G A C A	III
908-97*	C C . . . . . . C G **A** T . **C** . . . . . . T A G A C A	III
U41006 P[8]Brazil	C C A . . . . **A** T . . . . T A G A C A	IV
M96825 Wa	C C . . . . **A** . . **C** . . . . . . T A G A C A	IV
U30716RVG9-vp4	C C . . . . **A** T . **C** . . . . . . T A G A C A	IV
D16353	C C . . . . **A** T . **C** . . . . . . T A G A C A	IV
USAMO15	C C . . . . **A** T . **C** . . . . . . T A G A C A	IV
USAOh11	C C . . . . A . C . **A** . . **C** . . . . . . T A G A C A	IV
M21014-KU	C C . . . . T A G A C A	IV

Abbreviations:
N: A T C or G
: C or T
R: A or G

from downstream of the initiation codon of the normal open reading frame (ORF), resulting in an unaltered translation product and a long 3′ terminal untranslated region (Fig. 4A). There is evidence that segmental rearrangement events occur at the level of plus-strand RNA synthesis (Kojima et al., 1996; Matthijnssens et al., 2006b), and several hypotheses about the molecular mechanism of their emergence have been formulated (Ballard et al., 1992; Gault et al., 2001; Gorziglia et al., 1989; Kojima et al., 1996, 2000; Matthijnssens et al., 2006b; Schnepf et al., 2008; Scott et al., 1989; Shen et al., 1994). It has been observed that several RV strains with rearranged genes may coexist with or even have a replication advantage over RV strains with standard gene segments (Patton et al., 1996; Troupin et al., 2010; Xu et al., 1996). Segment-internal recombination events may also lead to the formation of deletions and insertions (Bányai et al., 2009b; Matthijnssens et al., 2006a; Ni and Kemp, 1994; Taniguchi et al., 1996).

In addition, there are some data in the literature suggesting the occurrence of true intrasegmental (i.e., recombination between cognate genome segments of two RV strains) and intersegmental recombination (i.e., recombination between noncognate gene segments) (Cao et al., 2008; Parra et al., 2004; Phan et al., 2007; Suzuki et al., 1998). An example of an intersegmental recombination is shown in Fig. 4B (Cao et al., 2008). The mechanism of intersegmental recombination is not understood, given the compartmental structure of the RV particle. In any case, intersegmental recombination is very rare compared to genome rearrangement and reassortment events.

Zoonotic Transmission

Several animal species appear to harbor sets of RVs of preferred genotype combinations. In pigs, G5P[7] RVs are most frequently found, and to a lesser extent also G11P[7], G3P[7], and G4P[6] viruses (Matthijnssens et al., 2008c). In cattle, G6P[5], G8P[1], and G10P[11] RV strains are most prevalent (Matthijnssens et al., 2008c). Lapine RVs usually exhibit G3P[14] or G3P[22] genotype combinations (Martella et al., 2005; Matthijnssens et al., 2006a). Horses (G3P[12] and G14P[12]) (Browning and Begg, 1996) and cats and dogs (G3P[3] and G3P[9]) are also usually infected by particular RV genotypes (Tsugawa and Hoshino, 2008). The G-P genotype combinations of RVs of many other animal species remain to be explored. The existence of typical genotype combinations of RVs in different animal species has suggested the presence of host species barriers for RVs, although these appear to be far from absolute.

There is increasing evidence for zoonotic transmission of group A RVs to human hosts. This occurs either as transmission of whole viruses, as was described for RVs typically found in rabbits, cats and dogs, or ungulate species (Bányai et al., 2010; Matthijnssens et al., 2006a, 2009b; Steyer et al., 2008, 2010; Tsugawa and Hoshino, 2008), or by reassortment events in which one or several segments of animal RV genomes are incorporated into human RV strains which then circulate in the human population and may even become predominant, such as G9P[8] (G9 is thought to have a porcine origin) and G12P[6 or 8] strains worldwide, G10P[11] strains (thought to be of bovine origin) in India (Iturriza-Gómara

FIGURE 2 Point mutations in RV genes. Alignment of fragments of the VP4 gene (VP8* portion) and the reverse complementary sequence of the original primer 1T-1 and the degenerate primer 1T-1D is shown. Divisions are as follows: I, sequences from strains which were not typed by RT-PCR with the primer 1T-1; II, sequences from strains typed as P[8] with the 1T-1 primer; III, sequences from strains typed as P[8] with the new degenerate primer 1T-1D; and IV, sequences of P[8] strains obtained from GenBank or EMBL. Strains in division I could also be successfully typed as P[8] by the degenerate primer 1T-1D. Strains from the same geographical region are marked with an asterisk. Residues that match primer 1T-1 are denoted by dots. Substitutions in the P[8] primer-binding site that are conserved in all sequences are boldface. The reverse complement sequences of primers 1T-1 and 1T-1D are shown with the changes in boldface. Adapted from Iturriza-Gómara et al. (2000) with permission of the publisher.

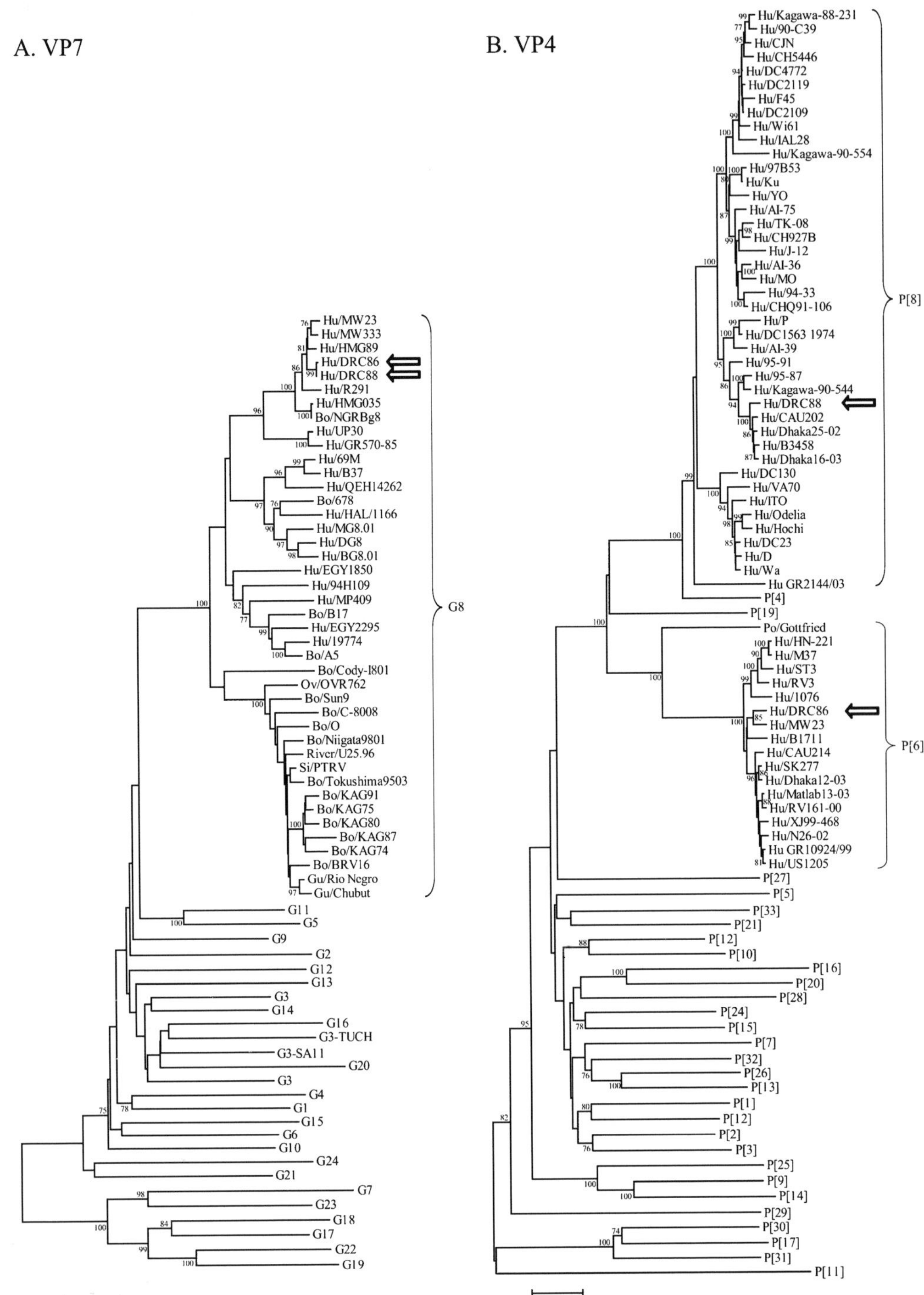

FIGURE 3 Gene reassortment of RVs. Phylogenetic analyses of the VP7 (A) and VP4 (B) gene segments of RV strains DRC88 (G8P[8]) and DRC86 (G8P[6]), isolated in the Democratic Republic of the Congo, are shown, indicating reassortment of the VP4 gene segment. RV strains DRC88 and DRC86 are indicated by arrows. Bootstrap values above 70 are shown.

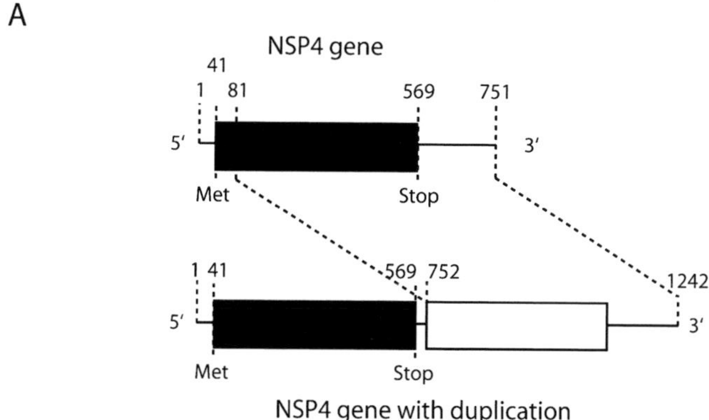

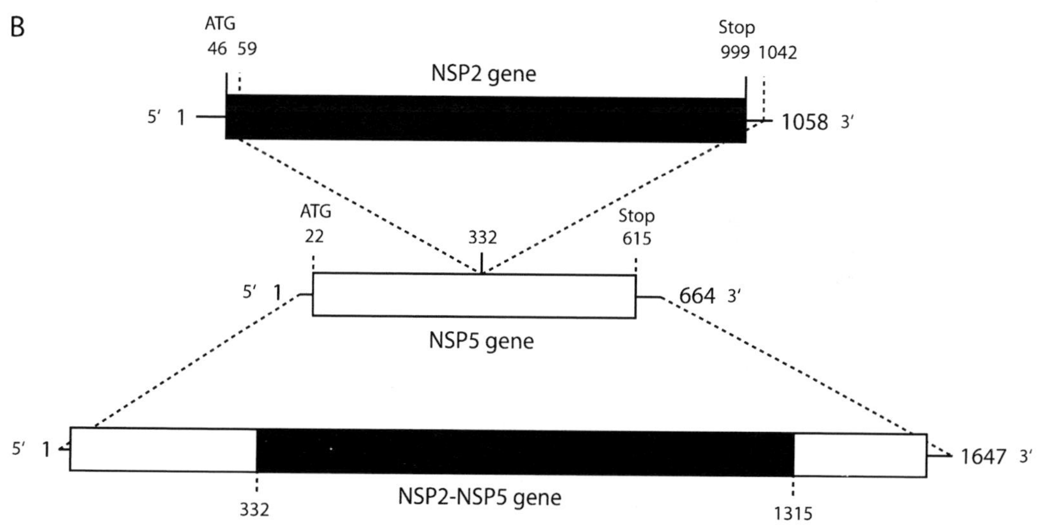

FIGURE 4 Intra- and intersegmental recombination. (A) Intrasegmental recombination (gene rearrangement). Diagram of the structures of normal and rearranged NSP4 gene of a human RV. Adapted from Ballard et al. (1992), with permission of the publisher. (B) Intersegmental recombination. Diagram of the structures of normal and recombined NSP2 and NSP5 genes of a human RV. Adapted from Cao et al. (2008) with permission of the publisher.

et al., 2004b; Matthijnssens et al., 2008c), and various others. The observation that RVs with certain gene constellations typical for animals such as rabbits, cattle, cats, and dogs appear to be mainly responsible for interspecies transmission from animals to humans may merely be a reflection of the fact that these animals (domestic, farm, or feral) live in close contact with humans rather than due to their having specific genetic features which would facilitate their transmission to humans. No specific viral properties which would render an animal RV more or less apt to successfully infect and spread in the human population have been distinguished. However, avian group A RVs have not been found to reassort with human group A RVs in vivo (further details are given below). Currently only two reports have presented evidence of interspecies transmissions among group C RVs. Chang and colleagues reported the isolation of a porcine group C RV in a coinfection with a group A RV in cattle, suggesting that a porcine group C RV had crossed the host-species barrier to a bovine host (Chang et al., 1999). More recently, Gabbay and colleagues reported the detection of nearly identical porcine group C RVs in several children in Brazil, suggesting that after an interspecies transmission of a porcine group C RV to the human host, the virus could be transmitted among humans (Gabbay et al., 2008). No interspecies transmissions for group B RV have been reported to date. The significance of zoonotic transmissions for human RV disease has recently been reviewed in detail (Martella et al., 2009; Matthijnssens et al., 2010b).

There is some evidence that the genetically diverse NSP1, the gene product of RNA segment 5, is partially associated with host specificity. The RV NSP1 protein interacts with the host interferon (IFN) response factors 3 and 7 (IRF3 and IRF7) and degrades them, thus blocking the IFN response (Barro and Patton, 2005, 2007; Graff et al., 2002, 2009). In cells unable to raise an IFN response, this effect is not seen (Feng et al., 2009). Mouse RV NSP1 exerts the IFN antagonist effect in mouse cells only, whereas the simian rhesus macaque RV (RRV) displays a host cell IFN-independent replication phenotype (Fenaux et al., 2006; Feng et al., 2008). Most RV NSP1 sequences seem to evolve with their homologous host species (Dunn et al., 1994; Matthijnssens et al., 2008a) and have therefore been considered to exert host cell-specific action. This conclusion was recently supported by showing that the 100 carboxy-terminal amino acids of NSP1 determine IRF3 degradation in a host cell-specific way (Sen et al., 2009).

NSP1 is the most variable of all RV genes (Matthijnssens et al., 2008a). Figure 5 shows the NSP1 phylogenetic tree, based on the entire ORF region, of more than 160 group A RV strains of human and various mammalian origins (Fig. 5A), together with an identity frequency graph (Fig. 5B). Pairwise comparison of the nucleotide identities among mammalian RV NSP1 gene sequences yields values as low as 47% (Fig. 5B). In comparison, for VP4 and VP7, identities reach only as low as 63% and 72%, respectively (Matthijnssens et al., 2008a). The high degree of genomic diversity of NSP1 genes of group A RVs may also be because this gene is not absolutely required for RV propagation in vitro (Taniguchi et al., 1996; Tian et al., 1993) and may therefore be subjected less to evolutionary pressure. On the other hand, RVs with defects in the NSP1 gene grow to lower infectivity titers, form smaller plaques, and suppress cellular protein synthesis less than RVs with fully functional NSP1 genes (Hundley et al., 1985; Taniguchi et al., 1996; Tian et al., 1993), suggesting support of viral growth via NSP1 by the mechanisms reviewed above (Barro and Patton, 2005; 2007; Feng et al., 2009; Graff et al., 2002, 2009). The two currently known avian NSP1 gene sequences (those of PO-13 and Ch-02V0002G3) are not included in the phylogenetic tree of Fig. 5, as their nucleotide (and deduced amino acid) sequences are too divergent to be properly aligned. As mentioned above, Trojnar et al. (2010) observed that the NSP1 gene sequences of group D avian RVs are quite closely related to those of mammalian group A RVs.

FIGURE 5 NSP1 gene diversity. (A) Phylogenetic tree of the NSP1 nucleotide sequence (entire ORF) of mammalian group A RVs. Bootstrap values (500 replicates) above 70 are shown. Designation of species of origin: Bo, bovine; Hu, human; Rh, rhesus monkey; Eq, equine; Po, porcine; Ov, ovine; La, lapine; Si, simian; Fe, feline; Ca, canine; Mu, murine; Gu, guanaco; An, antelope; Bu, buffalo. Some clusters of nearly identical human RVs in the A1 genotype were replaced by triangles and designated DC followed by the year of isolation for the sake of clarity. The closing braces on the right side of the dendrograms depict the 15 A-genotypes. Genotype A4 is found in avian group A RV isolates and is not included as being too diverse. (B) Pairwise identity frequency diagram.

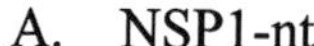
A. NSP1-nt

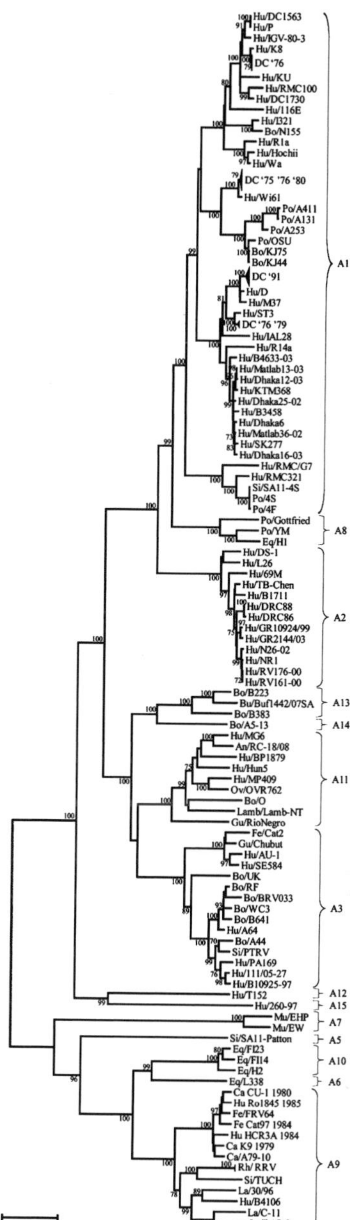
Hu/DC1563
Hu/P
Hu/IGV-80-3
Hu/K8
DC '76
Hu/KU
Hu/RMC100
Hu/DC1730
Hu/116E
Hu/I321
Bo/N155
Hu/R1a
Hu/Hochii
Hu/Wa
DC '75 '76 '80
Hu/Wi61
Po/A411
Po/A131
Po/A253
Po/OSU
Bo/KJ75
Bo/KJ44
DC '91
Hu/D
Hu/M37
Hu/ST3
DC '76 '79
Hu/IAL28
Hu/R14a
Hu/B4633-03
Hu/Matlab13-03
Hu/Dhaka12-03
Hu/KTM368
Hu/Dhaka25-02
Hu/B3458
Hu/Dhaka6
Hu/Matlab36-02
Hu/SK277
Hu/Dhaka16-03
Hu/RMC/G7
Hu/RMC321
Si/SA11-4S
Po/4S
Po/4F
A1
Po/Gottfried
Po/YM
Eq/H1
A8
Hu/DS-1
Hu/L26
Hu/69M
Hu/TB-Chen
Hu/B1711
Hu/DRC88
Hu/DRC86
Hu/GR10924/99
Hu/GR2144/03
Hu/N26-02
Hu/NR1
Hu/RV176-00
Hu/RV161-00
A2
Bo/B223
Bu/Buf1442/07SA
Bo/B383
A13
Bo/A5-13
A14
Hu/MG6
An/RC-18/08
Hu/BP1879
Hu/Hun5
Hu/MP409
Ov/OVR762
Bo/O
Lamb/Lamb-NT
Gu/RioNegro
A11
Fe/Cat2
Gu/Chubut
Hu/AU-1
Hu/SE584
Bo/UK
Bo/RF
Bo/BRV033
Bo/WC3
Bo/B641
Hu/A64
Bo/A44
Si/PTRV
Hu/PA169
Hu/111/05-27
Hu/B10925-97
A3
Hu/T152
A12
Hu/260-97
A15
Mu/EHP
Mu/EW
A7
Si/SA11-Patton
A5
Eq/FI23
Eq/FI14
Eq/H2
A10
Eq/L338
A6
Ca CU-1 1980
Hu Ro1845 1985
Fe/FRV64
Fe Cat97 1984
Hu HCR3A 1984
Ca K9 1979
Ca/A79-10
Rh/RRV
Si/TUCH
La/30/96
Hu/B4106
La/C-11
La/BAP-2
La/Alabama
A9
0.1 nt subst./nt

B.

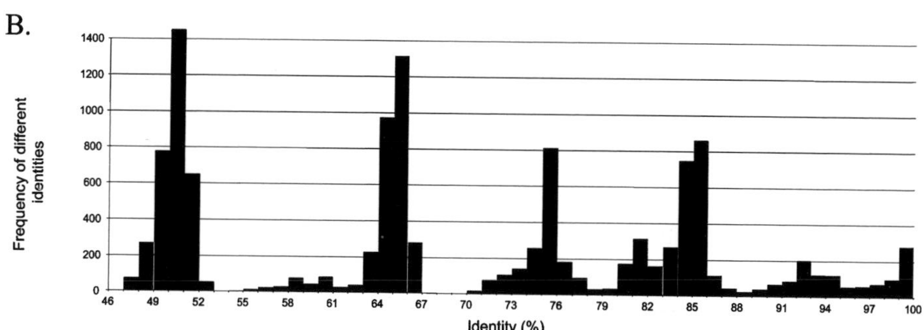
Frequency of different identities
1400
1200
1000
800
600
400
200
0
46
49
52
55
58
61
64
67
70
73
76
79
82
85
88
91
94
97
100
Identity (%)

Combination of Genetic Mechanisms

Genome rearrangements have been found in combination with point mutations (Shen et al., 1994), and reassortment is frequently combined with zoonotic transmission (Martella et al., 2006, 2009; Matthijnssens et al., 2008c, 2008d; Steyer et al., 2008). The different G-P combinations encountered in human and animal RVs are shown in Fig. 6, where it is indicated whether strains are usually found in humans or animals, are likely to be reassortants among cocirculating human RV strains or reassortants between human and animal RV strains, or are transmitted from animals to humans as the whole virus. Currently, 122 different G-P combinations are recognized in RVs isolated from humans and animals. This staggering number of different G-P genotype combinations does not represent anywhere near the entire picture, as G and P analyses are based on the composition of only 2 of the 11 genome segments. As all 11 RNA segments are able to reassort, the true genetic diversity of group A RVs is probably much higher. Whole-genome sequencing of more human and animal RV strains will without a doubt reveal a much greater genetic diversity of RVs, generated through interspecies transmission and reassortment events. The conditions of genome diversity of RVs are very reminiscent of those of influenza viruses (Webby et al., 2007).

Forces Driving RV Evolution

Several different mechanisms are exploited by RVs to generate genetic diversity. Mutations are the result of continuously occurring, more or less random mistakes by the error-prone polymerase (Hanada et al., 2004; Jenkins et al., 2002), resulting in a quasispecies, a swarm of closely related yet genetically different viruses (Martin and Domingo, 2008; Potgieter et al., 2009). Reassortment events are the result of the incorporation of gene segments from more than one parental RV strain into newly formed viral progeny particles, and interspecies transmissions are the result of the accidental transmission of an RV from one species to another. In addition, RV evolution is driven by a number of environmental factors, mainly host specific, which influence the success of viruses carrying any of these changes over the parental RV strain. Age of the host, immunodeficiencies of the host, and host immune responses, both humoral and innate, are all involved in the selection of new RV variants. This can occur at many levels such as virus attachment or entry and multiple subsequent steps of the viral replication cycle, including interaction with the host cell machinery and interference with host innate immunity (NSP1) (Barro and Patton, 2005, 2007; Desselberger, 1996; Estes and Kapikian, 2007; Feng et al., 2009; Graff et al., 2002, 2009; Martin and Domingo, 2008). While experimentally all these factors have been shown to play a role, it is difficult to disentangle their relative contributions in the in vivo epidemiological situation (Desselberger et al., 2001). HLA alleles do not seem to play a role in susceptibility to RV infection.

FURTHER UNDERSTANDING OF RV EVOLUTION ENABLED BY WHOLE-GENOME SEQUENCING

Whole-genome sequencing, resulting in the assignment of genotypes to all 11 individual RV RNA segments, has allowed further insights into RV evolution. Thus it was shown that human RV strains belonging to the Wa-like genogroup (G1P[8], G3P[8], G4P[8], and G9P[8]) share most, if not all, of their genotypes with porcine RV strains, R1-C1-M1-A1-N1-T1-E1-H1, corresponding to VP1 to VP3 and NSP1 to

FIGURE 6 G-P genotype combinations of group A RVs. A summary of the different G-P genotype combinations for the 25 G and 34 P genotypes (as of October 2010) is shown. Different color codes are used to differentiate the origin of RVs of a particular G-P combination. * indicates that only the partial VP4 gene sequence of the new G22 strains have been determined, and this sequence was considered to be distantly related to P[17] strains. ** indicates that the P genotype of the new G23 strain has not yet been determined. To the right of every row and under every column, the number of different combinations found is indicated.

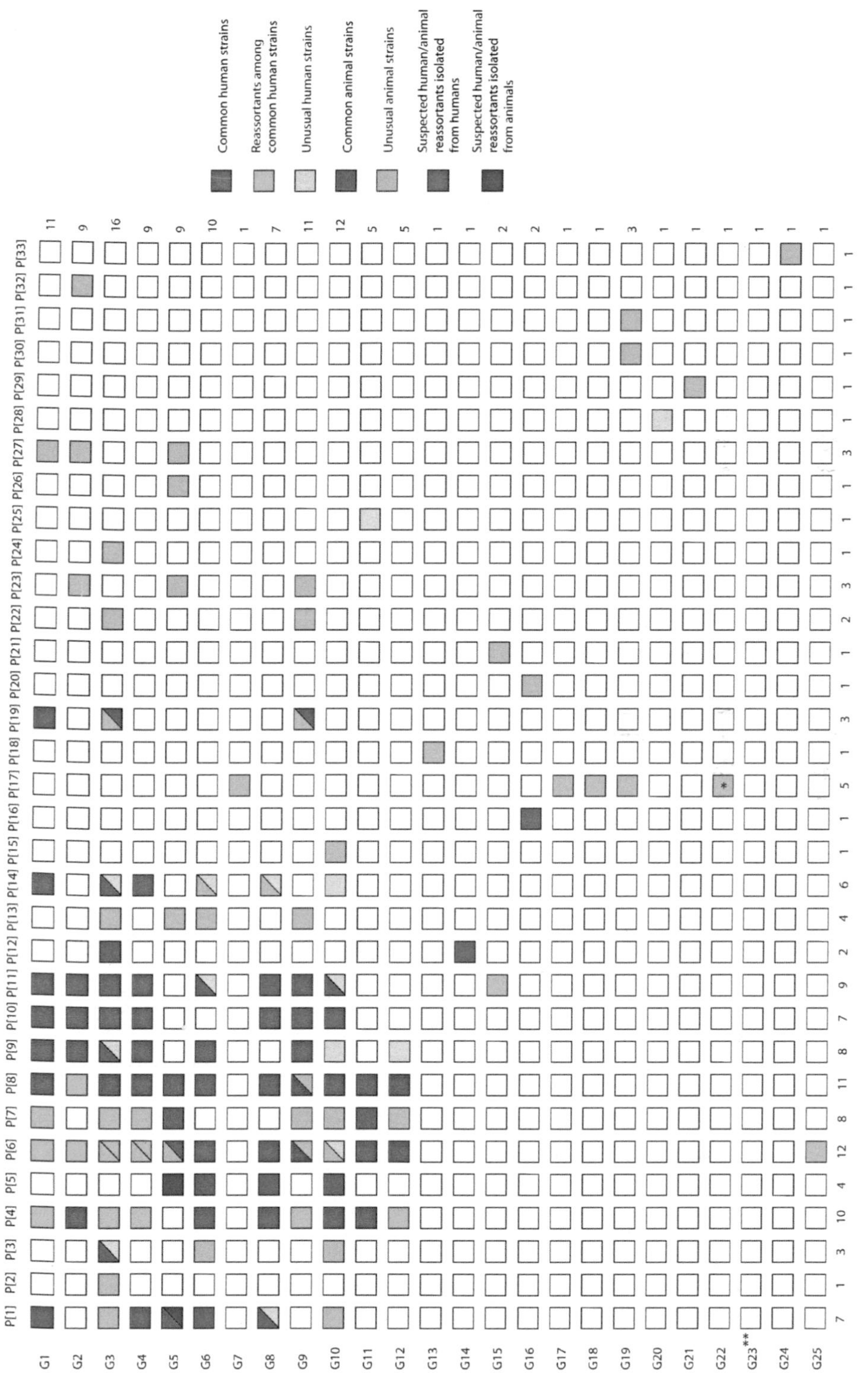

Common human strains

Reassortants among common human strains

Unusual human strains

Common animal strains

Unusual animal strains

Suspected human/animal reassortants isolated from humans

Suspected human/animal reassortants isolated from animals

	G1	G2	G3	G4	G5	G6	G7	G8	G9	G10	G11	G12	G13	G14	G15	G16	G17	G18	G19	G20	G21	G22	G23**	G24	G25
Total	11	9	16	9	9	10	1	7	11	12	5	5	1	1	2	2	1	1	3	1	1	1	1	1	1

	P[1]	P[2]	P[3]	P[4]	P[5]	P[6]	P[7]	P[8]	P[9]	P[10]	P[11]	P[12]	P[13]	P[14]	P[15]	P[16]	P[17]	P[18]	P[19]	P[20]	P[21]	P[22]	P[23]	P[24]	P[25]	P[26]	P[27]	P[28]	P[29]	P[30]	P[31]	P[32]	P[33]
Total	7	1	3	10	4	12	8	11	8	7	9	2	4	6	1	1	5	1	3	1	1	2	3	1	1	1	3	1	1	1	1	1	1

NSP5 genotypes (Fig. 7). Furthermore, human RV isolates related to the DS-1 strain share the majority of their genotypes, namely VP6, VP1, VP2, VP3, NSP2, and NSP4 (I2-R2-C2-M2-N2-E2), with those of bovine RV strains (Fig. 7), suggesting a common origin of human DS-1-like RV strains and bovine RVs although a few gene segments are likely to have been replaced by reassortment. In addition, it was shown that a number of unusual human RVs carrying the P[14] genotype might be the result of a number of individual interspecies transmissions from mammals belonging to the order Artiodactyla to humans (Bányai et al., 2009a; Banyai et al., 2010; Matthijnssens et al., 2009b; Steyer et al., 2010). A recent study of the complete genomes of nonhuman primate RVs (RRV) suggests a common origin of RRV and RVs isolated from cats or dogs, although again a few reassortments are likely to have taken place (Matthijnssens et al., 2009c). In yet another recent study, a number of unusual human G11 RV isolates (possibly of porcine origin) were investigated by whole-genome analyses. The data suggested that multiple reassortment events of G11 RV strains with cocirculating Wa-like human RVs had led to a G11P[8] RV with (except for G11) an entire human Wa-like genome backbone (Matthijnssens et al., 2010c). It is hypothesized that the mechanism of multiple reassortments of animal and human RVs is responsible for the successful emergence and spread of G9 and G12 genotypes in RVs with a human Wa-like genetic background (Matthijnssens et al., 2008c). Taken together, these observations have shown that genome diversity is not restricted to human RVs but is present as a continuum in RVs of many mammalian host species.

Whole-genome sequencing will also allow the study of gene linkage in reassortment events (Graham et al., 1987) in a much more comprehensive way than was previously possible.

GROUP A RVs

Birds are infected with RVs of groups A and D through G. So far, no human infections with an avian RV have been observed. However, one report described the isolation of an avian-like RV from a 3-day-old calf in Germany (Brussow et al., 1992). In addition, the terminal sequences of the RNA segments of avian group A RVs are very similar to those of mammalian group A RVs (Table 1), and in vitro reassortment between a mammalian and an avian group A RV has been achieved (Kool et al., 1992). Avian group A RVs have also been propagated in experimentally infected mice (Mori et al., 2001). The first complete genome analyses of an avian (pigeon) RV, strain PO-13 (G18P[17]), showed a high degree of genetic diversity between mammalian and avian group A RVs (Ito et al., 2001). The recent complete genome analysis of a second avian (chicken) group A RV, strain 02V0002G3 (G19P[30]), has confirmed that this virus is also very different from those infecting mammals, leading to the identification of novel genotypes for 8 of the 11 RNA segments (Trojnar et al., 2009) and suggesting that a putative common ancestor of avian and mammalian RVs may have existed a long time ago. Avian RVs were observed to reassort among themselves in nature very much as mammalian RVs do and also to be transmitted among avian species (Schumann et al., 2009). Natural reassortment of avian and mammalian group A RVs has not been observed, but the possibility should not be discarded outright, as the current detection methods for RVs in humans (and other mammals) may not contain the correct tools to pick up avian-mammalian interspecies transmissions.

FIGURE 7 Application of whole-genome analysis to the structural and nonstructural protein-encoding genes for known human, bovine, porcine, and avian group A RV strains. Green and red indicate Wa-like and DS-1-like gene segments, respectively. Yellow, blue, and purple represent the avian PO-13-like RV gene segments, some typical porcine VP4, VP7, and VP6 genotypes, and some typical bovine VP4 and VP7 genotypes, respectively. Updated from Matthijnssens et al., 2008a.

		VP7	VP4	VP6	VP1	VP2	VP3	NSP1	NSP2	NSP3	NSP4	NSP5
Wa	Human	G1	P[8]	I1	R1	C1	M1	A1	N1	T1	E1	H1
D	Human	G1	P[8]	I1	R1	C1	M1	A1	N1	T1	E1	H1
KU	Human	G1	P[8]	I1	R1	C1	M1	A1	N1	T1	E1	H1
Dhaka16-03	Human	G1	P[8]	I1	R1	C1	M1	*A1*	*N1*	*T1*	E1	*H1*
US6668	Human	G1	*P[8]*	I1	*R1*	*C1*	*M1*	A1	N1	T1	E1	H1
P	Human	G3	P[8]	I1	R1	C1	M1	A1	N1	T1	E1	H1
ST3	Human	G4	P[6]	I1	R1	C1	M1	A1	N1	T1	E1	H1
IAL28	Human	G5	P[8]	I1	R1	C1	M1	A1	N1	T1	E1	H1
6782/2000/ARN	Human	*G8*	*P[6]*	*I1*	*R1*	*C1*	*M1*	*A1*	*N1*	*T1*	*E1*	*H1*
6809/2000/ARN	Human	*G8*	*P[6]*	*I2*	*R1*	*C1*	*M1*	*A1*	*N1*	*T1*	*E1*	*H1*
6787/2000/ARN	Human	*G8*	*P[8]*	*I1*	*R1*	*C1*	*M1*	*A1*	*N1*	*T1*	*E1*	*H1*
6810/2000/ARN	Human	*G8*	*P[8]*	*I2*	*R1*	*C1*	*M1*	*A1*	*N1*	*T1*	*E1*	*H1*
6862/2000/ARN	Human	*G8*	*P[8]*	*I1*	*R1*	*C1*	*M1*	*A1*	*N1*	*T1*	*E1*	*H1*
WI61	Human	G9	P[8]	I1	R1	C1	M1	A1	N1	T1	E1	H1
B3458	Human	G9	P[8]	I1	R1	C1	M1	A1	N1	T1	E1	H1
116E	Human	G9	P[11]	I1	R1	C1	M1	A1	N1	T1	E1	H1
Dhaka6	Human	G11	P[25]	I1	R1	C1	M1	A1	N1	T1	E1	H1
KTM368	Human	G11	P[25]	I12	R1	C1	M1	A1	N1	T1	E1	H1
Dhaka12-03	Human	G12	P[6]	I1	R1	C1	M1	A1	N1	T1	E1	H1
Matlab13-03	Human	G12	P[6]	I1	R1	C1	M1	A1	N1	T2	E1	H1
B4633-03	Human	G12	P[8]	I1	R1	C1	M1	A1	N1	T1	E1	H1
DS-1	Human	G2	P[4]	I2	R2	C2	M2	A2	N2	T2	E2	H2
TB-Chen	Human	G2	P[4]	I2	R2	C2	M2	A2	N2	T2	E2	H2
06-030	Human	G2	P[4]	I2	R2	C2	M2	A2	N2	T2	E2	H2
06-152	Human	G2	P[4]	I2	R2	C2	M2	A2	N1	T2	E2	H2
06-242	Human	G2	P[6]	I2	R2	C2	M2	A2	N2	T2	E2	H2
B1711	Human	G6	P[6]	I2	R2	C2	M2	A2	N2	T2	E2	H2
DRC88	Human	G8	P[8]	I2	R2	C2	M2	A2	N2	T2	E2	H2
DRC86	Human	G8	P[6]	I2	R2	C2	M2	A2	N2	T2	E2	H2
69M	Human	G8	P[10]	I2	R2	C2	M2	A2	N2	T2	E2	H2
10924/99	Human	G9	P[6]	I2	R2	C2	M2	A2	N2	T2	E2	H2
N26-02	Human	G12	P[6]	I2	R2	C2	M2	A2	N1	T2	E6	H2
RV161-00	Human	G12	P[6]	I2	R2	C2	M2	A2	N2	T2	E1	H2
RV176-00	Human	G12	P[6]	I2	R2	C2	M2	A2	N2	T2	E6	H2
A131	Porcine	G3	P[7]	I5	R1	C2	M1	A1	N1	T1	E1	H1
Gottfried	Porcine	G4	P[6]	I1	R1	C1	M1	A8	N1	T1	E1	H1
OSU	Porcine	G5	P[7]	I5	R1	C1	M1	A1	N1	T1	E1	H1
A253	Porcine	G11	P[7]	I5	R1	C2	M1	A1	N1	T1	E1	H1
YM	Porcine	G11	P[7]	I5	R1	C1	M1	A8	N1	T1	E1	H1
RF	Bovine	G6	P[1]	I2	R2	C2	M2	A3	N2	T6	E2	H3
BRV033	Bovine	G6	P[1]	I2	R2	C2	M2	A3	N2	T6	E2	H3
WC3	Bovine	G6	P[5]	I2	R2	C2	M2	A3	N2	T6	E2	H3
Uk(tc)	Bovine	G6	P[5]	I2	R2	C2	M2	A3	N2	T7	E2	H3
PO-13	Pigeon	G18	P[17]	I4	R4	C4	M4	A4	N4	T4	E4	H4

NON-GROUP A RVs

Group B RVs seem to evolve at a much lower rate than group A RVs (Nagashima et al., 2008; Yang et al., 2004b). However, this statement must be seen in light of the fact that much less sequencing work has been carried out on these viruses compared to group A RVs. Group C RVs are also relatively closely related to one another (Mitui et al., 2009; Yamamoto et al., 2011). Recently, several novel, non-group-A to -C RVs (strains J19 and B219) have been isolated in China which phylogenetically are closer to group B than to groups A and C RVs but are distant enough to justify classification in a new group (Jiang et al., 2008; Nagashima et al., 2008; Yang et al., 2004a). The genetic diversity and evolution of group A through C and NADRV viruses have recently been reviewed (Matthijnssens et al., 2010b).

RV VACCINATION AND GENOTYPE DISTRIBUTION OF WILD-TYPE RVs

Since 2006, two RV vaccines have been licensed in various countries, and millions of doses have been distributed in universal mass vaccination (UMV) programs (Angel et al., 2007; Vesikari, 2008). The first positive effects on a population basis were noted in the United States (Centers for Disease Control and Prevention, 2008; Tate et al., 2009), with the annual peak of the RV epidemic being delayed and flattened out. Also in the United States, multiple individual hospitals reported marked reductions in the number of RV-associated AGE cases (Clark et al., 2009; Matthijnssens et al., 2009a). RV vaccination was introduced in Australia on 1 July 2007. The schedule is universally funded by the federal government, but the individual states are responsible for implementation. Some of the states use Rotarix (G1P[8]; monovalent), while others use RotaTeq (G1-G4, P[8]; pentavalent). There was a reduction of severe RV-associated AGE of approximately 70% in all states. However, postvaccination differences in the prevalence of wt RV strains were observed: G2 and G9 strains were found more frequently in states using Rotarix, and G3 strains were found more frequently in states using RotaTeq (Kirkwood et al., 2009). The conclusion that the differences were more likely due to natural annual fluctuations than to lack of protection is probably correct.

In Brazil, where Rotarix has been in use since 2006, a high prevalence of wt G2P[4] RV strains was observed in 2007 and 2008, and it was speculated that this finding may be associated with Rotarix vaccination (Carvalho-Costa et al., 2009; Leite et al., 2008). However, it is too early to make a valid judgment as similar elevated levels of circulating wt G2P[4] RV have been observed simultaneously in neighboring South American countries where no UMV program against RV disease was in place (Matthijnssens et al., 2009a). Vaccine coverage of more than 85% of all newborns was reached quickly after vaccine introduction in 2006 in Belgium. The average percentage of RV-positive cases in all children admitted with gastroenteritis at a university hospital was 19.0%. This percentage dropped to 12.4%, 9.6%, and 6.4% in the three seasons after vaccine introduction. In addition, the RV season was shortened and delayed (Zeller et al., 2010). The prevalence of the G2 genotype sharply increased in the 2006–2007 RV season compared to the previous seasons and remained high (30 to 40%) in the 2007–2008 and 2008–2009 seasons. It is, however, unclear if the predominance of G2 genotypes is related to vaccine introduction or is attributable to normal genotype fluctuations. In June 2009, the World Health Organization recommended the use of RV vaccination in developing countries, based on early result of clinical trials in Africa and South East Asia (SAGE, 2009).

Several years of UMV against RV disease have to be surveyed before an opinion on the epidemiological consequences can be formed. As both RV vaccines exert only moderate protection against infection of infants with RVs, those viruses will continue to circulate in humans. However, it is hoped that the RV vaccines will to some extent mimic natural infections and that a protective effect against RV disease from subsequent wt RV infections will be the outcome, similar to the prospective observations of Velazquez et al. (1996).

REFERENCES

Abe, M., N. Ito, S. Morikawa, M. Takasu, T. Murase, T. Kawashima, Y. Kawai, J. Kohara, and M. Sugiyama. 2009. Molecular epidemiology of rotaviruses among healthy calves in Japan: isolation of a novel bovine rotavirus bearing new P and G genotypes. *Virus Res.* **144:**250–257.

Adah, M. I., A. Rohwedder, O. D. Olaleyle, and H. Werchau. 1997. Nigerian rotavirus serotype G8 could not be typed by PCR due to nucleotide mutation at the 3′ end of the primer binding site. *Arch Virol.* **142:**1881–1887.

Ahmed, M. U., S. Urasawa, K. Taniguchi, T. Urasawa, N. Kobayashi, F. Wakasugi, A. I. Islam, and H. A. Sahikh. 1991. Analysis of human rotavirus strains prevailing in Bangladesh in relation to nationwide floods brought by the 1988 monsoon. *J. Clin. Microbiol.* **29:**2273–2279.

Angel, J., M. A. Franco, and H. B. Greenberg. 2007. Rotavirus vaccines: recent developments and future considerations. *Nat. Rev. Microbiol.* **5:**529–539.

Aoki, S. T., E. C. Settembre, S. D. Trask, H. B. Greenberg, S. C. Harrison, and P. R. Dormitzer. 2009. Structure of rotavirus outer-layer protein VP7 bound with a neutralizing Fab. *Science* **324:**1444–1447.

Araujo, I. T., R. M. Assis, A. M. Fialho, J. D. Mascarenhas, M. B. Heinemann, and J. P. Leite. 2007. Brazilian P[8],G1, P[8],G5, P[8],G9, and P[4],G2 rotavirus strains: nucleotide sequence and phylogenetic analysis. *J. Med. Virol.* **79:**995–1001.

Armah, G. E., A. D. Steele, M. D. Esona, V. A. Akran, L. Nimzing, and G. Pennap. 2010. Diversity of rotavirus strains circulating in west Africa from 1996 to 2000. *J. Infect. Dis.* **202**(Suppl,)**:**S64–S71.

Ball, J. M., P. Tian, C. Q. Zeng, A. P. Morris, and M. K. Estes. 1996. Age-dependent diarrhea induced by a rotaviral nonstructural glycoprotein. *Science* **272:**101–104.

Ballard, A., M. A. McCrae, and U. Desselberger. 1992. Nucleotide sequences of normal and rearranged RNA segments 10 of human rotaviruses. *J. Gen. Virol.* **73:**633–638.

Bányai, K., V. Martella, P. Molnar, I. Mihaly, M. Van Ranst, and J. Matthijnssens. 2009a. Genetic heterogeneity in human G6P[14] rotavirus strains detected in Hungary suggests independent zoonotic origin. *J. Infect.* **59:**213–215.

Bányai, K., J. Matthijnssens, G. Szucs, P. Forgach, K. Erdelyi, M. van Ranst, E. Lorusso, N. Decaro, G. Elia, and V. Martella. 2009b. Frequent rearrangement may explain the structural heterogeneity in the 11th genome segment of lapine rotaviruses—short communication. *Acta Vet. Hung.* **57:**453–461.

Bányai, K., H. Papp, E. Dandar, P. Molnar, I. Mihaly, M. Van Ranst, V. Martella, and J. Matthijnssens. 2010. Whole genome sequencing and phylogenetic analysis of a zoonotic human G8P[14] rotavirus strain. *Infect. Genet. Evol.* **10:**1140–1144.

Barro, M., and J. T. Patton. 2005. Rotavirus nonstructural protein 1 subverts innate immune response by inducing degradation of IFN regulatory factor 3. *Proc. Natl. Acad. Sci. USA* **102:**4114–4119.

Barro, M., and J. T. Patton. 2007. Rotavirus NSP1 inhibits expression of type I interferon by antagonizing the function of interferon regulatory factors IRF3, IRF5, and IRF7. *J. Virol.* **81:**4473–4481.

Berkova, Z., S. E. Crawford, G. Trugnan, T. Yoshimori, A. P. Morris, and M. K. Estes. 2006. Rotavirus NSP4 induces a novel vesicular compartment regulated by calcium and associated with viroplasms. *J. Virol.* **80:**6061–6071.

Bishop, R. F. 1996. Natural history of human rotavirus infection. *Arch. Virol. Suppl.* **12:**119–128.

Blackhall, J., A. Fuentes, and G. Magnusson. 1996. Genetic stability of a porcine rotavirus RNA segment during repeated plaque isolation. *Virology* **225:**181–190.

Block, S. L., T. Vesikari, M. G. Goveia, S. B. Rivers, B. A. Adeyi, M. J. Dallas, J. Bauder, J. W. Boslego, and P. M. Heaton. 2007. Efficacy, immunogenicity, and safety of a pentavalent human-bovine (WC3) reassortant rotavirus vaccine at the end of shelf life. *Pediatrics* **119:**11–18.

Boyce, M., C. C. Celma, and P. Roy. 2008. Development of reverse genetics systems for bluetongue virus: recovery of infectious virus from synthetic RNA transcripts. *J. Virol.* **82:**8339–8348.

Boyce, M., and P. Roy. 2007. Recovery of infectious bluetongue virus from RNA. *J. Virol.* **81:**2179–2186.

Brandt, C. D., H. W. Kim, W. J. Rodriguez, J. O. Arrobio, B. C. Jeffries, E. P. Stallings, C. Lewis, A. J. Miles, R. M. Chanock, A. Z. Kapikian, and R. H. Parrott. 1983. Pediatric viral gastroenteritis during eight years of study. *J. Clin. Microbiol.* **18:**71–78.

Browning, G. F., and A. P. Begg. 1996. Prevalence of G and P serotypes among equine rotaviruses in the faeces of diarrhoeic foals. *Arch. Virol.* **141:**1077–1089.

Brussow, H., O. Nakagomi, G. Gerna, and W. Eichhorn. 1992. Isolation of an avianlike group A rotavirus from a calf with diarrhea. *J. Clin. Microbiol.* **30:**67–73.

Cao, D., M. Barro. and Y. Hoshino. 2008. Porcine rotavirus bearing an aberrant gene stemming from an intergenic recombination of the NSP2 and NSP5 genes is defective and interfering. *J. Virol.* **82:**6073–6077.

Carvalho-Costa, F. A., I. T. Araujo, R. M. Santos de Assis, A. M. Fialho, C. M. de Assis Martins, M. N. Boia, and J. P. Leite. 2009. Rotavirus genotype distribution after vaccine introduction, Rio de Janeiro, Brazil. *Emerg. Infect. Dis.* **15:**95–97.

Caul, E. O., C. R. Ashley, J. M. Darville, and J. C. Bridger. 1990. Group C rotavirus associated with fatal enteritis in a family outbreak. *J. Med. Virol.* **30:**201–205.

Centers for Disease Control and Prevention. 2008. Delayed onset and diminished magnitude of rotavirus activity—United States, November 2007–May 2008. *MMWR Morb. Mortal. Wkly. Rep.* **57:**697–700.

Chang, K. O., P. R. Nielsen, L. A. Ward, and L. J. Saif. 1999. Dual infection of gnotobiotic calves with bovine strains of group A and porcine-like group C rotaviruses influences pathogenesis of the group C rotavirus. *J. Virol.* **73:**9284–9293.

Charpilienne, A., J. Lepault, F. Rey, and J. Cohen. 2002. Identification of rotavirus VP6 residues located at the interface with VP2 that are essential for capsid assembly and transcriptase activity. *J. Virol.* **76:**7822–7831.

Chen, J. Z., E. C. Settembre, S. T. Aoki, X. Zhang, A. R. Bellamy, P. R. Dormitzer, S. C. Harrison, and N. Grigorieff. 2009. Molecular interactions in rotavirus assembly and uncoating seen by high-resolution cryo-EM. *Proc. Natl. Acad. Sci. USA* **106:**10644–10648.

Cheung, W., M. Gill, A. Esposito, C. F. Kaminski, N. Courousse, S. Chwetzoff, G. Trugnan, N. Keshavan, A. Lever, and U. Desselberger. 2010. Rotaviruses associate with cellular lipid droplet components to replicate in viroplasms, and compounds disrupting or blocking lipid droplets inhibit viroplasm formation and viral replication. *J. Virol.* **84:**6782–6798.

Clark, H. F., D. Lawley, L. A. Mallette, M. J. Dinubile, and R. L. Hodinka. 2009. Decline in cases of rotavirus gastroenteritis presenting to the Children's Hospital of Philadelphia after introduction of pentavalent rotavirus vaccine. *Clin. Vaccine Immunol.* **16:**382–386.

Collins, P. J., V. Martella, C. Buonavoglia, and H. O'Shea. 2010. Identification of a G2-like porcine rotavirus bearing a novel VP4 type, P[32]. *Vet. Res.* **41:**73.

Contin, R., F. Arnoldi, M. Campagna, and O. R. Burrone. 2010. Rotavirus NSP5 orchestrates recruitment of viroplasmic proteins. *J. Gen. Virol.* **91:**1782–1793.

Cunliffe, N. A., J. R. Gentsch, C. D. Kirkwood, J. S. Gondwe, W. Dove, O. Nakagomi, T. Nakagomi, Y. Hoshino, J. S. Bresee, R. I. Glass, M. E. Molyneux, and C. A. Hart. 2000. Molecular and serologic characterization of novel serotype G8 human rotavirus strains detected in Blantyre, Malawi. *Virology* **274:**309–320.

Desselberger, U. 1996. Genome rearrangements of rotaviruses. *Arch. Virol. Suppl.* **12:**37–51.

Desselberger, U., M. Iturriza-Gómara, and J. J. Gray. 2001. Rotavirus epidemiology and surveillance. *Novartis Found. Symp.* **238:**125–147; discussion 147–152.

Devitt, C. M., and D. L. Reynolds. 1993. Characterization of a group D rotavirus. *Avian Dis.* **37:**749–755.

Dunn, S. J., T. L. Cross, and H. B. Greenberg. 1994. Comparison of the rotavirus nonstructural protein NSP1 (NS53) from different species by sequence analysis and northern blot hybridization. *Virology* **203:**178–183.

Esona, M., S. Mijatovic-Rustempasic, C. Conrardy, S. Tong, I. Kuzmin, B. Agwanda, R. F. Breiman, K. Banyai, M. Niezgoda, C. E. Rupprecht, J. R. Gentsch. and M. D. Bowen. 2010a. Reassortant group A rotavirus from straw-colored fruit bat (Eidolon hevlum). *Emerg. Infect. Dis.* **16:**1844–1852.

Esona, M. D., D. Steele, T. Kerin, G. Armah, I. Peenze, A. Geyer, N. Page, J. Nyangao, V. A. Agbaya, A. Trabelsi, B. Tsion, M. Aminu, T. Sebunya, J. Dewar, R. Glass, and J. Gentsch. 2010b. Determination of the G and P types of previously nontypeable rotavirus strains from the African Rotavirus Network, 1996–2004: identification of unusual G types. *J. Infect. Dis.* **202**(Suppl.):S49–S54.

Estes, M., and A. Kapikian. 2007. Rotaviruses, p. 1917–1974. *In* D. M. Knipe, P. M. Howley, D. E. Griffin, R. A. Lamb, M. A. Martin, B. Roizman, and S. E. Straus (ed.), *Fields Virology*, 5th ed., Kluwer Health/Lippincott Williams & Wilkins, Philadelphia, PA.

Fenaux, M., M. A. Cuadras, N. Feng, M. Jaimes, and H. B. Greenberg. 2006. Extraintestinal spread and replication of a homologous EC rotavirus strain and a heterologous rhesus rotavirus in BALB/c mice. *J. Virol.* **80:**5219–5232.

Feng, N., B. Kim, M. Fenaux, H. Nguyen, P. Vo, M. B. Omary, and H. B. Greenberg. 2008. Role of interferon in homologous and heterologous rotavirus infection in the intestines and extraintestinal organs of suckling mice. *J. Virol.* **82:**7578–7590.

Feng, N., A. Sen, H. Nguyen, P. Vo, Y. Hoshino, E. M. Deal, and H. B. Greenberg. 2009. Variation in antagonism of the interferon response to rotavirus NSP1 results in differential infectivity in mouse embryonic fibroblasts. *J. Virol.* **83:**6987–6994.

Gabbay, Y. B., A. A. Borges, D. S. Oliveira, A. C. Linhares, J. D. Mascarenhas, C. R. Barardi, C. M. Simoes, Y. Wang, R. I. Glass, and B. Jiang. 2008. Evidence for zoonotic transmission of group C rotaviruses among children in Belem, Brazil. *J. Med. Virol.* **80:**1666–1674.

Garbarg-Chenon, A., F. Bricout, and J. C. Nicolas. 1986. Serological characterization of human reassortant rotaviruses. *J. Virol.* **59:**510–513.

Gault, E., N. Schnepf, D. Poncet, A. Servant, S. Teran, and A. Garbarg-Chenon. 2001. A human rotavirus with rearranged genes 7 and 11 encodes a modified NSP3 protein and suggests an additional mechanism for gene rearrangement. *J. Virol.* **75:**7305–7314.

Gentsch, J. R., P. A. Woods, M. Ramachandran, B. K. Das, J. P. Leite, A. Alfieri, R. Kumar, M. K. Bhan, and R. I. Glass. 1996. Review of G and P typing results from a global collection of rotavirus strains: implications for vaccine development. *J. Infect. Dis.* **174** (Suppl. 1)**:**S30–S36.

Ghosh, S., N. Kobayashi, S. Nagashima, M. Chawla-Sarkar, T. Krishnan, B. Ganesh, and T. N. Naik. 2010. Molecular characterization of the VP1, VP2, VP4, VP6, NSP1 and NSP2 genes of bovine group B rotaviruses: identification of a novel VP4 genotype. *Arch. Virol.* **155:**159–167.

Ghosh, S., V. Varghese, S. Samajdar, S. K. Bhattacharya, N. Kobayashi, and T. N. Naik. 2006. Molecular characterization of a porcine Group A rotavirus strain with G12 genotype specificity. *Arch. Virol.* **151:**1329–1344.

Gleizes, O., U. Desselberger, V. Tatochenko, C. Rodrigo, N. Salman, Z. Mezner, C. Giaquinto, and E. Grimprel. 2006. Nosocomial rotavirus infection in European countries: a review of the epidemiology, severity and economic burden of hospital-acquired rotavirus disease. *Pediatr. Infect. Dis. J.* **25:**S12–S21.

Gombold, J. L., and R. F. Ramig. 1986. Analysis of reassortment of genome segments in mice mixedly infected with rotaviruses SA11 and RRV. *J. Virol.* **57:**110–116.

Gorziglia, M., K. Nishikawa, and N. Fukuhara. 1989. Evidence of duplication and deletion in super short segment 11 of rabbit rotavirus Alabama strain. *Virology* **170:**587–590.

Gouvea, V., L. de Castro, M. C. Timenetsky, H. Greenberg, and N. Santos. 1994. Rotavirus serotype G5 associated with diarrhea in Brazilian children. *J. Clin. Microbiol.* **32:**1408–1409.

Graff, J. W., K. Ettayebi, and M. E. Hardy. 2009. Rotavirus NSP1 inhibits NFkappaB activation by inducing proteasome-dependent degradation of beta-TrCP: a novel mechanism of IFN antagonism. *PLoS Pathog.* **5:**e1000280.

Graff, J. W., D. N. Mitzel, C. M. Weisend, M. L. Flenniken, and M. E. Hardy. 2002. Interferon regulatory factor 3 is a cellular partner of rotavirus NSP1. *J. Virol.* **76:**9545–9550.

Graham, A., G. Kudesia, A. M. Allen, and U. Desselberger. 1987. Reassortment of human rotavirus possessing genome rearrangements with bovine rotavirus: evidence for host cell selection. *J. Gen. Virol.* **68:**115–122.

Greenberg, H., V. McAuliffe, J. Valdesuso, R. Wyatt, J. Flores, A. Kalica, Y. Hoshino, and N. Singh. 1983. Serological analysis of the subgroup protein of rotavirus, using monoclonal antibodies. *Infect. Immun.* **39:**91–99.

Hanada, K., Y. Suzuki, and T. Gojobori. 2004. A large variation in the rates of synonymous substitution for RNA viruses and its relationship to a diversity of viral infection and transmission modes. *Mol. Biol. Evol.* **21:**1074–1080.

Haynes, J. S., D. L. Reynolds, J. A. Fagerland, and A. S. Fix. 1994. Morphogenesis of enteric lesions induced by group D rotavirus in ringneck pheasant chicks (Phasianus colchicus). *Vet. Pathol.* **31:**74–81.

Hundley, F., B. Biryahwaho, M. Gow, and U. Desselberger. 1985. Genome rearrangements of bovine rotavirus after serial passage at high multiplicity of infection. *Virology* **143:**88–103.

Ito, H., M. Sugiyama, K. Masubuchi, Y. Mori, and N. Minamoto. 2001. Complete nucleotide sequence of a group A avian rotavirus genome and a comparison with its counterparts of mammalian rotaviruses. *Virus Res.* **75:**123–138.

Iturriza-Gómara, M., T. Dallman, K. Banyai, B. Bottiger, J. Buesa, S. Diedrich, L. Fiore, K. Johansen, M. Koopmans, N. Korsun, D. Koukou, A. Kroneman, B. Laszlo, M. Lappalainen, L. Maunula, A. M. Marques, J. Matthijnssens, S. Midgley, Z. Mladenova, S. Nawaz, M. Poljsak-Prijatelj, P. Pothier, F. M. Ruggeri, A. Sanchez-Fauquier, A. Steyer, I. Sidaraviciute-Ivaskeviciene, V. Syriopoulou, A. N. Tran, V. Usonis, M. van Ranst, A. de Rougement, and J. Gray. 2011. Rotavirus genotypes co-circulating in Europe between 2006 and 2009 as determined by EuroRotaNet, a pan-European collaborative strain surveillance network. *Epidemiol. Infect.* **139:**895–909.

Iturriza-Gómara, M., U. Desselberger, and J. Gray. 2003. Molecular epidemiology of rotaviruses: genetic mechanisms associated with diversity, p. 317–344. *In* U. Desselberger and J. Gray (ed.), *Viral Gastroenteritis*. Elsevier, Amsterdam, The Netherlands.

Iturriza-Gómara, M., J. Green, D. W. Brown, U. Desselberger, and J. J. Gray. 2000. Diversity within the VP4 gene of rotavirus P[8] strains: implications for reverse transcription-PCR genotyping. *J. Clin. Microbiol.* **38:**898–901.

Iturriza-Gómara, M., B. Isherwood, U. Desselberger, and J. Gray. 2001. Reassortment in vivo: driving force for diversity of human rotavirus strains isolated in the United Kingdom between 1995 and 1999. *J. Virol.* **75:**3696–3705.

Iturriza-Gómara, M., G. Kang, and J. Gray. 2004a. Rotavirus genotyping: keeping up with an evolving population of human rotaviruses. *J. Clin. Virol.* **31:**259–265.

Iturriza-Gómara, M., G. Kang, A. Mammen, A. K. Jana, M. Abraham, U. Desselberger, D. Brown, and J. Gray. 2004b. Characterization of G10P[11] rotaviruses causing acute gastroenteritis in neonates and infants in Vellore, India. *J. Clin. Microbiol.* **42:**2541–2547.

Iturriza-Gómara, M., C. Wong, S. Blome, U. Desselberger, and J. Gray. 2002a. Molecular characterization ofVP6 genes of human rotavirus isolates: correlation of genogroups with subgroups and evidence of independent segregation. *J. Virol.* **76:**6596–6601.

Iturriza-Gómara, M., C. Wong, S. Blome, U. Desselberger, and J. Gray. 2002b. Rotavirus subgroup characterisation by restriction endonuclease digestion of a cDNA fragment of the VP6 gene. *J. Virol. Methods* **105:**99–103.

Jenkins, G. M., A. Rambaut, O. G. Pybus, and E. C. Holmes. 2002. Rates of molecular evolution in RNA viruses: a quantitative phylogenetic analysis. *J. Mol. Evol.* **54:**156–165.

Jiang, B., P. H. Dennehy, S. Spangenberger, J. R. Gentsch, and R. I. Glass. 1995. First detection of group C rotavirus in fecal specimens of children with diarrhea in the United States. *J. Infect. Dis.* **172:**45–50.

Jiang, S., S. Ji, Q. Tang, X. Cui, H. Yang, B. Kan, and S. Gao. 2008. Molecular characterization of a novel adult diarrhoea rotavirus strain J19 isolated in China and its significance for the evolution and origin of group B rotaviruses. *J. Gen. Virol.* **89:**2622–2629.

Kirkwood, C. D., K. Boniface, R. F. Bishop, and G. L. Barnes. 2009. Australian Rotavirus Surveillance Program annual report, 2008/2009. *Commun. Dis. Intell.* **33:**382–388.

Kobayashi, N., T. N. Naik, Y. Kusuhara, T. Krishnan, A. Sen, S. K. Bhattacharya, K. Taniguchi, M. M. Alam, T. Urasawa, and S. Urasawa. 2001. Sequence analysis of genes encoding structural and nonstructural proteins of a human group B rotavirus detected in Calcutta, India. *J. Med. Virol.* **64:**583–588.

Kobayashi, T., A. A. Antar, K. W. Boehme, P. Danthi, E. A. Eby, K. M. Guglielmi, G. H. Holm, E. M. Johnson, M. S. Maginnis, S. Naik, W. B. Skelton, J. D. Wetzel, G. J. Wilson, J. D. Chappell, and T. S. Dermody. 2007. A plasmid-based reverse genetics system for animal double-stranded RNA viruses. *Cell Host Microbe* **1:**147–157.

Kojima, K., K. Taniguchi, M. Kawagishi-Kobayashi, S. Matsuno, and S. Urasawa. 2000. Rearrangement generated in double genes, NSP1 and NSP3, of viable progenies from a human rotavirus strain. *Virus Res.* **67:**163–171.

Kojima, K., K. Taniguchi, T. Urasawa, and S. Urasawa. 1996. Sequence analysis of normal and rearranged NSP5 genes from human rotavirus strains isolated in nature: implications for the occurrence of the rearrangement at the step of plus strand synthesis. *Virology* **224:**446–452.

Komoto, S., M. Kugita, J. Sasaki, and K. Taniguchi. 2008. Generation of recombinant rotavirus with an antigenic mosaic of cross-reactive neutralization epitopes on VP4. *J. Virol.* **82:**6753–6757.

Komoto, S., J. Sasaki, and K. Taniguchi. 2006. Reverse genetics system for introduction of site-specific mutations into the double-stranded RNA genome of infectious rotavirus. *Proc. Natl. Acad. Sci. USA* **103:**4646–4651.

Kool, D. A., S. M. Matsui, H. B. Greenberg, and I. H. Holmes. 1992. Isolation and characterization of a novel reassortant between avian Ty-1 and simian RRV rotaviruses. *J. Virol.* **66:**6836–6839.

Krishnan, T., A. Sen, J. S. Choudhury, S. Das, T. N. Naik, and S. K. Bhattacharya. 1999. Emergence of adult diarrhoea rotavirus in Calcutta, India. *Lancet* **353:**380–381.

Kuga, K., A. Miyazaki, T. Suzuki, M. Takagi, N. Hattori, K. Katsuda, M. Mase, M. Sugiyama, and H. Tsunemitsu. 2009. Genetic diversity and classification of the outer capsid glycoprotein VP7 of porcine group B rotaviruses. *Arch. Virol.* **154:**1785–1795.

Lawton, J. A., M. K. Estes, and B. V. Prasad. 1997. Three-dimensional visualization of mRNA release from actively transcribing rotavirus particles. *Nat. Struct. Biol.* **4:**118–121.

Lawton, J. A., M. K. Estes, and B. V. Prasad. 1999. Comparative structural analysis of transcriptionally competent and incompetent rotavirus-antibody complexes. *Proc. Natl. Acad. Sci. USA* **96:**5428–5433.

Leite, J. P., F. A. Carvalho-Costa, and A. C. Linhares. 2008. Group A rotavirus genotypes and the ongoing Brazilian experience: a review. *Mem. Inst. Oswaldo Cruz* **103:**745–753.

Lepault, J., I. Petitpas, I. Erk, J. Navaza, D. Bigot, M. Dona, P. Vachette, J. Cohen, and F. A. Rey. 2001. Structural polymorphism of the major capsid protein of rotavirus. *EMBO J.* **20:**1498–1507.

Li, Z., M. L. Baker, W. Jiang, M. K. Estes, and B.V. Prasad. 2009. Rotavirus architecture at subnanometer resolution. *J. Virol.* **83:**1754–1766.

Linhares, A. C., F. R. Velazquez, I. Perez-Schael, X. Saez-Llorens, H. Abate, F. Espinoza, P. Lopez, M. Macias-Parra, E. Ortega-Barria, D. M. Rivera-Medina, L. Rivera, N. Pavia-Ruz, E. Nunez, S. Damaso, G. M. Ruiz-Palacios, B. De Vos, M. O'Ryan, P. Gillard, and A. Bouckenooghe. 2008. Efficacy and safety of an oral live attenuated human rotavirus vaccine against rotavirus gastroenteritis during the first 2 years of life in Latin American infants: a randomised, double-blind, placebo-controlled phase III study. *Lancet* **371:**1181–1189.

Lopez, S., and C. F. Arias. 2004. Multistep entry of rotavirus into cells: a Versaillesque dance. *Trends Microbiol.* **12:**271–278.

Lu, X., S. M. McDonald, M. A. Tortorici, Y. J. Tao, R. Vasquez-Del Carpio, M. L. Nibert, J. T. Patton, and S. C. Harrison. 2008. Mechanism for coordinated RNA packaging and genome replication by rotavirus polymerase VP1. *Structure* **16:**1678–1688.

Maes, P., J. Matthijnssens, M. Rahman, and M. Van Ranst. 2009. RotaC: a web-based tool for the complete genome classification of group A rotaviruses. *BMC Microbiol.* **9:**238.

Martella, V., K. Bányai, M. Ciarlet, M. Iturriza-Gómara, E. Lorusso, S. De Grazia, S. Arista, N. Decaro, G. Elia, A. Cavalli, M. Corrente, A. Lavazza, R. Baselga, and C. Buonavoglia. 2006. Relationships among porcine and human P[6] rotaviruses: evidence that the different human P[6] lineages have originated from multiple interspecies transmission events. *Virology* **344:**509–519.

Martella, V., K. Banyai, J. Matthijnssens, C. Buonavoglia. and M. Ciarlet. 2009. Zoonotic aspects of rotaviruses. *Vet. Microbiol.* **140:**246–255.

Martella, V., M. Ciarlet, A. Lavazza, A. Camarda, E. Lorusso, V. Terio, D. Ricci, F. Cariola, M. Gentile, A. Cavalli, M. Camero, N. Decaro, and C. Buonavoglia. 2005. Lapine rotaviruses of the genotype P[22] are widespread in Italian rabbitries. *Vet. Microbiol.* **111:**117–124.

Martella, V., V. Terio, S. Arista, G. Elia, M. Corrente, A. Madio, A. Pratelli, M. Tempesta, A. Cirani, and C. Buonavoglia. 2004. Nucleotide variation in the VP7 gene affects PCR genotyping of G9 rotaviruses identified in Italy. *J. Med. Virol.* **72:**143–148.

Martin, V., and E. Domingo. 2008. Influence of the mutant spectrum in viral evolution: focused selection of antigenic variants in a reconstructed viral quasispecies. *Mol. Biol. Evol.* **25:**1544–1554.

Mathieu, M., I. Petitpas, J. Navaza, J. Lepault, E. Kohli, P. Pothier, B. V. Prasad, J. Cohen, and F. A. Rey. 2001. Atomic structure of the major capsid protein of rotavirus: implications for the architecture of the virion. *EMBO J.* **20:**1485–1497.

Matsuo, E., C. C. Celma, and P. Roy. 2010. A reverse genetics system of African horse sickness virus reveals existence of primary replication. *FEBS Lett.* **584:**3386–3391.

Matthijnssens, J., J. Bilcke, M. Ciarlet, V. Martella, K. Banyai, M. Rahman, M. Zeller, P. Beutels, P. Van Damme, and M. Van Ranst. 2009a. Rotavirus disease and vaccination: impact on genotype diversity. *Future Microbiol.* **4:**1303–1316.

Matthijnssens, J., M. Ciarlet, E. Heiman, I. Arijs, T. Delbeke, S. M. McDonald, E. A. Palombo, M. Iturriza-Gómara, P. Maes, J. T. Patton, M. Rahman, and M. Van Ranst. 2008a. Full genome-based classification of rotaviruses reveals a common origin between human Wa-like and porcine rotavirus strains and human DS-1-like and bovine rotavirus strains. *J. Virol.* **82:**3204–3219.

Matthijnssens, J., M. Ciarlet, M. Rahman, H. Attoui, K. Banyai, M. K. Estes, J. R. Gentsch, M. Iturriza-Gómara, C. D. Kirkwood, V. Martella, P. P. Mertens, O. Nakagomi, J. T. Patton, F. M. Ruggeri, L. J. Saif, N. Santos, A. Steyer, K. Taniguchi, U. Desselberger, and M. Van Ranst. 2008b. Recommendations for the classification of group A rotaviruses using all 11 genomic RNA segments. *Arch. Virol.* **153:**1621–1629.

Matthijnssens, J., E. Heylen, M. Zeller, M. Rahman, P. Lemey, and M. Van Ranst. 2010a. Phylodynamic analyses of rotavirus genotypes G9 and G12 underscore their potential for swift global spread. *Mol. Biol. Evol.* **27:**2431–2436.

Matthijnssens, J., V. Martella, and M. Van Ranst. 2010b. Priority Paper Evaluation: Genomic evolution, host-species barrier, reassortment and classification of rotaviruses. *Future Virol.* **5:**385–390.

Matthijnssens, J., C. A. Potgieter, M. Ciarlet, V. Parreño, V. Martella, K. Bányai, L. Garaicoechea, E. A. Palombo, L. Novo, M. Zeller, S. Arista, G. Gerna, M. Rahman, and M. Van Ranst. 2009b. Are human P[14] rotavirus strains the result of interspecies transmissions from sheep or other ungulates that belong to the mammalian order Artiodactyla? *J. Virol.* **83:**2917–2929.

Matthijnssens, J., M. Rahman, M. Ciarlet, and M. Van Ranst. 2008c. Emerging human rotavirus genotypes, p. 171–219. *In* E. A. Palombo and C. D. Kirkwood (ed.), *Viruses in the Environment.* Research Signpost, Trivandrum, India.

Matthijnssens, J., M. Rahman, M. Ciarlet, M. Zeller, E. Heylen, T. Nakagomi, R. Uchida, Z. Hassan, T. Azim, O. Nakagomi, and M. Van Ranst. 2010c. Reassortment of human rotavirus gene segments into G11 rotavirus strains. *Emerg. Infect. Dis.* **16:**625–630.

Matthijnssens, J., M. Rahman, V. Martella, Y. Xuelei, S. De Vos, K. De Leener, M. Ciarlet, C. Buonavoglia, and M. Van Ranst. 2006a. Full genomic analysis of human rotavirus strain B4106 and lapine rotavirus strain 30/96 provides evidence for interspecies transmission. *J. Virol.* **80:**3801–3810.

Matthijnssens, J., M. Rahman, and M. Van Ranst. 2006b. Loop model: mechanism to explain partial gene duplications in segmented dsRNA viruses. *Biochem. Biophys. Res. Commun.* **340:**140–144.

Matthijnssens, J., M. Rahman. and M. Van Ranst. 2008d. Two out of the 11 genes of an unusual human G6P[6] rotavirus isolate are of bovine origin. *J. Gen. Virol.* **89:**2630–2635.

Matthijnssens, J., M. Rahman, X. Yang, T. Delbeke, I. Arijs, J. P. Kabue, J. J. Muyembe, and M. Van Ranst. 2006c. G8 rotavirus strains isolated in the Democratic Republic of Congo belong to the DS-1-like genogroup. *J. Clin. Microbiol.* **44:**1801–1809.

Matthijnssens, J., Z. F. Taraporewala, H. Yang, S. Rao, L. Yuan, D. Cao, Y. Hoshino, P. P. Mertens, G. R. Carner, M. McNeal, K. Sestak, M. Van Ranst, and J. T. Patton. 2009c. Simian rotaviruses possess divergent gene constellations originating from interspecies transmission and reassortment. *J. Virol.* **84:**2013–2026.

Maunula, L., and C. H. Von Bonsdorff. 2002. Frequent reassortments may explain the genetic heterogeneity of rotaviruses: analysis of Finnish rotavirus strains. *J. Virol.* **76:**11793–11800.

McClain, B., E. Settembre, B. R. Temple, A. R. Bellamy, and S. C. Harrison. 2010. X-ray crystal structure of the rotavirus inner capsid particle at 3.8 A resolution. *J. Mol. Biol.* **397:**587–599.

McDonald, S. M., J. Matthijnssens, J. K. McAllen, E. Hine, L. Overton, S. Wang, P. Lemey, M. Zeller, M. Van Ranst, D. J. Spiro, and J. T. Patton. 2009. Evolutionary dynamics of human rotaviruses: balancing reassortment with preferred genome constellations. *PLoS Pathog.* **5:**e1000634.

Mitui, M. T., G. Bozdayi, B. Dalgic, I. Bostanci, A. Nishizono, and K. Ahmed. 2009. Molecular characterization of a human group C rotavirus detected first in Turkey. *Virus Genes* **39:**157–164.

Mori, Y., M. Sugiyama, M. Takayama, Y. Atoji, T. Masegi, and N. Minamoto. 2001. Avian-to-mammal transmission of an avian rotavirus: analysis of its pathogenicity in a heterologous mouse model. *Virology* **288:**63–70.

Mwenda, J. M., K. M. Ntoto, A. Abebe, C. Enweronu-Laryea, I. Amina, J. McHomvu, A. Kisakye, E. M. Mpabalwani, I. Pazvakavambwa, G. E. Armah, L. M. Seheri, N. M. Kiulia, N. Page, M. A. Widdowson, M. A. and A. D. Steele. 2010. Burden and epidemiology of rotavirus diarrhea in selected African countries: preliminary results from the African Rotavirus Surveillance Network. *J. Infect. Dis.* **202**(Suppl.):S5–S11.

Nagashima, S., N. Kobayashi, M. Ishino, M. M. Alam, M. U. Ahmed, S. K. Paul, B. Ganesh, M. Chawla-Sarkar, T. Krishnan, T. N. Naik, and Y. H. Wang. 2008. Whole genomic characterization of a human rotavirus strain B219 belonging to a novel group of the genus Rotavirus. *J. Med. Virol.* **80:**2023–2033.

Nakagomi, O., and T. Nakagomi. 1991. Genetic diversity and similarity among mammalian rotaviruses in relation to interspecies transmission of rotavirus. *Arch. Virol.* **120:**43–55.

Nakagomi, O., T. Nakagomi, K. Akatani, and N. Ikegami. 1989. Identification of rotavirus genogroups by RNA-RNA hybridization. *Mol. Cell. Probes* **3:**251–261.

Nakagomi, T., and O. Nakagomi. 1989. RNA-RNA hybridization identifies a human rotavirus that is genetically related to feline rotavirus. *J. Virol.* **63:**1431–1434.

Ni, Y., and M. C. Kemp. 1994. Subgenomic S1 segments are packaged by avian reovirus defective interfering particles having an S1 segment deletion. *Virus Res.* **32:**329–342.

O'Ryan, M. L., G. Hermosilla, and G. Osorio. 2009. Rotavirus vaccines for the developing world. *Curr. Opin. Infect. Dis.* **22:**483–489.

Page, N., M. Esona, M. Seheri, J. Nyangao, P. Bos, J. Mwenda, and D. Steele. 2010. Characterization of genotype G8 strains from Malawi, Kenya, and South Africa. *J. Med. Virol.* **82:**2073–2081.

Parashar, U. D., C. J. Gibson, J. S. Bresee, and R. I. Glass. 2006. Rotavirus and severe childhood diarrhea. *Emerg. Infect. Dis.* **12:**304–306.

Parra, G. I., K. Bok, M. Martinez, and J. A. Gomez. 2004. Evidence of rotavirus intragenic recombination between two sublineages of the same genotype. *J. Gen. Virol.* **85:**1713–1716.

Patton, J. T., M. Wentz, J. Xiaobo, and R. F. Ramig. 1996. *cis*-acting signals that promote genome replication in rotavirus mRNA. *J. Virol.* **70:**3961–3971.

Pedley, S., J. C. Bridger, D. Chasey, and M. A. McCrae. 1986. Definition of two new groups of atypical rotaviruses. *J. Gen. Virol.* **67:**131–137.

Pesavento, J. B., M. K. Estes, and B. V. Prasad. 2003. Structural organization of the genome in rotavirus, p. 115–128. *In* U. Desselberger and J. Gray (ed.), *Viral Gastroenteritis*. Elsevier, Amsterdam, The Netherlands.

Phan, T. G., S. Okitsu, N. Maneekarn, and H. Ushijima. 2007. Evidence of intragenic recombination in G1 rotavirus VP7 genes. *J. Virol.* **81:**10188–10194.

Potgieter, A. C., N. A. Page, J. Liebenberg, I. M. Wright, O. Landt, and A. A. van Dijk. 2009.

Improved strategies for sequence-independent amplification and sequencing of viral double-stranded RNA genomes. *J. Gen. Virol.* **90:**1423–1432.

Prasad, B.V., R. Rothnagel, C. Q. Zeng, J. Jakana, J. A. Lawton, W. Chiu, and M. K. Estes. 1996. Visualization of ordered genomic RNA and localization of transcriptional complexes in rotavirus. *Nature* **382:**471–473.

Rahman, M., S. Banik, A. S. Faruque, K. Taniguchi, D. A. Sack, M. Van Ranst, and T. Azim. 2005a. Detection and characterization of human group C rotaviruses in Bangladesh. *J. Clin. Microbiol.* **434:**460–4465.

Rahman, M., Z. M. Hassan, H. Zafrul, F. Saiada, S. Banik, A. S. Faruque, T. Delbeke, J. Matthijnssens, M. Van Ranst, and T. Azim. 2007a. Sequence analysis and evolution of group B rotaviruses. *Virus Res.* **125:**219–225.

Rahman, M., J. Matthijnssens, T. Goegebuer, K. De Leener, L. Vanderwegen, I. van der Donck, L. Van Hoovels, S. De Vos, T. Azim, and M. Van Ranst. 2005b. Predominance of rotavirus G9 genotype in children hospitalized for rotavirus gastroenteritis in Belgium during 1999–2003. *J. Clin. Virol.* **33:**1–6.

Rahman, M., J. Matthijnssens, X. Yang, T. Delbeke, I. Arijs, K. Taniguchi, M. Iturriza-Gómara, N. Iftekharuddin, T. Azim, and M. Van Ranst. 2007b. Evolutionary history and global spread of the emerging G12 human rotaviruses. *J. Virol.* **81:**2382–2390.

Rahman, M., R. Sultana, G. Podder, A. S. Faruque, J. Matthijnssens, K. Zaman, R. F. Breiman, D. A. Sack, M. Van Ranst, and T. Azim. 2005c. Typing of human rotaviruses: nucleotide mismatches between the VP7 gene and primer are associated with genotyping failure. *Virol. J.* **2:**24.

Ramachandran, M., J. R. Gentsch, U. D. Parashar, S. Jin, P. A. Woods, J. L. Holmes, C. D. Kirkwood, R. F. Bishop, H. B. Greenberg, S. Urasawa, G. Gerna, B. S. Coulson, K. Taniguchi, J. S. Bresee, and R. I. Glass. 1998. Detection and characterization of novel rotavirus strains in the United States. *J. Clin. Microbiol.* **36:**3223–3229.

Ruiz-Palacios, G. M., I. Perez-Schael, F. R. Velazquez, H. Abate, T. Breuer, S. C. Clemens, B. Cheuvart, F. Espinoza, P. Gillard, B. L. Innis, Y. Cervantes, A. C. Linhares, P. Lopez, M. Macias-Parra, E. Ortega-Barria, V. Richardson, D. M. Rivera-Medina, L. Rivera, B. Salinas, N. Pavia-Ruz, J. Salmeron, R. Ruttimann, J. C. Tinoco, P. Rubio, E. Nunez, M. L. Guerrero, J. P. Yarzabal, S. Damaso, N. Tornieporth, X. Saez-Llorens, R. F. Vergara, T. Vesikari, A. Bouckenooghe, R. Clemens, B. De Vos, and M. O'Ryan. 2006. Safety and efficacy of an attenuated vaccine against severe rotavirus gastroenteritis. *N. Engl. J. Med.* **354:**11–22.

SAGE. 2009. Meeting of the immunization Strategic Advisory Group of Experts; April 2009—conclusions and recommendations. *Wkly. Epidemiol. Rec.* **84:**220–236.

Sanekata, T., M. U. Ahmed, A. Kader, K. Taniguchi, and N. Kobayashi. 2003. Human group B rotavirus infections cause severe diarrhea in children and adults in Bangladesh. *J. Clin. Microbiol.* **41:**2187–2190.

Santos, N., and Y. Hoshino. 2005. Global distribution of rotavirus serotypes/genotypes and its implication for the development and implementation of an effective rotavirus vaccine. *Rev. Med. Virol.* **15:**29–56.

Santos, N., E. M. Volotao, C. C. Soares, M. C. Albuquerque, F. M. da Silva, V. Chizhikov, and Y. Hoshino. 2003. VP7 gene polymorphism of serotype G9 rotavirus strains and its impact on G genotype determination by PCR. *Virus Res.* **93:**127–138.

Schnepf, N., C. Deback, A. Dehee, E. Gault, N. Parez, and A. Garbarg-Chenon. 2008. Rearrangements of rotavirus genomic segment 11 are generated during acute infection of immunocompetent children and do not occur at random. *J. Virol.* **82:**3689–3696.

Schumann, T., H. Hotzel, P. Otto, and R. Johne. 2009. Evidence of interspecies transmission and reassortment among avian group A rotaviruses. *Virology* **386:**334–343.

Scott, G. E., O. Tarlow, and M. A. McCrae. 1989. Detailed structural analysis of a genome rearrangement in bovine rotavirus. *Virus Res.* **14:**119–127.

Sen, A., N. Feng, K. Ettayebi, M. E. Hardy, and H. B. Greenberg. 2009. IRF3 inhibition by rotavirus NSP1 is host cell and virus strain dependent but independent of NSP1 proteasomal degradation. *J. Virol.* **83:**10322–10335.

Shen, S., B. Burke, and U. Desselberger. 1994. Rearrangement of the VP6 gene of a group A rotavirus in combination with a point mutation affecting trimer stability. *J. Virol.* **68:**1682–1688.

Simmonds, M. K., G. Armah, R. Asmah, I. Banerjee, S. Damanka, M. Esona, J. R. Gentsch, J. J., Gray, C. Kirkwood, N. Page, and M. Iturriza-Gomara. 2008. New oligonucleotide primers for P-typing of rotavirus strains: strategies for typing previously untypeable strains. *J. Clin. Virol.* **42:**368–373.

Solberg, O. D., M. E. Hasing, G. Trueba, and J. N. Eisenberg. 2009. Characterization of novel VP7, VP4, and VP6 genotypes of a previously untypeable group A rotavirus. *Virology* **385:**58–67.

Steyer, A., M. Bajzelj, M. Iturriza-Gomara, Z. Mladenova, N. Korsun, and M. Poljsak-Prijatelj. 2010. Molecular analysis of human group A rotavirus G10P[14] genotype in Slovenia. *J. Clin. Virol.* **49:**121–125.

Steyer, A., M. Poljsak-Prijatelj, D. Barlic-Maganja, and J. Marin. 2008. Human, porcine and bovine rotaviruses in Slovenia: evidence of interspecies transmission and genome reassortment. *J. Gen. Virol.* **89:**1690–1698.

Suzuki, Y., T. Gojobori, and O. Nakagomi. 1998. Intragenic recombinations in rotaviruses. *FEBS Lett.* **427:**183–187.

Taniguchi, K., K. Kojima, and S. Urasawa. 1996. Nondefective rotavirus mutants with an NSP1 gene which has a deletion of 500 nucleotides, including a cysteine-rich zinc finger motif-encoding region (nucleotides 156 to 248), or which has a nonsense codon at nucleotides 153–155. *J. Virol.* **70:**4125–4130.

Tao, H. 1988. Rotavirus and adult diarrhea. *Adv. Virus Res.* **35:**193–218.

Tate, J. E., C. A. Panozzo, D. C. Payne, M. M. Patel, M. M. Cortese, A. L. Fowlkes, and U. D. Parashar. 2009. Decline and change in seasonality of US rotavirus activity after the introduction of rotavirus vaccine. *Pediatrics* **124:**465–471.

Tian, Y., O. Tarlow, A. Ballard, U. Desselberger, and M. A. McCrae. 1993. Genomic concatemerization/deletion in rotaviruses: a new mechanism for generating rapid genetic change of potential epidemiological importance. *J. Virol.* **67:**6625–6632.

Trask, S. D., Z. F. Taraporewala, K. W. Boehme, T. S. Dermody, and J. T. Patton. 2010. Dual selection mechanisms drive efficient single-gene reverse genetics for rotavirus. *Proc. Natl. Acad. Sci. USA* **107:**18652–18657.

Trojnar, E., P. Otto, and R. Johne. 2009. The first complete genome sequence of a chicken group A rotavirus indicates independent evolution of mammalian and avian strains. *Virology* **386:**325–333.

Trojnar, E., P. Otto, B. Roth, J. Reetz, and R. Johne. 2010. The genome segments of a group D rotavirus possess group A-like conserved termini but encode group-specific proteins. *J. Virol.* **84:**10254–10265.

Troupin, C., A. Dehee, A. Schnuriger, P. Vende, D. Poncet, A. and Garbarg-Chenon. 2010. Rearranged genomic RNA segments offer a new approach to the reverse genetics of rotaviruses. *J. Virol.* **84:**6711–6719.

Tsugawa, T., and Y. Hoshino. 2008. Whole genome sequence and phylogenetic analyses reveal human rotavirus G3P[3] strains Ro1845 and HCR3A are examples of direct virion transmission of canine/feline rotaviruses to humans. *Virology* **230:**344–353.

Unicomb, L. E., G. Podder, J. R. Gentsch, P. A. Woods, K. Z. Hasan, A. S. Faruque, M. J. Albert, and R. I. Glass. 1999. Evidence of high-frequency genomic reassortment of group A rotavirus strains in Bangladesh: emergence of type G9 in 1995. *J. Clin. Microbiol.* **37:**1885–1891.

Ursu, K., P. Kisfali, D. Rigo, E. Ivanics, K. Erdelyi, A. Dan, B. Melegh, V. Martella, and K. Banyai. 2009. Molecular analysis of the VP7 gene of pheasant rotaviruses identifies a new genotype, designated G23. *Arch. Virol.* **154:**1365–1369.

Velazquez, F. R., D. O. Matson, J. J. Calva, L. Guerrero, A. L. Morrow, S. Carter-Campbell, R. I. Glass, M. K. Estes, L. K. Pickering, and G. M. Ruiz-Palacios. 1996. Rotavirus infections in infants as protection against subsequent infections. *N. Engl. J. Med.* **335:**1022–1028.

Vesikari, T. 2008. Rotavirus vaccines. *Scand. J. Infect. Dis.* **40:**691–695.

Vesikari, T., D. O. Matson, P. Dennehy, P. Van Damme, M. Santosham, Z. Rodriguez, M. J. Dallas, J. F. Heyse, M. G. Goveia, S. B. Black, H. R. Shinefield, C. D. Christie, S. Ylitalo, R. F. Itzler, M. L. Coia, M. T. Onorato, B. A. Adeyi, G. S. Marshall, L. Gothefors, D. Campens, A. Karvonen, J. P. Watt, K. L. O'Brien, M. J. DiNubile, H. F. Clark, J. W. Boslego, P. A. Offit, and P. M. Heaton. 2006. Safety and efficacy of a pentavalent human-bovine (WC3) reassortant rotavirus vaccine. *N. Engl. J. Med.* **354:**23–33.

Ward, R. L., D. I. Bernstein, E. C. Young, J. R. Sherwood, D. R. Knowlton, and G. M. Schiff. 1986. Human rotavirus studies in volunteers: determination of infectious dose and serological response to infection. *J. Infect. Dis.* **154:**871–880.

Ward, R. L., O. Nakagomi, D. R. Knowlton, M. M. McNeal, T. Nakagomi, J. D. Clemens, D. A. Sack, and G. M. Schiff. 1990. Evidence for natural reassortants of human rotaviruses belonging to different genogroups. *J. Virol.* **64:**3219–3225.

Webby, R. J., R. G. Webster, and J. A. Richt. 2007. Influenza viruses in animal wildlife populations. *Curr. Top. Microbiol. Immunol.* **315:**67–83.

Xu, Z., W. Tuo, K. I. Clark, and G. N. Woode. 1996. A major rearrangement of the VP6 gene of a strain of rotavirus provides replication advantage. *Vet. Microbiol.* **52:**235–247.

Yamamoto, D., S. Ghosh, B. Ganesh, T. Krishnan, M. Chawla-Sarkar, M. M. Alam, T. S. Aung, and N. Kobayashi. 2010. Analysis of genetic diversity and molecular evolution of human group B rotaviruses based on whole genome segments. *J. Gen. Virol.* **91:**1772–1781.

Yamamoto, D., S. Ghosh, M. Kuzuya, Y. Wang, X. Zhou, M. Chawla-Sarkar, S. K. Paul, M. Ishino. and N. Kobayashi. 2011. Whole genomic characterization of human group C rotaviruses:

identification of two lineages in the VP3 gene. *J. Gen. Virol.* **92:**361–369.

Yang, H., E. V. Makeyev, Z. Kang, S. Ji, D. H. Bamford, and A. A. van Dijk. 2004a. Cloning and sequence analysis of dsRNA segments 5, 6 and 7 of a novel non-group A, B, C adult rotavirus that caused an outbreak of gastroenteritis in China. *Virus Res.* **106:**15–26.

Yang, J. H., N. Kobayashi, Y. H. Wang, X. Zhou, Y. Li, D. J. Zhou, Z. H. Hu, M. Ishino, M. M. Alam, T. N. Naik, and M. U. Ahmed. 2004b. Phylogenetic analysis of a human group B rotavirus WH-1 detected in China in 2002. *J. Med. Virol.* **74:**662–667.

Yoder, J. D., and P. R. Dormitzer. 2006. Alternative intermolecular contacts underlie the rotavirus VP5* two- to three-fold rearrangement. *EMBO J.* **25:**1559–1568.

Yoder, J. D., S. D. Trask, T. P. Vo, M. Binka, N. Feng, S. C. Harrison, H. B. Greenberg, and P. R. Dormitzer. 2009. VP5* rearranges when rotavirus uncoats. *J. Virol.* **83:**11372–11377.

Zeller, M., M. Rahman, E. Heylen, S. De Coster, S. De Vos, I. Arijs, L. Novo, N. Verstappen, M. Van Ranst, and J. Matthijnssens. 2010. Rotavirus incidence and genotype distribution before and after national rotavirus vaccine introduction in Belgium. *Vaccine* **28:**7507–7513.

Zhang, X., E. Settembre, C. Xu, P. R. Dormitzer, R. Bellamy, S. C. Harrison, and N. Grigorieff. 2008. Near-atomic resolution using electron cryomicroscopy and single-particle reconstruction. *Proc. Natl. Acad. Sci. USA* **105:**1867–1872.

GENOME PLASTICITY OF PAPILLOMAVIRUSES

Hans-Ulrich Bernard

14

GENETIC FEATURES OF PAPILLOMAVIRUSES

Figure 1 shows the genome organization of the best-studied papillomavirus, human papillomavirus type 16 (HPV-16), the most frequent papillomavirus found in anogenital cancer of humans. The HPV-16 genome is typical for the vast majority of all papillomaviruses. It has a double-stranded circular DNA genome of 7,905 bp. A long control region contains most *cis*-responsive elements that regulate transcription and replication. A single promoter (which can be complemented by other transcription initiation sites) induces transcription around the whole genome, beginning with the oncogenes E6 and E7. These transcripts are processed by differential splicing into a variety of mRNAs with diverging genetic content. The protein products of the oncogenes E6 and E7 have pleiotropic functions. In the case of HPV-16, binding and inactivation of the cell cycle regulators and tumor suppressors RB and p53 have been particularly well studied. A consequence of these functions is the reactivation of the replication machinery of suprabasal epithelial cells that normally do not undergo mitosis, leading to a molecular environment favorable for viral replication. In a pathogenic context, the same activity contributes to the amplification of cancer cells. The products of the next two genes downstream of E6 and E7, namely, E1 and E2, are the principal regulators of replication and transcription and have several binding sites in the long control region. E5, the small gene downstream of E2, encodes a membrane-bound transforming protein. The two late genes, L2 and L1, encode the major (L1) and a minor (L2) capsid proteins (for a review and references, see zur Hausen [2002]).

TAXONOMY, BIOLOGY, AND PATHOGENICITY OF PAPILLOMAVIRUSES

Papillomavirus isolates are historically described as "types." A papillomavirus type is defined as a complete virus genome whose L1 nucleotide sequence (and the rest of the genome) is at least 10% different from that of any other human papillomavirus type. Currently there are 189 formally described papillomavirus types, 125 of which are found in humans (de Villiers et al., 2004; Bernard et al., 2010). While

Hans-Ulrich Bernard, Department of Molecular Biology and Biochemistry and Program of Public Health, University of California Irvine, Irvine, CA 92697.

Genome Plasticity and Infectious Diseases,
Edited by J. Hacker, U. Dobrindt, and R. Kurth,

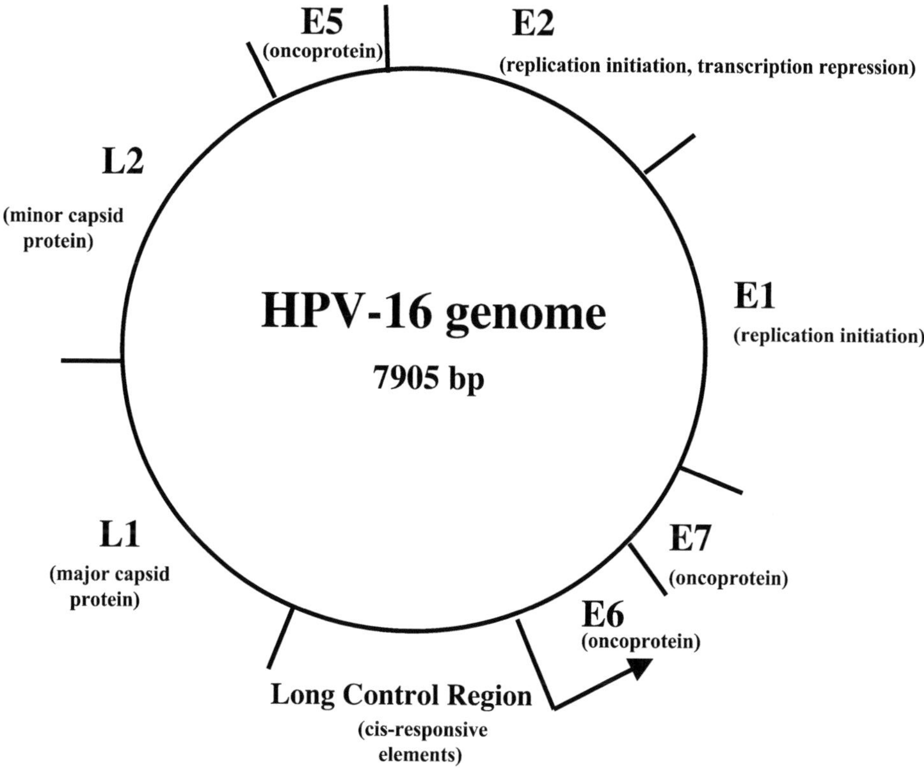

FIGURE 1 The genome of human papillomavirus type 16 (HPV-16) represents a genetic organization that is typical for all papillomaviruses. The function of early (E) and late (L) genes is described elsewhere in this chapter.

this definition of papillomavirus types appears somewhat arbitrary, they clearly represent natural taxa, as genomes intermediate between two types have never been found.

Papillomaviruses infect epithelial cells and do not undergo a productive viral replication in any other cell type. It is thought that the viral infection typically becomes established in basal cells, the lowest layer of epithelia. Papillomaviruses may persist in epithelial cells without causing morphological effects or may trigger an expansion of suprabasal cell populations that can lead to a variety of neoplastic growths. If the lesion is derived from the skin, many of these neoplasias are referred to by the vernacular name "wart." Most papillomavirus types are specific for either cutaneous or mucosal epithelia. Depending on the virus type, they also give rise to pathologically distinct lesions. For example, infections of the genital mucosa by human papillomavirus types 6 and 11 can give rise to genital warts, while human papillomavirus types 16 and 18 induce flat and inconspicuous lesions, which, however, can progress to anogenital cancer. Human papillomavirus type 2 is the cause of the widespread common warts of the skin. Pathologically similar skin lesions are caused by most of the other papillomaviruses identified in mammals, birds, and reptiles. These biological features of papillomaviruses allow us to predict their replication rate, which is normally not higher than that of the proliferating epithelium, i.e., roughly once per day. Papillomaviruses do not undergo rapid amplification with concomitant lysis of the host cell, as it is typical for most other DNA and RNA viruses. However, at the time they are shed with peripheral epithelial cells, they have increased the copy number of their genomes, about 100 DNA molecules per cell probably being typical. This requires an increased replication rate in differentiating epithelial cells; this is, however, much lower than that of viruses whose normal life cycle involves inflammation and cellular lysis of the target tissues.

GENOMIC STABILITY OF PAPILLOMAVIRUSES IN LABORATORY SETTINGS

In contrast to RNA viruses, papillomaviruses replicate based on the same mechanisms and enzymes that support replication of the chromosomes of the host cell. The proofreading capability of these reactions and the slow molecular evolution of the hosts suggest a priori a very low rate of nucleotide exchanges in papillomavirus genomes. As a consequence, the nucleotide sequence of papillomaviruses does not rapidly evolve as is typical for RNA viruses. This statement is based mainly on genomic sampling of natural papillomavirus isolates, as discussed below. The change in viral genomes over short periods, e.g., days to a few years, is studied for many viruses in the laboratory by repeated infections of cell cultures or laboratory animals and subsequent genomic and biological characterization of the newly replicated viral genomes. Unfortunately, there are only a few laboratory systems for papillomavirus growth, and none of these is widely used. Successful infection and amplification of human papillomaviruses in cell culture remained restricted to a few laboratories (Meyers et al., 1997). In the 1980s, there was extensive research on the maintenance of bovine papillomavirus type 1 in mouse fibroblasts, involving amplification and maintenance of the viral genome but not virus production (Sarver et al., 1981). The only papillomavirus well studied in laboratory animal infection experiments is cottontail rabbit papillomavirus (Jeckel et al., 2002). While none of these experimental systems aimed specifically at studying papillomavirus evolution, there was never any observation of obvious genomic alterations. While this statement is based on fortuitous observations, it suggests that papillomavirus genomes are not exposed to substantial rates of nucleotide exchanges over periods of days to a few years.

DIVERSIFICATION OF PAPILLOMAVIRUSES IN HUMANS SINCE THE EMERGENCE OF *HOMO SAPIENS*

A large number of epidemiological studies have compared the medically important human papillomavirus types throughout the world (reviewed by Bernard et al. [2006]), beginning with seminal reports in 1993 that the cancer-associated types HPV-16 and HPV-18 can be isolated in all geographic locations and all human groups with largely the same nucleotide sequence. Surprisingly, however, there are minor variations (up to 2% of the nucleotide sequence) of each virus type that conspicuously cluster in specific geographic regions and specific ethnic groups (Ho et al., 1993). The most compelling interpretation of these findings is a model that all human papillomavirus types existed in humans from the very beginning of our species, i.e., about 100,000 years ago, with sequences nearly identical to those of extant papillomaviruses. They possibly spread and evolved in linkage with the ethnic groups as these settled the world, and during this process they developed geographic clusters of variants of all papillomavirus types. Papillomavirus genomes apparently change by only 1 to 2% of their nucleotide sequence over periods ranging from a few tens of thousands to a few hundreds of thousands of years, or maximally 10^{-7} per nucleotide per year. A more precise and even lower rate of evolution of about 10^{-8} nucleotide change per year was calculated from the linked evolution of papillomaviruses with various feline hosts (see below and Rector et al. [2007]).

ANCIENT DIVERSITY OF PAPILLOMAVIRUSES IN HUMANS

Humans are presently known to carry at least 125 different human papillomavirus types, i.e., virus genomes differing by more than 10% from one another. In phylogenetic trees, these 125 human papillomaviruses form minor and major clusters that, under present taxonomic rules, are identified as "species" and "genera." On the higher taxonomic level of the genus, the human papillomaviruses belong to five remotely related genera, *Alphapapillomavirus, Betapapillomavirus, Gammapapillomavirus, Mupapillomavirus,* and *Nupapillomavirus*. From what was just said about the generation of variants of each type, it must be concluded that the evolution of human papillomavirus species and genera occurred over an even longer timescale than 100,000 years. Estimates based on the linked evolution of papillomaviruses with their hosts, discussed in the next paragraph, lead to the assumption that the 125 different types of human papillomaviruses separated several tens of millions of years ago. It has to be concluded that humans and our primate ancestors were always infected with these five lineages (genera) of papillomaviruses and that it took millions of years to establish the intrahost diversity of the 125 types and of yet unknown but probably countless relatives in all primate species.

THE TAXONOMIC DIVERSITY OF PAPILLOMAVIRUSES IS SHAPED BY LINKED EVOLUTION OF THE VIRUS WITH THE HOST SPECIES

Papillomaviruses have been detected in all carefully examined vertebrate species, and always in the form of new types that were substantially (i.e., in much more than 10% of their nucleotide sequence) different from all previously identified types. Each papillomavirus type was found to be specific for each host species. The sole exception involves some papillomaviruses from hoofed animals (ungulates) that were apparently transferred due to close physical contact between different ungulate species on farms. No papillomavirus was ever found in more than one free-living host species, and host species and papillomavirus types are clearly closely linked. Interestingly, papillomaviruses of related animal host species (e.g., primates, cats, and rodents) are often related to one another in spite of their significant diversity. Examples are (i) clusters of related macaque papillomaviruses that all belong to the alphapapillomaviruses, which otherwise contain only human and ape papillomaviruses (Chan et al., 1997); (ii) the genus *Deltapapillomavirus,* which consists of isolates from remotely related ungulates such as cattle, various species of deer, and sheep (de Villiers et al., 2004); and (iii) papillomaviruses from cats as diverse as lynxes, lions, and snow leopards (Rector et al., 2007). From this correlation, one concludes that the linkages between papillomaviruses and their hosts are apparently not random but the outcome of a continuous process, a linked evolution of the virus and the host over millions of years. Whether this process was based on molecular barriers or just on the most likely infectious pathways has never been studied. The most extreme examples of papillomavirus-host linkage are the three and two papillomaviruses which have so far been identified in birds and reptiles, respectively, and which form phylogenetic outgroups to all mammalian papillomaviruses and to one another. As the evolutionary pathway leading to the extant reptiles, birds, and mammals split more than 100 million years ago, one has to conclude that the principal organization of the papillomavirus genome, namely, a gene sequence as shown for HPV-16 (Fig. 1) is as ancient as these phylogenetic splits.

OVERALL STABILITY OF THE ORGANIZATION OF PAPILLOMAVIRUS GENOMES

The phylogenetic interpretations listed above were based on nucleotide alignments, most often of the L1 genes. In intertype comparisons, L1 genes as well as L2, E1, and E2 genes can be readily aligned as they contain a high fraction of conserved sequence motifs, and insertions and deletions between these sequences are small (for alignments of papillomavirus sequences, see Farmer et al. [1995] and the related website http://www.stdgen.lanl.gov). Not only are sequence motifs within these four genes highly conserved, but so is the relative arrangement of the genes themselves, which is the same in all 189 known papillomavirus genomes (see, for example, Fig. 3 in

Fauquet et al. [2005]). The molecular strategies encoded in the replication initiator E1, the transcription/replication regulator E2, the major capsid protein L1, and the minor capsid protein L2, with its important role in the infection process (Sapp and Day, 2009), are apparently very successful and indispensable to the papillomavirus life cycle. This restriction may not apply to the transforming proteins E5, E6, and E7, although they are so central to the carcinogenic process induced by HPV-16 and HPV-18. The majority of papillomaviruses have these genes, but one or two of the genes are lacking in many animal (see, e.g., Jackson et al. [1991]) and even three human (Chen et al., 2007) papillomavirus types. Whenever E6 or E7 is absent, it is likely that it has been lost from these papillomaviruses rather than gained by all others, because the reptile papillomaviruses, likely representing the most ancestral genomes, have both genes (Herbst et al., 2009).

On a yet older evolutionary level, the replication initiator contains a helicase motif that is shared with replication proteins of several unrelated viruses including the polyomaviruses (Clertant and Seif, 1984; Rebrikov et al., 2002). The most likely interpretation of this finding is the existence of a replication protein, possibly going back all the way to the origin of life, that remained conserved while genes assembled around it to give rise to diverse groups of viruses.

MEDICAL CONSIDERATIONS EMERGING FROM THE LOW PLASTICITY OF PAPILLOMAVIRUS GENOMES

The stability of papillomavirus genomes has been useful for the design of DNA diagnostic tests for cervical cancer. For the last 60 years, cervical cancer and its precursors have been diagnosed by a cytological staining procedure called the Pap smear. This diagnosis has been very important for public health, as it has helped to detect and remove cancer precursors in millions of women. In spite of this positive role, it is now increasingly amended and may in the future even be replaced by more powerful DNA diagnostic procedures, such as the Hybridcapture test. Such a development would be unthinkable if papillomavirus genomes readily mutated.

The genomic stability of papillomaviruses was also a prerequisite to development of the prophylactic vaccines Gardasil and Cervarix against infection with HPV-16 and HPV-18, which have sometimes been heralded as vaccinations against cervical cancer. The stability of the HPV-16 and HPV-18 genomes makes it unlikely that new viral variants will emerge in response to vaccination. Since mutations are extremely rare events, it is hard to see how mutants that would modify the immunological properties of these infectious agents could be generated. As an alternative possibility, it has been speculated whether suppression of papillomavirus infections as a consequence of the immunization campaign targeting HPV-16 and HPV-18 may open an avenue for more frequent infections by other carcinogenic papillomavirus types (e.g. HPV-31, HPV-33, and HPV-35), which are currently rare. While this possibility cannot be completely excluded, it appears unlikely, as there is no evidence that papillomaviruses compete with one another, and consequently the elimination of one papillomavirus type does not open an "ecological" niche for another virus that did not exist previously.

There are important aspects of the epidemic and endemic spread of papillomavirus infections that are yet poorly understood: Does the rich reservoir of pathogenically similar papillomaviruses, including variants of the same type, lead to independent epidemics? Such a scenario could resemble the frequent infection of humans with the more than 100 serotypes of rhinoviruses, although the affected individuals are immune to a variety of other rhinovirus strains from previous infections. It is quite conceivable that certain variants of HPV-16 that originated in the native American Indian population but are now common throughout Latin America explain the much higher incidence of anogenital cancer in this part of the world than in Europe or North America (Bernard et al., 2006).

REFERENCES

Bernard, H. U., I. E. Calleja-Macias, and S. T. Dunn. 2006. Genome variation of human papillomavirus types: phylogenetic and medical implications. *Int. J. Cancer* **118:**1071–1076.

Bernard, H. U., R. D. Burk, Z. Chen, K. van Doorslaer, M. van Ranst, H. zur Hausen, and E. M. de Villiers. 2010. Classification of papillomaviruses (PVs) based on 189 PV types and proposal of taxonomic amendments. *Virology* **401:**70–79.

Chan, S. Y., H. U. Bernard, M. Ratterree, T. A. Birkebak, A. J. Faras, and R. S. Ostrow. 1997. Genomic diversity and evolution of papillomaviruses in rhesus monkeys. *J. Virol.* **71:**4938–4943.

Chen, Z., M. Schiffman, R. Herrero, R. Desalle, and R. D. Burk. 2007. Human papillomavirus (HPV) types 101 and 103 isolated from cervicovaginal cells lack an E6 open reading frame (ORF) and are related to gamma-papillomaviruses. *Virology* **360:**447–453.

Clertant, P., and I. Seif. 1984. A common function for polyoma virus large-T and papillomavirus E1 proteins? *Nature* **311:**276–279.

de Villiers, E. M., C. Fauquet, T. R. Broker, H. U. Bernard, and H. zur Hausen. 2004. Classification of papillomaviruses. *Virology* **324:**17–27.

Farmer, A. D., C. E. Calef, K. Millman, and G. L. Myers. 1995. The human papillomavirus database. *J. Biomed. Sci.* **2:**90–104. http://www.stdgen.lanl.gov.

Fauquet, C. M., M. A. Mayo, J. Maniloff, U. Desselberger, and L. A. Ball (ed.). 2005. *Virus Taxonomy: Eighth Report of the International Committee on Taxonomy of Viruses*, p. 239–255. Academic Press, New York, NY.

Herbst, L. H., J. Lenz, K. Van Doorslaer, Z. Chen, B. A. Stacy, J. F. Wellehan, C. A. Manire, and R. D. Burk. 2009. Genomic characterization of two novel reptilian papillomaviruses, Chelonia mydas papillomavirus 1 and Caretta caretta papillomavirus 1. *Virology* **383:**131–135.

Ho, L., S. Y. Chan, R. D. Burk, B. C. Das, K. Fujinaga, J. P. Icenogle, T. Kahn, N. Kiviat, W. Lancaster, P. Mavromara, V. Labropoulou, S. Mitrani-Rosenbaum, B. Norrild, M. R. Pillai, J. Stoerker, K. Syrjaenen, S. Syrjaenen, S. K. Tay, L. L. Villa, C. M. Wheeler, A. L. Williamson and H. U. Bernard. 1993. The genetic drift of human papillomavirus type 16 is a means of reconstructing prehistoric viral spread and movement of ancient human populations. *J. Virol.* **67:**6413–6423.

Jackson, M. E., W. D. Pennie, R. E. McCaffery, K. T. Smith, G. J. Grindlay, and M. S. Campo. 1991. The B subgroup bovine papillomaviruses lack an identifiable E6 open reading frame. *Mol. Carcinog.* **4:**382–387.

Jeckel, S., E. Huber, F. Stubenrauch, and T. Iftner. 2002. A transactivator function of cottontail rabbit papillomavirus e2 is essential for tumor induction in rabbits. *J. Virol.* **76:**11209–11215.

Meyers, C., T. J. Mayer, and M. A. Ozbun. 1997. Synthesis of infectious human papillomavirus type 18 in differentiating epithelium transfected with viral DNA. *J. Virol.* **71:**7381–7386.

Rebrikov, D. V., E. A. Bogdanova, M. E. Bulina, and S. A. Lukyanov. 2002. A new planarian extrachromosomal virus-like element revealed by subtractive hybridization. *Mol. Biol.* **36:**813–820.

Rector, A., P. Lemey, R. Tachezy, S. Mostmans, S. J. Ghim, K. Van Doorslaer, M. Roelke, M. Bush, R. J. Montali, J. Joslin, R. D. Burk, A. B. Jenson, J. P. Sundberg, B. Shapiro, and M. Van Ranst. 2007. Ancient papillomavirus-host cospeciation in Felidae. *Genome Biol.* **8:**R57.

Sapp, M., and P. M. Day. 2009. Structure, attachment and entry of polyoma- and papillomaviruses. *Virology* **384:**400–409.

Sarver, N., P. Gruss, M. F. Law, G. Khoury, and P. M. Howley. 1981. Bovine papilloma virus deoxyribonucleic acid: a novel eucaryotic cloning vector. *Mol. Cell. Biol.* **1:**486–496.

zur Hausen, H. 2002. Papillomaviruses and cancer: from basic studies to clinical application. *Nat. Rev. Cancer* **2:**342–350.

GENOME PLASTICITY OF HERPESVIRUSES: CONSERVATIVE YET FLEXIBLE

Mirko Trilling, Vu Thuy Khanh Le, and Hartmut Hengel

15

AN INTRODUCTION TO HERPESVIRUSES AND THEIR LIFESTYLE

Herpesviruses represent a particular successful family of viral pathogens shaped during vertebrate evolution. They are found in the large majority of vertebrate host species, and many hosts harbor multiple members of the herpesvirus family. Due to their ability to achieve latency, herpesvirus genomes are carried for the entire lifetime of the infected host. Extrapolations of evolutionary rates suggested that the common ancestor of all herpesviruses arose approximately 180 million to 220 million years ago (McGeoch et al., 1995), indicating that herpesviruses and their natural hosts share a very long history of reciprocal coevolution and cospeciation. Herpesvirus virions contain a double-stranded DNA (dsDNA) genome of 108 kbp (bovine herpesvirus 4) to 248.5 kbp (anguillid herpesvirus 1) (Table 1) in length. To date, eight different human herpesviruses (HHV) are known (listed in Table 2). Among human-pathogenic herpesviruses, human cytomegalovirus (HCMV) has the longest genome at ~230 kbp. The viral genome is embedded in three characteristic structures: the icosahedral capsid, the proteinaceous tegument, and the membrane envelope, constituting the virion of ca. 120 to 260 nm (a model of a herpesvirus particle is shown in Fig. 1). The virion is a highly complex assembly built from at least 58 viral proteins as determined for the mouse cytomegalovirus (Kattenhorn et al., 2004), the viral DNA genome, and additional viral RNAs (Bresnahan and Shenk, 2000). Importantly, selected host proteins (such as actin, annexin, CD55, and CD59) become "deliberately" incorporated into herpesvirus particles as well (Baldick and Shenk, 1996; Kattenhorn et al., 2004; Michelson et al., 1996; Spear et al., 1995; Varnum et al., 2004; Wright et al., 1995).

Based on virion morphology criteria, herpesviruses have been found in a variety of vertebrate classes, such as mammals, reptiles, fish, and birds, and even in invertebrates such as oysters (Davison et al., 2005; Farley et al., 1972). Herpesviruses are subdivided into the alpha-, beta-, and gammaherpesvirus subfamilies based on their pathogenesis, tissue and cell tropism, duration of viral replication cycle, and DNA sequence relatedness. This subdivision matches

Mirko Trilling, Vu Thuy Khanh Le and Hartmut Hengel, Institute for Virology, Heinrich-Heine-University, Düsseldorf, Germany.

Genome Plasticity and Infectious Diseases,
Edited by J. Hacker, U. Dobrindt, and R. Kurth,

TABLE 1 Selection of herpesviruses of nonhuman primates, mammals, birds, and fish

Designation	Abbreviation	Vernacular name (synonyms)	Subfamily and genus	% G+C	Genome size (kbp)
Cercopithecine herpesvirus 8 (macacine herpesvirus 3)	Ce-HV-6	Rhesus monkey CMV	β	49	221
Pongine herpesvirus 4 (panine herpesvirus 2)	PoHV-4	Chimpanzee CMV	β	62	241
Bovine herpesvirus 4	BoHV-4	Movar herpesvirus	γ	41	109
Murid herpesvirus 1	MuHV-1	Mouse CMV	β	59	235
Murid herpesvirus 4	MuHV-4	Murine gamma herpesvirus 68	γ	47	135
Suid herpesvirus 1	SuHV-1	Pseudorabies virus, Aujeszky disease virus	α	74	143
Gallid herpesvirus 2	GaHV-2	Marek's disease virus 1	α	47	180
Anguillid herpesvirus 1	AngHV-1	Japanese eel herpesvirus		53	248.5

genome-based phylogenetic analysis as visualized by sequence alignment in a phylogenetic tree of the herpesvirus DNA polymerase protein sequences (Fig. 2). A systematic taxonomy of herpesviruses has recently been presented (Davison, 2010). A general feature of herpesviruses is the establishment of latent infection as a molecularly defined state of infection in distinct target cells of the natural host. The concerted action of all branches of the immune system is required to control viral replication without achieving true sterile immunity. Combined depletion of defined branches of the immune system (e.g., T-cell subsets, NK cells, B cells, and gamma interferon) leads to rapid reactivation of virus production from latent herpesvirus genomes (Polic et al., 1998). Therefore, an immune serostatus implies not only preceding infection of the host but also the invariable presence of replication-competent latent herpesvirus genomes. For mammalian herpesviruses it has been shown that reactivation of latent genomes is initiated in response to various stress stimuli and/or immunocompromising conditions. Although differing considerably among the known human herpesviruses, seroprevalence is mostly very high, indicating rates of infection between 60 and 90% for the

TABLE 2 Herpesviruses of humans

Designation	Abbreviation	Vernacular name (synonyms)	Subfamily and genus	% G+C	Genome size (kbp)
Human herpesvirus 1	HHV-1	Herpes simplex virus 1	α	68.3	152
Human herpesvirus 2	HHV-2	Herpes simplex virus 2	α	70	155
Human herpesvirus 3	HHV-3	Varicella-zoster virus	α	45	125
Human herpesvirus 4	HHV-4	Epstein-Barr virus	γ	60	172/184
Human herpesvirus 5	HHV-5	Cytomegalovirus	β	57	236
Human herpesvirus 6A	HHV-6A	HHV-6 variant A	β	43	159/170
Human herpesvirus 6B	HHV-6B	HHV-6 variant B	β	43	162/168
Human herpesvirus 7	HHV-7		β	36	145
Human herpesvirus 8	HHV-8	Kaposi's sarcoma-associated herpesvirus	γ	59	170/210

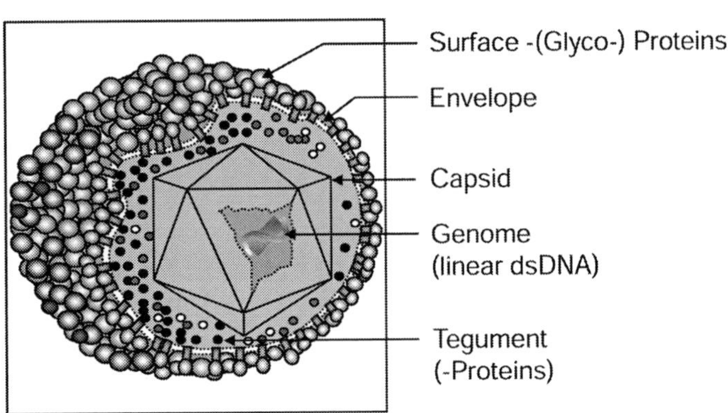

FIGURE 1 Model of herpesvirus virion morphology. The linear dsDNA genome is enclosed in the icosahedral capsid, which is surrounded by the proteinaceous tegument and embedded in the membrane envelope derived from the host cell. The virion membrane contains several virus-encoded as well as host-derived transmembrane proteins.

majority of herpesviruses (e.g., Epstein-Barr virus [EBV], varicella-zoster virus [VZV], herpes simplex virus type 1 [HSV-1], and HCMV) in adults (Wrensch et al., 2001). Therefore, the majority of humans are coinfected and harbor several herpesvirus genomes. By definition, latent infections are not apparent, but upon reactivation of productive infection, life-threatening disease complications may occur. While immuocompromised individuals have a strong disposition to overt disease, herpesvirus infections can have fatal outcomes even in apparently healthy immunocompetent individuals (Rafailidis et al., 2008; Rustgi et al., 1983). In addition, some gammaherpesviruses, like EBV and human herpesvirus 8 (HHV-8)/Kaposi's sarcoma-associated herpesvirus (KSHV), can cause malignant tumors.

PRODUCTIVE VERSUS LATENT HERPESVIRUS INFECTION

Herpesviruses are the only known viruses capable of deploying two separate transcriptional programs upon infection of a target cell: productive (and usually lytic) infection and latent infection. Most susceptible target cells are prone to productive genome replication during which all herpesvirus genes are expressed in a strict cascade order. The first transcripts become sufficiently induced by cellular transcription factors (a reason why herpesvirus genomes are infectious when transfected in permissive cells) and are termed immediate-early or α genes. The second wave of viral proteins requires induction and/or transactivation by immediate-early proteins, and the genes are called early or β genes. The last class of genes mostly encodes structural components of the next generation of viral particles. These genes are named late or γ genes. Late genes necessitate genome amplification by the viral DNA polymerase and are therefore significantly repressed in the presence of pharmacologic inhibitors of viral genome replication. Conversely, in specific target cells, herpesvirus infection results in latency, a nonlytic state of infection restricting viral gene expression to a very few transcripts avoiding any production of viral progeny but maintaining genetically intact DNA genomes. According to current concepts, the two states are mutually exclusive at the level of an individually infected cell but not at the level of the infected host organism. Latent infection can secondarily progress to virus production.

Latency, therefore, is one of the most fascinating autapomorphies of the *Herpesviridae*. This unique invention of two separate but linked viral states in infected cells leads to an increased transcriptional plasticity, allowing the establishment of lifelong genome persistence, and is likely to be one major reason for the evolutionary success of the herpesvirus bauplan. Since latently infected cells exist only in very small numbers in nature, the three known steps of genome latency (i.e., establishment, maintenance, and reactivation) (Wagner and Bloom, 1997) defy easy experimental analysis and are understood only at a rudimentary level. The viral genome remains sequestered in an episomal

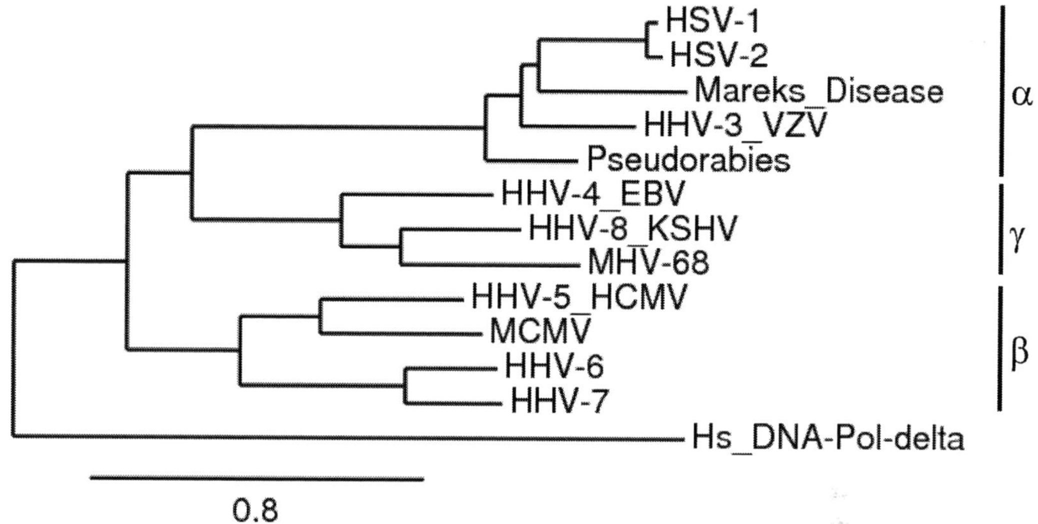

FIGURE 2 Phylogenetic tree based on alignment of the primary amino acid sequences of DNA polymerases of the indicated herpesviruses demonstrates a relationship between the eight human-pathogenic herpesviruses (HSV-1, HSV-2, VZV, EBV, HCMV, HHV-6, HHV-7, and KSHV) and relevant animal herpesviruses (i.e. Marek's disease virus, pseudorabies virus, MHV-68, and MCMV). The sequence of the *Homo sapiens* DNA polymerase delta serves as an outgroup. The alignment and phylogenetic tree were constructed using the www.phylogeny.fr online tool (Dereeper et al., 2008). The legend depicts the protein sequence divergence.

form in the nucleus of the latently infected cell. Although the copy number of latent genomes present in the nucleus is usually low, replication of the viral DNA might occur to maintain the genome in dividing cells. If the host experiences stressful conditions (typical stimuli are emotional stress, UV light, cortisol, and cytokines due to infections) which might impede the survival prospects of virus progeny, the herpesvirus genome can readily be reactivated and initiate a productive infection mode by switching the transcriptional program to give rise to a new generation of particles and to reach out for new hosts. The question if and how productively infected cells can revert to a latent state of infection is a matter of debate. An oversimplified model proposes that latency results from a failure to initiate an acute infection mode upon insufficient amounts of viral immediate-early proteins and/or tegument resident transactivator proteins (or their cellular counterparts) reaching the nucleus. Under these circumstances the herpesvirus starts to express a limited number of so-called latency-associated transcripts, including nontranslated RNAs (like EBERs of EBV) and microRNAs.

GENETIC FEATURES CONTRIBUTING TO THE PLASTICITY OF HERPESVIRUS GENOMES

This section explains leading genetic paradigms combined with selected findings from certain herpesviruses, to put the most important principles of herpesvirus genome plasticity and also their limitations into a broader perspective.

Genome Length

Genomes of herpesvirus family members vary significantly in size from relatively small (e.g., VZV, about 125 kbp) to relatively large (e.g., CMVs, about 230 kbp) (Tables 1 and 2). Interestingly, some herpesviruses rapidly delete or mutate particular gene regions during repetitive cell culture passaging, as demonstrated by the HCMV laboratory strains HCMV-AD169 and HCMV-Towne, which have lost approx. 15 and 13 kbp, respectively (corresponding to about 20 and 15 open reading frames [ORFs], respectively) of the unique long (UL) region during continuous passage in fibroblasts without severely affecting the overall genome length (Fig. 3). These strains harbor a large duplication of the terminal repeat long (TRL) region, which is subsequently assigned as internal repeat long (IRL) region (Cha et al., 1996). Presumably, optimal genome length has to be maintained in a narrow range since DNA cleavage at the *cis*-acting packaging signals is suppressed until a "headful" (i.e., capsidful) amount of the genome has entered the capsid (Cockrell et al., 2009). Longer or shorter genomes would lead to packaging of mutated genomes containing deletions and duplications, respectively. Accordingly, it has been found for guinea pig CMV that the genome has to be retained within a range of +8.8 kbp, otherwise the mutant reacts with eventual deletions to readjust the appropriate genome size (Cui et al., 2009) suggesting that upper boundaries exist for herpesvirus genome length. The lower boundaries seem to be more flexible, since it has been described that mouse CMV (MCMV) tolerates the deletion of 32 genes, equal to 31.3 kbp of genomic sequence (Cicin-Sain et al., 2007). As discussed by Roizman (1980), the variations in herpesvirus genome length, together with the almost identical capsid size of all herpesviruses, lead to a conundrum. The question arises whether all herpesviruses are in principle capable of packing genomes of the maximal length (i.e., HCMV DNA of ~230 kbp) or if CMVs have evolved additional mechanisms to optimize packaging efficiency.

Base Composition

The G+C versus A+T content of herpesviral genomes varies significantly among different herpesviruses, even between alphaherpesvirus subfamily members, which share similar pathobiology and a concordant genome organization: VZV has a low G+C content (~46%), whereas HSV-1 has a high G+C content of approximately 68% (Tables 1 and 2). This difference is reflected not by an overall change in amino acid composition of homologous proteins, but by a changed codon usage due to a significant shift of the G+C content in the third wobble codon site (Schachtel et al., 1991). This difference raises the apparent question concerning the causative selective pressure leading to such discrepancies in codon usage and G+C content. This enigma has been widely discussed but is probably unfeasible for experimental analysis. Genomes with a high G+C content seem to be overrepresented in the alphaherpesvirus subfamily. It was speculated that the selective pressure driving this high G+C content might result from an intrinsic protection mechanism directed against insertion of L1 retrotransposons, which are known to favor AT-rich sequences for insertion (Brown et al., 2007). For EBV, another observation has been made concerning the G+C content in the third codon site: the G+C content is significantly lower in latency-associated genes than in genes expressed during lytic EBV infection. This can be explained on the basis of differences in mutation rates, different selection pressure between latency and productive infection, or even a different origin of these two classes of genes (Karlin et al., 1990).

For murine gammaherpesvirus 68 (MHV-68), it has been shown that the G+C content varies between the unique portion of the

FIGURE 3 Comparative genomic organization and gene content of prototypic human herpesviruses, herpes simplex virus (top), human cytomegalovirus clinical isolates and laboratory strain AD169 (middle), and Epstein-Barr virus (bottom). For more detailed descriptions, see the text. *a* and *b* depict repetitive sequences of the L-terminal *a* sequence (a_L) or the S-terminal sequence (a_S) and the L-terminal *b* sequence, respectively, and their inverted repeats *(a′* and *b′)* with zero to several *(n)* or one to several *(m)* copies. Additionally, the *c* sequence and the inverted repeat *c′* are shown. *b* and *b′* are synonymous with *TRL* and *IRL*, respectively, and *c* and *c′* are synonymous with *TRS* and *IRS*, respectively. Abbreviations: *TRL*, terminal repeat long; *IRL*, internal repeat long; *IRS*, internal repeat short; *TRS*, terminal repeat short; *UL*, unique long gene segment; *US*, unique short gene segment; *TR*, terminal direct repeat; *IR*, internal direct repeat; *oriLyt*, origin of lytic replication; *oriLyt* (L), origin of lytic replication in L component *(UL); oriLyt*(S1/2), origin of lytic replication in the S component *(TRS/IRS); oriP*, origin of plasmid replication; MIEP, major immediate-early promoter.

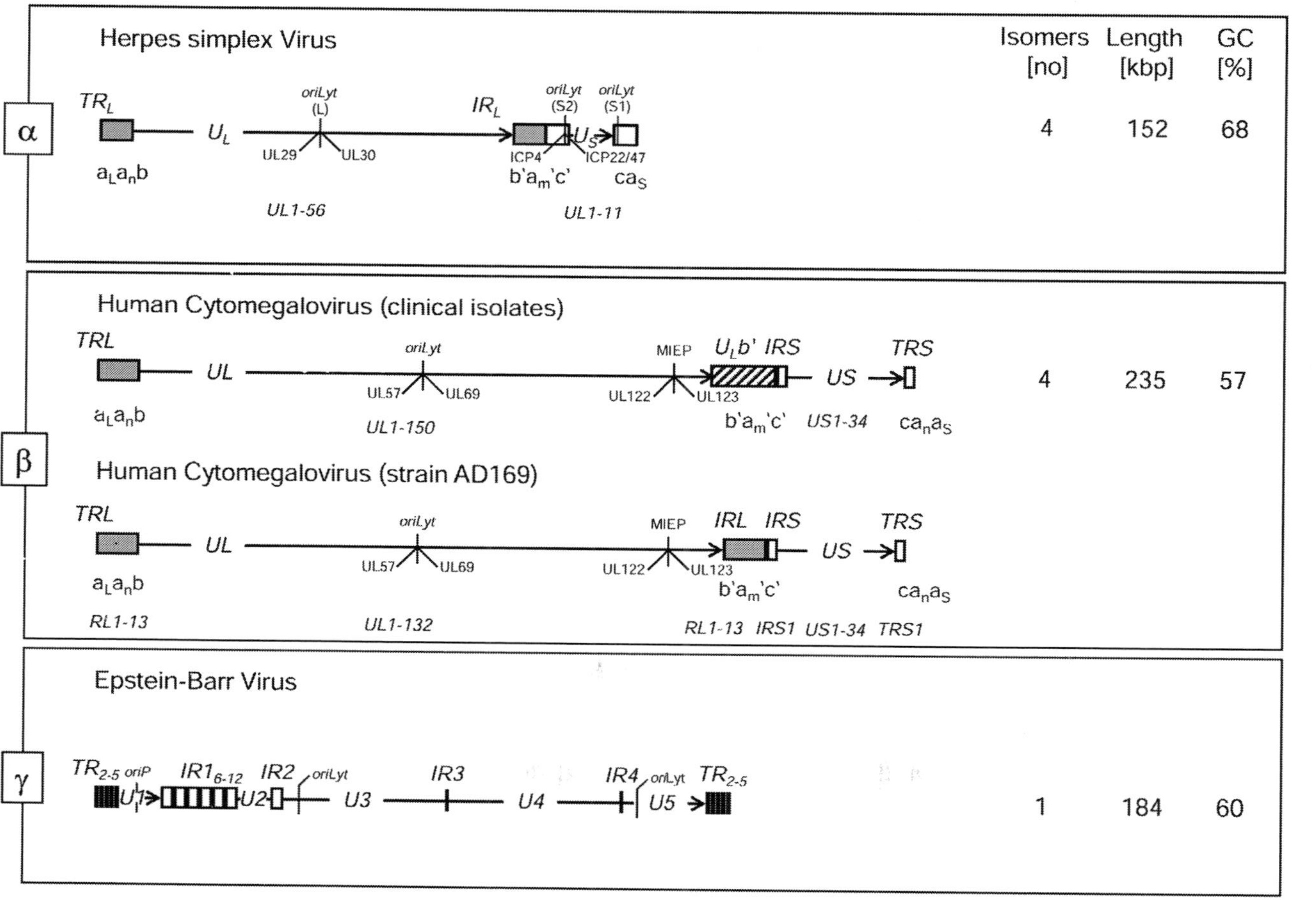

α
Herpes simplex Virus
Isomers [no]
Length [kbp]
GC [%]
TR_L
U_L
oriLyt (L)
UL29
UL30
IR_L
oriLyt (S2)
oriLyt (S1)
U_S
ICP4
ICP22/47
a_La_nb
b'a_m'c'
ca_S
UL1-56
UL1-11
4
152
68
β
Human Cytomegalovirus (clinical isolates)
TRL
UL
oriLyt
UL57
UL69
MIEP
UL122
UL123
U_Lb' IRS
US
TRS
a_La_nb
UL1-150
b'a_m'c'
US1-34
ca_na_S
4
235
57
Human Cytomegalovirus (strain AD169)
TRL
UL
oriLyt
UL57
UL69
MIEP
UL122
UL123
IRL IRS
US
TRS
a_La_nb
b'a_m'c'
ca_na_S
RL1-13
UL1-132
RL1-13 IRS1 US1-34 TRS1
γ
Epstein-Barr Virus
TR_{2-5} oriP
U_1
$IR1_{6-12}$
U2
IR2
oriLyt
U3
IR3
U4
IR4
oriLyt
U5
TR_{2-5}
1
184
60

genome (G+C content of ~46%) and the terminal repeats (G+C content of ~78%) (Virgin et al., 1997). The discrepancy between the G+C content of the unique regions and the terminal repeats also seems to be present in other gammaherpesviruses like HHV-8 (~53.5% in the unique region versus ~84.5% in terminal repeats) (Russo et al., 1996), again highlighting differential mutation rates in individual genome regions.

Herpesvirus DNA Repair and Proofreading

Herpesviruses are equipped with virus-encoded DNA repair proteins and additionally recruit elements of the host-derived DNA repair machinery to preserve their genome integrity. With this machinery, herpesviruses can control the mutation rate of their genomes—at least to a certain degree—on their own. Herpesviral DNA polymerases have an intrinsic 3′-5′ exonuclease activity leading to proofreading to ensure high fidelity when synthesizing the DNA genome (Boehmer and Lehman, 1997). The HSV-1 polymerase (pUL30) also exhibits apurinic/apyrimidinic and 5′-deoxyribosephosphate lyase activity (Bogani and Boehmer, 2008). Moreover, herpesviruses express uracil DNA glycosylases (pUL2 in HSV-1 and HSV-2; homologous proteins can be found in a variety of herpesviruses), which excise the base after deamination of cytosine to uracil to avoid accidental conversion from CG to AT base pairs (Boehmer and Lehman, 1997). These features define a high degree of DNA sequence integrity on the one hand and sufficient genome plasticity on the other.

Episome versus Insertion

Particle resident herpesvirus genomes are long linear dsDNA molecules which are flanked by terminal inverted repeats (Fig. 3). The linear molecules circularize within the cell to allow DNA replication by a rolling-circle mechanism, leading to concatemeric genomes which are subsequently trimmed to the appropriate length. Herpesvirus genome replication occurs in the nucleus of the infected cell but usually does not lead to integration into the cellular chromosomes. Likewise, during latency, herpesvirus genomes remain episomal. Remarkably, for some herpesviruses integration into host chromosomes has been observed, as in Marek's disease virus, EBV, and HHV-6 (Arbuckle et al., 2010). Marek's disease virus is a herpesvirus which causes serious damage in the poultry industry. Interestingly, it regularly integrates into host chromosomes and can also be reactivated from these sites (Delecluse and Hammerschmidt, 1993; Delecluse et al., 1993). EBV is also able to integrate into the host chromosomes (Hurley et al., 1991; Lawrence et al., 1988). Integrated and episomal genomes coexist in individual cells (Delecluse and Hammerschmidt, 1993), and the sites of integration seems not to be randomly selected (Lestou et al., 1993). In the past such integration events have been considered sporadic and anecdotal events, but recent findings suggest that the frequency of HHV-6 integration is in the range of up to 1% of the global population (Morissette and Flamand, 2010), and genome-integrated HHV-6 can be transmitted even along the germ line (Arbuckle et al., 2010). Therefore, it is tempting to speculate that the integration site might affect neighboring host genes and might change the viral life cycle in individual cells.

Molecular Piracy: Acquisition and Integration of Host Genes

As pointed out above, herpesviruses have an intimately shared evolutionary history with their hosts and are thus highly adapted to one particular host species and perhaps to isolated subpopulations thereof. As observed in other DNA viruses like the *Poxviridae,* herpesviruses seem to steal genes from their host species and use them for their own purposes, a strategy called molecular piracy. One prominent example is the expression of virus-encoded interleukin-10 (IL-10) homologs by HCMV and EBV. HCMV even expresses two different cmvIL-10 transcripts, one being expressed during latency (Jenkins et al., 2004). IL-10 is an effective immunosuppressive cytokine required to down-regulate overt immune responses and to avoid autoimmunity. Herpesviruses like EBV and HCMV seem to have acquired the genes directly from their hosts, since cmvIL-10 contains two introns which are homologous to the first and third introns of the human IL-10 gene, indicating that the sequences are indeed related (Kotenko et al., 2000). ebvIL-10 does not harbor any introns, suggesting that the two viruses acquired their IL-10 genes independently. Among herpesviruses, HHV-8 seems to be "the unchallenged master of molecular piracy" (Choi et al., 2001). HHV-8 expresses multiple proteins with homologies to immune factors, including complement binding proteins (ORF 4), an IL-6-like cytokine (ORF K2), three chemokines (ORFs K4, K4.1, and K6), a bcl-2 homolog (ORF 16), homologs to interferon regulatory factors (ORF K9), a vCyclin (ORF 72), and a FLICE-inhibitory protein (ORF K13) (reviewed by Choi et al. [2001]).

Herpesvirus MicroRNAs

MicroRNAs are small noncoding RNAs which are capable of modulating posttranscriptional gene expression through both inhibition of translation and regulation of mRNA stability by short stretches of complementary Watson-Crick pairing to respective target mRNAs, frequently within the 3′ untranslated region (Baek et al., 2008; Grimson et al., 2007; Selbach et al., 2008). Recently, it has become evident that herpesviruses (among other virus families) express a virus-specific set of microRNAs (Pfeffer et al., 2004, 2005) which are capable of affecting the transcription of viral as well as host genes (Stern-Ginossar et al., 2007) and significantly affecting viral replication in specific tissues (Dolken et al., 2010). Unfortunately, only a few studies concerning the inter- and intraspecies conservation of herpesviral microRNAs have been conducted. Two recent studies compared the virus-encoded microRNAs of HSV-1 and HSV-2, which share nine positional and/or sequence microRNA homologs. The sequence conservation was quite diverse between individual microRNA pairs, ranging from 52% to 74% (including changes in the seed region) to an astonishing 91% for miR-H7 (Jurak et al., 2010; Umbach et al., 2010). Interestingly, especially in the seed region (the major determinant for target specificity), a high degree of identity was found and interpreted as a hint for conservation of the microRNA targets (Jurak et al., 2010). In a new deep-sequencing study focusing on four different gallid and meleagrid herpesviruses, it was found that these viruses share the loci but not the sequence of the microRNAs. None of the microRNAs detected was homologous to any microRNAs of other herpesviruses, indicating a high degree of variability of microRNA sequences (Waidner et al., 2009). The authors found the majority of microRNA loci within the repeated *IRL/TRL* and the *IRS/TRS* regions (Waidner et al., 2009), which exhibit higher mutation rates than the unique sequences (see below). Consistently, Umbach and colleagues found HSV-encoded microRNAs in a deep-sequencing approach to be located within the *IRS/IRL* region (Umbach et al., 2009) while in MCMV a cluster of microRNA genes was found in the *m01* gene region at the border of the viral genome (Dolken et al., 2007). Such a biased distribution of microRNA-coding regions contrasts with the widely distributed HCMV gene regions encoding microRNAs (Stern-Ginossar et al., 2009).

Isomerization of Herpesvirus Genomes

Herpesvirus genomes contain both unique and repeated sequences (Fig. 3). The genomes of HSV, VZV, and HCMV are binary covalently linked compositions of unique long (UL) and unique short (US) regions which are surrounded by internal and terminal repeated regions, *IRL/TRL* and *IRS/TRS*, respectively (Fig. 3). It has been shown that the orientation of the unique regions with respect to each other is variable, leading to four different isomers (Delius and Clements, 1976; Hayward et al., 1975). For HSV and HCMV, the abundance of all four isomers is similar and experiments with genetically arrested isomer mutants indicate that all forms are infectious and have to be considered functionally equivalent (Jenkins and Roizman, 1986). It is not known whether individual isomeric forms have growth advantages under certain in vivo conditions. The isomerization seems to be temporally linked with the concatemerization, indicating that the rearrangement occurs during (or briefly after) the rolling-circle replication (McVoy and Adler, 1994). Studies using bacterial artificial chromosome plasmid (BACmid)-derived virus genomes show that clonal genomes undergo rapid reisomerization when infectious HCMV is reconstituted from BACmid DNA (Borst et al., 1999). The insertion of an additional *IRL*- and *IRS*-containing *UL-US* junction sequence leads to a complex pattern of rearrangements when the inserted sequences are in inverted orientation to the original viral sequences (Mocarski et al., 1980). The inversion machinery requires seven viral proteins, i.e., the minimal set of viral DNA synthesis enzymes, to allow inversion of foreign nonherpesvirus sequences like transposons (Weber et al., 1988). These findings raise the question of whether herpesvirus-infected cells are prone to genomic rearrangements between inverted, homologous, or repeated regions of the host chromosomes due to the nuclear presence of such a herpesviral recombination machinery.

Some closely related herpesviruses with colinear genomes do not share a similar *UL/US* genome organization and isomerizations: HCMV shows isomeric genome organization, but the related MCMV does not. Internal insertion of a sequence containing both terminal repeats into the MCMV genome induces the rearrangement of the genome, leading to four equimolar isomers (McVoy and Ramnarain, 2000). This indicates that the machinery supporting the inversion is either fully conserved by MCMV or can be complemented by host-derived factors. For VZV it has been shown that the four isomers also occur, albeit with significantly biased likelihoods. The *UL* region is found in one predominant orientation (95 to 98%), whereas the *US* region is found in both orientations with equimolar concentrations (Kinchington et al., 1985). The minor *UL* inversion is not due to an inefficient rearrangement machinery, since superinfection with HSV or pseudorabies virus does not induce additional *UL* isomerization (Hayakawa and Hyman, 1987). EBV does not have inverted repeat regions and shows no isomerization, but it contains four additional classes of direct internal repeats (*IR1* through *IR4*), which subdivide the linear genome into five unique stretches (*U1* through *U5*) (Fig. 3). The whole genome is flanked by two to five 0.5-kbp variable terminal direct repeats (TR) (Cheung and Kieff, 1982). The homogeneity or heterogeneity of the *TR* regions allowed a determination of virus ancestry between different strains or isolates (Raab-Traub and Flynn, 1986).

IMPLICATIONS OF HERPESVIRUS PLASTICITY FOR CURRENT RESEARCH

Nonclonal Virus Preparations: Isolates, Strains, and Variants

Herpesvirus preparations grown in cell culture (i.e., wild isolates or laboratory strains) usually comprise a complex mixture of genetically diverse virus variants. A notable example is the VZV vaccine strain Oka-V, used to vaccinate against VZV diseases, i.e., varicella and herpes zoster. The originally patient-derived parental virus (Oka-P) was attenuated by serial passages in human embryo lung cells and guinea pig embryo fibroblast cell cultures at low temperature. It was further plaque purified, but after expansion, development, and final preparation of the variants it was still not clonal (Tillieux et al., 2008). In fact, Oka-V contains genetically distinct variants, which became apparent during sequencing of the immediate-early gene *ORF 62* and the entire Oka genome(s) (Gomi et al., 2000, 2002). As a consequence of the genetic microheterogeneity, licensed vaccine preparations differ among different manufacturers, resulting in disparate vaccine effectiveness (Spackova et al., 2010). This clinical finding highlights the complex nature of herpesvirus preparations. Moreover, some herpesviruses, like MCMV, form infectious multicapsid particles containing multiple genomes (Chong and Mims, 1981; Hudson et al., 1976; Kurz et al., 1997), making it even more difficult to obtain clonal viruses from mixed source material. It is tempting to speculate that many herpesviruses acquired and actively maintain mutated genomes with different "alleles," particularly in gene regions which are under diverse and variable selection pressure in vivo to extend the herpesviral gene pool and improve flexible responses to specific but also variable selection pressure of the host population. Decreasing costs of DNA sequencing will hopefully allow future global sequence analysis and deep-sequencing approaches, thus revealing more information on herpesvirus genome diversity and its biological consequences. This should clarify whether primary infections are initiated with very few seeding virus genomes that diversify their gene pool over time or whether a few genomes become selected during replication from larger numbers of infecting genomes. A recent study indicates that in the majority of HCMV primary infections only one dominant virus strain—as defined by sequencing of four genes, two of which with pronounced sequence hypervariability—can be detected at various sites of virus shedding (Murthy et al., 2011).

During the last decade the genomes of almost all human-pathogenic and a variety of nonhuman herpesviruses have been cloned into BACmids, allowing fast, reproducible, and efficient genetic manipulation (Wagner et al., 2002). A problematic situation could arise from the fact that many laboratories have set up the BACmid-based technologies and label clonal viruses reconstituted from BACmids of wild-type viruses as "wt virus." The BACmid technology is based on a single clonal DNA copy which is derived from a BAC cassette insertion event into the viral genome. The resulting BACmid is than introduced into *Escherichia coli* and individual colonies are selected for genetic manipulation. Consequently, only one individual herpesvirus genome becomes the ancestor for all descending monoclonal viruses. Although this technology has become one of the most important inventions in herpesvirus genetics, allowing rapid and precise manipulation of the viral genome, it nevertheless might have unforeseen implications by strongly reducing the herpesvirus gene pool and create "nonplastic" situations, particularly when viruses are analyzed in vivo.

HOMOLOGOUS RECOMBINATION UPON COINFECTION

It is widely documented that the immune host can readily be superinfected by the same herpesvirus. Using an elegant genetic approach, Cicin-Sain et al. (2005) demonstrated that two different MCMV viruses, one expressing a *cre* recombinase expression cassette and the other carrying a green fluorescent protein (GFP) gene which was interrupted by a *floxP*-site-flanked stop cassette, can even coinfect the very same target cell in vivo. Upon coinfection of one cell, the *cre* recombinase removes the stop cassette within the sister MCMV genome and thereby activates expression of GFP, leading to genetically stable labeling of the viral progeny. A frequency of ~2% recombined GFP-positive viruses was observed, indicating an astonishingly high frequency of double infections of individual cells in vivo (Cicin-Sain et al., 2005). Earlier studies already indicated that simultaneous mixed inoculation of mice with two different avirulent HSV strains can generate deadly recombinants in vivo (Javier et al., 1986). Natural infections of patients confirm the presence of more than one genotype of a given herpesvirus, highlighting the potential impact of homologous recombination for pathogenesis in vivo. For HCMV, 8 of 10 stillborn infants who succumbed to a CMV infection harbored more than one HCMV genotype (differentiated based on *UL144* and *US28* polymorphisms), indicating that coinfections do play an important role for HCMV pathogenicity (Arav-Boger et al., 2002). Additionally, a minimal estimate of ~46% coinfections with different HCMV genotypes was assessed in AIDS patients (Baldanti et al., 1998) and confirmed in transplant recipients based on genotyping of *UL33* and *UL55*/gB (Deckers et al., 2009). From these observations the apparent question arises whether the human host acquires different HCMV variants mainly upon exposure to new HCMV genotypes or whether the viral variants evolve de novo in the infected individual as a result of diverse selection processes in vivo.

INTRASPECIES CONSERVATION VERSUS VARIATION OF HERPESVIRUS GENOMES

Herpesviruses have highly conserved genomes. For MCMV a mutation rate of ~1.4×10^{-7} per bp per day during in vitro cultivation and ~1×10^{-7} per bp per day after in vivo passage have been found (Cheng et al., 2010). Accordingly, unrelated individuals are shedding herpesviruses which differ with regard to their endonuclease restriction fragment pattern (Roizman and Tognon, 1983). Moreover, mobility shift heterogeneities of viral proteins as demonstrated in electrophoretic separation techniques confirmed that herpesviruses differ to some extent with respect to their genetic material (Pereira et al., 1976). Further biochemical methods allowed differentiation between variable herpesviral proteins and nonvariable host cell proteins based on electrophoretic migration patterns when comparing HCMV-encoded IgG-Fc receptors which display an obvious strain-dependent heterogeneity, reflecting their genetic plasticity (Atalay et al., 2002).

Notable variations in the herpesvirus genomes seem to be clustered in defined gene regions which are located outside of the conserved gene blocks encoding conserved core proteins often shared among many herpesvirus family members. Therefore, genetic variations are seemingly more frequent at the termini of the linear genomes affecting "nonessential" genes, which are dispensable for genome replication but involved in tissue tropism and immune modulation. Consistent with this notion, extensive sequence variations between different MCMV low-passage strains have been mapped to the termini (Smith et al., 2008) and the *m02* gene family in particular (*m02* through *m16*) (Corbett et al., 2007). In a global sequence comparison of four different isolates, the majority of the genes are identical between strains, and 151 of 190 coding regions have >98 % amino acid similarity. Nevertheless, variations do occur: the most variable regions have been found to be the left and right termini, namely, the sequences *m01* through *m19* and *m144* through *m170* (Smith et al., 2008). Astonishingly, even though located within the central part of the genome, distinct genes have been found to exhibit some variability (like *M55* and *m124*). The *m02*-through-*m16* gene region is not essential for MCMV replication in cell culture but is required for efficient replication in the presence of NK cells in vivo (Oliveira et al., 2002) and is also involved in the subversion of T-cell responses (Hengel et al., 1999). The variations do not affect the sequences coding for crucial protein domains like transmembrane domains, but mainly relate to the extracellular parts of the encoded glycoproteins arguing for shaping evolution. This might suggest that these potentially immune-evasive genes take part in an evolutionary arms race between the virus and the immune system and an increased likelihood to be altered is favored by the virus. Another straightforward interpretation would be that, due to alternating linearization and (re)circularization events during every infection cycle, the mutation rate is higher closer to this "resealable" region. One might speculate that herpesviruses make use of such effects and that genes which are under positive selection become located in these regions on purpose to gain higher mutation rates whereas the viral core genes are located in the more conservative central parts of the genome. Concordant with this idea, a clustering of nonessential genes at the termini of the genome has been observed in other CMVs such as HCMV (Yu et al., 2003). Other gene regions which might represent a hot spot for mutations are located at the junctions between the *UL* and the *RL* region, since here the isomerization indicates ongoing and frequent recombination events which presumably increase the likelihood of mutations due to imperfect recombination. Consistent with this notion, the comparison between the two HCMV strains HCMV-Towne and HCMV-AD169 has revealed a disruption of homology at the boundaries of *UL-IRL* and the junctions of *IRL-US* and *IRS-US*, respectively (Wang et al., 2009). A comparison of the HCMV-Toledo strain with strain AD169 also revealed increased divergence in genome fragments comprising the *UL-RL* boundaries (Brondke et al., 2007).

Nevertheless, even within defined HCMV gene regions, like the *ULb'* region, striking individual differences can be found. An alignment of protein sequences documents a high degree of conservation of pUL138, whereas the neighboring genes encoding pUL139 and pUL146 are markedly divergent (Fig. 4). Whether this difference is a consequence of differing high degrees of purifying selection due to unequal importance for current evolutionary success, depends on the multifunctional tasks of the variable proteins, or reflects the genetic plasticity of the relevant interaction partners in the host population is still unknown.

ADAPTIVE MUTATIONS IN HERPESVIRUSES AND MAINTENANCE OF VIRAL FITNESS IN VIVO

The adaptability of few "nonessential" herpesviral genes has been experimentally analyzed with respect to their consequences for pathogenesis, virulence, and viral fitness in the natural host. Analysis of MCMV pathogenesis and replication efficacy indicated that inbred mouse strains differ significantly with respect to their MCMV susceptibility. C57BL/6 mice are relatively resistant to MCMV, whereas BALB/c mice are more susceptible. This difference could be linked to the so called *cmv1* gene locus located on mouse chromosome 6, which maps to the NK cell complex (NKC). The resistance of C57BL/6 mice is due to the expression of the activating Ly49H NK cell receptor (Daniels et al., 2001; Dokun et al., 2001; Lee et al., 2001). Ly49H recognizes a viral determinant, the *m157*-encoded MHC-like glycoprotein, and thereby mediates NK cell activation, eliciting a very strong selective pressure against MCMV replication (Arase et al., 2002; Smith et al., 2002). Consistent with viral activation of host NK cells, the deletion of the *m157* gene from the MCMV genome by BACmid-based mutagenesis increased the virulence of the virus compared to the wt virus in Ly49H(+) mice (Bubic et al., 2004). After six sequential passages in resistant mice, five individual virus isolates were analyzed. Each of them showed a mutation leading to an abrogation of Ly49H activation either by DNA insertions or by deletions within the *m157* gene, allowing the mutated viruses to replicate in *cmv1*^{r} mice as efficiently as in BALB/c mice (Voigt et al., 2003). These data indicate that MCMV can rapidly mutate to evade a selective pressure elicited by the immune system, in particular by NK cells. An obvious question is why MCMV expresses Ly49H activating *m157* although it is able to evade from this selective pressure within six passages in vivo. A potential answer might come from the finding that *m157* activates not only the activatory Ly49H but also the inhibitory NK cell receptor Ly49I, which is widely found in mice (Arase et al., 2002).

A strong antiviral selection pressure arises in patients upon long-term treatment with antiviral drugs. Under such regimes, resistant mutants have an obvious replication advantage compared to wt genomes, even when the mutation compromises the optimal function of the mutated enzyme to a certain degree, impairing replication fitness (Field and Biron, 1994). Basically two groups of antiviral drugs are used against herpesviruses: (i) nucleoside analogs like ganciclovir (GCV) or acyclovir (ACV) and (ii) direct DNA polymerase inhibitors like phosphonoformate (foscarnet) and phosphonoacetate. ACV is a prodrug which has to be activated by viral enzymes. The compound is converted to a monophosphate by the viral thymidine kinase (TK) before subsequent di- and triphosphorylation by cellular kinases takes place, and only the triphosphate can serve as a nucleotide analog blocking polymerase function. TK-deficient viruses are therefore resistant to ACV. HSV and VZV mutants which are resistant to ACV as a result of absent or impaired TK expression have been recovered from patients after ACV therapy (Burns et al., 1982; Linnemann et al., 1990; Pahwa et al., 1988). Additionally, virus mutants have been found which do express functional TK enzymes capable of phosphorylating thymidine but not ACV. Interestingly, the TK$^-$ virus mutants were less virulent in mice.

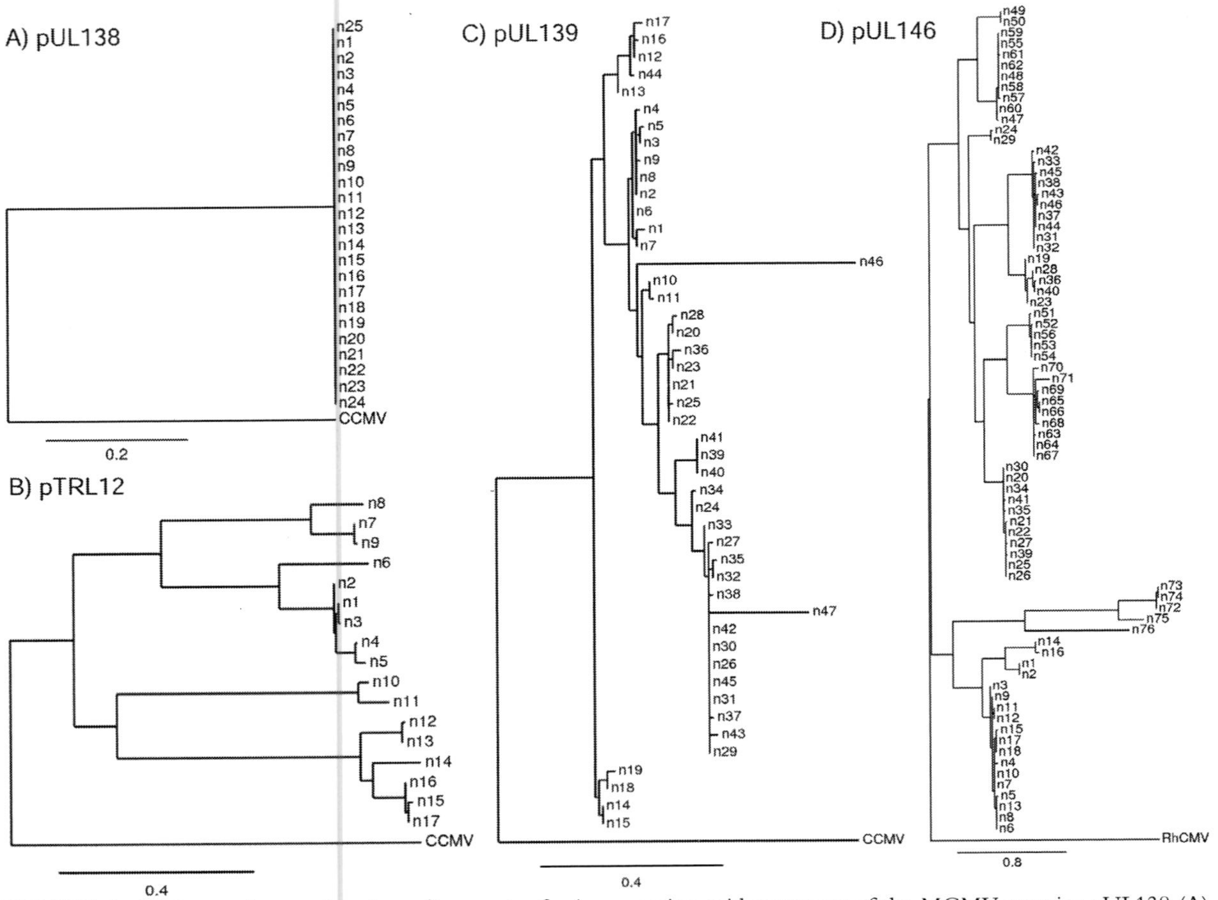

FIGURE 4 Phylogenetic trees based on alignments of primary amino acid sequences of the MCMV proteins pUL138 (A), pTRL12 (B), pUL139 (C), and pUL146 (D) indicate significant differences concerning variability of individual viral proteins, even at adjacent positions in the viral genome, like the *ULb′* region. For all four proteins, all currently available protein sequences (status January 2011) from the NCBI server have been compared. The sequences of the homologous chimpanzee or rhesus CMV (CCMV or rhCMV, respectively) proteins serve as the outgroup. The alignment and phylogenetic tree were constructed with the www.phylogeny.fr online tool (Dereeper et al., 2008). The legend depicts the protein sequence divergence.

These examples highlight the ability of herpesviruses to rapidly mutate under selecting conditions, indicating a remarkable potential of genetic plasticity and adaptability within a handful of in vivo passages. During nonselecting episodes, large fractions of the viral genome are astonishingly stable and almost no mutations are observed throughout the whole genome. This discrepancy between conservative periods with high genomic uniformity on the one hand and periods of quick adaptation to new and stringent selective pressures on the other hand raises a conundrum. Two possible explanations might solve this seeming paradox. One would be the ability of herpesviruses to regulate or control their own mutation rate (or DNA repair) to a certain degree. Some of the virus-encoded proofreading enzymes and/or the viral repair enzymes might have differential activation states. Such a flexible mutation rate could also be achieved passively. Assuming that antiviral effects often reduce viral gene transcription (directly by abrogating viral genome replication and thereby abrogating viral late-gene expression or indirectly by, e.g., NK-dependent interferon production, which has been shown to affect viral late-gene expression), it is tempting to speculate that the transcription-coupled DNA repair, which is present in the nucleus of the host cells and basically depends on stalled RNA-polymerase complexes, differs under these two conditions, leading to increased mutation rates for nontranscriptional active genomes. This is a scenario which also might apply to latent genomes compared to genomes in lytic replication cycles.

Another possible explanation could be that herpesviruses are extremely well adapted to the longstanding host and almost any mutation implies immediate costs of reduced replication fitness, bringing herpesviruses into a constant state of purifying and stabilizing selection. In view of the densely packaged genomes full of partially overlapping and also complementary ORFs with their respective promoters, enhancer, and control regions, there appears to be little scope for silent mutations. This would mean that herpesviruses acquire mutations, albeit at a low frequency due to their high genetic fidelity, but mutant viruses suffer from disadvantages compared to the competing wt virus. Only during episodes of altered selective pressure (e.g., antiviral drug treatment or modified immune selection) does this change dramatically, leading to fast and efficient emergence of genetic adaptation.

REFERENCES

Arase, H., E. S. Mocarski, A.E. Campbell, A. B. Hill, and L. L. Lanier. 2002. Direct recognition of cytomegalovirus by activating and inhibitory NK cell receptors. *Science* **296:**1323–1326.

Arav-Boger, R., R. E. Willoughby, R. F. Pass, J. C. Zong, W. J. Jang, D. Alcendor, and G. S. Hayward. 2002. Polymorphisms of the cytomegalovirus (CMV)-encoded tumor necrosis factor-alpha and beta-chemokine receptors in congenital CMV disease. *J. Infect. Dis.* **186:**1057–1064.

Arbuckle, J. H., M. M. Medveczky, J. Luka, S. H. Hadley, A. Luegmayr, D. Ablashi, T. C. Lund, J. Tolar, M. K. De, J. G. Montoya, A. L. Komaroff, P. F. Ambros, and P. G. Medveczky. 2010. The latent human herpesvirus-6A genome specifically integrates in telomeres of human chromosomes in vivo and in vitro. *Proc. Natl. Acad. Sci. USA* **107:**5563–5568.

Atalay, R., Z. Zimmermann, M. Wagner, E. Borst, C. Benz, M. Messerle, and H. Hengel. 2002. Identification and expression of human cytomegalovirus transcription units coding for two distinct Fc gamma receptor homologs. *J. Virol.* **76:**8596–8608.

Baek, D., J. Villen, C. Shin, F. D. Camargo, S. P. Gygi, and D. P. Bartel. 2008. The impact of microRNAs on protein output. *Nature* **455:**64–71.

Baldanti, F., A. Sarasini, M. Furione, M. Gatti, G. Comolli, M. G. Revello, and G. Gerna. 1998. Coinfection of the immunocompromised but not the immunocompetent host by multiple human cytomegalovirus strains. *Arch. Virol.* **143:**1701–1709.

Baldick, C. J., Jr., and T. Shenk. 1996. Proteins associated with purified human cytomegalovirus particles. *J. Virol.* **70:**6097–6105.

Boehmer, P. E., and I. R. Lehman. 1997. Herpes simplex virus DNA replication. *Annu. Rev. Biochem.* **66:**347–384.

Bogani, F., and P. E. Boehmer. 2008. The replicative DNA polymerase of herpes simplex virus 1 exhibits apurinic/apyrimidinic and 5′-deoxyribose phosphate lyase activities. *Proc. Natl. Acad. Sci. USA* **105:**11709–11714.

Borst, E. M., G. Hahn, U. H. Koszinowski, and M. Messerle. 1999. Cloning of the human cytomegalovirus (HCMV) genome as an infectious bacterial artificial chromosome in *Escherichia coli:* a new approach for construction of HCMV mutants. *J. Virol.* **73:**8320–8329.

Bresnahan, W. A., and T. Shenk. 2000. A subset of viral transcripts packaged within human cytomegalovirus particles. *Science* **288:**2373–2376.

Brondke, H., B. Schmitz, and W. Doerfler. 2007. Nucleotide sequence comparisons between several strains and isolates of human cytomegalovirus reveal alternate start codon usage. *Arch. Virol.* **152:**2035–2046.

Brown, J. C. 2007. High G+C content of herpes simplex virus DNA: proposed role in protection against retrotransposon insertion. *Open Biochem. J.* **1:**33–42.

Bubic, I., M. Wagner, A. Krmpotic, T. Saulig, S. Kim, W. M. Yokoyama, S. Jonjic, and U. H. Koszinowski. 2004. Gain of virulence caused by loss of a gene in murine cytomegalovirus. *J. Virol.* **78:**7536–7544.

Burns, W. H., R. Saral, G. W. Santos, O. L. Laskin, P. S. Lietman, C. McLaren, and D. W. Barry. 1982. Isolation and characterisation of resistant herpes simplex virus after acyclovir therapy. *Lancet* **i:**421–423.

Cha, T. A., E. Tom, G. W. Kemble, G. M. Duke, E. S. Mocarski, and R. R. Spaete. 1996. Human cytomegalovirus clinical isolates carry at least 19 genes not found in laboratory strains. *J. Virol.* **70:**78–83.

Cheng, T. P., M. C. Valentine, J. Gao, J. T. Pingel, and W. M. Yokoyama. 2010. Stability of murine cytomegalovirus genome after in vitro and in vivo passage. *J. Virol.* **84:**2623–2628.

Cheung, A., and E. Kieff. 1982. Long internal direct repeat in Epstein-Barr virus-DNA. *J. Virol.* **44:** 286–294.

Choi, J. K., R. E. Means, B. Damania, and J. U. Jung. 2001. Molecular piracy of Kaposi's sarcoma associated herpesvirus. *Cytokine Growth Factor Rev.* **12:**245–257.

Chong, K. T., and C. A. Mims. 1981. Murine cytomegalovirus particle types in relation to sources of virus and pathogenicity. *J. Gen. Virol.* **57:**415–419.

Cicin-Sain, L., I. Bubic, M. Schnee, Z. Ruzsics, C. Mohr, S. Jonjic, and U. H. Koszinowski. 2007. Targeted deletion of regions rich in immune-evasive genes from the cytomegalovirus genome as a novel vaccine strategy. *J. Virol.* **81:**13825–13834.

Cicin-Sain, L., R. Podlech, M. Messerle, M. J. Reddehase, and U. H. Koszinowski. 2005. Frequent coinfection of cells explains functional in vivo complementation between cytomegalovirus variants in the multiply infected host. *J. Virol.* **79:**9492–9502.

Cockrell, S. K., M. E. Sanchez, A. Erazo, and F. L. Homa. 2009. Role of the UL25 protein in herpes simplex virus DNA encapsidation. *J. Virol.* **83:**47–57.

Corbett, A. J., C. A. Forbes, D. Moro, and A. A. Scalzo. 2007. Extensive sequence variation exists among isolates of murine cytomegalovirus within members of the m02 family of genes. *J. Gen. Virol.* **88:**758–769.

Cui, X. H., A. McGregor, M. R. Schleiss, and M. A. McVoy. 2009. The impact of genome length on replication and genome stability of the herpesvirus guinea pig cytomegalovirus. *Virology* **386:**132–138.

Daniels, K. A., G. Devora, W. C. Lai, C. L. O'Donnell, M. Bennett, and R. M. Welsh. 2001. Murine cytomegalovirus is regulated by a discrete subset of natural killer cells reactive with monoclonal antibody to Ly49H. *J. Exp. Med.* **194:**29–44.

Davison, A. J. 2010. Herpesvirus systematics. *Vet. Microbiol.* **143:**52–69.

Davison, A. J., B. L. Trus, N. Q. Cheng, A. C. Steven, M. S. Watson, C. Cunningham, R. M. Le Deuff, and T. Renault. 2005. A novel class of herpesvirus with bivalve hosts. *J. Gen. Virol.* **86:**41–53.

Deckers, M., J. Hofmann, K. A. Kreuzer, H. Reinhard, A. Edubio, H. Hengel, S. Voigt, and B. Ehlers. 2009. High genotypic diversity and a novel variant of human cytomegalovirus revealed by combined UL33/UL55 genotyping with broad-range PCR. *Virol. J.* **6:**210.

Delecluse, H. J., and W. Hammerschmidt. 1993. Status of Marek's disease virus in established lymphoma cell-lines: herpesvirus integration is common. *J. Virol.* **67:**82–92.

Delecluse, H. J., S. Schuller, and W. Hammerschmidt. 1993. Latent Marek's disease virus can be activated from its chromosomally integrated state in herpesvirus-transformed lymphoma cells. *EMBO J.* **12:**3277–3286.

Delius, H., and J. B. Clements. 1976. A partial denaturation map of herpes simplex virus type 1 DNA: evidence for inversions of the unique DNA regions. *J. Gen. Virol.* **33:**125–133.

Dereeper, A., V. Guignon, G. Blanc, S. Audic, S. Buffet, F. Chevenet, J. F. Dufayard, S. Guindon, V. Lefort, M. Lescot, J. M. Claverie, and O. Gascuel. 2008. Phylogeny.fr: robust phylogenetic analysis for the non-specialist. *Nucleic Acids Res.* **36:**W465–W469.

Dokun, A. O., S. Kim, H. R. C. Smith, H. S. P. Kang, D. T. Chu, and W. M. Yokoyama. 2001. Specific and nonspecific NK cell activation during virus infection. *Nat. Immunol.* **2:**951–956.

Dolken, L., A. Krmpotic, S. Kothe, L. Tuddenham, M. Tanguy, L. Marcinowski, Z. Ruzsics, N. Elefant, Y. Altuvia, H. Margalit, U. Koszinowski, S. Jonjic, and S. Pfeffer. 2010. Cytomegalovirus microRNAs facilitate persistent virus infection in salivary glands. *PLoS Pathog.* **6:**e1001150.

Dolken, L., J. Perot, V. Cognat, A. Alioua, M. John, J. Soutschek, Z. Ruzsics, U. Koszinowski, O. Voinnet, and S. Pfeffer. 2007. Mouse cytomegalovirus microRNAs dominate the cellular small RNA profile during lytic infection and show features of posttranscriptional regulation. *J. Virol.* **81:** 13771–13782.

Farley, C. A., W. S. Foster, W. G. Banfield, and G. Kasnic. 1972. Oyster herpes-type virus. *Science* **178:**759–760.

Field, A. K., and K. K. Biron. 1994. The end of innocence revisited: resistance of herpesviruses to antiviral drugs. *Clin. Microbiol. Rev.* **7:**1–13.

Gomi, Y., T. Imagawa, M. Takahashi, and K. Yamanishi. 2000. Oka varicella vaccine is distinguishable from its parental virus in DNA sequence of open reading frame 62 and its transactivation activity. *J. Med. Virol.* **61:**497–503.

Gomi, Y., H. Sunamachi, Y. Mori, K. Nagaike, M. Takahashi, and K. Yamanishi. 2002. Comparison of the complete DNA sequences of the Oka varicella vaccine and its parental virus. *J. Virol.* **76:** 11447–11459.

Grimson, A., K. K. Farh, W. K. Johnston, P. Garrett-Engele, L. P. Lim, and D. P. Bartel. 2007. MicroRNA targeting specificity in mammals: determinants beyond seed pairing. *Mol. Cell* **27:**91–105.

Hayakawa, Y., and R. W. Hyman. 1987. Isomerization of the UL region of varicella-zoster virus DNA. *Virus Res.* **8:**25–31.

Hayward, G. S., R. J. Jacob, S. C. Wadsworth, and B. Roizman. 1975. Anatomy of herpes simplex virus DNA: evidence for four populations of molecules that differ in the relative orientations of their long and short components. *Proc. Natl. Acad. Sci. USA* **72:**4243–4247.

Hengel, H., U. Reusch, A. Gutermann, H. Ziegler, S. Jonjic, P. Lucin, and U. H. Koszinowski. 1999. Cytomegaloviral control of MHC class I function in the mouse. *Immunol. Rev.* **168:**167–176.

Hudson, J. B., V. Misra, and T. R. Mosmann. 1976. Properties of the multicapsid virions of murine cytomegalovirus. *Virology* **72:**224–234.

Hurley, E. A., S. Agger, J. A. McNeil, J. B. Lawrence, A. Calendar, G. Lenoir, and D. A. Thorley-Lawson. 1991. When Epstein-Barr virus persistently infects B-cell lines, it frequently integrates. *J. Virol.* **65:**1245–1254.

Javier, R. T., F. Sedarati, and J. G. Stevens. 1986. Two avirulent herpes simplex viruses generate lethal recombinants in vivo. *Science* **234:**746–748.

Jenkins, C., A. Abendroth, and B. Slobedman. 2004. A novel viral transcript with homology to human interleukin-10 is expressed during latent human cytomegalovirus infection. *J. Virol.* **78:**1440–1447.

Jenkins, F. J., and B. Roizman. 1986. Herpes simplex virus 1 recombinants with noninverting genomes frozen in different isomeric arrangements are capable of independent replication. *J. Virol.* **59:**494–499.

Jurak, I., M. F. Kramer, J. C. Mellor, A. L. van Lint, F. P. Roth, D. M. Knipe, and D. M. Coen. 2010. Numerous conserved and divergent microRNAs expressed by herpes simplex viruses 1 and 2. *J. Virol.* **84:**4659–4672.

Karlin, S., B. E. Blaisdell, and G. A. Schachtel. 1990. Contrasts in codon usage of latent versus productive genes of Epstein-Barr virus: data and hypotheses. *J. Virol.* **64:**4264–4273.

Kattenhorn, L. M., R. Mills, M. Wagner, A. Lomsadze, V. Makeev, M. Borodovsky, H. L. Ploegh, and B. M. Kessler. 2004. Identification of proteins associated with murine cytomegalovirus virions. *J. Virol.* **78:**11187–11197.

Kinchington, P. R., W. C. Reinhold, T. A. Casey, S. E. Straus, J. Hay, and W. T. Ruyechan. 1985. Inversion and circularization of the varicella-zoster virus genome. *J. Virol.* **56:**194–200.

Kotenko, S. V., S. Saccani, L. S. Izotova, O. V. Mirochnitchenko, and S. Pestka. 2000. Human cytomegalovirus harbors its own unique IL-10 homolog (cmvIL-10). *Proc. Natl. Acad. Sci. USA* **97:**1695–1700.

Kurz, S., H. P. Steffens, A. Mayer, J. R. Harris, and M. J. Reddehase. 1997. Latency versus persistence or intermittent recurrences: evidence for a latent state of murine cytomegalovirus in the lungs. *J. Virol.* **71:**2980–2987.

Lawrence, J. B., C. A. Villnave, and R. H. Singer. 1988. Sensitive, high-resolution chromatin and chromosome mapping in situ: presence and orientation of 2 closely integrated copies of EBV in a lymphoma line. *Cell* **52:**51–61.

Lee, S. H., S. Girard, D. Macina, M. Busa, A. Zafer, A. Belouchi, P. Gros, and S. M. Vidal. 2001. Susceptibility to mouse cytomegalovirus is associated with deletion of an activating natural killer cell receptor of the C-type lectin superfamily. *Nat. Genet.* **28:**42–45.

Lestou, V. S., M. Debraekeleer, S. Strehl, G. Ott, H. Gadner, and P. F. Ambros. 1993. Nonrandom integration of Epstein-Barr virus in lymphoblastoid cell lines. *Genes Chromosomes Cancer* **8:**38–48.

Linnemann, C. C., Jr., K. K. Biron, W. G. Hoppenjans, and A. M. Solinger. 1990. Emergence of acyclovir-resistant varicella zoster virus in an AIDS patient on prolonged acyclovir therapy. *AIDS* **4:**577–579.

McGeoch, D. J., S. Cook, A. Dolan, F. E. Jamieson, and E. A. Telford. 1995. Molecular phylogeny and evolutionary timescale for the family of mammalian herpesviruses. *J. Mol. Biol.* **247:**443–458.

McVoy, M. A., and S. P. Adler. 1994. Human cytomegalovirus DNA replicates after early circularization by concatemer formation, and inversion occurs within the concatemer. *J. Virol.* **68:**1040–1051.

McVoy, M. A., and D. Ramnarain. 2000. Machinery to support genome segment inversion exists in a herpesvirus which does not naturally contain invertible elements. *J. Virol.* **74:**4882–4887.

Michelson, S., P. Turowski, L. Picard, J. Goris, M. P. Landini, A. Topilko, B. Hemmings, C. Bessia, A. Garcia, and J. L. Virelizier. 1996. Human cytomegalovirus carries serine/threonine protein phosphatases PP1 and a host-cell derived PP2A. *J. Virol.* **70:**1415–1423.

Mocarski, E. S., L. E. Post, and B. Roizman. 1980. Molecular engineering of the herpes simplex virus genome: insertion of a second L-S junction into the genome causes additional genome inversions. *Cell* **22:**243–255.

Morissette, G., and L. Flamand. 2010. Herpesviruses and chromosomal integration. *J. Virol.* **84:**12100–12109.

Murthy, S., G. S. Hayward, S. Wheelan, M. S. Forman, J. H. Ahn, R. F. Pass, and R. Rav-Boger. 2011. Detection of a single identical cytomegalovirus (CMV) strain in recently seroconverted young women. *PLoS One* **6:**e15949.

Oliveira, S. A., S. H. Park, P. Lee, A. Bendelac, and T. E. Shenk. 2002. Murine cytomegalovirus m02 gene family protects against natural killer cell-mediated immune surveillance. *J. Virol.* **76:**885–894.

Pahwa, S., K. Biron, W. Lim, P. Swenson, M. H. Kaplan, N. Sadick, and R. Pahwa. 1988. Continuous varicella-zoster infection associated with acyclovir resistance in a child with AIDS. *JAMA* **260:**2879–2882.

Pereira, L., E. Cassai, R. W. Honess, B. Roizman, M. Terni, and A. Nahmias. 1976. Variability in structural polypeptides of herpes simplex virus 1 strains: potential application in molecular epidemiology. *Infect. Immun.* **13:**211–220.

Pfeffer, S., A. Sewer, M. Lagos-Quintana, R. Sheridan, C. Sander, F. A. Grasser, L. F. van Dyk, C. K. Ho, S. Shuman, M. Chien, J. J. Russo, J. Ju, G. Randall, B. D. Lindenbach, C. M. Rice, V. Simon, D. D. Ho, M. Zavolan, and T. Tuschl. 2005. Identification of microRNAs of the herpesvirus family. *Nat. Methods* **2:**269–276.

Pfeffer, S., M. Zavolan, F. A. Grasser, M. Chien, J. J. Russo, J. Ju, B. John, A. J. Enright, D. Marks, C. Sander, and T. Tuschl. 2004. Identification of virus-encoded microRNAs. *Science* **304:**734–736.

Polic, B., H. Hengel, A. Krmpotic, J. Trgovcich, I. Pavic, P. Lucin, S. Jonjic, and U. H. Koszinowski. 1998. Hierarchical and redundant lymphocyte subset control precludes cytomegalovirus replication during latent infection. *J. Exp. Med.* **188:**1047–1054.

Raab-Traub, N. and K. Flynn. 1986. The structure of the termini of the Epstein-Barr virus as a marker of clonal cellular proliferation. *Cell* **47:**883–889.

Rafailidis, P. I., E. G. Mourtzoukou, I. C. Varbobitis, and M. E. Falagas. 2008. Severe cytomegalovirus infection in apparently immunocompetent patients: a systematic review. *Virol. J.* **5:**47.

Roizman, B. 1980. Genome variation and evolution among herpes viruses. *Ann. N. Y. Acad. Sci.* **354:**472–483.

Roizman, B., and M. Tognon. 1983. Restriction endonuclease patterns of herpes simplex virus DNA: application to diagnosis and molecular epidemiology. *Curr. Top. Microbiol. Immunol.* **104:**273–286.

Russo, J. J., R. A. Bohenzky, M. C. Chien, J. Chen, M. Yan, D. Maddalena, J. P. Parry, D. Peruzzi, I. S. Edelman, Y. Chang, and P. S. Moore. 1996. Nucleotide sequence of the Kaposi sarcoma-associated herpesvirus (HHV8). *Proc. Natl. Acad. Sci. USA* **93:**14862–14867.

Rustgi, V. K., R. A. Sacher, P. O'Brien, and V. F. Garagusi. 1983. Fatal disseminated cytomegalovirus infection in an apparently normal adult. *Arch. Intern. Med.* **143:**372–373.

Schachtel, G. A., P. Bucher, E. S. Mocarski, B. E. Blaisdell, and S. Karlin. 1991. Evidence for selective evolution in codon usage in conserved amino-acid segments of human alphaherpesvirus proteins. *J. Mol. Evol.* **33:**483–494.

Selbach, M., B. Schwanhausser, N. Thierfelder, Z. Fang, R. Khanin, and N. Rajewsky. 2008. Widespread changes in protein synthesis induced by microRNAs. *Nature* **455:**58–63.

Smith, H. R. C., J. W. Heusel, I. K. Mehta, S. Kim, B. G. Dorner, O. V. Naidenko, K. Iizuka, H. Furukawa, D. L. Beckman, J. T. Pingel, A. A. Scalzo, D. H. Fremont, and W. M. Yokoyama. 2002. Recognition of a virus-encoded ligand by a natural killer cell activation receptor. *Proc. Natl. Acad. Sci. USA* **99:**8826–8831.

Smith, L. M., A. R. McWhorter, L. L. Masters, G. R. Shellam, and A. J. Redwood. 2008. Laboratory strains of murine cytomegalovirus are genetically similar to but phenotypically distinct from wild strains of virus. *J. Virol.* **82:**6689–6696.

Spackova, M., M. Wiese-Posselt, M. Dehnert, D. Matysiak-Klose, U. Heininger, and A. Siedler. 2010. Comparative varicella vaccine effectiveness during outbreaks in day-care centres. *Vaccine* **28:**686–691.

Spear, G. T., N. S. Lurain, C. J. Parker, M. Ghassemi, G. H. Payne, and M. Saifuddin. 1995. Host cell-derived complement control proteins CD55 and CD59 are incorporated into the virions of two unrelated enveloped viruses. Human T cell leukemia/lymphoma virus type I (HTLV-I) and human cytomegalovirus (HCMV). *J. Immunol.* **155:**4376–4381.

Stern-Ginossar, N., N. Elefant, A. Zimmermann, D. G. Wolf, N. Saleh, M. Biton, E. Horwitz, Z. Prokocimer, M. Prichard, G. Hahn, D. Goldman-Wohl, C. Greenfield, S. Yagel, H. Hengel, Y. Altuvia, H. Margalit, and O. Mandelboim. 2007. Host immune system gene targeting by a viral miRNA. *Science* **317:**376–381.

Stern-Ginossar, N., N. Saleh, M. D. Goldberg, M. Prichard, D. G. Wolf, and O. Mandelboim. 2009. Analysis of human cytomegalovirus-encoded microRNA activity during infection. *J. Virol.* **83:**10684–10693.

Tillieux, S. L., W. S. Halsey, E. S. Thomas, J. J. Voycik, G. M. Sathe, and V. Vassilev. 2008. Complete DNA sequences of two Oka strain varicella-zoster virus genomes. *J. Virol.* **82:**11023–11044.

Umbach, J. L., M. A. Nagel, R. J. Cohrs, D. H. Gilden, and B. R. Cullen. 2009. Analysis of human alphaherpesvirus microRNA expression in latently infected human trigeminal ganglia. *J. Virol.* **83:**10677–10683.

Umbach, J. L., K. Wang, S. Tang, P. R. Krause, E. K. Mont, J. I. Cohen, and B. R. Cullen. 2010. Identification of viral microRNAs expressed in human sacral ganglia latently infected with herpes simplex virus 2. *J. Virol.* **84:**1189–1192.

Varnum, S. M., D. N. Streblow, M. E. Monroe, P. Smith, K. J. Auberry, L. Pasa-Tolic, D. Wang, D. G. Camp, K. Rodland, S. Wiley, W. Britt, T. Shenk, R. D. Smith, and J. A. Nelson. 2004. Identification of proteins in human cytomegalovirus (HCMV) particles: the HCMV proteome. *J. Virol.* **78:**10960–10966.

Virgin, H. W., P. Latreille, P. Wamsley, K. Hallsworth, K. E. Weck, A. J. DalCanto, and S. H. Speck. 1997. Complete sequence and genomic analysis of murine gammaherpesvirus 68. *J. Virol.* **71:**5894–5904.

Voigt, V., C. A. Forbes, J. N. Tonkin, M. A. Degli-Esposti, H. R. C. Smith, W. M. Yokoyama, and A. A. Scalzo. 2003. Murine cytomegalovirus m157 mutation and variation leads to immune evasion of natural killer cells. *Proc. Natl. Acad. Sci. USA* **100:**13483–13488.

Wagner, E. K., and D. C. Bloom. 1997. Experimental investigation of herpes simplex virus latency. *Clin. Microbiol. Rev.* **10:**419–443.

Wagner, M., Z. Ruzsics, and U. H. Koszinowski. 2002. Herpesvirus genetics has come of age. *Trends Microbiol.* **10:**318–324.

Waidner, L. A., R. W. Morgan, A. S. Anderson, E. L. Bernberg, S. Kamboj, M. Garcia, S. M. Riblet, M. Ouyang, G. K. Isaacs, M. Markis, B. C. Meyers, P. J. Green, and J. Burnside. 2009. MicroRNAs of gallid and meleagrid herpesviruses show generally conserved genomic locations and are virus specific. *Virology* **388:**128–136.

Wang, A., L. Ren, G. Abenes, and R. Hai. 2009. Genome sequence divergences and functional variations in human cytomegalovirus strains. *FEMS Immunol. Med. Microbiol.* **55:**23–33.

Weber, P. C., M. D. Challberg, N. J. Nelson, M. Levine, and J. C. Glorioso. 1988. Inversion events in the HSV-1 genome are directly mediated by the viral DNA replication machinery and lack sequence specificity. *Cell* **54:**369–381.

Wrensch, M., A. Weinberg, J. Wiencke, R. Miike, G. Barger, and K. Kelsey. 2001. Prevalence of antibodies to four herpesviruses among adults with glioma and controls. *Am. J. Epidemiol.* **154:**161–165.

Wright, J. F., A. Kurosky, E. L. Pryzdial, and S. Wasi. 1995. Host cellular annexin II is associated with cytomegalovirus particles isolated from cultured human fibroblasts. *J. Virol.* **69:**4784–4791.

Yu, D., M. C. Silva, and T. Shenk. 2003. Functional map of human cytomegalovirus AD169 defined by global mutational analysis. *Proc. Natl. Acad. Sci. USA* **100:**12396–12401.

PARASITIC AND FUNGAL INFECTIONS

GENOME DIVERSITY, POPULATION GENETICS, AND EVOLUTION OF MALARIA PARASITES

Xin-zhuan Su and Deirdre A. Joy

16

MALARIA AND MALARIA PARASITES

The parasites that cause malaria are protozoa of the genus *Plasmodium*, family Plasmodidae, order Coccidia. Malaria parasites infect an impressively broad range of vertebrate hosts, with over 100 species identified in mammals, reptiles, and birds. The majority of malaria parasites are transmitted by mosquitoes; human malaria parasites are transmitted by anopheline mosquitoes exclusively. Four species of malaria infect humans: *Plasmodium falciparum*, *Plasmodium vivax*, *Plasmodium malariae*, and *Plasmodium ovale*. Human outbreaks of the monkey malaria parasite *Plasmodium knowlesi* have also been reported (Singh et al., 2004); this parasite can therefore be considered a human parasite, as well.

Malaria parasites infect hundreds of millions of people and cause approximately 1 million deaths each year (Snow et al., 2005; World Health Organization, 2008). Children infected with *P. falciparum*, primarily in Africa, account for the vast majority of deaths. Although *P. vivax* is generally not fatal, it is the most widespread human malaria parasite and, as a result, inflicts heavy health and economic losses on communities and entire countries (Carter and Mendis, 2002).

The malaria parasite has a complex life cycle that includes two types of asexual reproduction, known as schizogony, in the vertebrate (mammal, reptile, or bird) host and insect vector, in addition to sexual reproduction (or sporogony) in the insect vector (Fig. 1). When a mosquito bites a human, sporozoites are released into the bloodstream. The sporozoites quickly invade liver cells and begin the first round of schizogony, producing thousands of merozoites that enter the bloodstream, where they invade red blood cells (RBC). The parasites begin another round of schizogony within RBC, producing up to 32 merozoites in a mature schizont within 2 to 3 days. The mature schizonts then rupture and release merozoites into the bloodstream, where they reinvade other RBC. While this process is under way, a small proportion of parasites switch to sexual stages called gametocytes. It takes up to 2 weeks, depending on the malaria species, to develop into a mature gametocyte that can survive in the mosquito midgut. In the midgut, gametocytes quickly

Xin-zhuan Su, Laboratory of Malaria and Vector Research, National Institute of Allergy and Infectious Diseases, National Institutes of Health, Bethesda, MD 20892. *Deirdre A. Joy*, Parasitology and International Programs Branch, National Institute of Allergy and Infectious Diseases, National Institutes of Health, Bethesda, MD 20892.

Genome Plasticity and Infectious Diseases,
Edited by J. Hacker, U. Dobrindt, and R. Kurth,

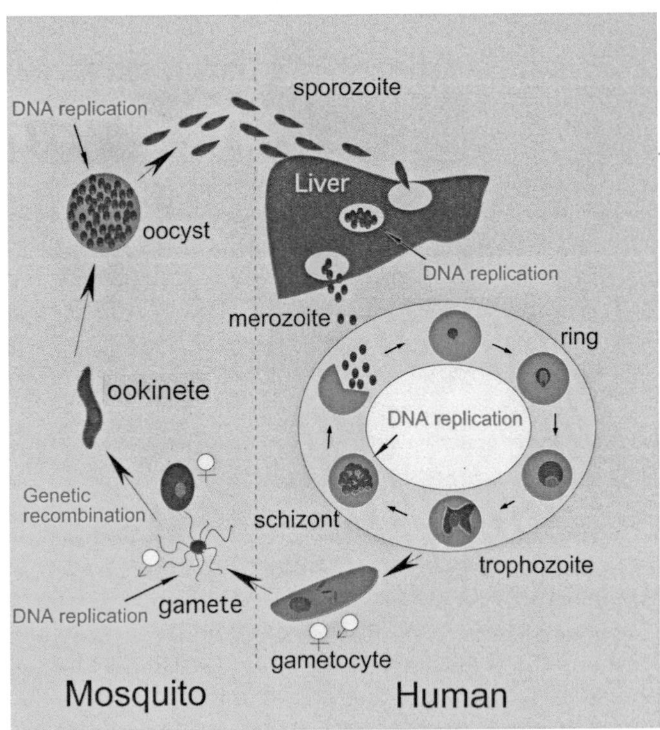

FIGURE 1 Cartoon of the *Plasmodium falciparum* life cycle, showing stages of DNA replication and genetic recombination.

produce male and female gametes that fuse to form a diploid zygote, known as the ookinete. This brief diploid stage provides an opportunity for recombination between genetically distinct parasite isolates, or outcrossing, and can generate genetic diversity. The mobile ookinetes subsequently penetrate the midgut epithelium and encyst on the outer wall of the midgut to develop into oocycsts. Thousands of sporozoites are produced in a single oocyst through yet another round of sporogony. Once released, the sporozoites eventually migrate to the mosquito salivary gland and are injected into a new human host when a mosquito bites again.

Millions of individual parasites are typically present in a single host; however, a mosquito bite delivers only a limited number of sporozoites. Multiple cycles of replications in the liver and subsequently in RBC are needed to reach a parasitemia that can be detected under a microscope. DNA replication errors may occur during these replications. Accumulation of DNA replication errors in each cycle may result in a parasite population in which some genome regions differ among individual parasites, increasing the ability of the population as a whole to respond to pressures from antimalarial drugs or host immunity.

MALARIA GENOMES

All malaria parasites that infect vertebrate hosts have a haploid genome of ~23 to 35 Mb and 14 chromosomes (Carlton, 2003; Carlton et al., 2002, 2005; Gardner et al., 2002; Hall et al., 2005). Malaria parasite genomes sequenced to date contain ~5,500 to 12,000 predicted genes, although the numbers of genes will most certainly change as the accuracy of genome annotation continues to improve. Despite the concerted efforts and hard work of many scientists, the computer-predicted gene models of malaria parasites require further verification using experimental data (cDNA sequences). Indeed, alignment of cDNA sequences with the predicted gene sequences in the *P. falciparum* genome showed that approximately one-quarter of the predicted genes had errors in their gene models (Lu et al., 2007; Wakaguri et al., 2009).

In contrast to the relatively similar genome size among malaria parasite species, the G+C content of the genome varies widely. *P. falciparum* and *Plasmodium reichenowi* (a parasite in chimpanzees) genomes are highly AT rich at ~80%; the three rodent malaria parasites *Plasmodium yoelii yoelii, Plasmodium chabaudi chabaudi,* and *Plasmodium berghei* have an A+T content of ~75%; and *P. vivax* has an A+T content of 62% (Carlton et al., 2005). Approximately 50% of the genomes consist of coding regions, and 50% to 55% of the genes have one or more introns. Although the genomes of malaria parasites differ from each other in G+C content, there is a high degree of conservation in gene synteny; the location of many genes and gene order are preserved over large regions of the chromosomes among many species of malaria parasites (Janse et al., 1994; Carlton et al., 1998). This is well illustrated in a composite chromosome map of rodent malaria parasites developed based on gene synteny between the rodent parasites and *P. falciparum* (Kooij et al., 2005). At least for *P. falciparum*, most genes carry relatively long 5′ (~300-bp) and 3′ (~200-bp) untranslated regions and have an average of two to six transcription start sites per gene (Watanabe et al., 2002; Wakaguri et al., 2009). Useful information on gene prediction, expression, polymorphism, and more can be found at http://www.plasmoDB.org and at http://fullmal.hgc.jp.

THE HIGHLY DIVERSE GENOME OF THE *P. FALCIPARUM* PARASITE

As is true for many microorganisms, *Plasmodium* genomes exhibit diversity at several levels, with variations in chromosome size, gene copy number, number of simple sequence repeats, and number of single nucleotide polymorphisms (SNP) (Fig. 2). They also contain many diverse gene families, and the expression of these genes can be regulated in response to immune and other pressures.

The study of genome diversity and plasticity, particularly at chromosome ends, is a robust area of research within the malaria community (Lanzer et al., 1995; Kemp et al., 1990). Within a species, chromosome size is highly variable.

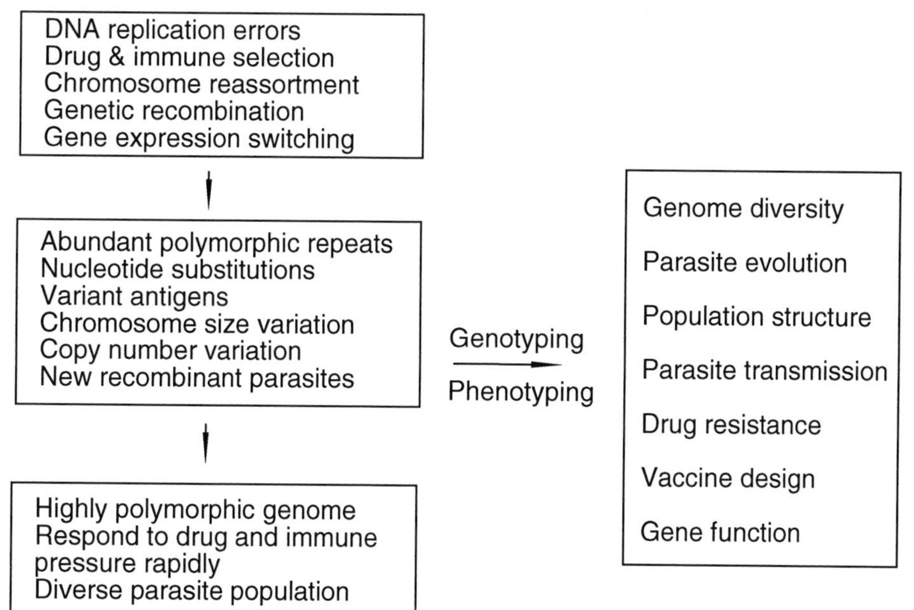

FIGURE 2 Diversity generation, types of polymorphism, effects of genetic variation, and potential applications.

Pulsed-field gel electrophoresis was able to detect chromosome size variation of up to 20% between *P. falciparum* isolates (Kemp et al., 1985; Wellems et al., 1988). Gene amplification, chromosomal end deletion, and unequal recombination occur frequently, even among parasites grown in in vitro culture, all of which likely contribute to differences in chromosome size (Bottius et al., 1998; Scherf and Mattei, 1992). Variation in chromosome size has also been observed in rodent malaria parasite species (Janse and Waters, 1993). Chromosomal deletion is associated with gametocyte development and possibly with cytoadherence (Day et al., 1993; Kemp et al., 1992) and is likely to play a role in antigenic variation, because many antigen gene families are located at subtelomere regions in malaria parasites.

Another class of polymorphisms contributing to genome diversity and plasticity is deletions and insertions (indels) of short repetitive DNA sequences, known as microsatellites (MS) or minisatellites depending on the size of the repeated unit. Change in MS size is believed to result from slippage of DNA polymerase during replication (Kroutil and Kunkel, 1999). Polymorphic MS are extremely abundant in the AT-rich *P. falciparum* genome, especially in noncoding regions, with a frequency of about 1 MS per kb (Su and Wellems, 1996; Su et al., 1999). The majority of MS in *P. falciparum* are AT-rich repeats such as $(A/T)_n$, $(TA)_n$, or $(TAA)_n$. A collection of 90 worldwide *P. falciparum* field isolates was found to have on average 15 alleles per MS locus (Wootton et al., 2002; Joy et al., 2006). MS are apparently much less abundant in *P. vivax* and *P. yoelii* (Feng et al, 2003; Li et al., 2009). Additionally, there are large numbers of genes containing polymorphic multi-amino-acid repeats (Hughes, 2004). The repeat arrays often differ in size among parasites of the same species. Some of these genes, such as the circumsporozoite surface protein gene *(csp)* in both *P. falciparum* and *P. vivax* and the *P. falciparum Pf11-1* gene (Scherf et al., 1993), may be under host immune pressure to diversify with regard to number of repeats due to antibody recognition (Walliker et al., 1998; Putaporntip et al., 2009). A third repetitive element that figures prominently in malaria parasite genomes comprises the large and highly polymorphic gene families that can make up 10% to 15% of the genome. For example, each individual *P. falciparum* parasite has ~60 *var* gene copies and more than 200 copies of hypervariable *rifin*, *stevor*, and *Pfmc*-2TM genes (Gardner et al., 2002; Templeton, 2009). These genes differ among parasites not only in sequences but also in the number of gene copies and expression patterns. Given two *P. falciparum* parasites carrying unique sets of 60 *var* genes, the number of progeny having a unique set of *var* genes would be expected to be quite large after chromosomal assortment and recombination. When one considers this in the context of Africa, where large numbers of parasite strains are present, it is clear that the number of possible different *var* genes is enormous. Indeed, high *var* gene recombination frequencies and signatures of *var* gene conversion have been detected in *P. falciparum* field isolates (Freitas-Junior et al., 2000; Trimnell et al., 2006). The *var* genes encode a family of large erythrocyte membrane proteins (PfEMP1) that play an important role in immune evasion and disease pathogenesis (Howard et al., 1988; Baruch et al., 1995; Smith et al., 1995; Su et al., 1995).

Gene copy number variation (CNV) is yet another factor contributing to genome diversity in malaria parasites. In *P. falciparum*, CNV has been detected for many genes by using high-density microarray and/or real-time PCR (Kidgell et al., 2006; Ribacke et al., 2007; Jiang et al., 2008a, 2008b; Nair et al., 2008). CNV has been documented for the gene encoding a homolog of the human P-glycoprotein (*pfmdr1*) and for the gene encoding the first enzyme in the *Plasmodium* folate biosynthesis pathway, GTP-cyclohydrolase I, both of which show evidence of gene amplification (Cowman et al., 1994; Nair et al., 2008). Both genes have also been shown to be under drug selection, and amplification of the genes may be associated with responses to many drugs (Cowman et al., 1994; Hayton and Su, 2004; Price et al., 2004; Nair et al., 2007, 2008; Preechapornkul et al., 2009). Conversely, deletions of chromosomal segments and genes have also been reported (Pologe and Ravetch, 1986; Biggs et al., 1989; Kidgell et al., 2006; Ribacke et al., 2007; Jiang et al., 2008a, 2008b). CNV plays an important role in parasite response to antimalarial drugs and environmental changes.

Recent large-scale studies have shown that *P. falciparum* has a high frequency of SNP, with one SNP in less than 500 bp of DNA sequence (Kidgell et al., 2006; Jeffares et al., 2007; Mu et al., 2007; Volkman et al., 2007; Jiang et al., 2008b). Of interest, the genomes of *P. falciparum* and *P. vivax* have more nonsynonymous substitutions than synonymous substitutions, perhaps due in part to both host immune and drug selection (Mu et al., 2002; Feng et al., 2003), although the high proportion of genes encoding proteins with low-complexity domains and the nucleotide composition of the genomes may also contribute to the high nonsynonymous substitution rate (Hey, 1999; Mu et al., 2002). These observations and studies clearly show that the genome of *P. falciparum* is highly polymorphic, a key feature that allows the parasite to thrive in hostile environments.

HIGH RECOMBINATION RATE AND GENOME DIVERSITY

Malaria parasites have relatively high recombination rates compared with other organisms studied, such as humans and mice. This high recombination rate constitutes another means of generating and maintaining allelic diversity. Recombination rates in *P. falciparum* have been estimated both from genetic crosses and from field populations. A map unit of ~17 kb/cM was obtained from crossover counts among 35 progeny of a genetic cross (Dd2 × HB3) (Wellems et al., 1990; Su et al., 1999). The actual value is closer to 15 kb/cM when the correct genome size (23 Mb) is used instead of the 27 Mb used in the initial calculation of recombination frequency. For a different genetic cross (GB4 × 7G8), the map unit was estimated to be 36 kb/cM (Hayton et al., 2008), approximately twice that of the Dd × HB3 cross. Although the numbers of progeny from these two crosses was comparable (35 from Dd2 × HB cross; 32 from the GB4 × 7G8 cross), the numbers of MS markers used in typing the progeny differed considerably (901 in the Dd2 × HB3 cross and 281 in the GB4 × 7G8 cross). Higher marker density in the Dd2 × HB3 cross partly explains the differences in map unit estimates; and it seems reasonable to expect that the map unit for the GB4 × 7G8 cross would decrease if the progeny were typed using more markers. Similarly, the mean map unit was estimated to be 13.7 kb/cM for the rodent malaria parasite *P. c. chabaudi* based on a study of 22 independent progeny from a genetic cross between AS and AJ strains using 819 amplified fragment-length polymorphism (AFLP) markers (Martinelli et al., 2005). Map units have value primarily when approximately the same numbers of progeny and markers are used for the analysis of each cross.

Recombination rates are high and can vary in the field due to differences in transmission intensity and the probability of infections with multiple genotypes (Conway et al., 1999); these rates have been shown to vary both among different parasite populations and across a chromosome in *P. falciparum* (Mu et al., 2005a; Volkman et al., 2007). Compared with those of southeast Asia and South America, African parasite populations have the highest detectable recombination rate, likely due to higher transmission intensity, which in turn can increase the probability of multiple genotype infections within a single individual (Mu et al., 2005a; Volkman et al., 2007).

Recombination hot spots are commonly observed among progeny of a genetic cross and in field populations, with many recombination hot spots occurring at chromosome ends (Mu et al., 2005a; Su et al., 1999). *P. falciparum* chromosome ends, or telomeres, contain a high proportion of genes implicated in host interactions and are likely to be under strong immune-mediated diversifying selection. Selection pressure may also promote high recombination rates in other genomic regions (Reed and Tishkoff, 2006). Frequent recombination may accelerate the emergence of parasites with different levels of virulence by shuffling genomic content and producing unique genomes.

GENOTYPING AND MEASUREMENT OF GENOME DIVERSITY

Over the years, many methods have been employed to genotype malaria parasites. These methods include isoenzyme electrophoresis (Carter and Voller, 1975), restriction fragment length polymorphism (Wellems et al., 1990), AFLP (Grech et al., 2002), MS typing (Su and Wellems, 1996), and SNP typing (Mu et al., 2003; Neafsey et al., 2008). MS and SNP typing are currently the preferred methods for *P. falciparum* because of simplicity and the potential for high-throughput analysis. MS have also been used quite extensively to type *P. vivax*. In contrast, AFLP typing has been the predominant method used with rodent malaria parasites.

MS typing is typically done through amplification of DNA fragments containing small repeat units (2- to 6-mer) and size separation of PCR products in a DNA sequencing gel or capillaries. The PCR products can be labeled with fluorescent dyes or radioactive isotopes (Ferdig and Su, 2000). A single-labeled-primer method was recently introduced for use with *P. yoelii*, greatly reducing primer labeling costs (Li et al., 2007). Separating PCR products using a QIAxcel (Qiagen, Valencia, CA) instrument or similar equipment bypasses the PCR product labeling step altogether. Due to these reductions in cost, this machine may be ideal for MS typing at field sites in regions of endemic infection.

Although MS typing can be quite fast and efficient, the development of various high-throughput methods has made SNPs the markers of choice for genotyping. High-density tiling arrays with up to 4.8 million oligonucleotides covering ~76% of the *P. falciparum* genome, including 90% of the predicted coding regions, have been used to detect SNP and CNV (Kidgell et al., 2006; Jiang et al., 2008b; Dharia et al., 2009). Thousands of unique SNPs and regions of deletion/insertion were detected from each field isolate. The advantages of a high-density tiling array include the ability to detect novel mutations; the disadvantages are the time and computing capacity required to analyze the large data set generated from millions of probes for each parasite DNA sample. Microarray chips are still quite expensive, costing $300 to $600 per chip. A second type of microarray detects known SNPs identified from large-scale genome sequencing of multiple parasite isolates. A microarray using molecular inversion probe technology (Hardenbol et al., 2003; Absalan and Ronaghi, 2007) has been successfully developed to interrogate ~3,500 SNPs in the *P. falciparum* genome (Mu et al., 2010). This approach involves one PCR amplification step before hybridization of the parasite DNA to the chip and therefore may need less DNA than is required for tiling arrays. Other arrays include the Affymetrix 3,000 SNP assay array, employing a standard Affymetrix 500K array design with 56 probes to interrogate one SNP. This allows roughly half the SNPs to be detected with 100% accuracy (Neafsey et al., 2008). Recently, an array using a different technology (NimbleGen CGH platform) was employed to detect SNP and CNV, although the long oligos in this array make it insensitive to SNP (Tan et al., 2009). Finally, with the increasing availability of high-throughput genome sequencing (Solexa/Illumina, SOLiD/ABI, 454/Roche, and HeliScope/Helicos) and rapid decrease in sequencing costs, the possibility of using genome-wide sequencing to genotype parasites is now imminent (Bennett et al., 2005).

GENOME DIVERSITY AND ESTIMATES OF THE AGE AND CLONALITY OF *P. FALCIPARUM*

The degree and extent of genome diversity is tightly linked to parasite origins and evolutionary history. The "malaria's Eve" hypothesis was proposed approximately 10 years ago to explain both the observed absence of synonymous substitutions in some *P. falciparum* genes and the lack of correlation between the strength of linkage disequilibrium (LD) and nucleotide distances in the *csp* gene (Rich et al., 1997, 1998). This hypothesis posits that the *P. falciparum* genome is quite homogeneous and that the population is effectively clonal. Subsequent studies provided additional evidence in support of this hypothesis (Conway et al., 2000; Tishkoff et al., 2001; Volkman et al., 2001). The low frequency of synonymous substitution (P = 0.0004) in the *P. falciparum* mitochondrial genome suggested that the parasite had recently emerged from a single ancestral progenitor (Conway et al., 2000). The presence of small numbers of SNPs in 25 introns from 10 housekeeping genes on chromosomes 2 and 3 also supports a young parasite population, with only a few SNPs found in 4,217-bp intron sequences from eight global isolates (Volkman et al., 2001). Mitochondrial SNPs from a worldwide collection of parasites point to a recent (~10,000 years ago) and rapid *P. falciparum* population expansion in Africa that may have coincided with agricultural changes and mosquito speciation events (Coluzzi, 1999; Tishkoff et al., 2001; Joy et al., 2003), yet paradoxically, as discussed above, the *P. falciparum* genome is quite diverse. In addition to size polymorphisms such as chromosome size variation, gene deletion and amplification, and highly polymorphic MS, SNPs are much more abundant than previously thought. Based on the large numbers of SNPs identified from recent large-scale genome sequencing, the most recent common ancestor of *P. falciparum* parasites was estimated to have existed ~50,000 to 300,000 years ago (Hughes and Verra, 2002; Mu et al., 2002, 2007; Joy et al., 2003; Jeffares et al., 2007; Volkman et al., 2007). The different findings regarding the age of *P. falciparum* can be reconciled in light of the fact that recent population bottlenecks and expansions at various scales are also likely to have occurred through drug selection, migration and expansion of human populations, or mosquito speciation (Tishkoff et al., 2001; Coluzzi et al., 2002; Wootton et al., 2002; Su et al., 2003).

GENOME DIVERSITY AND *P. FALCIPARUM* POPULATION STRUCTURE

Understanding the population structure of malaria is essential for predicting and detecting the spread of drug resistance and other adaptive variation. It is crucial that samples used in association studies be assessed for population structure, because undetected structure can lead to erroneous associations between alleles and phenotypes. This is because allele frequencies in different populations are likely to differ.

The population structure of *P. falciparum* has been alternatively described as effectively clonal, epidemic, or panmictic (Day et al., 1992; Razakandrainibe et al., 2005). Clonal and epidemic population structures share the characteristic of having low genetic diversity, in contrast to a panmictic population, where genetic diversity is high and sexual recombination is frequent. A study comparing *P. falciparum* population structure on different continents by using MS typing found that *P. falciparum* was panmictic in Africa with frequent recombination (Anderson et al., 2000); in contrast, high levels of LD were associated with low diversity in regions of low endemicity in South America (Anderson et al., 2000; Tami et al., 2002). Many more studies examining *P. falciparum* population genetics on both global and local scales have followed, most recently with genome-wide SNP markers. A survey of SNPs across chromosome 3 has confirmed that *P. falciparum* populations primarily cluster by continent (Mu et al., 2005a). A separate study of 137 SNPs across 20 genomic regions among 66 parasites from Africa, Asia, and Latin America further confirmed population differentiation among continental groups (Volkman et al., 2007).

GENETIC MAPPING

MS have been used successfully to genotype malaria parasites for a variety of studies. MS typing of progeny from a genetic cross led to the identification of a locus containing the gene encoding *P. falciparum* chloroquine resistant transporter (*pfcrt*) (Su et al., 1997), as well as a gene that was linked to *P. falciparum* invasion of *Aotus* monkeys (Hayton et al., 2008). The *pfcrt* locus was again identified with the help of MS when field isolates were genotyped and a region of reduced MS heterozygosity was detected in the chromosome region where the *pfcrt* gene resides (Wootton et al., 2002). Indeed, identifying regions of reduced MS diversity could become a strategy for searching for genes under drug selection (Anderson, 2004; Su and Wootton, 2004). Typing MS markers flanking a known drug resistance gene has already been widely employed to study drug-selective sweeps, origins of drug-resistant parasites, and population structure (Anderson and Day, 2000; Anderson et al., 2000; Wootton et al., 2002; Nair et al., 2003; Roper et al., 2003, 2004; McCollum et al., 2007; Pearce et al., 2009). As new classes of drugs are introduced to fight malaria, MS markers will continue to be very useful tools for monitoring the origin and spread of drug-resistant parasites.

Genome-wide polymorphic SNPs can also be applied to mapping genes or mutations that are associated with parasite phenotypes of interest. Various high-throughput genotyping methods have made it possible to interrogate the entire parasite genome, making these studies truly genome-wide (Su et al., 2007). A proof of principle of genome-wide association in *P. falciparum* was detection of the association between the *pfcrt* locus and chloroquine resistance by using MS markers (Wootton et al., 2002). Unfortunately, there are relatively few parasite phenotypes that can be easily studied using genome-wide association, with the exception of drug resistance, growth characteristics, and possibly virulence (Su and Wootton, 2004). Although there is currently great interest in mapping disease phenotypes such as severe malaria, this has nonetheless proven challenging, as disease phenotypes are likely the result of interactions between the parasite and host genomes as well as the environment. Discovery and characterization of malaria phenotypes will be critical for genome-wide association studies. A recent report in which a large number of chemical compounds were screened for their ability to produce differential chemical phenotypes in the parasite provides a powerful new high-throughput approach for studying gene function and identifying novel targets for antimalarial drugs (Yuan et al., 2009).

GENOME DIVERSITY, VACCINE DEVELOPMENT, AND DRUG RESISTANCE

Malaria control has relied primarily on antimalarial drugs and other interventions such as bed nets, although an effective vaccine to prevent infection is the ultimate goal. Unfortunately, the complex life cycle and highly diverse genome of the malaria parasite have greatly complicated efforts to develop an effective vaccine. One goal of studying genome diversity is to uncover information that will facilitate vaccine and drug development. A large number of vaccine candidate proteins or surface antigens from malaria parasites have been identified, and many of them are being tested for protection (Walther, 2006; Vekemans and Ballou, 2008). Because of their interaction with the host immune system, the majority of these vaccine candidates are highly polymorphic, which in turn presents a formidable problem for vaccine development. For example, the *P. falciparum* apical membrane antigen (PfAMA1) is a protein expressed on the surface of the apical end of merozoites and is one of the prime targets of the host immune response. PfAMA1 is highly polymorphic, and hundreds of PfAMA1 haplotypes have thus far been identified (Polley and Conway, 2001; Duan et al., 2008). Because the host immune response to this and other antigens is often allele specific (Cortes et al., 2005), a vaccine with one or a few specific PfAMA1 alleles is unlikely to protect individuals from infection by parasites with alleles not contained in the vaccine. Another highly polymorphic antigen is PfEMP1, which is expressed on the surface of infected RBCs. The protein is encoded by a diverse *var* gene family comprising approximately 60 diverse genes (Baruch et al., 1995; Smith et al., 1995; Su et al., 1995). To evade the host immune response to PfEMP1, malaria parasites undergo antigenic variation in which each individual parasite expresses a unique copy of the *var* genes (Chen et al., 1998; Deitsch et al., 1999). Differences in gene expression add another dimension to genome variation and make it even more challenging to develop a protective vaccine. Approaches that may overcome the issue of antigenic polymorphism in vaccine design include the use of relatively conserved antigens, if they can be found, or employment of whole, attenuated parasites (VanBuskirk et al., 2009).

A highly diverse genome may pose still other challenges to malaria control. For example, a genetically diverse parasite population may respond more rapidly to drug pressure than a homogeneous population, simply because a more diverse genome is more likely to contain resistance alleles by chance. Although there has been no solid evidence to prove this hypothesis in the field, parasites from the Thai-Cambodian border appear to have a propensity to rapidly develop resistance to almost all antimalarial drugs used in the region (Na-Bangchang and Congpuong, 2007). It has been shown that a parasite already resistant to chloroquine and other common antimalarial agents became resistant to newer drugs more quickly than did a parasite sensitive to chloroquine (Rathod et al., 1997). This suggests that exposure of malarial parasites to multiple antimalarial drugs may have selected for genetic traits that favor the initiation of resistance to novel unrelated antimalarial agents (this is known as accelerated resistance to multiple drugs [ARMD]) (Rathod et al., 1997). Genes encoding transporters such as *pfmdr1*, *pfmrp*, and *pfcrt* could play an important role in ARMD (Reed et al., 2000; Johnson et al., 2004; Sidhu et al., 2006; Raj et al., 2008).

GENOME DIVERSITY AND POPULATION STRUCTURE OF *P. VIVAX*

The *P. vivax* genome is at least as diverse as that of *P. falciparum*, according to estimates of the nucleotide substitution rate across a 200-kb DNA segment sampled from five *P. vivax* isolates, although the frequency of MS is much lower than that of *P. falciparum*, probably in part due to the lower A+T content of the *P. vivax* genome (Feng et al., 2003). One study using eight MS markers showed extremely low levels of diversity among isolates, suggestive of a severe and recent population bottleneck (Leclerc et al., 2004); however, low marker heterogeneity was later shown to be an artifact of marker choice. It is known that MS marker heterogeneity is positively correlated with the average number of MS repeats. The markers chosen for this study were biased downward with regard to repeat number, and consequently they lacked variability (Imwong et al., 2006). Subsequent studies employing the complete mitochondrial genome (Jongwutiwes et al., 2005; Mu et al., 2005b) and different MS loci (Imwong et al., 2007; Joy et al., 2008; Karunaweera et al., 2008) found that the genetic diversity of *P. vivax* is equal to that of *P. falciparum*, if not greater. Similar to *P. falciparum*, the *P. vivax* genome also contains large families of variant antigens (Janssen et al., 2002; del Portillo et al., 2004; Carlton et al., 2008). Expression of some gene family members appeared to be "random" (Cunningham et al., 2009), and expression for subsets of genes predicted to encode proteins associated with virulence and host pathogen interaction appeared to be strain specific (Bozdech et al., 2008). Karyotype polymorphism among *P. vivax* field isolates has also been observed (Langsley et al., 1988). This level of genomic diversity is consistent with a worldwide distribution.

As markers for *P. vivax* have been developed, investigators have also explored the population structure of this parasite. Population diversity and population structure both within and between geographic areas of Africa, China, India, Indonesia, the Philippines, Papua New Guinea, the Solomon Islands, and Thailand were analyzed using the polymorphic regions of the genes encoding *P. vivax* apical membrane antigen 1 (PvAMA1) and merozoite surface protein 1 (PvMSP1) (Figtree et al., 2000). Significant differences in allele frequencies between different regions were present, but the differences were small compared with the diversity within populations. The evidence for continental subdivision of *P. vivax* populations has not been as compelling as for *P. falciparum*. Although there are exceptions (Imwong et al., 2007), most studies have detected only minor continental structuring in *P. vivax* (Mu et al., 2005b; Cornejo and Escalante, 2006; Karunaweera et al., 2008). Some structuring by continent is expected, because geographically separated populations cannot freely mate and recombine. A possible explanation for the pattern seen in *P. vivax* may be that continental structure is obscured by noise created by a unique aspect of *P. vivax* biology. During infection of a human host, *P. vivax* undergoes a period of dormancy in the liver. The dormant liver stage (the hypnozoite) can reactivate and cause a relapse of the illness long after the primary blood-stage episode has been treated and cleared. The length of the relapse period differs among geographic regions and is probably related to temperature and perhaps also to seasonal availability of vectors. Shorter latent periods (3 to 5 weeks) and more frequent relapse episodes are characteristics of infection with *P. vivax* from tropical regions, while longer latent periods (5 to 10 months) and fewer incidences are more characteristic of infection with *P. vivax* from temperate regions. Relapse, especially where it is long lasting, probably acts to obscure geographic associations as infected humans move between geographic regions (Karunaweera et al., 2008).

On both regional and local scales, the population structure of *P. vivax* appears to be similar to that of *P. falciparum* in many respects; however, some differences have emerged (Imwong et al., 2007). Whereas *P. falciparum* exhibits low genetic diversity, high LD, and infrequent multiclone infections in low-transmission areas, *P. vivax* in low-transmission regions of Brazil, Columbia, and Sri Lanka exhibits a combination of high genetic diversity and high multilocus LD (Ferreira et al., 2007; Imwong et al., 2007; Karunaweera et al., 2008). A possible explanation for this pattern is the presence of more than one distinct parasite population. High multilocus LD would be expected if population structure was present but undetected because alleles from the same subpopulation would be associated with each other more often than expected by chance.

In southern Mexico, more than one distinct *P. vivax* population was detected, and each population was preferentially transmitted by a single local mosquito vector (Gonzalez-Ceron et al., 2000; Joy et al., 2008). An earlier study identified two distinct *P. vivax* populations, designated Old World and New World types, and demonstrated that they, too, differed markedly with respect to mosquito vector compatibility (Li et al., 2001). Vector-parasite compatibilities may play an important role in generating population structure in *P. vivax*.

SUMMARY

Malaria parasites are highly diverse organisms whose ability to adapt to, and survive in, variable and often harsh host environments is enhanced through genetic variation. An understanding of the genome diversity of malaria parasites provides valuable insights into parasite evolution, population structure, dynamics of transmission, mechanisms of drug resistance, immune evasion, and parasite development. The recent development of high-throughput methods for characterizing genomic variations will greatly enhance our understanding of the parasite genome and the genetic diversity contained therein.

ACKNOWLEDGMENTS

This work was supported by the Intramural Research Program of the Division of Intramural Research, National Institute of Allergy and Infectious Diseases (NIAID), National Institutes of Health.

We declare no conflicts of interest relevant to this chapter.

We thank NIAID intramural editor Brenda Rae Marshall for assistance.

REFERENCES

Absalan, F., and M. Ronaghi. 2007. Molecular inversion probe assay. *Methods Mol. Biol.* **396:**315–330.

Anderson, T. J., 2004. Mapping drug resistance genes in *Plasmodium falciparum* by genome-wide association. *Curr. Drug Targets Infect. Disord.* **4:**65–78.

Anderson, T. J., and K. P. Day. 2000. Geographical structure and sequence evolution as inferred from the *Plasmodium falciparum* S-antigen locus. *Mol. Biochem. Parasitol.* **106:**321–326.

Anderson, T. J., B. Haubold, J. T. Williams, J. G. Estrada-Franco, L. Richardson, R. Mollinedo, M. Bockarie, J. Mokili, S. Mharakurwa, N. French, J. Whitworth, I. D. Velez, A. H. Brockman, F. Nosten, M. U. Ferreira, and K. P. Day.

2000. Microsatellite markers reveal a spectrum of population structures in the malaria parasite *Plasmodium falciparum*. *Mol. Biol. Evol.* **17:**1467–1482.

Baruch, D. I., B. L. Pasloske, H. B. Singh, X. Bi, X. C. Ma, M. Feldman, T. F. Taraschi, and R. J. Howard. 1995. Cloning the *P. falciparum* gene encoding PfEMP1, a malarial variant antigen and adherence receptor on the surface of parasitized human erythrocytes. *Cell* **82:**77–87.

Bennett, S. T., C. Barnes, A. Cox, L. Davies, and C. Brown. 2005. Toward the 1,000 dollars human genome. *Pharmacogenomics* **6:**373–382.

Biggs, B. A., D. J. Kemp, and G. V. Brown. 1989. Subtelomeric chromosome deletions in field isolates of *Plasmodium falciparum* and their relationship to loss of cytoadherence *in vitro*. *Proc. Natl. Acad. Sci. USA* **86:**2428–2432.

Bottius, E., N. Bakhsis, and A. Scherf. 1998. *Plasmodium falciparum* telomerase: *de novo* telomere addition to telomeric and nontelomeric sequences and role in chromosome healing. *Mol. Cell. Biol.* **18:**919–925.

Bozdech, Z., S. Mok, G. Hu, M. Imwong, A. Jaidee, B. Russell, H. Ginsburg, F. Nosten, N. P. Day, N. J. White, J. M. Carlton, and P. R. Preiser. 2008. The transcriptome of *Plasmodium vivax* reveals divergence and diversity of transcriptional regulation in malaria parasites. *Proc. Natl. Acad. Sci. USA* **105:**16290–16295.

Carlton, J. 2003. The *Plasmodium vivax* genome sequencing project. *Trends Parasitol.* **19:**227–231.

Carlton, J. M., J. H. Adams, J. C. Silva, S. L. Bidwell, H. Lorenzi, E. Caler, J. Crabtree, S. V. Angiuoli, E. F. Merino, P. Amedeo, Q. Cheng, R. M. Coulson, B. S. Crabb, H. A. Del Portillo, K. Essien, T. V. Feldblyum, C. Fernandez-Becerra, P. R. Gilson, A. H. Gueye, X. Guo, S. Kang'a, T. W. Kooij, M. Korsinczky, E. V. Meyer, V. Nene, I. Paulsen, O. White, S. A. Ralph, Q. Ren, T. J. Sargeant, S. L. Salzberg, C. J. Stoeckert, S. A. Sullivan, M. M. Yamamoto, S. L. Hoffman, J. R. Wortman, M. J. Gardner, M. R. Galinski, J. W. Barnwell, and C. M. Fraser-Liggett. 2008. Comparative genomics of the neglected human malaria parasite *Plasmodium vivax*. *Nature* **455:**757–763.

Carlton, J. M., S. V. Angiuoli, B. B. Suh, T. W. Kooij, M. Pertea, J. C. Silva, M. D. Ermolaeva, J. E. Allen, J. D. Selengut, H. L. Koo, J. D. Peterson, M. Pop, D. S. Kosack, M. F. Shumway, S. L. Bidwell, S. J. Shallom, S. E. van Aken, S. B. Riedmuller, T. V. Feldblyum, J. K. Cho, J. Quackenbush, M. Sedegah, A. Shoaibi, L. M. Cummings, L. Florens, J. R. Yates, J. D. Raine, R. E. Sinden, M. A. Harris, D. A. Cunningham, P. R. Preiser, L. W. Bergman, A. B. Vaidya, L. H. van Lin, C. J. Janse, A. P. Waters, H. O. Smith, O R. White, S. L. Salzberg, J. C. Venter, C. M. Fraser, S. L. Hoffman, M. J. Gardner, and D. J. Carucci. 2002. Genome sequence and comparative analysis of the model rodent malaria parasite *Plasmodium yoelii yoelii*. *Nature* **419:**512–519.

Carlton, J., J. Silva, and N. Hall. 2005. The genome of model malaria parasites, and comparative genomics. *Curr. Issues Mol. Biol.* **7:**23–37.

Carlton, J. M., R. Vinkenoog, A. P. Waters, and D. Walliker. 1998. Gene synteny in species of *Plasmodium*. *Mol. Biochem. Parasitol.* **93:**285–294.

Carter, R., and K. N. Mendis. 2002. Evolutionary and historical aspects of the burden of malaria. *Clin. Microbiol. Rev.* **15:**564–594.

Carter, R., and A. Voller. 1975. The distribution of enzyme variation in populations of *Plasmodium falciparum* in Africa. *Trans. R. Soc. Trop. Med. Hyg.* **69:**371–376.

Chen, Q., V. Fernandez, A. Sundstrom, M. Schlichtherle, S. Datta, P. Hagblom, and M. Wahlgren. 1998. Developmental selection of *var* gene expression in *Plasmodium falciparum*. *Nature* **394:**392–395.

Coluzzi, M. 1999. The clay feet of the malaria giant and its African roots: hypotheses and inferences about origin, spread and control of *Plasmodium falciparum*. *Parassitologia* **41:**277–283.

Coluzzi, M., A. Sabatini, A. della Torre, M. A. di Deco, and V. Petrarca. 2002. A polytene chromosome analysis of the *Anopheles gambiae* species complex. *Science* **298:**1415–1418.

Conway, D. J., C. Fanello, J. M. Lloyd, B. M. al-Joubori, A. H. Baloch, S. D. Somanath, C. Roper, A. M. Oduola, B. Mulder, M. M. Povoa, B. Singh, and A. W. Thomas. 2000. Origin of *Plasmodium falciparum* malaria is traced by mitochondrial DNA. *Mol. Biochem. Parasitol.* **111:**163–171.

Conway, D. J., C. Roper, A. M. Oduola, D. E. Arnot, P. G. Kremsner, M. P. Grobusch, C. F. Curtis, and B. M. Greenwood. 1999. High recombination rate in natural populations of *Plasmodium falciparum*. *Proc. Natl. Acad. Sci. USA* **96:**4506–4511.

Cornejo, O. E., and A. A. Escalante. 2006. The origin and age of *Plasmodium vivax*. *Trends Parasitol.* **22:**558–563.

Cortes, A., M. Mellombo, R. Masciantonio, V. J. Murphy, J. C. Reeder, and R. F. Anders. 2005. Allele specificity of naturally acquired antibody responses against *Plasmodium falciparum* apical membrane antigen 1. *Infect. Immun.* **73:**422–430.

Cowman, A. F., D. Galatis, and J. K. Thompson. 1994. Selection for mefloquine resistance in

Plasmodium falciparum is linked to amplification of the *pfmdr1* gene and cross-resistance to halofantrine and quinine. *Proc. Natl. Acad. Sci. USA* **91:** 1143–1147.

Cunningham, D., J. Fonager, W. Jarra, C. Carret, P. Preiser, and J. Langhorne. 2009. Rapid changes in transcription profiles of the *Plasmodium yoelii* yir multigene family in clonal populations: lack of epigenetic memory? *PLoS One* **4:**e4285.

Day, K .P., F. Karamalis, J. Thompson, D. A. Barnes, C. Peterson, H. Brown, G. V. Brown, and D. J. Kemp. 1993. Genes necessary for expression of a virulence determinant and for transmission of *Plasmodium falciparum* are located on a 0.3-megabase region of chromosome 9. *Proc. Natl. Acad. Sci. USA* **90:**8292–8296.

Day, K. P., J. C. Koella, S. Nee, S. Gupta, and A. F. Read. 1992. Population genetics and dynamics of *Plasmodium falciparum*: an ecological view. *Parasitology* **104:**S35–52.

Deitsch, K. W., A. del Pinal, and T. E. Wellems. 1999. Intra-cluster recombination and *var* transcription switches in the antigenic variation of *Plasmodium falciparum. Mol. Biochem. Parasitol.* **101:** 107–116.

del Portillo, H. A., M. Lanzer, S. Rodriguez-Malaga, F. Zavala, and C. Fernandez-Becerra. 2004. Variant genes and the spleen in *Plasmodium vivax* malaria. *Int. J. Parasitol.* **34:** 1547–1554.

Dharia, N. V., A. B. Sidhu, M. B. Cassera, S. J. Westenberger, S. E. Bopp, R. T. Eastman, D. Plouffe, S. Batalov, D. J. Park, S. K. Volkman, D. F. Wirth, Y. Zhou, D. A. Fidock, and E. A. Winzeler. 2009. Use of high-density tiling microarrays to identify mutations globally and elucidate mechanisms of drug resistance in *Plasmodium falciparum. Genome Biol.* **10:**R21.

Duan, J., J. Mu, M. A. Thera, D. Joy, S. L. Kosakovsky Pond, D. Diemert, C. Long, H. Zhou, K. Miura, A. Ouattara, A. Dolo, O. Doumbo, X. Z. Su, and L. Miller. 2008. Population structure of the genes encoding the polymorphic *Plasmodium falciparum* apical membrane antigen 1: implications for vaccine design. *Proc. Natl. Acad. Sci. USA* **105:**7857–7862.

Feng, X., J. M. Carlton, D. A. Joy, J. Mu, T. Furuya, B. B. Suh, Y. Wang, J. W. Barnwell, and X. Z. Su. 2003. Single-nucleotide polymorphisms and genome diversity in *Plasmodium vivax. Proc. Natl. Acad. Sci. USA* **100:**8502–8507.

Ferdig, M. T., and X.-Z. Su. 2000. Microsatellite markers and genetic mapping in *Plasmodium falciparum. Parasitol. Today* **7:**307–312.

Ferreira, M. U., N. D. Karunaweera, M. da Silva-Nunes, N. S. da Silva, D. F. Wirth, and D. L. Hartl. 2007. Population structure and transmission dynamics of *Plasmodium vivax* in rural Amazonia. *J. Infect. Dis.* **195:**1218–1226.

Figtree, M., C. J. Pasay, R. Slade, Q. Cheng, N. Cloonan, J. Walker, and A. Saul. 2000. *Plasmodium vivax* synonymous substitution frequencies, evolution and population structure deduced from diversity in AMA 1 and MSP 1 genes. *Mol. Biochem. Parasitol.* **108:**53–66.

Freitas-Junior, L. H., E. Bottius, L. A. Pirrit, K. W. Deitsch, C. Scheidig, F. Guinet, U. Nehrbass, T. E. Wellems, and A. Scherf. 2000. Frequent ectopic recombination of virulence factor genes in telomeric chromosome clusters of *P. falciparum. Nature* **407:**1018–1022.

Gardner, M. J., N. Hall, E. Fung, O. White, M. Berriman, R. W. Hyman, J. M. Carlton, A. Pain, K. E. Nelson, S. Bowman, I. T. Paulsen, K. James, J. A. Eisen, K. Rutherford, S. L. Salzberg, A. Craig, S. Kyes, M. S. Chan, V. Nene, S. J. Shallom, B. Suh, J. Peterson, S. Angiuoli, M. Pertea, J. Allen, J. Selengut, D. Haft, M. W. Mather, A. B. Vaidya, D. M. Martin, A. H. Fairlamb, M. J. Fraunholz, D. S. Roos, S. A. Ralph, G. I. McFadden, L. M. Cummings, G. M. Subramanian, C. Mungall, J. C. Venter, D. J. Carucci, S. L. Hoffman, C. Newbold, R. W. Davis, C. M. Fraser, and B. Barrell. 2002. Genome sequence of the human malaria parasite *Plasmodium falciparum. Nature* **419:**498–511.

Gonzalez-Ceron, L., M. H. Rodriguez, F. V. Santillan, J. E. Hernandez, and R. A. Wirtz. 2000. Susceptibility of three laboratory strains of *Anopheles albimanus* (Diptera: Culicidae) to coindigenous *Plasmodium vivax* circumsporozoite protein phenotypes in southern Mexico. *J. Med. Entomol.* **37:** 331–334.

Grech, K., A. Martinelli, S. Pathirana, D. Walliker, P. Hunt, and R. Carter. 2002. Numerous, robust genetic markers for *Plasmodium chabaudi* by the method of amplified fragment length polymorphism. *Mol. Biochem. Parasitol.* **123:**95–104.

Hall, N., M. Karras, J. D. Raine, J. M. Carlton, T. W. Kooij, M. Berriman, L. Florens, C. S. Janssen, A. Pain, G. K. Christophides, K. James, K. Rutherford, B. Harris, D. Harris, C. Churcher, M. A. Quail, D. Ormond, J. Doggett, H, E. Trueman, J. Mendoza, S. L. Bidwell, M. A. Rajandream, D. J. Carucci, J. R. Yates III, F. C. Kafatos, C. J. Janse, B. Barrell, C. M. Turner, A. P. Waters, and R. E. Sinden. 2005. A comprehensive survey of the *Plasmodium* life cycle by genomic, transcriptomic, and proteomic analyses. *Science* **307:**82–86.

Hardenbol, P., J. Baner, M. Jain, M. Nilsson, E. A. Namsaraev, G. A. Karlin-Neumann, H. Fakhrai-Rad, M. Ronaghi, T. D. Willis, U. Landegren, and R. W. Davis. 2003. Multiplexed genotyping with sequence-tagged molecular inversion probes. *Nat. Biotechnol.* **21:**673–678.

Hayton, K., D. Gaur, A. Liu, J. Takahashi, B. Henschen, S. Singh, L. Lambert, T. Furuya, R. Bouttenot, M. Doll, F. Nawaz, J. Mu, L. Jiang, L. H. Miller, and T. E. Wellems. 2008. Erythrocyte binding protein PfRH5 polymorphisms determine species-specific pathways of *Plasmodium falciparum* invasion. *Cell Host Microbe* **4:**40–51.

Hayton, K., and X.-Z. Su. 2004. Genetic and biochemical aspects of drug resistance in malaria parasites. *Curr. Drug Targets Infect. Disord.* **4:**1–10.

Hey, J. 1999. Parasite populations: the puzzle of *Plasmodium*. *Curr. Biol.* **9:**R565–567.

Howard, R. J., J. W. Barnwell, E. P. Rock, J. Neequaye, D. Ofori-Adjei, W. L. Maloy, J. A. Lyon, and A. Saul. 1988. Two approximately 300 kilodalton *Plasmodium falciparum* proteins at the surface membrane of infected erythrocytes. *Mol. Biochem. Parasitol.* **27:**207–223.

Hughes, A. L. 2004. The evolution of amino acid repeat arrays in *Plasmodium* and other organisms. *J. Mol. Evol.* **59:**528–535.

Hughes, A. L., and F. Verra. 2002. Extensive polymorphism and ancient origin of *Plasmodium falciparum*. *Trends Parasitol.* **18:**348–351.

Imwong, M., S. Nair, S. Pukrittayakamee, D. Sudimack, J. T. Williams, M. Mayxay, P. N. Newton, J. R. Kim, A. Nandy, L. Osorio, J. M. Carlton, N. J. White, N. P. Day, and T. J. Anderson. 2007. Contrasting genetic structure in *Plasmodium vivax* populations from Asia and South America. *Int. J. Parasitol.* **37:**1013–1022.

Imwong, M., D. Sudimack, S. Pukrittayakamee, L. Osorio, J. M. Carlton, N. P. Day, N. J. White, and T. J. Anderson. 2006. Microsatellite variation, repeat array length, and population history of *Plasmodium vivax*. *Mol. Biol. Evol.* **23:**1016–1018.

Janse, C. J., J. M. Carlton, D. Walliker, and A. P. Waters. 1994. Conserved location of genes on polymorphic chromosomes of four species of malaria parasites. *Mol. Biochem. Parasitol.* **68:**285–296.

Janse, C. J., and A. P. Waters. 1993. Genome organization, chromosome translocation and size polymorphism in rodent malaria parasites. *Parassitologia* **35**(Suppl.):51–53.

Janssen, C. S., M. P. Barrett, C. M. Turner, and R. S. Phillips. 2002. A large gene family for putative variant antigens shared by human and rodent malaria parasites. *Proc. Biol. Sci.* **269:**431–436.

Jeffares, D. C., A. Pain, A. Berry, A. V. Cox, J. Stalker, C. E. Ingle, A. Thomas, M. A. Quail, K. Siebenthall, A. C. Uhlemann, S. Kyes, S. Krishna, C. Newbold, E. T. Dermitzakis, and M. Berriman. 2007. Genome variation and evolution of the malaria parasite *Plasmodium falciparum*. *Nat. Genet.* **39:**120–125.

Jiang, H., J. J. Patel, M. Yi, J. Mu, J. Ding, R. Stephens, R. A. Cooper, M. T. Ferdig, and X.-Z. Su. 2008a. Genome-wide compensatory changes accompany drug- selected mutations in the *Plasmodium falciparum crt* gene. *PLoS One* **3:**e2484.

Jiang, H., M. Yi, J. Mu, L. Zhang, A. Ivens, L. J. Klimczak, Y. Huyen, R. M. Stephens, and X.-Z. Su. 2008b. Detection of genome wide polymorphisms in the AT rich *Plasmodium falciparum* genome using a high density microarray. *BMC Genomics* **9:**398.

Johnson, D. J., D. A. Fidock, M. Mungthin, V. Lakshmanan, A. B. Sidhu, P. G. Bray, and S. A. Ward. 2004. Evidence for a central role for PfCRT in conferring *Plasmodium falciparum* resistance to diverse antimalarial agents. *Mol. Cell* **15:**867–877.

Jongwutiwes, S., C. Putaporntip, T. Iwasaki, M. U. Ferreira, H. Kanbara, and A. L. Hughes. 2005. Mitochondrial genome sequences support ancient population expansion in *Plasmodium vivax*. *Mol. Biol. Evol.* **22:**1733–1739.

Joy, D. A., X. Feng, J. Mu, T. Furuya, K. Chotivanich, A. U. Krettli, M. Ho, A. Wang, N. J. White, E. Suh, P. Beerli, and X.-Z. Su. 2003. Early origin and recent expansion of *Plasmodium falciparum*. *Science* **300:**318–321.

Joy, D. A., L. Gonzalez-Ceron, J. M. Carlton, A. Gueye, M. Fay, T. F. McCutchan, and X.-Z. Su. 2008. Local adaptation and vector-mediated population structure in *Plasmodium vivax malaria*. *Mol. Biol. Evol.* **25:**1245–1252.

Joy, D. A., J. Mu, H. Jiang, and X.-Z. Su. 2006. Genetic diversity and population history of *Plasmodium falciparum* and *Plasmodium vivax*. *Parassitologia* **48:**561–566.

Karunaweera, N. D., M. U. Ferreira, A. Munasinghe, J. W. Barnwell, W. E. Collins, C. L. King, F. Kawamoto, D. L. Hartl, and D. F. Wirth. 2008. Extensive microsatellite diversity in the human malaria parasite *Plasmodium vivax*. *Gene* **410:**105–112.

Kemp, D. J., L. M. Corcoran, R. L. Coppel, H. D. Stahl, A. E. Bianco, G. V. Brown, and R. F. Anders. 1985. Size variation in chromosomes from independent cultured isolates of *Plasmodium falciparum*. *Nature* **315:**347–350.

Kemp, D. J., A. F. Cowman, and D. Walliker. 1990. Genetic diversity in *Plasmodium falciparum*. *Adv. Parasitol.* **29:**75–149.

Kemp, D. J., J. Thompson, D. A. Barnes, T. Triglia, F. Karamalis, C. Petersen, G. V. Brown, and K. P. Day. 1992. A chromosome 9 deletion in *Plasmodium falciparum* results in loss of cytoadherence. *Mem. Inst. Oswaldo Cruz* **87:**85–89.

Kidgell, C., S. K. Volkman, J. Daily, J. O. Borevitz, D. Plouffe, Y. Zhou, J. R. Johnson, K. Le Roch, O. Sarr, O. Ndir, S. Mboup, S. Batalov,

D. F. Wirth, and E. A. Winzeler. 2006. A systematic map of genetic variation in *Plasmodium falciparum*. *PLoS Pathog.* **2:**e57.

Kooij, T. W., J. M. Carlton, S. L. Bidwell, N. Hall, J. Ramesar, C. J. Janse, and A. P. Waters. 2005. A *Plasmodium* whole-genome synteny map: indels and synteny breakpoints as foci for species-specific genes. *PLoS Pathog.* **1:**e44.

Kroutil, L. C., and T. A. Kunkel. 1999. Deletion errors generated during replication of CAG repeats. *Nucleic Acids Res.* **27:**3481–3486.

Langsley, G., J. Patarapotikul, S. Handunnetti, E. Khouri, K. N. Mendis, and P. H. David. 1988. *Plasmodium vivax*: karyotype polymorphism of field isolates. *Exp. Parasitol.* **67:**301–306.

Lanzer, M., K. Fischer, and S. M. Le Blancq. 1995. Parasitism and chromosome dynamics in protozoan parasites: is there a connection? *Mol. Biochem. Parasitol.* **70:**1–8.

Leclerc, M. C., P. Durand, C. Gauthier, S. Patot, N. Billotte, M. Menegon, C. Severini, F. J. Ayala, and F. Renaud. 2004. Meager genetic variability of the human malaria agent *Plasmodium vivax*. *Proc. Natl. Acad. Sci. USA* **101:**14455–14460.

Li, J., W. E. Collins, R. A. Wirtz, D. Rathore, A. Lal, and T. F. McCutchan. 2001. Geographic subdivision of the range of the malaria parasite *Plasmodium vivax*. *Emerg. Infect. Dis.* **7:**35–42.

Li, J., Y. Zhang, S. Liu, L. Hong, M. Sullivan, T. F. McCutchan, J. M. Carlton, and X. Z. Su. 2009. Hundreds of microsatellites for genotyping *Plasmodium yoelii* parasites. *Mol. Biochem. Parasitol.* **166:**153–158.

Li, J., Y. Zhang, M. Sullivan, L. Hong, L. Huang, F. Lu, T. F. McCutchan, and X. Z. Su. 2007. Typing *Plasmodium yoelii* microsatellites using a simple and affordable fluorescent labeling method. *Mol. Biochem. Parasitol.* **155:**94–102.

Lu, F., H. Jiang, J. Ding, J. Mu, J. G. Valenzuela, J. M. Ribeiro, and X. Z. Su. 2007. cDNA sequences reveal considerable gene prediction inaccuracy in the *Plasmodium falciparum* genome. *BMC Genomics* **8:**255.

Martinelli, A., P. Hunt, R. Fawcett, P. V. Cravo, D. Walliker, and R. Carter. 2005. An AFLP-based genetic linkage map of *Plasmodium chabaudi chabaudi*. *Malar. J.* **4:**11.

McCollum, A. M., K. Mueller, L. Villegas, V. Udhayakumar, and A. A. Escalante. 2007. Common origin and fixation of *Plasmodium falciparum* dhfr and dhps mutations associated with sulfadoxine-pyrimethamine resistance in a low-transmission area in South America. *Antimicrob. Agents Chemother.* **51:**2085–2091.

Mu, J., P. Awadalla, J. Duan, K. M. McGee, D. A. Joy, G. A. McVean, and X.-Z. Su. 2005a. Recombination hotspots and population structure in *Plasmodium falciparum*. *PLoS Biol.* **3:**e335.

Mu, J., P. Awadalla, J. Duan, K. M. McGee, J. Keebler, K. Seydel, G. A. McVean, and X.-Z. Su. 2007. Genome-wide variation and identification of vaccine targets in the *Plasmodium falciparum* genome. *Nat. Genet.* **39:**126–130.

Mu, J., J. Duan, K. Makova, D. A. Joy, C. Q. Huynh, O. H. Branch, W.-H. Li, and X.-Z. Su. 2002. Chromosome-wide SNPs reveal an ancient origin for *Plasmodium falciparum*. *Nature* **418:**323–326.

Mu, J., R. A. Myers, H. Jiang, S. Liu, S. Ricklefs, M. Waisberg, K. Chotivanich, P. Wilairatana, S. Krudsood, N. J. White, R. Udomsangpetch, L. Cui, M. Ho., F. Ou, H. Li, J. Song, G. Li, X. Wang, S. Seila, S. Sokunthea, D. Socheat, D. E. Sturdevant, S. F. Porcella, R. M. Fairhurst, T. E. Wellems, P. Awadalla, and S.-Z. Su. 2010. *Plasmodium falciparum* genome-wide scans for positive selection, recombination hot spots and resistance to antimalarial drugs. *Nat. Genet.* **42:**268–271.

Mu, J., D. A. Joy, J. Duan, Y. Huang, J. Carlton, J. Walker, J. Barnwell, P. Beerli, M. A. Charleston, O. G. Pybus, and X.-Z. Su. 2005b. Host switch leads to emergence of *Plasmodium vivax* malaria in humans. *Mol. Biol. Evol.* **22:**1686–1693.

Na-Bangchang, K., and K. Congpuong. 2007. Current malaria status and distribution of drug resistance in east and southeast Asia with special focus to Thailand. *Tohoku J. Exp. Med.* **211:**99–113.

Nair, S., B. Miller, M. Barends, A. Jaidee, J. Patel, M. Mayxay, P. Newton, F. Nosten, M. T. Ferdig, and T. J. Anderson. 2008. Adaptive copy number evolution in malaria parasites. *PLoS Genet.* **4:**e1000243.

Nair, S., D. Nash, D. Sudimack, A. Jaidee, M. Barends, A. C. Uhlemann, S. Krishna, F. Nosten, and T. J. Anderson. 2007. Recurrent gene amplification and soft selective sweeps during evolution of multidrug resistance in malaria parasites. *Mol. Biol. Evol.* **24:**562–573.

Nair, S., J. T. Williams, A. Brockman, L. Paiphun, M. Mayxay, P. N. Newton, J. P. Guthmann, F. M. Smithuis, T. T. Hien, N. J. White, F. Nosten, and T. J. Anderson. 2003. A selective sweep driven by pyrimethamine treatment in southeast Asian malaria parasites. *Mol. Biol. Evol.* **20:**1526–1536.

Neafsey, D. E., S. F. Schaffner, S. K. Volkman, D. Park, P. Montgomery, D. A. Milner, Jr., A. Lukens, D. Rosen, R. Daniels, N. Houde, J. F. Cortese, E. Tyndall, C. Gates, N. Stange-Thomann, O. Sarr, D. Ndiaye, O. Ndir, S. Mboup, M. U. Ferreira, S. D. Moraes, A. P. Dash, C. E. Chitnis, R. C. Wiegand, D. L.

Hartl, B. W. Birren, E. S. Lander, P. C. Sabeti, and D. F. Wirth. 2008. Genome-wide SNP genotyping highlights the role of natural selection in *Plasmodium falciparum* population divergence. *Genome Biol.* **9:**R171.

Pearce, R. J., H. Pota, M. S. Evehe, E.-H. Bâ, G. Mombo-Ngoma, A. L. Malisa, R. Ord, W. Inojosa, A. Matondo, D. A. Diallo, W. Mbacham, I. V. van den Broek, T. D. Swarthout, A. Getachew, S. Dejene, M. P. Grobusch, F. Njie, S. Dunyo, M. Kweku, S. Owusu-Agyei, D. Chandramohan, M. Bonnet, J. P. Guthmann, S. Clarke, K. I. Barnes, E. Streat, S. T. Katokele, P. Uusiku, C. O. Agboghoroma, O. Y, Elegba, B. Cissé, I. E. A-Elbasit, H. A. Giha, S. P. Kachur, C. Lynch, J. B. Rwakimari, P. Chanda, P., M. Hawela, B. Sharp, I. Naidoo, and C. Roper. 2009. Multiple origins and regional dispersal of resistant dhps in African *Plasmodium falciparum* malaria. *PLoS Med.* **6:** e1000055.

Polley, S. D., and D. J. Conway. 2001. Strong diversifying selection on domains of the *Plasmodium falciparum* apical membrane antigen 1 gene. *Genetics* **158:**1505–1512.

Pologe, L. G., and J. V. Ravetch. 1986. A chromosomal rearrangement in a *P. falciparum* histidine-rich protein gene is associated with the knobless phenotype. *Nature* **322:**474–477.

Preechapornkul, P., M. Imwong, K. Chotivanich, W. Pongtavornpinyo, A. M. Dondorp, N. P. Day, N. J. White, and S. Pukrittayakamee. 2009. *Plasmodium falciparum pfmdr1* amplification, mefloquine resistance, and parasite fitness. *Antimicrob. Agents Chemother.* **53:**1509–1515.

Price, R. N., A. C. Uhlemann, A. Brockman, R. McGready, E. Ashley, L. Phaipun, R. Patel, K. Laing, S. Looareesuwan, N. J. White, F. Nosten, and S. Krishna. 2004. Mefloquine resistance in *Plasmodium falciparum* and increased *pfmdr1* gene copy number. *Lancet* **364:**438–447.

Putaporntip, C., S. Jongwutiwes, and A. L. Hughes. 2009. Natural selection maintains a stable polymorphism at the circumsporozoite protein locus of *Plasmodium falciparum* in a low endemic area. *Infect. Genet. Evol.* **9:**567–573.

Raj, D. K., J. Mu, H. Jiang, J. Kabat, S. Singh, M. Sullivan, M. P. Fay, T. F. McCutchan, and X. Z. Su. 2008. Disruption of a *Plasmodium falciparum* multidrug resistance-associated protein (PfMRP) alters its fitness and transport of antimalarial drugs and glutathione. *J. Biol. Chem.* **284:**7687–7696.

Rathod, P. K., T. McErlean, and P. C. Lee. 1997. Variations in frequencies of drug resistance in *Plasmodium falciparum*. *Proc. Natl. Acad. Sci. USA* **94:** 9389–9393.

Razakandrainibe, F. G., P. Durand, J. C. Koella, T. De Meeus, F. Rousset, F. J. Ayala, and F. Renaud. 2005. "Clonal" population structure of the malaria agent *Plasmodium falciparum* in high-infection regions. *Proc. Natl. Acad. Sci. USA* **102:**17388–17393.

Reed, F. A., and S. A. Tishkoff. 2006. Positive selection can create false hotspots of recombination. *Genetics* **172:**2011–2014.

Reed, M. B., K. J. Saliba, S. R. Caruana, K. Kirk, and A. F. Cowman. 2000. Pgh1 modulates sensitivity and resistance to multiple antimalarials in *Plasmodium falciparum*. *Nature* **403:**906–909.

Ribacke, U., B. W. Mok, V. Wirta, J. Normark, J. Lundeberg, F. Kironde, T. G. Egwang, P. Nilsson, and M. Wahlgren. 2007. Genome wide gene amplifications and deletions in *Plasmodium falciparum*. *Mol. Biochem. Parasitol.* **155:**33–44.

Rich, S. M., R. R. Hudson, and F. J. Ayala. 1997. *Plasmodium falciparum* antigenic diversity: evidence of clonal population structure. *Proc. Natl. Acad. Sci. USA* **94:**13040–13045.

Rich, S. M., M. C. Licht, R. R. Hudson, and F. J. Ayala. 1998. Malaria's Eve: evidence of a recent population bottleneck throughout the world populations of *Plasmodium falciparum*. *Proc. Natl. Acad. Sci. USA* **95:**4425–4430.

Roper, C., R. Pearce, B. Bredenkamp, J. Gumede, C. Drakeley, F. Mosha, D. Chandramohan, and B. Sharp. 2003. Antifolate antimalarial resistance in southeast Africa: a population-based analysis. *Lancet* **361:**1174–1181.

Roper, C., R. Pearce, S. Nair, B. Sharp, F. Nosten, and T. Anderson. 2004. Intercontinental spread of pyrimethamine-resistant malaria. *Science* **305:**1124.

Scherf, A., C. Behr, J. L. Sarthou, M. Pla, C. Rogier, J. F. Trape, L. P. da Silva, and P. Dubois. 1993. Immune response in mouse and malaria-exposed humans to peptides derived from Pf11-1, a highly repetitive megadalton protein of *Plasmodium falciparum*. *Eur. J. Immunol.* **23:**1574–1581.

Scherf, A., and D. Mattei. 1992. Cloning and characterization of chromosome breakpoints of *Plasmodium falciparum*: breakage and new telomere formation occurs frequently and randomly in subtelomeric genes. *Nucleic Acids Res.* **20:**1491–1496.

Sidhu, A. B., A. C. Uhlemann, S. G. Valderramos, J. C. Valderramos, S. Krishna, and D. A. Fidock. 2006. Decreasing *pfmdr1* copy number in *Plasmodium falciparum* malaria heightens susceptibility to mefloquine, lumefantrine, halofantrine, quinine, and artemisinin. *J. Infect. Dis.* **194:**528–535.

Singh, B., L. Kim Sung, A. Matusop, A. Radhakrishnan, S. S. Shamsul, J. Cox-Singh, A. Thomas, and D. J. Conway. 2004. A large focus of naturally acquired *Plasmodium knowlesi* infections in human beings. *Lancet* **363:**1017–1024.

Smith, J. D., C. E. Chitnis, A. G. Craig, D. J. Roberts, D. E. Hudson-Taylor, D. S. Peterson, R. Pinches, C. I. Newbold, and L. H. Miller. 1995. Switches in expression of *Plasmodium falciparum var* genes correlate with changes in antigenic and cytoadherent phenotypes of infected erythrocytes. *Cell* **82:**101–110.

Snow, R. W., C. A. Guerra, A. M. Noor, H. Y. Myint, and S. I. Hay. 2005. The global distribution of clinical episodes of *Plasmodium falciparum* malaria. *Nature* **434:**214–217.

Su, X.-Z., M. T. Ferdig, Y. Huang, C. Q. Huynh, A. Liu, J. You, J. C. Wootton, and T. E. Wellems. 1999. A genetic map and recombination parameters of the human malaria parasite *Plasmodium falciparum. Science* **286:**1351–1353.

Su, X.-Z., K. Hayton, and T. E. Wellems. 2007. Genetic linkage and association analyses for trait mapping in *Plasmodium falciparum. Nat. Rev. Genet.* **8:**497–506.

Su, X.-Z., V. M. Heatwole, S. P. Wertheimer, F. Guinet, J. A. Herrfeldt, D. S. Peterson, J. A. Ravetch, and T. E. Wellems. 1995. The large diverse gene family *var* encodes proteins involved in cytoadherence and antigenic variation of *Plasmodium falciparum*-infected erythrocytes. *Cell* **82:** 89–100.

Su, X.-Z., L. A. Kirkman, H. Fujioka, and T. E. Wellems. 1997. Complex polymorphisms in an approximately 330 kDa protein are linked to chloroquine-resistant *P. falciparum* in southeast Asia and Africa. *Cell* **91:**593–603.

Su, X.-Z., J. Mu, and D. A. Joy. 2003. The "Malaria's Eve" hypothesis and the debate concerning the origin of the human malaria parasite *Plasmodium falciparum. Microbes Infect.* **5:**891–896.

Su, X.-Z., and T. E. Wellems. 1996. Toward a high-resolution *Plasmodium falciparum* linkage map: polymorphic markers from hundreds of simple sequence repeats. *Genomics* **33:**430–444.

Su, X.-Z., and J. C. Wootton. 2004. Genetic mapping in the human malaria parasite *Plasmodium falciparum. Mol. Microbiol.* **53:**1573–1582.

Tami, A., H. Grundmann, C. Sutherland, J. S. McBride, D R. Cavanagh, E. Campos, G. Snounou, C. Barnabe, M. Tibayrenc, and D. C. Warhurst. 2002. Restricted genetic and antigenic diversity of *Plasmodium falciparum* under mesoendemic transmission in the Venezuelan Amazon. *Parasitology* **124:**569–581.

Tan, J. C., J. J. Patel, A. Tan, J. C. Blain, T. J. Albert, N. F. Lobo, and M. T. Ferdig. 2009. Optimizing comparative genomic hybridization probes for genotyping and SNP detection in *Plasmodium falciparum. Genomics* **93:**543–550.

Templeton, T. J. 2009. The varieties of gene amplification, diversification and hypervariability in the human malaria parasite, *Plasmodium falciparum. Mol. Biochem. Parasitol.* **166:**109–116.

Tishkoff, S. A., R. Varkonyi, N. Cahinhinan, S. Abbes, G. Argyropoulos, G. Destro-Bisol, A. Drousiotou, B. Dangerfield, G. Lefranc, J. Loiselet, A. Piro, M. Stoneking, A. Tagarelli, G. Tagarelli, E. H. Touma, S. M. Williams, and A. G. Clark. 2001. Haplotype diversity and linkage disequilibrium at human G6PD: recent origin of alleles that confer malarial resistance. *Science* **293:**455–462.

Trimnell, A., S. Kraemer, S. Mukherjee, D. J. Phippard, J. H. Janes, E. Flamoe, X.-z. Su, P. Awadalla, and J. D. Smith. 2006. Global genetic diversity and evolution of *var* genes associated with placental and severe childhood malaria. *Mol. Biol. Parasitol.* **148:**169–180.

VanBuskirk, K. M., M. T. O'Neill, P. De La Vega, A. G. Maier, U. Krzych, J. Williams, M. G. Dowler, J. B. Sacci, Jr., N. Kangwanrangsan, T. Tsuboi, N. M. Kneteman, D. G. Heppner, Jr., B. A. Murdock, S. A. Mikolajczak, A. S. Aly, A. F. Cowman, and S. H.Kappe. 2009. Preerythrocytic, live-attenuated *Plasmodium falciparum* vaccine candidates by design. *Proc. Natl. Acad. Sci. USA* **106:**13004–13009.

Vekemans, J., and W. R. Ballou. 2008. *Plasmodium falciparum* malaria vaccines in development. *Expert Rev. Vaccines* **7:**223–240.

Volkman, S. K., A. E. Barry, E. J. Lyons, K. M. Nielsen, S. M. Thomas, M. Choi, S. S. Thakore, K. P. Day, D. F. Wirth, and D. L. Hartl. 2001. Recent origin of *Plasmodium falciparum* from a single progenitor. *Science* **293:**482–484.

Volkman, S. K., P. C. Sabeti, D. DeCaprio, D. E. Neafsey, S. F. Schaffner, D. A. Milner, Jr., J. P. Daily, O. Sarr, D. Ndiaye, O. Ndir, S. Mboup, M. T. Duraisingh, A. Lukens, A. Derr, N. Stange-Thomann, S. Waggoner, R. Onofrio, L. Ziaugra, E. Mauceli, S. Gnerre, D. B. Jaffe, J. Zainoun, R. C. Wiegand, B. W. Birren, D. L. Hartl, J. E. Galagan, E. S. Lander, and D. F. Wirth. 2007. A genome-wide map of diversity in *Plasmodium falciparum. Nat. Genet.* **39:**113–119.

Wakaguri, H., Y. Suzuki, M. Sasaki, S. Sugano, and J. Watanabe. 2009. Inconsistencies of genome annotations in apicomplexan parasites revealed by 5′-end-one-pass and full-length sequences of oligo-capped cDNAs. *BMC Genomics* **10:**312.

Walliker, D., H. Babiker, and L. Ranford-Cartwright. 1998. The genetic structure of malaria populations, p. 235–253. *In* I. W. Sherman (ed.), *Malaria: Parasite Biology, Pathogenesis, and Protection.* ASM Press, Washington, DC.

Walther, M. 2006. Advances in vaccine development against the pre-erythrocytic stage of *Plasmodium falciparum* malaria. *Expert Rev. Vaccines* **5:**81–93.

Watanabe, J., M. Sasaki, Y. Suzuki, and S. Sugano. 2002. Analysis of transcriptomes of human malaria parasite *Plasmodium falciparum* using full-length enriched library: identification of novel genes and diverse transcription start sites of messenger RNAs. *Gene* **291:**105–113.

Wellems, T., A. M. J. Oduola, B. Fenton, R. Desjardins, L. J. Panton, and V. E. do Rosario. 1988. Chromosome size variation occurs in cloned *Plasmodium falciparum* on *in vitro* cultivation. *Rev. Bras. Genet.* **11:**813–825.

Wellems, T. E., L. J. Panton, I. Y. Gluzman, V. E. do Rosario, R. W. Gwadz, A. Walker-Jonah, and D. J. Krogstad. 1990. Chloroquine resistance not linked to *mdr*-like genes in a *Plasmodium falciparum* cross. *Nature* **345:**253–255.

Wootton, J. C., X. Feng, M. T. Ferdig, R. A. Cooper, J. Mu, D. I. Baruch, A. J. Magill, and X.-Z. Su. 2002. Genetic diversity and chloroquine selective sweeps in *Plasmodium falciparum*. *Nature* **418:** 320–323.

World Health Organization. 2008. *World Malaria Report 2008.* World Health Organization, Geneva, Switzerland.

Yuan, J., R. L. Johnson, R. Huang, J. Wichterman, H, Jiang, K. Hayton, D. A. Fidock, T. E. Wellems, J. Inglese, C. P. Austin, and X. Z. Su. 2009. Genetic mapping of targets mediating differential chemical phenotypes in *Plasmodium falciparum*. *Nat. Chem. Biol.* **5:**765–771.

THE FUNDAMENTAL CONTRIBUTION OF GENOME HYPERVARIABILITY TO THE SUCCESS OF A EUKARYOTIC PATHOGEN, *Trypanosoma brucei*

J. David Barry

17

As a parasite that causes a variety of chronic human and livestock diseases in Africa and elsewhere, the trypanosome needs to overcome a number of grand challenges mounted, directly or indirectly, by its wide range of hosts. Fundamental to the success of this single-cell, eukaryotic parasite in overcoming such challenges are extraordinary adaptations in its genome. These adaptations are major and dynamic, correlate directly with parasitism, and lie at different scales, from major chromosomal features to, at a finer scale, localized and enhanced mutation within and around genes. In general, the adaptations are all to do with the generation, diversification, and regulation of hypervariant, multigene families, the most important of which encodes thousands of variant surface glycoprotein (VSG) isoforms. This silent archive of *VSG* genes also has subtle means of expanding its coding potential, probably massively, beyond one VSG per gene—a prominent example of the "implicit genome" (Caporale, 2006). Having such a large gene family, allied with efficient mechanisms for its expansion and diversification, appears to have created the inevitable spinoff of at least one gene variant that has escaped from encoding VSG and has neofunctionalized, contributing a novel phenotype and broadening the parasitic potential of the trypanosome. All in all, heavy investment in mechanisms for genome diversification has paid off well for the trypanosome.

The dominant parasitological feature providing selective pressure for genome evolution is antigenic variation, a sophisticated system which, just like the genome adaptations, operates at, and links between, several scales. So broad are the scope and complexity of antigenic variation—it links causally with persistence in host individuals and populations, with transmission, which is the strongest driver of pathogen evolution, and with host range—that these days the process increasingly is being studied through complementation of experimental analyses with ecological methods, in a systems biology approach (Lythgoe et al., 2007; Gjini et al, 2010). To understand how the various interlinked processes in antigenic variation contribute to and are served by genome adaptations, it is necessary first to describe what we know, phenotypically and genotypically, about this variation system.

J. David Barry, Wellcome Trust Centre for Molecular Parasitology, Institute of Infection, Immunity and Inflammation, University of Glasgow, Glasgow G12 8TA, United Kingdom.

Genome Plasticity and Infectious Diseases,
Edited by J. Hacker, U. Dobrindt, and R. Kurth,

WHAT IS ANTIGENIC VARIATION?

Biology of Antigenic Variation

Antigenic variation is a process that leads to diversity in a protective antigen displayed by a population of micropathogens in the course of a single infection. By enabling evasion of immunity, the process contributes to prolongation of individual infections and provides several important benefits for the parasite, including enhancement of transmission between hosts, interstrain competition in the field (Futse et al., 2008), and possibly, we are beginning to realize, subtle but powerful mechanisms for successfully infecting a very broad host range. Antigenic variation is a form of a wider phenomenon of enhanced phenotypic variation, in which rare individuals within a population preemptively switch to an alternative phenotype, which can confer benefit under appropriate circumstances (Moxon et al., 1994; Barry and McCulloch, 2001). Best understood are phase variation systems in bacteria, where simple toggling between two alternative phenotypes can modulate important events like invasion or survival of assault by the host. The genes responsible for the phenotype switch spontaneously, at a relatively high rate (typically 10^{-3} switch/cell/generation). Such hypermutable genes (phase variation is considered mutational because it confers a heritable change when switched) are known as contingency loci, and a variety of hypermutation mechanisms exist, including many that are "accidental" (i.e., spontaneous and stochastic) rather than specifically regulated, although there are now a few cases of regulated switching (Metruccio et al., 2009). Antigenic variation has the specific property that, because immune responses persist, new variants are required cumulatively, so that extensive diversity is often required. Antigenic variation is a phenotypic phenomenon, driven by stochastic processes, but all too often attempts are made to classify it genotypically, according to how switching occurs. This has led to a confusing view that there is a "real" system, termed "sensu stricto," and other types, and that there are "programmed" (in the sense of being based on existing genetic information) and random types. All antigenic variation is real, and "programming" can give the false impression that variation is not stochastic. So, if classification is needed, it would be better applied at the phenotype level.

Trypanosoma brucei lives extracellularly in its mammalian hosts, a lifestyle that provokes potent and lethal antibody responses which, at their height, might be expected to eliminate all accessible trypanosomes. Most antibodies, however, and all protective antibodies, are directed against the parasite's major VSG, and some circulating trypanosomes, having switched clonally to expression of an alternative VSG through antigenic variation, are not recognized by the protective antibodies and can proliferate freely. Dense VSG packing on the cell surface ensures that other antibodies do not access their target antigens, including necessarily invariant macromolecules. The hallmarks of trypanosome antigenic variation (reviewed in detail by Barry and McCulloch [2001]) are typical of similar systems in other pathogens: a major protective antigen, spontaneous switching, a multitude of variants most of the time, and a degree of order in appearance of variants. Normally, each parasitemia peak contains a number of detectable variants, ranging from 5 or 6 (in slowly switching laboratory strains) to >20 (in more wild-type strains), although occasionally there can be one major variant in a peak. The total number of variants a trypanosome is capable of expressing probably will never be known, as many different combinations of many different *VSG* genes can be created temporarily. Characterization of trypanosome clones isolated from infections has revealed a minimum of 101 variants, while the outcome of genome analysis implies inestimably large numbers. The overall switching rate for *T. brucei* has been calculated as ~10^{-2} to ~10^{-5} switch/cell/generation. In common with antigenic variation in other pathogens, there is an intriguingly imprecise order in expression of variants, sometimes called "semipredictable," that sees some variants tending to appear early in infection and others arising progressively later. Statistical analysis has shown that early variants have low variance in timing of appearance, at least when measured by timing of specific antibody appearance (Morrison et al., 2005), and later variants have greater variance (Marcello and Barry, 2007a). Thus, early variants are more predictable than later variants. The order is thought to be a mechanism for prolonging infection, with antibodies acting to remove early variants before later ones can emerge, in a rolling fashion. Thus, we can consider antigenic variation as producing a "stochastic swarm" of variants, but with a degree of regulation that prevents them appearing in overwhelming multiplicity. Key areas of research at present are to understand and identify how this balance is achieved, and how the trypanosome can orchestrate differential expression of many variants. The stochasticity and rate of the switching process lie at the heart of chronic infection, and, as we shall see, these features are specified primarily in DNA sequences.

VSG and the Surface Coat

The VSG (Fig. 1) is structured as a professional, defensive protein rather than an immunologically variable, functional protein such as an enzyme or receptor (Schwede and Carrington, 2010). Its major role is to form a densely packed coat that blocks host intervention, and it comprises fully ~10% of the cell's soluble protein. It has an amino-terminal variable domain of 350 to 400 amino acids that bears the variable, protective epitopes, and a carboxy-terminal domain of 40 to 80 residues that carries the plasma membrane-inserted glycosylphosphatidylinositol anchor. There are two N-terminal domain groups, both with about 800 members encoded in the half- to two-thirds-sequenced genome (Berriman et al., 2005; Marcello and Barry, 2007b). The C-terminal domain forms six groups that range in frequency, within the sequenced genome, from 1.5% to 36% (Marcello and Barry, 2007b). It is apparent, from what is observed in expressed and silent *VSG* genes, that the N- and C-terminal domain groups can associate in any combination. A major feature of the VSG is that, through assessment by homology or (to a limited extent) functional studies, it appears not to have biochemical or receptor functions. It is likely to have originated as a dimeric surface protein, such as a receptor, and to have lost its original function in favor of its present role in forming a densely packed, sterically blocking coat. Release from narrowly defined function has liberated the protein from purifying selection for an active or recognition site and has allowed considerable diversification. This diversity is best illustrated by the fact that, among nearly 2,000 determined potential *VSG* sequences in the trypanosome genome strain (two-thirds are pseudogenes but, as argued below, contain much intact sequence), the peptide identity for the N-terminal domain has a mode of only ~10% (A group) or 15% (B group) (range, <1% to >90%) (J. D. Barry, unpublished data). Nevertheless, there are some structural constraints. The "VSG fold" that dominates the variable domain is a coiled coil, the long alpha helices of which, allied with a degree of conservation of cysteine positioning, provide conservation of the elongated proportions that appear to produce a coat of uniform thickness. The paradox of low identity but conserved structure can be explained by alpha helices being determined by the characteristic heptad spacing of hydrophobic and oppositely charged residues, rather than by specific residues. In addition to this highly variable gene set, an unknown number of temporary, mosaic *VSG* genes can be formed, generating new, combinatorial versions of what is encoded by the silent genes. Overall, then, the combination of lack of function and prominence of alpha helix allows this protein to retain its structure but vary enormously in sequence, which is ideal for antigenic variation and has allowed dramatic expansion of the global VSG family, both within the single genome and between strains (Marcello and Barry, 2007b; Hutchinson et al., 2007).

The basis of antigenic variation is the peptide diversity in the N-terminal domain, rather than differences in glycosylation. As antigens VSGs are highly immunogenic, and as variants they are highly diverse. The host sees the N-terminal domain, of which only a small region is visible due to the dense packing of the coat. As with many other pathogen surface antigens, the protective epitopes are conformational and

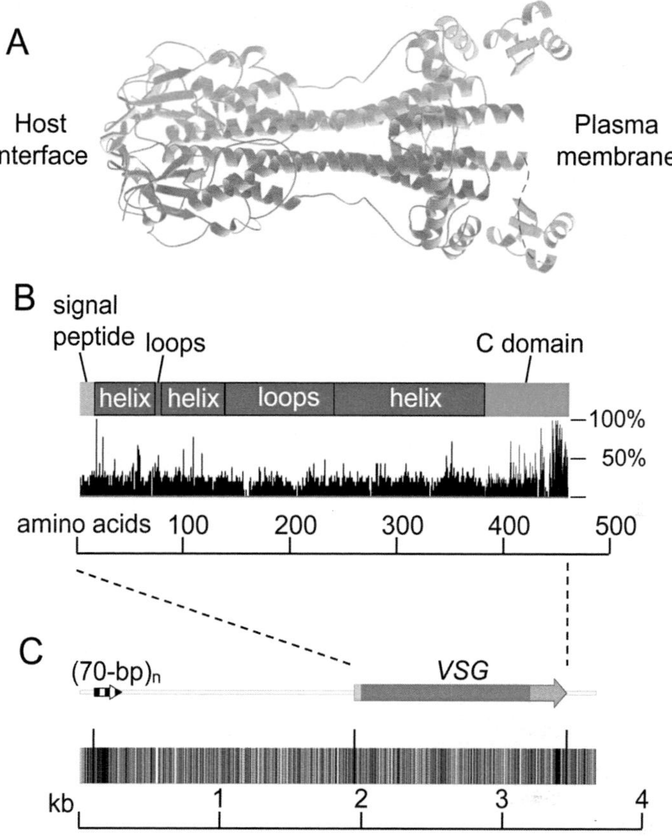

FIGURE 1 The VSG protein and *VSG* gene cassette. (A) Quaternary structure of the ILTat 1.24 VSG dimer (image courtesy of Mark Carrington), with the N-terminal domain (monomers purple or green) to the left and the C-terminal domain (both monomers orange) to the right. (B) Diagram of the VSG primary structure, showing signal peptide (light blue), the N-terminal domain (purple) with secondary structure indicated, and the C-terminal domain (orange). Accompanying the primary structure is an identity histogram of ILTat 1.24 and the six top ClustalW hits in the genome strain queried with the ILTat 1.24 VSG (N- and C-terminal domains queried separately), showing that conservation is greatest at the downstream end of the C-terminal domain. (C) Silent *VSG* cassette, in which the coding sequence is color-coded to match the protein diagrams. The 70-bp tract delimiting the upstream end of the cassette is indicated by a hatched arrow. Beneath is a Jalview (Waterhouse et al., 2009) image of the alignment of two cassettes retrieved by ILTat 1.24 querying of the genome strain in geneDB (http://old.genedb.org/genedb/tryp/index.jsp), stretching 2,000 bp upstream and 200 bp downstream of the coding sequence. Extended vertical lines denote the cassette ends and the *VSG* start codon. The only significant identity is at the cassette flanks.

therefore have evaded structural identification. There is extensive circumstantial evidence, however, that those epitopes are associated with loops decorating the N-terminal end of the variable domain (Miller et al., 1984; Hall and Esser, 1984) (Fig. 1). It is therefore puzzling, at first sight, that the whole length of this domain is hypervariable. Until the recent availability of many *VSG* gene sequences allowed deeper interrogation of variability, comparisons had led to suggestions of local hypervariability that were biased by sample size limitation (Field and Boothroyd, 1996). It is now becoming clearer that hypervariability appears to be slightly greater in the regions of those surface loops (Hutchinson et al., 2007), in keeping with their proposed role of harboring protective and variable epitopes. Overall, however, the wide variability of sequence (Marcello and Barry, 2007b) and of T-cell epitopes (Dagenais et al., 2009) across the domain cannot easily be explained at the phenotypic level. A likely explanation is that the mechanisms for sequence diversification act across the whole N-terminal domain and are sufficiently rapid to nearly obscure the effects of antibody-mediated diversifying selection and to obscure other positive selection acting at the primary structural level. This explanation sits well with what is required for evolution of these antigens. Although there are thousands of genes, many are likely to be expressed very rarely, if at all, and even the most frequently expressed members of the archive have only brief spells of expression. Evolution applies fairly evenly across the archive, as can be seen from phylogenetic analysis of the array genes (Marcello and Barry, 2007b); the archive evolves in concert, rather than as a collection of individuals each acting as an independent evolutionary unit. This pattern of even evolution can be explained by selection acting directly, not on *VSG* genes themselves, but rather on mechanisms for rapid generation of diversity. The *VSG* genes then would diversify at common rates, under secondary selection, in consequence of those mechanisms. Such broad, concerted evolution requires broadly acting mechanisms, which might be facilitated by the sequestration of *VSG* into distinct genome compartments.

CONTRIBUTION OF THE GENOME TO ANTIGENIC VARIATION

Antigenic Variation Loci

Antigenic variation in African trypanosomes is based on a pool of silent information, in the form of an archive of silent *VSG* genes that are called into service individually in a spontaneous manner. Although this information strategy is common to a number of pathogenic bacteria and parasites, what sets the trypanosome apart is the enormous scale of the archive. Bacterial antigenic variation archives normally have fewer than 10 or 20 silent genes (Futse et al., 2008), other parasites have tens or occasionally hundreds (Prucca and Lujan, 2009; Lau, 2009), but trypanosomes have thousands (Berriman et al., 2005). Even allowing for relative genome size and complexity, the trypanosome is very lavishly endowed with silent antigen genes; crude estimation predicts that in one strain there are nearly as many *VSG* genes as other genes (J. D. Barry, unpublished observations)! The genome accommodates the archive in a number of discrete compartments, each of which is associated with activities for the expression and/or evolution of the *VSG* family. It is generally accepted that expansion of a genome has no metabolic cost to an organism (Lynch, 2007), so growth of the archive is unlikely to be subject to heavy restriction. The basic genetic unit of antigenic variation is the silent *VSG* cassette (Michels et al., 1983) (Fig. 1C), characterized by a common 5′ flank comprising <16 imperfect "70-bp" repeats, one motif of which is an intrinsically, physically unstable run of TAA repeats (Ohshima et al., 1996). There is then a spacer, followed by the intronless coding sequence, and terminating in common sequences which stretch from within the 3′ end of the coding sequence, encoding the partially conserved C′ domain, to further conservation in the 3′ untranslated region (UTR). Figure 1C shows alignment of two intact *VSG* cassettes, revealing that they have appreciable similarity at only their ends.

Based on BlastP comparative analysis of predicted proteins, *T. brucei* and its closest sequenced relatives, *Trypanosoma cruzi* and *Leishmania major* (all three are in the order Trypanosomatida), share ~6,000 genes in the haploid genome (El Sayed et al., 2005). These core genes, including effectively all those recognizable in other eukaryotes, occupy the central regions of the 11 pairs of conventional chromosomes, which range in size from ~1 to >5 Mb (Berriman et al., 2005; Melville et al., 1998). Each species also has substantial species-specific gene families, which in the African trypanosome is mainly the *VSG* set, comprising up to ~1,800 *VSG* genes and pseudogenes in the diploid genome of the sequenced strain (Berriman et al., 2005; Marcello and Barry, 2007b). The unusual size and various requirements of the *VSG* archive have resulted in two prominent and unusual features of the trypanosome genome at the gross level. The first feature is partitioning of the genome into different *VSG* gene-containing compartments (Fig. 2), some of which are unconventional in eukaryotic genomes and each of which has distinct functional roles in antigenic variation, and the second feature is the exclusive use of subtelomeres, with probably not a single of the many hundreds of authentic *VSG* genes located in a chromosome core (Marcello and Barry, 2007b).

Most, perhaps ~1,600, of the silent gene cassettes are arranged as densely packed tandem arrays in several, but not all, of the subtelomeres of the megabase chromosomes (Berriman et al., 2005). The arrays contain few genes other than *VSG* and, generally, are orientated toward the centromere, although the larger ones are punctuated by subarrays in the opposite orientation. Some 92% of the full-length *VSG* genes in the arrays have upstream 70-bp repeats, ranging from 1 repeat unit for most genes up to 15 units (Marcello and Barry, 2007b). About two-thirds of array genes are pseudogenes, having frameshifts and premature stop codons and/or lacking start codons. It is apparent that the array genome compartment has two functions: to harbor and to diversify silent genes. Uniquely to the African trypanosomes that use antigenic variation, there is also a set of minichromosomes, which in *T. brucei* number ~100 and are 30 to 150 kb long (Wickstead et al., 2004). Apparently the sole use of the minichromosomes is as a repository for *VSG* genes, which are arranged as one gene at some but not all subtelomeres, immediately adjacent to the telomere. Hence, the minichromosomal set contains up to ~200 silent *VSG* genes, and the few that have been characterized are intact. The core of the minichromosomes comprises mainly a repetitive sequence, outside which lie typical *VSG*-bearing subtelomeres, flanked in the one characterized case by 35 of the 70-bp repeats (Shah et al., 1987; N. Robinson and J. D. Barry, unpublished data). Functions of the minichromosomal compartment arguably are to harbor silent genes and to provide a pool of telomere-adjacent *VSG* genes for rapid activation. There are also several intermediate chromosomes, of 200 to 900 kb, that are partially related to the minichromosomes. Besides the array and minichromosomal *VSG* sets, there is a set, known as *MVSG* (metacyclic *VSG*), that is used in the metacyclic population transmitted from the tsetse fly to mammals (Graham et al., 1999; Bringaud et al., 2001). Finally, there is a set of potential transcription units, known as bloodstream expression sites (BES), adjacent to the telomeres of some of the megabase chromosomes (Young et al., 2008; Hertz-Fowler et al., 2008) and numbering 5 to 15 per genome, depending on the strain. The main function of BES is to provide transcription loci for *VSG*.

Regulation of *VSG*

With respect to the archive, the two main requirements for the trypanosome are regulation, such that *VSG* genes are expressed singly, strongly, and differentially, and evolution, such that diversification is rapid but does not compromise the specific needs of antigenic variation. The different genomic compartments contribute to these requirements in specific ways.

Trypanosomes and their relatives are unusually biased toward posttranscriptional mechanisms for differential control of gene expression. The bias is unavoidable, because virtually all protein-coding genes are arranged as long directional arrays that are polycistrons, in which genes are transcribed from common transcription start regions, with a major promoter at the start of clusters and possibly some additional promoters within (Siegel et al., 2009). Although such an arrangement is reminiscent of bacterial operons, trypanosome gene clusters differ in that the component genes do not have related

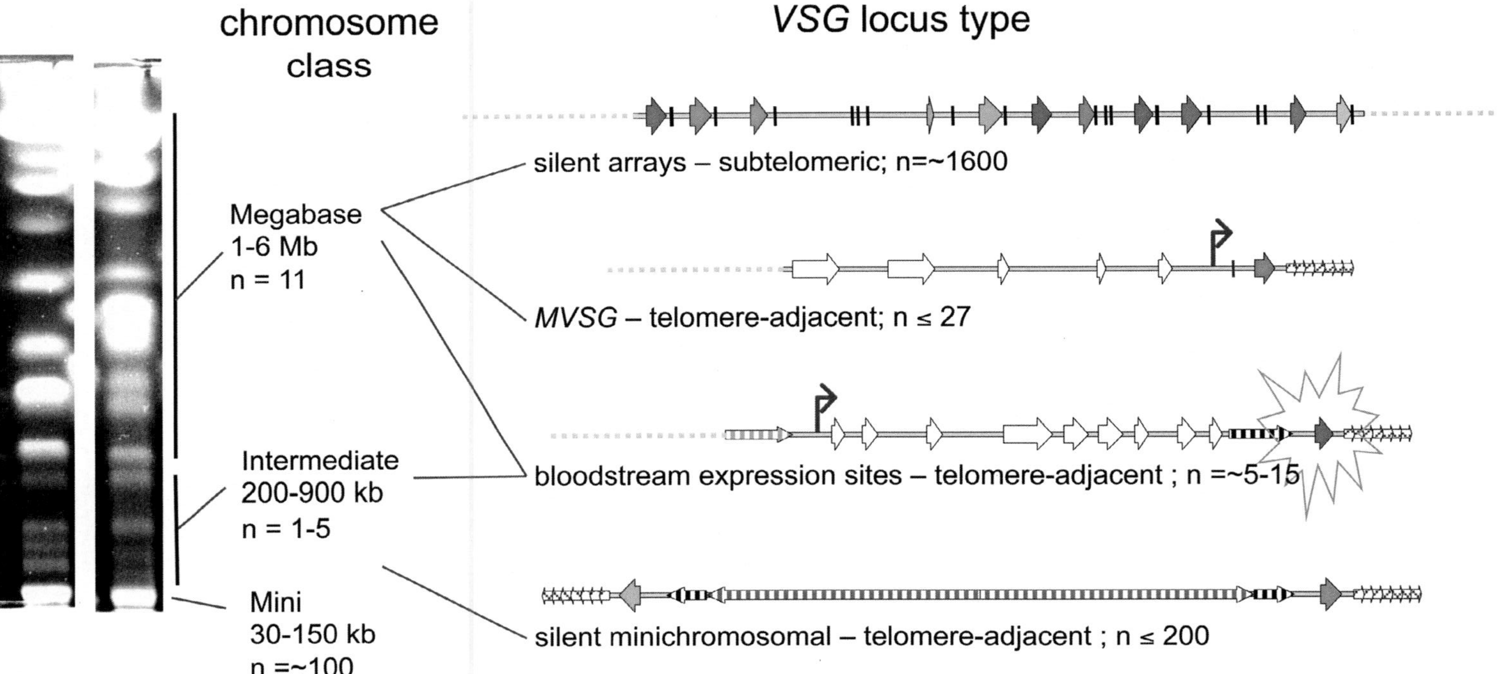

FIGURE 2 The genome. To the left are images of ethidium bromide-stained pulsed-field gel separations of genomic DNA of two strains of *T. brucei* (images courtesy of Sara Melville); the positions and sizes of, and numbers within, each chromosome size class are shown alongside. To the right are maps of typical loci from the four genome compartments inhabited by *VSG*. On the maps, solid-colored arrows indicate *VSG*s, white arrows indicate other open reading frames, black vertically hatched arrows indicate 70-bp repeat tracts (shown as vertical lines when there are very few repeats in the tract), colored vertically hatched arrows indicate other repeat tracts (which have no direct role in antigenic variation), multiply repeated arrows with blue X's indicate telomere repeat tracts, right-angled arrows indicate promoters, and the flash symbol indicates active *VSG*. The karyotypic locations of the *VSG* genome compartments are indicated.

function and in general are not transcribed conditionally. Instead, the directional gene clusters appear to be transcribed constitutively. As not all gene products are required constitutively, differential expression is attained mainly through 3′-UTR-mediated regulation of mRNA stability and secondarily at the level of translation and possibly other processes (Haanstra et al., 2008). Despite this regulatory strategy being successful, it is not readily compatible with the needs of antigenic variation, and specifically the tightly regulated expression of only one member of the large archive at a time. The *VSG* mRNA is highly abundant, amounting to nearly 10% of all mRNA, and it would be logistically difficult to transcribe hundreds of *VSG* genes and then control to this specificity at a later step, regardless of which molecular mechanisms could be proposed. The solution to this problem is that minichromosomal and array-based silent archive genes do not have promoters. Instead, they can be expressed only from the specialized BES loci. As for all other trypanosome protein-coding genes, the expression sites are polycistronic, with other, unrelated genes but a common promoter (Siegel et al., 2009). There are, however, two prominent features of the BES that distinguish them from standard trypanosome polycistons and are conducive to the requirements of antigenic variation. The BES are transcribed by RNA polymerase I (polI) (Gunzl et al., 2003), which is highly processive, providing a high transcript yield, and are regulated between life cycle stages through control of initiation and elongation of transcription (Vanhamme et al., 2000). Transcription by polI normally would be unproductive for protein-coding genes, as only RNA polymerase II (polII) provides the essential 5′ cap to mRNA. However, the polycistronic nature of transcription in trypanosomes requires a distinct mechanism that would cap each mRNA after excision from the long precursor transcript, and that is provided by a *trans*-splicing process operating posttranscriptionally (Blumenthal, 1998). In principle, therefore, any RNA polymerase could transcribe protein-coding genes in trypanosomes, and the *VSG* system apparently has exploited this loophole to recruit the highly processive polI. The BES promoter displays differential activity between life cycle stages, and the relatively low level of transcription that does occur in the "wrong" life cycle stage terminates near the promoter, preventing production of *VSG* mRNA (Vanhamme et al., 2000).

Mechanisms for singular and differential expression of *VSG* center on the BES, which emphasizes the pivotal role of the expression site in antigenic variation. Within the bloodstream stage, there must be a means of ensuring that only one BES is active at any time. Normally, polI is detectable only in the nucleolus, where it transcribes rRNA genes. In *T. brucei*, however, there is an extra, small focus of polI, the "expression site body" (ESB), which colocalizes with the promoter of the active BES, while inactive (i.e., slightly active) BES promoters appear to be located at the periphery of the nucleolus (Navarro et al., 2007). Occasionally there is a switch in transcription between two BES (Fig. 3), which involves exchange into the ESB. The other way that *VSG* genes are expressed differentially is the switch itself, the fundamental step in antigenic variation. Clearly transcriptional switching between BES is one way to achieve a *VSG* switch, between the two *VSG* occupying those BES. That type of switch, however, cannot account for the enormous range of variants arising in infection. Instead, most *VSG* switching is driven by recombination, with complete or partial copying of an archive *VSG* into the BES (Fig. 3).

VSG Switching

It appears that, despite the possibility for transcriptional switching, one BES remains active throughout at least the early weeks of infection (Robinson et al., 1999). It sits in the ESB, continually receiving information copied from the archive by recombination reactions. Recent, significant experiments have revealed initiating events in such switches. Through the agency of an artificially introduced yeast endonuclease cleaving at its specific target site engineered into the trypanosome genome, induction of a double-strand break (DSB) adjacent to

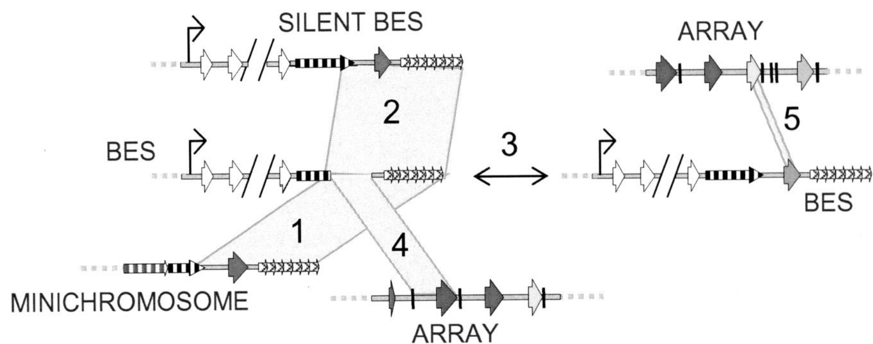

FIGURE 3 *VSG* switching. Maps of the genome compartments are as in Fig. 2, and the five types of switch that have been observed in vivo in normally switching trypanosomes are depicted, in order of their probability in the switching hierarchy. Two BES are shown centrally, the left one with the *VSG* and some of its flanks deleted following a spontaneous break that initiates recombinational switching. (1) A minichromosome donates a duplicate running from its 70-bp repeat tract to perhaps the end of the chromosome; (2) a silent BES donates as for switch type 1; (3) there is a reversible transcriptional switch between two BES (note that this mechanism would not be prompted by the break-deletion events in the active BES); (4) a cassette is duplicated from an intact array gene, replacing the cassette in the active BES—the 3′ limit of duplication could be anywhere from the start of the C-terminal domain-encoding sequence to within the 3′ UTR of the *VSG;* (5) one or more segments from one or more array (pseudo) *VSG*s segmentally convert the *VSG* in the BES.

the downstream end of the 70-bp repeats in the BES precipitated a flurry of switching (Boothroyd et al., 2009). Crucially, it was shown in parallel that trypanosomes without an introduced nuclease naturally display breaks within the 70 bp of the active BES, but not elsewhere, including an inactive BES (Boothroyd et al., 2009). Whether the corresponding, mythical trypanosome endonuclease exists is open to debate, an alternative possibility being that the inherent physical instability of 70-bp repeats (Ohshima et al., 1996), of which there are tens or hundreds in the BES, introduces DSB during DNA replication. Whatever the DSB-generating agent, the 70-bp repeats are now center stage in the switching process, formally supporting what had long been inferred from the oft-repeated observation that, particularly under natural switching conditions, the repeats form the upstream end of the segment duplicated into the BES (Michels et al., 1983; Barry, 1997). In model organisms, generation of a DSB often is followed by creation of a gap, which must be repaired from an intact region of high sequence similarity to avoid provoking cell death. Presumably the expressed *VSG* is deleted, leaving a gap from the 70-bp repeats. This is repaired by duplication from an intact *VSG* cassette, running from its 70-bp repeats. The cassette therefore can be seen as a fundamental unit in antigenic variation. It is not always the case, however, that both ends of the cassette become involved in the duplication process. When the donor gene is telomere-adjacent, duplication can run possibly to the very end of the chromosome (Boothroyd et al., 2009; de Lange et al., 1983), akin to break-induced replication, in which case the downstream flank appears not to play a role.

Silent *VSG* genes compete with each other as donors, which is the basis for ordered expression of variants. Deciphering patterns of hierarchy is not straightforward, as experiments tend to focus on only early events and relatively few variants. From what is known about early infection peaks, each variant has surprisingly low variance in time of activation in different infections (Morrison et al., 2005). One determinant of hierarchy appears to be the genome compartments, with the telomere-adjacent loci having highest probability for activation (Robinson et al., 1999; Pays, 1989). Minichromosomal, *MVSG*, and BES genes duplicate into the BES early (in infections initiated by syringe injection of bloodstream trypanosomes; when the infection is tsetse fly transmitted, MVSGs initiate infection) (Fig. 3), and statistically these locus types appear to have different probability ranges (Morrison et al., 2005). Array genes follow and in general are first seen in infection after at least 2 weeks (Marcello and Barry, 2007b). Although telomere proximity per se might qualify as a mechanistic basis for high-probability switching, due to the tendency of telomeres to interact genetically, it seems likely also that the flanks of *VSG* genes contribute to hierarchical activation. Although these genome compartment groups contribute to hierarchy at a gross level, there is finer specification of activation probability, to the individual gene level. How this is specified might be apparent from the broadly similar antigenic variation system in *Borrelia hermsii*, where it has been established that flanks on either side of the antigen genes fine-tune the timing of duplication into the expression site, by a combination of degree of identity and spacing from the gene (Barbour et al., 2006). In the trypanosome, the 70-bp repeats are candidates for providing similar fine-tuning function, given their homology to the putative switch-initiating DSB sites in the BES, and their fairly marked degeneracy.

In the case of intact array genes, duplication into the BES involves both flanks of the cassette (Fig. 3). Sometimes the downstream flank delimiting the duplication is the relatively short homology region as displayed in Fig. 1C, but sometimes the C-terminal domain-encoding region acts as the 3′ limit of duplication, resulting in the incoming gene gaining much or all of this domain-encoding sequence from the gene that was already being expressed (Marcello and Barry, 2007b; Pays et al., 1985). The scant evidence available is that intact array genes are first activated after at least 2 weeks of infection (Marcello and Barry, 2007b; Timmers et al., 1987; Lee and Van der Ploeg, 1987). Very soon afterward, the phenomenon of mosaic gene formation becomes apparent (Marcello and Barry, 2007b). At this stage, infections are still at an early phase, with the typical chronic phase still to take hold, so there is a requirement for many more variants. Initial signs are that the large set of *VSG* pseudogenes has the potential to contribute enormously to infections, by a capacity to generate, stochastically, a very broad range of expressed mosaic *VSGs* (Thon et al., 1989; Barbet and Kamper, 1993). About 40% of array *VSG* N-terminal domains have one or more high-identity partners in the archive, and expression of an intact array gene can be followed by creation of a mosaic that is a hybrid of the initially expressed allele and a high-identity partner pseudogene (Marcello and Barry, 2007b). Even later in infection, it seems possible that partially related pseudogenes could also create mosaics at a lower frequency due to their lesser degree of identity. Serological and structural studies are required to ascertain whether successively arising mosaics are sufficiently novel to escape antibodies against the initially expressed allele. The segmental conversion events typical of *VSG* mosaics resemble what happens in the evolution of other multigene families, most notably the human major histocompatibility complex family, so there is ample precedent for mosaicism creating novel function. Curiously, however, this is a subject hardly studied, despite its importance. Segmental variants do appear to be immunologically distinct in antigenic variation in bacteria (Futse et al., 2005), and one study provides reasonably strong evidence for mosaicism creating novel function for major histocompatibility complex alleles (Pease et al., 1983). Early switching, therefore, activates existing information, while later switching transiently can generate novel *VSG*, via a highly evolved mechanism.

VSG EVOLUTION

Patterns and Mechanisms of Evolution

At the core of evolution of the *VSG* archive within the single genome, and indeed more broadly across the range of archives in different strains and subspecies in the field, is strong selection for diversification within VSG proteins, particularly in epitopes, balanced by a degree of structural constraint. As argued above, it is more likely that evolution has selected diversifying mechanisms that act broadly across the archive than that all *VSG* genes are exposed individually to direct selection. In addition, the rate of evolution of *VSG* genes greatly exceeds that of other genes, and the intimate relationship between mutation, DNA RRR (replication, recombination, repair) processes, and chromatin raises complications for dealing differentially between the *VSG* and core genes. It is little wonder that *VSG* and other genes occupy separate genome compartments. In particular, subtelomeres constitute a hyperevolutionary chromosome domain, containing multivariant, multigene families (Freitas-Junior et al., 2000; Verstrepen and Fink, 2009) and acting as sites for generation of new genes in organisms as diverse as rice (Fan et al., 2008) and the bacterium *Streptomyces* (Bentley et al., 2002a, 2002b). Unlike chromosome core regions, which recombine extremely rarely with cores of other chromosomes and, in mitotic growth, rarely recombine even with the core of the second homolog of the same chromosome (LaFave and Sekelsky, 2009; Lee et al., 2009), subtelomeres of different chromosomes are considered to recombine promiscuously with each other (Freitas-Junior et al., 2000; Linardopoulou et al., 2005). However, improved imaging resolution and data processing techniques are now revealing the promiscuity to be more restricted and transient than previously thought (Therizols et al., 2010), but the sharing of tracts of identity among subtelomeres of distinct chromosomes reveals that it does occur. *T. brucei* is the most striking case of colonization of subtelomeres by a gene family, in one strain the right subtelomere making up three-quarters of chromosome 1 (Callejas et al., 2006). Study of the assembled subtelomere haplotypes allows inference of how diversification has occurred. Basically, *VSG* diversification operates at different scales. Commonly, gene conversion processes have caused duplication of whole *VSG*, sometimes as stretches of several genes, commonly as single genes, and sometimes as gene segments (Marcello and Barry, 2007b). Featuring prominently within the *VSG* arrays are inversions and duplications of long segments flanked by sequences of (relics of) the retrotransposon *ingi*, which is restricted to subtelomeric regions (Berriman et al., 2005). These segments contain several *VSG* genes, and their inversion disrupts the normal orientation of the arrays toward the centromere. Many of the rearrangements of whole *VSG* are flanked by the 70-bp repeats and/or by the common 3′ end of *VSG*; the cassette flank sequences therefore have dual recombinational roles, in gene switching during antigenic variation and in archive diversification (Marcello and Barry, 2007b).

Much as these larger-scale events shuffle the archive, their real importance lies in the creation of *VSG* duplicates. As revealed above, it is the existence of high-identity duplicates that appears to drive the initial appearance of mosaic, expressed *VSG*, and the involvement of 40% of *VSG* genes in such partnerships is likely to give mosaicism some prominence in antigenic variation. However, archive diversification is an opposing and critical evolutionary force on the archive. It appears that a basic evolutionary protocol operates on the archive, counterbalancing duplication and diversification in dynamic equilibrium: an ever-changing archive with constant general structure (Fig. 4). The diversification processes are more subtle than the large-scale duplication mechanisms. Base substitutions arise throughout *VSG* genes and their flanks, which sometimes are nonsynonymous, causing amino acid substitutions (Marcello and Barry, 2007b). Importantly, short indels of a few bases also occur, creating frameshifting: pseudogene formation (Pays et al., 2007) (Fig. 4). Pseudogenes can also be created by substitution in start or stop codons. As *VSG* pseudogenes are incapable of activation on their own and can contribute to antigenic variation only through the stochastic process of mosaic formation, they are not restricted to yielding only one distinct VSG but can produce potentially multiple, distinct VSG. A superficial survey of *VSG* arrays suggests that mutations are random (Fig. 4), in keeping with the view that selection is not operating on individual

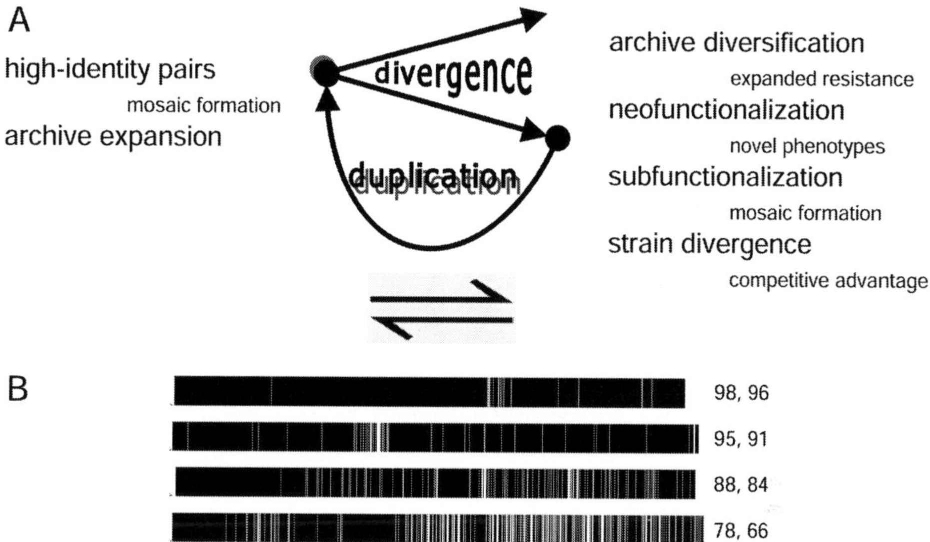

FIGURE 4 *VSG* evolution. (A) The basic evolutionary protocol operating on the *VSG* array. Benefits to the trypanosome of gene duplication are shown to the left, and benefits of divergence are shown to the right. (B) Divergence of recently duplicated *VSG* N-terminal domains. ClustalW nucleotide alignments of high-identity N-terminal domains identified in the genome strain are displayed as Jalview images (Waterhouse et al., 2009). Each image shows identity as black and difference as white. The percent peptide and nucleotide identities of each pair are shown. The highest-identity pair shows some base substitutions (point mutations) and short indels, as well as one cluster of substitutions or a segmental conversion from another gene. Similar substitutions, short indels, and a segmental conversion are evident in the second pair, while the remaining two pairs show too many differences to allow interpretation. Examination of many such pairs shows no particular preference in the position of mutations.

array genes but, rather, across the array chromosome compartment. Nevertheless, a degree of increased diversity in the presumed epitope regions can be discerned, as expected (Hutchinson et al., 2007).

The other types of *VSG* locus also display signs of change through recombination, although fewer data are available. BES are sequence mosaics, with different regions that have undergone conversion events (Hertz-Fowler et al., 2008), which has possible evolutionary consequences for *ESAG*, the other genes in expression sites. Nothing is known about events in the minichromosomal *VSG* set. The *MVSG* loci contain only the gene and its promoter, but the gene does get replaced with another, through recombination (perhaps by gene conversion) at various sites in the locus (Graham et al., 1999; Bringaud et al., 2001). This event, although not altering the coding sequence, is important in gradual turnover of the surface coat set displayed by the metacyclic population; this has important implications for overcoming herd immunity (Barry et al., 1990).

Little more than speculation can be offered as to how the range of mutations in silent *VSG* occurs; it is difficult to study experimentally effects that take place on (hyper)evolutionary timescales. It may be that standard RRR mechanisms operate in both chromosome cores and subtelomeres, with subtle control differences allowing distinct outcomes. On the other hand, there could be novel mechanisms operating in subtelomeres. The only RRR activities shown to influence the archive are two proteins involved in the main eukaryotic homologous recombination pathway, which is based on RAD51. When either *MRE11* or *BRCA2* is deleted from the genome, the megabase chromosomes undergo a dramatic reduction in size (Robinson et al., 2002; Hartley and McCulloch, 2008). Whereas one examined BES *VSG* gene persisted in the *mre11* null mutant, a study of one family of five silent *VSG* genes showed that the presumed array members, but not a telomere-adjacent member, displayed a tendency for deletion. Subsequent detailed mapping across the cores of two diploid chromosomes has shown the loss of a marker at only one of the eight core ends and not internally (A. Browitt and J. D. Barry, unpublished data). One possible implication is that homologous recombination in the subtelomere array compartment of the genome is modified, although there are other possibilities. As yet, nothing is known about which RRR activities affect the within-*VSG* base substitutions, indels, and segmental conversions.

Consequences of *VSG* Evolution

There clearly are exuberant mutagenic processes that expand and diversify the archive, increasing the trypanosome's arsenal for resisting the adaptive immune system. These processes also generate distinct *VSG* serodemes, allowing strains to compete with each other in the field. There are other substantial evolutionary consequences of the trypanosome's duplication-diversification evolutionary protocol (Fig. 4). Gene neofunctionalization, in which the two alleles of a duplicated gene end up with distinct function, is the fundamental process in organisms for development of new traits (Teshima and Innan, 2008). The related phenomenon of subfunctionalization, where the two alleles degenerate to a state of interdependence but together yield the original activity (He and Zhang, 2005), arguably can also be important in evolution. In one type of subfunctionalization, promoter activities can diverge, resulting in, for example, the appearance of tissue specificity of protein activity; having both forms of the protein can be essential. The trypanosome is exquisitely equipped for gaining new traits in these ways, by having a huge archive of genes that individually are rarely used and nonessential, are duplicated frequently, and are exposed to hypermutation mechanisms. There are indeed signs that occasionally *VSG* genes have escaped and developed neofunction. A number of trypanosome surface proteins have the characteristic VSG fold, which could arise by convergent evolution, imposed by a need to fit in the densely packed coat, or by neofunctionalization, reflecting evolution in a lineage. One protein that almost certainly has arisen from VSG acts as a critical determinant of the human infectivity of the subspecies *T. brucei rhodesiense*. Apolipoprotein L1 (apoL1) in human plasma is lytic to *T. brucei brucei*, which infects other mammals, including livestock. In *T. b. rhodesiense*, a VSG fragment known as SRA (serum resistance-associated) protein, which locates to the endosomal system rather than the cell surface, binds the internalized apoL1, preventing lysis (Pays and Vanhollebeke, 2008). The *SRA* gene lies in a BES and can be activated differentially through BES switching. It can be argued that the formation of *VSG* pseudogenes is a form of subfunctionalization, as a pseudogene can contribute functionally to antigenic variation, but only through interaction with an intact *VSG* or an intact segment of another pseudo-*VSG*. Other proteins related to VSG but having distinct function, including the transferrin receptor family (Carrington and Boothroyd, 1996; Bitter et al., 1998) and possibly those encoded by the *VR* (*VSG*-related) genes (Marcello and Barry, 2007a), appear to be ancestral to the VSG of *T. brucei* (A. Jackson, M. Berriman, and C. Hertz-Fowler, personal communication).

CONCLUSIONS

The phenotypic needs of the trypanosome, living extracellularly in the highly challenging environment of mammalian blood, are well served by a robustly defensive molecular phenotype. Underlying the phenotype is a tightly regulated and stochastically switching genetic system. In turn, that system relies on an enormous and highly dynamic silent gene archive. Genome compartmentalization helps in the marshalling and evolution of the gene archive. There is clear evidence for several different types of mutation, and it is predicted that mutational mechanisms have been adapted in both rate and localization to yield hypermutation of the silent archive. As a spinoff of the archive, novel genes and associated novel phenotypes can arise.

ACKNOWLEDGMENTS

I thank Richard McCulloch for reading the manuscript and Mark Carrington and Sara Melville for kind provision of images.

I also thank the Wellcome Trust for funding.

REFERENCES

Barbet, A. F., and S. M. Kamper. 1993. The importance of mosaic genes to trypanosome survival. *Parasitol. Today* **9:**63–66.

Barbour, A. G., Q. Dai, B. I. Restrepo, H. G. Stoenner, and S. A. Frank. 2006. Pathogen escape from host immunity by a genome program for antigenic variation. *Proc. Natl. Acad. Sci. USA* **103:**18290–18295.

Barry, J. D. 1997. The relative significance of mechanisms of antigenic variation in African trypanosomes. *Parasitol. Today* **13:**212–218.

Barry, J. D., and R. McCulloch. 2001. Antigenic variation in trypanosomes: enhanced phenotypic variation in a eukaryotic parasite. *Adv. Parasitol.* **49:**1–70.

Barry, J. D., S. V. Graham, K. R. Matthews, P. G. Shiels, and O. A. Shonekan. 1990. Stage-specific mechanisms for activation and expression of variant surface glycoprotein genes in *Trypanosoma brucei*. *Biochem. Soc. Trans.* **18:**708–710.

Bentley, D., M. Holden, M. Sebaihia, A. M. Cerdeno-Tarraga, and J. Parkhill. 2002a. Genome giants. *Trends Microbiol.* **10:**309–310.

Bentley, S. D., K. F. Chater, A. M. Cerdeno-Tarraga, G. L. Challis, N. R. Thomson, K. D. James, D. E. Harris, M. A. Quail, H. Kieser, D. Harper, A. Bateman, S. Brown, G. Chandra, C. W. Chen, M. Collins, A. Cronin, A. Fraser, A. Goble, J. Hidalgo, T. Hornsby, S. Howarth, C. H. Huang, T. Kieser, L. Larke, L. Murphy, K. Oliver, S. O'Neil, E. Rabbinowitsch, M. A. Rajandream, K. Rutherford, S. Rutter, K. Seeger, D. Saunders, S. Sharp, R. Squares, S. Squares, K. Taylor, T. Warren, A. Wietzorrek, J. Woodward, B. G. Barrell, J. Parkhill, and D. A. Hopwood. 2002b. Complete genome sequence of the model actinomycete Streptomyces coelicolor A3(2). *Nature* **417:**141–147.

Berriman, M., E. Ghedin, C. Hertz-Fowler, G. Blandin, H. Renauld, D. C. Bartholomeu, N. J. Lennard, E. Caler, N. E. Hamlin, B. Haas, U. Bohme, L. Hannick, M. A. Aslett, J. Shallom, L. Marcello, L. Hou, B. Wickstead, U. C. Alsmark, C. Arrowsmith, R. J. Atkin, A. J. Barron, F. Bringaud, K. Brooks, M. Carrington, I. Cherevach, T. J. Chillingworth, C. Churcher, L. N. Clark, C. H. Corton, A. Cronin, R. M. Davies, J. Doggett, A. Djikeng, T. Feldblyum, M. C. Field, A. Fraser, I. Goodhead, Z. Hance, D. Harper, B. R. Harris, H. Hauser, J. Hostetler, A. Ivens, K. Jagels, D. Johnson, J. Johnson, K. Jones, A. X. Kerhornou, H. Koo, N. Larke, S. Landfear, C. Larkin, V. Leech, A. Line, A. Lord, A. MacLeod, P. J. Mooney, S. Moule, D. M. Martin, G. W. Morgan, K. Mungall, H. Norbertczak, D. Ormond, G. Pai, C. S. Peacock, J. Peterson, M. A. Quail, E. Rabbinowitsch, M. A. Rajandream, C. Reitter, S. L. Salzberg, M. Sanders, S. Schobel, S. Sharp, M. Simmonds, A. J. Simpson, L. Tallon, C. M. Turner, A. Tait, A. R. Tivey, S. Van Aken, D. Walker, D. Wanless, S. Wang, B. White, O. White, S. Whitehead, J. Woodward, J. Wortman, M. D. Adams, T. M. Embley, K. Gull, E. Ullu, J. D. Barry, A. H. Fairlamb, F. Opperdoes, B. G. Barrell, J. E. Donelson, N. Hall, C. M. Fraser, S. E. Melville, and N. M. El Sayed. 2005. The genome of the African trypanosome *Trypanosoma brucei*. *Science* **309:**416–422.

Bitter, W., H. Gerrits, R. Kieft, and P. Borst. 1998. The role of transferrin-receptor variation in the host range of *Trypanosoma brucei*. *Nature* **391:**499–502.

Blumenthal, T. 1998. Gene clusters and polycistronic transcription in eukaryotes. *Bioessays* **20:**480–487.

Boothroyd, C. E., O. Dreesen, T. Leonova, K. I. Ly, L. M. Figueiredo, G. A. Cross, and F. N. Papavasiliou. 2009. A yeast-endonuclease-generated DNA break induces antigenic switching in *Trypanosoma brucei*. *Nature* **459:**278–281.

Bringaud, F., N. Biteau, J. E. Donelson, and T. Baltz. 2001. Conservation of metacyclic variant surface glycoprotein expression sites among different trypanosome isolates. *Mol. Biochem. Parasitol.* **113:**67–78.

Callejas, S., V. Leech, C. Reitter, and S. Melville. 2006. Hemizygous subtelomeres of an African trypanosome chromosome may account for over 75% of chromosome length. *Genome Res.* **16:**1109–1118.

Caporale, L. H. 2006. *The Implicit Genome*. Oxford University Press, Oxford, United Kingdom.

Carrington, M., and J. Boothroyd. 1996. Implications of conserved structural motifs in disparate trypanosome surface proteins. *Mol. Biochem. Parasitol.* **81:**119–126.

Dagenais, T. R., K. P. Demick, J. D. Bangs, K. T. Forest, D. M. Paulnock, and J. M. Mansfield. 2009. T-cell responses to the trypanosome variant surface glycoprotein are not limited to hypervariable subregions. *Infect. Immun.* **77:**141–151.

de Lange, T., J. M. Kooter, P. A. M. Michels, and P. Borst. 1983. Telomere conversion in trypanosomes. *Nucleic Acids Res.* **11:**8149–8165.

El Sayed, N. M., P. J. Myler, G. Blandin, M. Berriman, J. Crabtree, G. Aggarwal, E. Caler, H. Renauld, E. A. Worthey, C. Hertz-Fowler, E. Ghedin, C. Peacock, D. C. Bartholomeu, B. J. Haas, A. N. Tran, J. R. Wortman, U. C. Alsmark, S. Angiuoli, A. Anupama, J. Badger, F. Bringaud, E. Cadag, J. M. Carlton, G. C. Cerqueira, T. Creasy, A. L. Delcher, A. Djikeng, T. M. Embley, C. Hauser, A. C. Ivens, S. K. Kummerfeld, J. B. Pereira-Leal, D. Nilsson, J. Peterson, S. L. Salzberg, J. Shallom, J. C. Silva, J. Sundaram, S. Westenberger, O. White, S. E. Melville, J. E. Donelson, B. Andersson, K. D. Stuart, and N. Hall. 2005. Comparative genomics of Trypanosomatid parasitic protozoa. *Science* **309:**404–409.

Fan, C., Y. Zhang, Y. Yu, S. Rounsley, M. Long, and R. A. Wing. 2008. The subtelomere of Oryza sativa chromosome 3 short arm as a hot bed of new gene origination in rice. *Mol. Plant* **1:**839–850.

Field, M. C., and J. C. Boothroyd. 1996. Sequence divergence in a family of variant surface glycoprotein genes from trypanosomes—coding region hypervariability and downstream recombinogenic repeats. *J. Mol. Evol.* **42:**500–511.

Freitas-Junior, L. H., E. Bottius, L. A. Pirrit, K. W. Deitsch, C. Scheidig, F. Guinet, U. Nehrbass, T. E. Wellems, and A. Scherf. 2000. Frequent ectopic recombination of virulence factor genes in telomeric chromosome clusters of *P. falciparum*. *Nature* **407:**1018–1022.

Futse, J. E., K. A. Brayton, D. P. Knowles, Jr., and G. H. Palmer. 2005. Structural basis for segmental gene conversion in generation of *Anaplasma marginale* outer membrane protein variants. *Mol. Microbiol.* **57:**212–221.

Futse, J. E., K. A. Brayton, M. J. Dark, D. P. Knowles, Jr., and G. H. Palmer. 2008. Superinfection as a driver of genomic diversification in antigenically variant pathogens. *Proc. Natl. Acad. Sci. USA* **105:**2123–2127.

Gjini, E., D. T. Haydon, J. D. Barry, and C. Cobbold. 2010. Critical interplay between parasite differentiation, host immunity, and antigenic variation in trypanosome infections. *Am. Nat.* **176:**424–439.

Graham, S. V., S. Terry, and J. D. Barry. 1999. A structural and transcription pattern for variant surface glycoprotein gene expression sites used in metacyclic stage *Trypanosoma brucei*. *Mol. Biochem. Parasitol.* **103:**141–154.

Gunzl, A., T. Bruderer, G. Laufer, B. Schimanski, L. C. Tu, H. M. Chung, P. T. Lee, and M. G. Lee. 2003. RNA polymerase I transcribes procyclin genes and variant surface glycoprotein gene expression sites in *Trypanosoma brucei*. *Eukaryot. Cell* **2:**542–551.

Haanstra, J. R., M. Stewart, V. D. Luu, A. van Tuijl, H. V. Westerhoff, C. Clayton, and B. M. Bakker. 2008. Control and regulation of gene expression: quantitative analysis of the expression of phosphoglycerate kinase in bloodstream form Trypanosoma brucei. *J. Biol. Chem.* **283:**2495–2507.

Hall, T., and K. Esser. 1984. Topologic mapping of protective and nonprotective epitopes on the variant surface glycoprotein of the WRATat 1 clone of *Trypanosoma brucei* rhodesiense. *J. Immunol.* **132:** 2059–2063.

Hartley, C. L., and R. McCulloch. 2008. Trypanosoma brucei BRCA2 acts in antigenic variation and has undergone a recent expansion in BRC repeat number that is important during homologous recombination. *Mol. Microbiol.* **68:**1237–1251.

He, X., and J. Zhang. 2005. Rapid subfunctionalization accompanied by prolonged and substantial neofunctionalization in duplicate gene evolution. *Genetics* **169:**1157–1164.

Hertz-Fowler, C., L. M. Figueiredo, M. A. Quail, M. Becker, A. Jackson, N. Bason, K. Brooks, C. Churcher, S. Fahkro, I. Goodhead, P. Heath, M. Kartvelishvili, K. Mungall, D. Harris, H. Hauser, M. Sanders, D. Saunders, K. Seeger, S. Sharp, J. E. Taylor, D. Walker, B. White, R. Young, G. A. Cross, G. Rudenko, J. D. Barry, E. J. Louis, and M. Berriman. 2008. Telomeric expression sites are highly conserved in *Trypanosoma brucei*. *PLoS One* **3:**e3527.

Hutchinson, O. C., K. Picozzi, N. G. Jones, H. Mott, R. Sharma, S. C. Welburn, and M. Carrington. 2007. Variant surface glycoprotein gene repertoires in Trypanosoma brucei have diverged to become strain-specific. *BMC Genomics* **8:**234.

LaFave, M. C., and J. Sekelsky. 2009. Mitotic recombination: why? when? how? where? *PLoS Genet.* **5:**e1000411.

Lau, A. O. 2009. An overview of the Babesia, Plasmodium and Theileria genomes: a comparative perspective. *Mol. Biochem. Parasitol.* **164:**1–8.

Lee, M. G., and L. H. T. Van der Ploeg. 1987. Frequent independent duplicative transpositions activate a single VSG gene. *Mol. Cell. Biol.* **7:** 357–364.

Lee, P. S., P. W. Greenwell, M. Dominska, M. Gawel, M. Hamilton, and T. D. Petes. 2009. A fine-structure map of spontaneous mitotic crossovers in the yeast Saccharomyces cerevisiae. *PLoS Genet.* **5:**e1000410.

Linardopoulou, E. V., E. M. Williams, Y. Fan, C. Friedman, J. M. Young, and B. J. Trask. 2005. Human subtelomeres are hot spots of interchromosomal recombination and segmental duplication. *Nature* **437:**94–100.

Lynch, M. 2007. *The Origins of Genome Architecture.* Sinauer Associates, Sunderland, MA.

Lythgoe, K. A., L. J. Morrison, A. F. Read, and J. D. Barry. 2007. Parasite-intrinsic factors can explain ordered progression of trypanosome antigenic variation. *Proc. Natl. Acad. Sci. USA* **104:** 8095–8100.

Marcello, L., and J. D. Barry. 2007a. From silent genes to noisy populations—dialogue between the genotype and phenotypes of antigenic variation. *J. Eukaryot. Microbiol.* **54:**14–17.

Marcello, L., and J. D. Barry. 2007b. Analysis of the VSG gene silent archive in *Trypanosoma brucei* reveals that mosaic gene expression is prominent in antigenic variation and is favored by archive substructure. *Genome Res.* **17:**1344–1352.

Melville, S. E., V. Leech, C. S. Gerrard, A. Tait, and J. M. Blackwell. 1998. The molecular karyotype of the megabase chromosomes of *Trypanosoma brucei* and the assignment of chromosome markers. *Mol. Biochem. Parasitol.* **94:**155–173.

Metruccio, M. M., E. Pigozzi, D. Roncarati, F. Berlanda Scorza, N. Norais, S. A. Hill, V. Scarlato, and I. Delany. 2009. A novel phase variation mechanism in the meningococcus driven by a ligand-responsive repressor and differential spacing of distal promoter elements. *PLoS Pathog.* **5:**e1000710.

Michels, P. A. M., A. Y. C. Liu, A. Bernards, P. Sloof, M. M. W. Vanderbijl, A. H. Schinkel, H. H. Menke, P. Borst, G. H. Veeneman, M. C. Tromp, and J. H. Vanboom. 1983. Activation of the genes for variant surface glycoprotein-117 and glycoprotein-118 in *Trypanosoma brucei. J. Mol. Biol.* **166:**537–556.

Miller, E. N., L. M. Allan, and M. J. Turner. 1984. Topological analysis of antigenic determinants on a variant surface glycoprotein of *Trypanosoma brucei. Mol. Biochem. Parasitol.* **13:**67–81.

Morrison, L. J., P. Majiwa, A. F. Read, and J. D. Barry. 2005. Probabilistic order in antigenic variation of *Trypanosoma brucei. Int. J. Parasitol.* **35:**961–972.

Moxon, E. R., P. B. Rainey, M. A. Nowak, and R. E. Lenski. 1994. Adaptive evolution of highly mutable loci in pathogenic bacteria. *Curr. Biol.* **4:** 24–33.

Navarro, M., X. Penate, and D. Landeira. 2007. Nuclear architecture underlying gene expression in *Trypanosoma brucei. Trends Microbiol.* **15:**263–270.

Ohshima, K., S. Kang, J. E. Larson, and R. D. Wells. 1996. TTA.TAA triplet repeats in plasmids form a non-H bonded structure. *J. Biol. Chem.* **271:**16784–16791.

Pays, E. 1989. Pseudogenes, chimaeric genes and the timing of antigen variation in African trypanosomes. *Trends Genet.* **5:**389–391.

Pays, E., and B. Vanhollebeke. 2008. Mutual self-defence: the trypanolytic factor story. *Microbes Infect.* **10:**985–989.

Pays, E., D. Salmon, L. J. Morrison, L. Marcello, and J. D. Barry. 2007. Antigenic variation in *Trypanosoma brucei,* p. 339–372. *In* D. Barry, R. McCulloch, J. Mottram, and A. Acosta-Serrano (ed.), *Trypanosomes: after the Genome.* Horizon Scientific Press, Wymondham, United Kingdom.

Pays, E., S. Houard, A. Pays, S. Van Assel, F. Dupont, D. Aerts, G. Huet-Duvillier, V. Gomes, C. Richet, P. Degand, et al. 1985. *Trypanosoma brucei*: the extent of conversion in antigen genes may be related to the DNA coding specificity. *Cell* **42:**821–829.

Pease, L. R., D. H. Schulze, G. M. Pfaffenbach, and S. G. Nathenson. 1983. Spontaneous H-2 mutants provide evidence that a copy mechanism analogous to gene conversion generates polymorphism in the major histocompatibility complex. *Proc. Natl. Acad. Sci. USA* **80:**242–246.

Prucca, C. G., and H. D. Lujan. 2009. Antigenic variation in Giardia lamblia. *Cell Microbiol.* **11:**1706–1715.

Robinson, N. P., N. Burman, S. E. Melville, and J. D. Barry. 1999. Predominance of duplicative *VSG* gene conversion in antigenic variation in African trypanosomes. *Mol. Cell. Biol.* **19:**5839–5846.

Robinson, N. P., R. McCulloch, C. Conway, A. Browitt, and J. D. Barry. 2002. Inactivation of Mre11 does not affect VSG gene duplication mediated by homologous recombination in *Trypanosoma brucei. J. Biol. Chem.* **277:**26185–26193.

Schwede, A., and M. Carrington. 2010. Bloodstream form trypanosome plasma membrane proteins: antigenic variation and invariant antigens. *Parasitology* **137:**2029–2039..

Shah, J. S., J. R. Young, B. E. Kimmel, K. P. Iams, and R. O. Williams. 1987. The 5′ flanking sequence of a *Trypanosoma brucei* variable surface glycoprotein gene. *Mol. Biochem. Parasitol.* **24:**163–174.

Siegel, T. N., D. R. Hekstra, L. E. Kemp, L. M. Figueiredo, J. E. Lowell, D. Fenyo, X. Wang, S. Dewell, and G. A. Cross. 2009. Four histone variants mark the boundaries of polycistronic transcription units in *Trypanosoma brucei. Genes Dev.* **23:**1063–1076.

Teshima, K. M., and H. Innan. 2008. Neofunctionalization of duplicated genes under the pressure of gene conversion. *Genetics* **178:**1385–1398.

Therizols, P., T. Duong, B. Dujon, C. Zimmer, and E. Fabre. 2010. Chromosome arm length and nuclear constraints determine the dynamic relationship of yeast subtelomeres. *Proc. Natl. Acad. Sci. USA* **107:**2025–2030.

Thon, G., T. Baltz, and H. Eisen. 1989. Antigenic diversity by the recombination of pseudogenes. *Genes Dev.* **3:**1247–1254.

Timmers, H. T. M., T. de Lange, J. M. Kooter, and P. Borst. 1987. Coincident multiple activations of the same surface antigen gene in *Trypanosoma brucei*. *J. Mol. Biol.* **194:**81–90.

Vanhamme, L., P. Poelvoorde, A. Pays, P. Tebabi, H. V. Xong, and E. Pays. 2000. Differential RNA elongation controls the variant surface glycoprotein gene expression sites of *Trypanosoma brucei*. *Mol. Microbiol.* **36:**328–340.

Verstrepen, K. J., and G. R. Fink. 2009. Genetic and epigenetic mechanisms underlying cell-surface variability in protozoa and fungi. *Annu. Rev. Genet.* **43:**1–24.

Waterhouse, A. M., J. B. Procter, D. M. Martin, M. Clamp, and G. J. Barton. 2009. Jalview Version 2—a multiple sequence alignment editor and analysis workbench. *Bioinformatics* **25:**1189–1191.

Wickstead, B., K. Ersfeld, and K. Gull. 2004. The small chromosomes of *Trypanosoma brucei* involved in antigenic variation are constructed around repetitive palindromes. *Genome Res.* **14:** 1014–1024.

Young, R., J. E. Taylor, A. Kurioka, M. Becker, E. J. Louis, and G. Rudenko. 2008. Isolation and analysis of the genetic diversity of repertoires of VSG expression site containing telomeres from *Trypanosoma brucei gambiense*, *T. b. brucei* and *T. equiperdum*. *BMC Genomics* **9:**385.

GENOME PLASTICITY IN *Candida albicans*

Claude Pujol and David R. Soll

18

Candida albicans is a common commensal of mammals and humans in particular. As a commensal it can colonize multiple body locations, but the gastrointestinal tract and the genitalia are favored. In the immunocompromised host, it often becomes infectious at the same body locations where it can be found as a commensal, but it can also invade deeper tissues and affect multiple internal organs. It is the most frequent source of fungal nosocomial infection, and mortality associated with disseminated candidiasis is estimated to range between 40 and 60%.

In commensals, phenotypic plasticity plays an important role that becomes critical during the infectious process. Phenotypic plasticity in *C. albicans* can be achieved through different mechanisms. *C. albicans* has the ability to adjust gene expression at the transcriptional level in response to signals from the environment without undergoing DNA reorganization. *C. albicans* also undergoes three major developmental programs: (i) the bud-hypha transition, which allows yeast cells to reversibly differentiate to a filamentous form (Sudbery et al., 2004); (ii) a 3153A-like switching system, which enables cells to interconvert between multiple phenotypes (Slutsky et al., 1985; Soll, 1992); and (iii) the white-opaque transition, which allows *MTL*-homozygous cells to reversibly switch between two cell types (Slutsky et al., 1987; Soll, 1992). Except for the white-opaque transition that requires homozygosis at the *MTL* locus (Miller and Johnson, 2002; Lockhart et al., 2002), developmental programs do not require genome plasticity and are modulated by environmental cues. This phenotypic plasticity seems to be sufficient to support the commensal and infectious life cycles of *C. albicans* in the mammalian host and allow cells to adapt to the different environments represented by the multiple body locations that *C. albicans* colonizes. Nevertheless, the genome of *C. albicans* can also undergo substantial plasticity, including (i) changes in transposable elements, (ii) genetic exchange and recombination through a parasexual cycle, (iii) karyotypic instability which can lead to chromosome translocation and aneuploidy, and (iv) loss of heterozygosity (LOH). While each of these mechanisms can potentially lead to phenotypic plasticity, their relevance in *C. albicans* biology has not been firmly established. Recent advances in our

Claude Pujol and David R. Soll, Department of Biology, The University of Iowa, Iowa City, IA 52242.

Genome Plasticity and Infectious Diseases,
Edited by J. Hacker, U. Dobrindt, and R. Kurth,

understanding of the development of antifungal drug resistance have, however, clearly revealed the advantage of genomic plasticity in rapid adaptation to new conditions. *C. albicans* responds to rapid environmental challenges through its built-in capacity to modulate its phenotype. Antifungals, however, may represent the single most significant challenge that these cells can encounter that will directly affect their survival and against which no intrinsic developmental program is already available for a rapid riposte. Advances in the understanding of genome plasticity in the framework of antifungal drug resistance have benefited from several factors. Antifungals are a source of strong selective pressure. They can easily be used for in vitro experiments. Resistant and susceptible isolates derived from the same parental strain can readily be obtained from treated patients. Most importantly, the clinical relevance of the establishment of resistance has greatly impacted this field. In this chapter we describe the different mechanisms of genome plasticity in *C. albicans* and their impact on phenotypic plasticity, with an emphasis on recent advances in antifungal drug resistance.

PLOIDY LEVEL

C. albicans was first demonstrated to be diploid by fluorescence-activated cell sorter analysis, UV resistance, and chemical mutagenesis experiments in 1979 (Olaiya and Sogin, 1979). Since then, the use of codominant markers has demonstrated the presence of typical heterozygous patterns at numerous loci for strains isolated worldwide. More recently, our understanding of the complexity of the *C. albicans* diploid genome has been greatly improved by the availability of the sequenced genomes of strains SC5314 and WO-1 (Jones et al., 2004; Butler et al., 2009). The large majority of *C. albicans* stains are diploid. This does not preclude the possibility of rare aneuploidies, tetraploidies, and even haploidies. Suzuki et al. (1982) described haploids and tetraploids, but their data were somewhat controversial since at least one isolate deemed to represent a haploid *C. albicans* strain, NUM43, was later reported to be *Candida gulliermondii* (Kanbe et al., 2003), a haploid species (Reedy et al., 2009). Comparative genome hybridization is a very sensitive technique that allows the detection of aneuploidy even over relatively short sequence tracts. This approach is a tremendous improvement over fluorescence-activated cell sorter analysis, which still remains the method of choice to assess the overall ploidy level of a cell. Its use in *C. albicans* has been spearheaded by Berman and colleagues (Selmecki et al., 2005), who demonstrated segmental aneuploidies, gains and losses of chromosome, and the creation of isochromosomes in an otherwise basically diploid genome background (Selmecki et al., 2005, 2006, 2008; Coste et al., 2006, 2007).

RETROTRANSPOSONS IN *C. ALBICANS*

Retrotransposons are mobile elements that can cause mutations and genomic rearrangements. Multiple long terminal repeat (LTR) retrotransposons and L1-like non-LTR retrotransposon elements have been found in *C. albicans* (Goodwin and Poulter, 2000; Goodwin et al., 2001). LTR retrotransposons have been classified into 34 families in *C. albicans*. Most are degenerate, and for about half of them only their LTR sequences have been maintained in the genome and hence lack any associated internal regions (Goodwin and Poulter, 2000). Some of the retrotransposons with internal sequences have been shown to be transcriptionally active, and for three families, apparently full-length retrotransposon elements have been retained and could be potentially active. It has been suggested that some of the degenerate elements could still be transposable by borrowing the machinery of active retrotransposons. The situation is similar for the Zorro elements of non-LTR retrotransposons (Goodwin et al., 2001). Among these, the Zorro-3 element in particular is active for retrotransposition (Goodwin et al., 2007). Elements from both classes of retrotransposons are present at low copy number, and some are thought to have transposed relatively recently (Goodwin and Poulter, 2000; Goodwin et al., 2001). The genetic divergence found in *C. albicans* suggests that the species could be at least three million years old (Lott et al., 2005;

Mishra et al., 2007). This suggests that what is meant by "recent" in the evolutionary history of *C. albicans* may represent the last thousand or hundred thousand years. To our knowledge, the Zorro-3 element is the only element that has been shown to transpose, and this was observed by using selectable markers. While there does not seem to be any example of observed natural transposition, retrotransposons may still play a role in the long-term evolution of *C. albicans*. Retrotransposons are often concentrated at subtelomeric sites and could play a role in telomere structure or silencing (Goodwin and Poulter, 2000; Goodwin et al., 2001). They can also be found in intergenic regions, including promoter regions, and there is at least one example of an LTR sequence inserted in a functional gene. The last 13 codons of *CBP1*, which encodes a corticosteroid-binding protein, are derived from an LTR sequence (Goodwin and Poulter, 2000). In conclusion, the genetic diversity generated by retrotransposons may potentially play a role in *C. albicans*, but definitive evidence is still lacking. Interestingly, recombination at or near LTR regions has recently been shown to be associated with LOH in *C. albicans* (Diogo et al., 2009).

MATING AND RECOMBINATION

Sexual reproduction is generally thought to be more beneficial than asexual reproduction due to its capacity to purge genomes of deleterious mutations, repair DNA damage, and generate genetic diversity through genetic exchange and recombination. Meiosis is central in promoting most of these processes. *C. albicans* can mate, but meiosis and sporulation have not yet been observed. The locus encoding mating types in *C. albicans*, *MTL* (for "mating type-like"), was first described in 1999 by Hull and Johnson. It consists of two idiomorphs, *MTL***a** and *MTL*α. The *MTL***a** locus contains two genes involved in the regulation of mating, **a**1 and **a**2, plus three additional genes with no known role in mating, *OBP1***a**, *PIK1***a**, and *PAP1***a** (Hull and Johnson, 1999; Tsong et al., 2003). *MTL*α also bears two genes involved in mating, α1 and α2, and the three genes *OBP1*α, *PIK1*α, and *PAP1*α. This configuration is different from that of the model organism *Saccharomyces cerevisiae* and evolved in species of the hemiascomycetes more closely related to *C. albicans* (Butler et al., 2009; Soll et al., 2009). The majority of natural strains of *C. albicans* (90 to 97%) are *MTL* heterozygotes (Lockhart et al., 2002; Legrand et al., 2004; Odds et al., 2007). In cells of these strains, the protein complex formed by the **a**1 and α2 gene products repress mating-specific genes and the master switch locus gene for white-opaque switching, *WOR1*. Meiosis has not been observed in *C. albicans*, but upon LOH at the *MTL* locus by gene conversion, mitotic crossover, or chromosome loss, mating-type **a** or α specificity is acquired (Wu et al., 2005, 2007; Coste et al., 2007). In *C. albicans*, this is not sufficient for cells to mate; they must first switch from the white to the opaque phenotype (Slutsky et al., 1987; Miller and Johnson, 2002; Lockhart et al., 2002, 2003b; Tsong et al., 2003), which requires *WOR1* expression (Srikantha et al., 2006; Zordan et al., 2006; Huang et al., 2006). In the white-opaque transition, cells undergo a spontaneous and reversible epigenetic switch between a small round (white) and a larger elongated (opaque) cell type (Slutsky et al., 1987). This transition is observed only in *MTL*-homozygous cells (Miller and Johnson, 2002; Lockhart et al., 2002). Opaque cells secrete mating-type-specific pheromones which induce a mating-specific response in opaque cells of opposite mating type, characterized by cell cycle arrest, cellular polarization, production of mating projections (shmoos), and mating (Bennett et al., 2003; Lockhart et al., 2003a, 2003b; Dignard et al., 2007; Yi et al., 2008). White cells do not produce pheromone and do not undergo a mating response in response to pheromone. Instead, pheromone induces cell-cell and cell-surface adhesion and the production of an enhanced biofilm that facilitates chemotropism and mating of opaque cells by stabilizing pheromone gradients (Daniels et al., 2006; Yi et al., 2008; Sahni et al., 2009). Mating has been demonstrated to occur in vivo in a murine candidemia model (Hull et al., 2000) and in a murine gastrointestinal model

(Dumitru et al., 2007). Mating in the host is facilitated by high CO_2 levels that stabilize the opaque phenotype (Huang et al., 2009), suggesting that mating may be favored in the gastrointestinal tract of the host.

The mating of two diploid cells generates tetraploid progeny. Meiosis has not been observed in *C. albicans*, and earlier comparative genomics data suggested that the absence of many genes important for meiosis may indicate the loss of this pathway (Tzung et al., 2001). This assumption has recently been challenged by the description of a meiotic sex cycle in the related species *Candida lusitaniae* which lacks even more of the genes deemed crucial for meiosis than does *C. albicans* (Reedy et al., 2009; Butler et al., 2009). Meiosis, therefore, may still be present in *C. albicans*, but the conditions that support it have not yet been found. Even in the absence of meiosis, however, tetraploid cells can undergo a reduction to the diploid state or near diploid state through a parasexual cycle (Bennett and Johnson, 2003; Forche et al., 2008). Bennett and Johnson (2003) showed that growth of tetraploid cells in specific media, sorbose medium or *S. cerevisiae* presporulation medium, can induce concerted and apparently random chromosome loss. While the large majority of tetraploid cells grown under these conditions rapidly die, a large proportion of the survivors lost chromosomes (Bennett and Johnson, 2003). Comparative genome hybridization and single-nucleotide polymorphism (SNP) analyses have demonstrated that recombination is sometimes associated with this ploidy reduction (Forche et al., 2008). Although recombination was relatively rare, it was concerted. Only one of seven presporulation-derived progeny and two of six sorbose-derived progeny that were analyzed had undergone recombination. In these three strains, recombination occurred at multiple locations on different chromosomes. This form of ploidy reduction provides a means of completing a parasexual cycle that has been shown to be useful in carrying out genetic analyses (Bennett and Johnson, 2003). Its role in nature, however, must still be confirmed.

Population Genetics Studies Indicate that Mating Is Rare in Nature

Population genetics analyses compare observed gene frequencies with the frequencies expected under a purely panmictic (sexual) situation where the segregation of alleles at a specific locus and recombination among loci should lead to a random distribution of alleles in a population. A snapshot of genetic diversity is used to infer the evolutionary history that led to it. As such, these methods are not precise and cannot readily be used to determine when sex may last have occurred. They do, however, give a general picture of the population structure of a species. By using this approach, Pujol et al. (1993) first demonstrated that *C. albicans* has a clonal population structure. Since then, multiple studies of diverse collections of *C. albicans* isolates collected worldwide have come to the same general consensus of a predominantly clonal population structure and suggest that sex, if still ongoing, is rare in *C. albicans* (reviewed by Pujol et al. [2005]). A number of studies have, however, also shown that recombination occurs and suggest that genetic exchange may still play an important role in driving genetic diversity in *C. albicans* (Gräser et al., 1996; Forche et al., 1999; Tavanti et al., 2004; Odds et al., 2007). Even so, the consequences of diploidy in *C. albicans* do not readily support this conclusion (Pujol et al., 2005; Cowen et al., 1999; Tavanti et al., 2004). In haploid genomes, recombination unquestionably reveals the occurrence of sex. In contrast, in a diploid genome, recombination can be generated by other means, e.g., gene conversion, mitotic crossover, loss of a homologous chromosome, or loss of diploidy over a limited sequence tract. A portion of recombination observed in *C. albicans* may have been generated by mating, but how much and when is still uncertain.

Another indication that mating is rare in *C. albicans* comes from the correlation among independent genetic markers, a strong indicator of the paucity of recombination. This led to the description of clades in *C. albicans*. Pujol et al. (1997) first showed that dendrograms generated by three independent methods, multilocus enzyme electrophoresis, random amplification of polymorphic DNA, and fingerprinting with the Ca3 DNA probe, identified the same three groups of genetically related isolates in a collection of strains from the United States. These groups were defined as clades I, II, and III. Clades defined by Ca3 fingerprinting were later shown to correlate with clades defined by multilocus sequence typing (MLST) analysis (Robles et al., 2004; Tavanti et al., 2005; Bougnoux et al., 2008), lending further support to the concept of a clonal population structure. These clades were not limited to the United States. They were found in other geographic locales including Europe and South Africa (Blignaut et al., 2002; Pujol et al., 2002), where new clades were also described. These general results were confirmed and extended to other regions of the globe by MLST analysis, which led to the description of a total of 17 major and minor clades (Odds et al., 2007). Strains from a clade could be found at different locations around the globe and coexisted with strains from other clades. Clades were stable geographically and temporally and revealed reproductive isolation since genetic exchange between strains from different clades appeared limited. This supported the hypothesis that mating might be rare between strains of different clades but frequent among strains from the same clade (Soll and Pujol, 2003). Indeed, population genetics analyses discriminated among the structures of large populations of strains, subdividing them into clades in *C. albicans*, but it was possible that reproductive isolation between clades masked sexuality inside the clades, and the clades therefore could represent cryptic species. This hypothesis was proved wrong by the demonstration that on average, 66% of the nucleotide positions polymorphic in an individual clade had a significant excess of heterozygotes in five major clades analyzed by MLST (Bougnoux et al., 2008), while deficits of heterozygotes were extremely rare. This excess of heterozygotes indicated that mating among strains from the same clade and self-mating were rare events in *C. albicans*.

Correlation between independent markers has also been assessed between mitochondrial and nuclear markers in two studies that led to conflicting conclusions (Anderson et al., 2001; Jacobsen et al., 2008b). Anderson et al. (2001) showed an overall good correlation between the two sets of markers and concluded that recombination (mating) was infrequent in *C. albicans*. Jacobsen et al. (2008b) found basically no correlation between the two sets of markers and concluded that mating in *C. albicans* is much more frequent than initially thought. Jacobsen et al. (2008b) proposed that the difference between the two studies was due to the difference in nuclear markers (both studies used the same mitochondrial regions). These authors suggested that the nuclear markers used by Anderson et al. (2001) were not as "comprehensive" (i.e., were less discriminative). This explanation is not satisfactory because if the nuclear markers used by Anderson et al. (2001) were not discriminative enough, they should have generated a "random" dendrogram with no correlation to the mitochondrial markers. Another major disparity exists between the two studies that may explain the distinct outcomes. The *C. albicans* strain samples used in the two studies were dissimilar. In the Anderson et al. (2001) study, strains were randomly selected, resulting in a collection of 45 *C. albicans* isolates with no geographic or temporal subdivisions and different clades. The authors did not base selection on the unrelatedness of strains. In contrast, in the Jacobsen et al. (2008b) study, strains were not randomly picked. Instead they were carefully selected from a worldwide collection spanning several decades to represent maximum genetic diversity as defined by their MLST analyses. Basically, 37 strains were selected to be as unrelated as possible. The consequence of this selection is that this analysis involved mostly strains from different clades that diverged from each other millions of years ago. Mishra et al. (2007) have estimated that the average divergence between *C. albicans* genetic groups is approximately 2 million years. As a consequence, the recombination and genetic exchanges demonstrated in this study are most likely due to ancient mating events in *C. albicans* and not due to recent mating events.

A last indication of clonality in *C. albicans* comes from the presence of two very distinct alleles for the *ALS9* gene (Zhao et al., 2003). The ALS gene family comprises eight genes that encode cell wall glycoproteins playing an important role in adhesion. Two extremely divergent alleles of *ALS9* are present in SC5314, a laboratory strain used for sequencing the *C. albicans* genome (available at http://www.candidagenome.org/). The two alleles diverge the most in their N-terminal regions, which are involved in adhesive interaction. This region is the most highly conserved among genes of the ALS gene family (Hoyer, 2001). In this region, divergence between the two *ALS9* alleles (11% and 16% at the nucleotide and amino acid levels, respectively) is of the same magnitude as that observed between some ALS genes. For example, nucleotide divergence of the N terminus of *ALS1* and *ALS5* is only 10%, and the amino acid divergence of this domain between Als1 and Als5, and between Als1 and Als3, is only 13% and 15%, respectively. The two types of alleles are present in 53% of 196 strains tested (Zhao et al., 2007) and in different clades (Zhao et al., 2003). This observation is reminiscent of the Meselson effect, demonstrated in the ancient asexual bdelloid rotifers (Welch and Meselson, 2000), which stipulates that in the absence of recombination, alleles at a locus accumulate mutations and become increasingly divergent. Divergence between the two types of alleles affects their function. *ALS9-2* plays a role in adhesion to endothelial cells, whereas *ALS9-1* does not (Zhao et al., 2007). It has been suggested that they may have acquired different functions (Zhao et al., 2003). Divergence of the *ALS9* alleles seems to be unusual in *C. albicans*, since this level of divergence has not been observed for other genes, except *PAP1*, *PIK1*, and *OBP1* at the *MTL* locus where recombination is hindered. It is hard to explain such a level of divergence if genetic exchange and recombination were frequent.

Population genetics studies suggest that mating is overall rare and hence does not play a major role in generating frequent and new genetic diversity in *C. albicans*. This does not mean that sex did not play an important role in the genesis of the present genetic diversity, since it is likely that sexuality may have been much more frequent in the past in *C. albicans* and that the different clades were derived from an ancestral population that frequently underwent mating (Bougnoux et al., 2008; Anderson et al., 2001). Despite this interpretation, mating is still functional and therefore is most likely important in the survival of *C. albicans*.

Is Mating Dispensable in *C. albicans*?

Mating and the mating machinery are, therefore, well conserved in *C. albicans*, suggesting that they are under strong selection, providing an advantage for this species. But if mating is a rare event, what is the selective pressure that maintains the machinery? Recent discoveries of the role of switching in the mating process may supply the answer to this question. Mating may play a role in pathogenesis, and the constant selective pressure on pathogenesis may result in the conservation of the mating machinery. The *MTL* genotype regulates the white-opaque transition, which represents a source of phenotypic plasticity and plays a differential role in virulence (Miller and Johnson, 2002; Kvaal et al., 1997, 1999). *MTL* heterozygosity itself impacts virulence (Lockhart et al., 2005; Ibrahim et al., 2005; Wu et al., 2007). In addition, part of the mating pathway has been co-opted to regulate biofilm formation, an important virulence trait, in *MTL*-homozygous white cells (Daniels et al., 2006; Yi et al., 2008; Sahni et al., 2009). It may well be that mating and its machinery are conserved because they confer a direct advantage in virulence.

The different potential advantages of sexuality and clonality (Goddard, 2007; Aanen and Hoekstra, 2007) and the special role played by ploidy (Zeyl, 2007) have recently been reviewed in detail with an emphasis on yeast. Theories abound, but the experimental evidence remains limited and sometimes contradictory. We will give a brief overview of some of the hypotheses that may particularly apply to *C. albicans*.

Some arguments suggest that *C. albicans* may have overcome the need for sex by different means in modern populations. One of the advantages of sexuality is to generate genetic diversity by mixing alleles to create new combinations that can confer an advantage when the environment changes. This may not be necessary in *C. albicans*, because strains are already adapted to their host environment. Their built-in phenotypic plasticity seems to be sufficient to rapidly adapt to the array of niches represented by the different body locations and changes in host physiology. In this regard, clonality would represent an advantage, since it would preserve the allelic combinations that work best.

Another important factor that needs to be integrated into the equation is the diploid status of *C. albicans*. The requirement of sex to repair DNA damage may be moot in a diploid because sequences on homologous chromosomes can be used as templates to repair DNA breaks by an effective homologous recombination mechanism (Ciudad et al., 2004). A similar argument can also be invoked for the purging of deleterious deletions. Mutations in a diploid genome arise at twice the frequency as in a haploid genome. This is true for both adaptive and deleterious mutations. Mutations should accumulate in a diploid genome because they are not efficiently removed. The sequenced genomes of SC5314 and WO-1 indicate a high level of heterozygosity (Jones et al., 2004; Butler et al., 2009), and excessive heterozygosity is present in clades (Bougnoux et al., 2008), supporting the idea that this is indeed the case. Deleterious mutations in *C. albicans* are known to exist. Recessive lethal alleles (Whelan and Soll, 1982) have been found in the genome. Deleterious mutations can be masked by the presence of a wild-type allele on the homologous chromosome (Whelan and Soll, 1982), and the diploid genome is therefore more resilient to harmful mutations. Diploidy in this context provides an advantage since it can store genetic variation. Mutations should accumulate as long as they are recessive enough to not be harmful. They can still be selected for, or purged from the genome by mitotic recombination and gene conversion, if they prove deleterious.

CHROMOSOME POLYMORPHISMS

The diploid genome size of *C. albicans* is approximately 29.7 to 32.8 Mbp, depending on the method and strain used (Jones et al., 2004; Doi et al., 1992; Chu et al., 1993). It is generally organized into eight pairs of homologous chromosomes that can range in size from 0.5 to 4 Mbp (Iwaguchi et al., 1990; Chu et al., 1993; Jones et al., 2004). The advent in the late 1980s of electrophoretic methods to separate chromosomes revealed that there was extensive variation in karyotype and chromosome size among *C. albicans* strains (Snell et al., 1987; Magee and Magee, 1987; Lasker et al., 1989; Iwaguchi et al., 1990; Asakura et al., 1991). Due to this diversity, karyotypes have been used in strain typing (Asakura et al., 1991; Barton et al., 1995; Wilson et al., 2001). A recent comparative genomics analysis of 11 hemiascomycetes demonstrated that *C. albicans* has the least conserved gene order and hence the highest rate of genome instability (Fischer et al., 2006). This instability had been suggested to be the source of morphological phenotypic switching (Rustchenko-Bulgac et al., 1990; Rustchenko-Bulgac, 1991), but causality was never demonstrated. While it is true that phenotypic switching and genome instability often occur concomitantly, they appear to be separate processes that can be enhanced by the same trigger (Barton and Scherer, 1994; Ramsey et al., 1994). The most common source of chromosomal variation is length polymorphism of the chromosome homologues containing the tandemly repeated ribosomal cistrons, chromosome R (Rustchenko-Bulgac, 1991; Iwaguchi et al., 1992; Rustchenko-Bulgac et al., 1993; Ramsey et al., 1994). The chromosome nomenclature in use is the one developed by Wickes et al. (1991), in which this chromosome is called R and the remaining chromosomes are numbered from 1 to 7 in order of decreasing size. This is true in the most common karyotype configuration, which is considered to be ancestral to the less frequent karyotypes, which are considered variant. Changes in the length of chromosome R are mainly due to variations in the number of ribosomal cistron repeats caused by sister chromatid exchange or mitotic crossover (Wickes et al., 1991; Iwaguchi et al., 1992).

RPS Loci and Chromosome Alterations

Another common source of chromosome polymorphism has been associated with the loci containing tandemly repeated RPS sequences. RPS sequences are flanked by a sequence named HOK on one side and by RB2 on the other (Chindamporn et al., 1998; Pujol et al., 1999). HOK-RPS-RB2 constitutes a unique structure named the major repeat sequence (MRS), present on all of the chromosomes but chromosome 3. MRSs represent approximately 10% of the genome (see Chibana and Magee [2009] for a more detailed review). On chromosomes 4 and 7 the MRS is present twice. Solo partial RB2 sequences are also present on all chromosomes except chromosome 6, and two solo partial HOK elements are present on chromosomes 2 and 4. All of these elements are located in close proximity to the centromeres, and orientation of the MRS is conserved relative to the centromere (Chibana and Magee, 2009). MRSs are also present in *C. dubliniensis*, the closest relative of *C. albicans* (Joly et al., 1999, 2002). The two species diverged approximately 20 million years ago (Mishra et al., 2007). Despite the strong conservation of the MRS, its function remains elusive.

Uhl et al. (2003) performed a transposon-based mutational analysis to identify genes affecting the bud-hypha transition in *C. albicans*. Among the mutants analyzed, 20% possessed a transposon insertion in RPSs that could be associated with either hyperfilamentation (73%) or hypofilamentation (27%). These mutants were not further analyzed. In addition, 5 of 163 unambiguous insertions were in, or close to, the open reading frame of different members of the *FGR6* gene family. These genes are found in the RB2 region of the MRS and are hence represented by 8 to 10 loci (Chibana and Magee, 2009; Uhl et al., 2003). These insertions were associated with both hyper- and hypofilamentation, depending on the specific locus affected and possibly the site of insertion. In conclusion, while the RPSs or RB2 subunits can affect filamentation, this relationship is still unsettled. In particular, it is not known how the number of RPS tandem repeats at different loci may affect dimorphism.

The length of RPS tandem arrays has been shown to influence chromosome segregation (Lephart et al., 2005). The propensity to undergo the loss of one of the chromosome 5 homologues by nondisjunction at mitosis increases with the number of RPS copies carried by that chromosome. This effect appears incidental and is unlikely to represent a function for which the MRS evolved. It nevertheless shows that the MRS plays a role in chromosome stability. This role does not seem to be essential since chromosome 3 does not carry an MRS. Insertions of URA3-containing sequences in the MRS (Barton and Scherer, 1994) or the RB2 region (Iwaguchi et al., 2004) induce an increase in chromosomal translocation and fragmentation. These engineered chromosome alterations suggest a link between the MRS and chromosome stability, and, indeed, the MRS has been shown to be the source of spontaneous chromosomal changes that can affect karyotypes. The MRS has been suggested to be a hot spot for mitotic recombination, but more recent evidence suggests that this is not the case (Lephart and Magee, 2006).

Recombination at the MRS can modify karyotypes in two different ways. Changes in the number of RPS tandem repeats can significantly alter the size of a chromosome, and recombination at the MRS between nonhomologous chromosomes can lead to chromosomal translocations. The polymorphisms found at MRS loci have been used to develop very sensitive and useful fingerprinting methods to type strains of *C. albicans* (see the review by Soll [2000]), the 27A (Scherer and Stevens, 1988) and the Ca3 (Soll et al., 1987; Sadhu et al., 1991) repetitive-sequence probes. Fine analysis of the Ca3 fingerprinting patterns has been particularly useful in the characterization of changes in the number of RPS repeats at the MRS. When used to probe Southern blots of EcoRI-digested DNA, Ca3 identified over 20 bands including monomorphic, moderately variable, and hypervariable bands (Schmid et al., 1990). The subset of hypervariable bands often shows differences between isolates that diverged very recently from the same strain, indicative of microevolution (Soll et al., 1991; Lockhart et al., 1995, 1996). The hypervariability of these bands is due to rapid changes in the number of RPS copies at MRS loci (Pujol et al., 1999). At most MRS loci, RPSs are not tandemly repeated and a single partial RPS element is found, but whenever multiple RPSs are present in an MRS, their number can fluctuate very rapidly by intrachromosomal recombination, either sister chromatid exchange or slipped misalignment during DNA replication (Pujol et al., 1999). Microevolutionary changes in the number of RPS tandem repeats can happen frequently both in vitro and in vivo (Soll et al., 1991; Lockhart et al., 1995, 1996; Pujol et al., 1999). In vivo, 14 hypervariable RPS tandem repeat bands were monitored in four strains over 3,000 generations and a total of 13 changes were observed for 8 of these bands (Pujol et al., 1999). When the difference in the number of tandem RPS repeats between two chromosome homologues is large enough, it can result in two distinct bands in a karyotype. This represents a common source of chromosome length polymorphism (Chibana et al., 2000; Lephart et al., 2005). The difference in the number of RPS units between the two homologues of chromosome 5 in strain NUM46 has been shown to vary from 1 RPS on one homologue to 39 RPSs on the other, a difference of 76 kb (Lephart et al., 2005).

A second source of genome plasticity associated with recombination at MRS loci is chromosome translocation. Several clinical strains of *C. albicans* have undergone translocations between chromosomes, in some cases between multiple chromosomes (Chu et al., 1993; Navarro-Garcia et al., 1995; Iwaguchi et al., 2001). The site of translocations in these strains mapped at, or near, the MRS, suggesting that recombination at homologous MRS sequences by mitotic crossover between nonhomologous chromosomes was responsible for these translocations. Chibana et al. (2000) performed a high-resolution analysis of some of these strains and unambiguously concluded that the sites of interchromosomal translocations corresponded to the MRS. Each of these translocations was reciprocal and did not appear to affect ploidy. This means that gene synteny was conserved up to the MRS and that there was no change in ploidy associated with these chromosomal rearrangements. In conclusion, these translocations do not seem to have the potential to affect phenotype. Nevertheless, the same phenomenon can also occur between two homologous chromosomes and lead to LOH over a large chromosomal region spanning from the MRS to the telomere. This seems to have been the case, for example, in strains P75063 and P37039, where no heterozygous SNPs could be found past the MRS on chromosome 5 (Wu et al., 2005, 2007). Diogo et al. (2009) have also identified a strain where recombination at the MRS led to LOH. Finally, the possibility exists that recombinations at the MRS can alter its structure and affect filamentation.

The effect of chromosomal translocation due to recombination at the MRS is even more dramatic in *C. dubliniensis*. This species, like *C. albicans*, is subdivided into distinct clades (Joly et al., 1999; Gee et al., 2002; McManus et al., 2008); strains from clade I are the most frequent and have thus been more extensively studied. In this species, the range of karyotypic variation is remarkable (Joly et al., 2002; Magee et al., 2008). The chromosomal polymorphisms are so extreme that it is often impossible to distinguish homologous chromosomes between most strains and only the use of DNA probes permits identification of homologous chromosomal fragments (Joly et al., 2002; Magee et al., 2008). These analyses indicate that most *C. dubliniensis* translocations, if not all, are due to recombination at an MRS between nonhomologous chromosomes. The analysis of chromosome 7 sequences in 10 strains showed that only 4 chromosomes over a total of 20 total homologues apparently maintained gene synteny between SfiI fragments F and G that are separated by a MRS (Joly et al., 2002). This indicated that 80% of chromosome 7 underwent recombination at the MRS between nonhomologous chromosomes, leading to translocations in these strains. This extreme chromosomal polymorphism is even more remarkable in *C. dubliniensis* since its genetic diversity, as assessed by MLST, is very limited compared to that of *C. albicans* (McManus et al., 2008). These data, together with the demonstration that length polymorphisms in bands containing tandem arrays of RPS elements are also more frequent in strains of *C. dubliniensis* passaged in vitro than in *C. albicans* strains, suggest that mitotic recombination is more frequent in *C. dubliniensis* (Joly et al., 2002). It has been proposed that the apparent excess of recombination in *C. dubliniensis* allows this species to adapt faster to new conditions but that it is deleterious in the long term as it can decrease genetic diversity by LOH. This may explain why *C. albicans* remains more pervasive (Joly et al., 2002; Sullivan et al., 2004).

Aneuploidy in *C. albicans*

While diploidy remains the common motif in *C. albicans*, strains from this species appear to possess an exceptional tolerance for aneuploidy. Both gain (Rustchenko et al., 1994; Perepnikhatka et al., 1999; Chen et al., 2004; Legrand et al., 2004; Selmecki et al., 2005, 2006; Coste et al., 2006, 2007; Legrand et al., 2008; Ramírez-Zavala et al., 2008; Diogo et al., 2009) and loss (Magee and Magee, 1997; Janbon et al., 1998; Perepnikhatka et al., 1999) of an entire chromosome and gain of a portion of a chromosome, segmental aneuploidy (Chibana et al., 2000; Legrand et al., 2004; Selmecki et al., 2005, 2006, 2008; Coste et al., 2007) that can be due to the formation of a chromosome 5 isochromosome (Selmecki et al., 2006, 2008; Coste et al., 2007), have been detected in many strains. Often, chromosome alterations can be associated with some sort of stress that can include heat shock (Hilton et al., 1985), genetic manipulations (Chen et al., 2004; Selmecki et al., 2005; Wellington and Rustchenko, 2005), growth in the presence of fluconazole (Perepnikhatka et al., 1999; Selmecki et al., 2006), or the use of carbon sources that are usually nonutilizable (Rustchenko et al., 1994; Janbon et al., 1998). Chromosome alterations may be inherent to the stress response and could play an important role in adaptation to environmental changes. The specific genes affected by chromosomal alterations that provide a selective advantage, however, are unknown.

Some chromosome alterations are associated with specific phenotypes. Chromosome 5 monosomy has, for example, been associated with the ability to grow on sorbose. The inoculation of *C. albicans* cells on medium containing sorbose often leads to the loss of one chromosome 5 before cells can grow (Rustchenko et al., 1994; Janbon et al., 1998; Andaluz et al., 2007). Chromosome 5 monosomy is associated with increased expression of *SOU1*, encoding an L-sorbose reductase located on a different chromosome (Janbon et al., 1998) that allows cells to utilize sorbose. However, the putative gene that is directly affected by this dosage effect and that regulates *SOU1* remains unknown. Trisomy of chromosome 1 in strain SC5314 has been demonstrated to impart lower virulence in a murine model of disseminated candidiasis (Chen et al., 2004). Most of these changes are transient. Strains trisomic for chromosome 1 tend to lose the extra chromosome when passaged in mice (Chen et al., 2004). Strains monosomic for chromosome 5 can grow on sorbose, but they duplicate the retained chromosome 5 homologue whenever grown in media lacking sorbose, regaining their wild-type phenotype (Janbon et al., 1998). Strains that gain fluconazole resistance by generating a chromosome 5 isochromosome can lose that isochromosome when grown on medium lacking fluconazole (Selmecki et al., 2006; also see below). It appears that at least some of these chromosome alterations associated with adaptation to new environmental conditions can later be lost when normal conditions are reestablished; this further suggests that chromosomal alterations can represent an important path for rapid adaptation but that they also can be detrimental, and selected against, during standard growth conditions. Because chromosomal alterations are more often observed in response to a stressful environment, it has not been clear if these phenomena can also play a role during commensalism and the normal life cycle of *C. albicans*. Recent work by Diogo et al. (2009) suggests that chromosome trisomy can be a relatively frequent phenomenon, at least in isolates recovered from individuals with Crohn's disease.

Fluconazole Resistance and Genome Plasticity

The development of fluconazole resistance in *C. albicans* represents a unique example in which the role of genome plasticity on gene function has been analyzed in exquisite detail and the relationship between genomic and phenotypic plasticity is best understood. Fluconazole is an azole antifungal commonly used to treat candidiasis. Azole compounds inhibit the lanosterol-14-α-demethylase encoded by *ERG11*. Inhibition of this cytochrome P450 enzyme in the ergosterol pathway leads to decreased ergosterol synthesis and growth inhibition. Fluconazole resistance is most often associated with increased expression of the ATP-binding cassette genes *CDR1* and *CDR2,* encoding efflux pumps (Akins, 2005). It is also associated with *ERG11* mutations and increased expression (Perea et al., 2001; Akins, 2005). The major facilitator efflux gene *MDR1* also plays an important role in fluconazole resistance (Akins, 2005).

Rustad et al. (2002) described an association between fluconazole resistance and homozygosity at the *MTL* locus. Among Flu^R strains, 22% were *MTL* homozygotes, compared to 2% of fluconazole-susceptible (Flu^S) strains. Resistance was soon shown not to be directly due to *MTL* homozygosity. It was proposed that this correlation indicated the presence of a gene important in Flu^R strains that was closely linked to the *MTL* locus (Pujol et al., 2003). This gene was later identified by Coste et al. (2004) as the transcription factor *TAC1* located on chromosome 5, between the *MTL* locus and the centromere, 14 kb from the *MTL*. *TAC1* is an inducer of both *CDR1* and *CDR2* (Coste et al., 2004, 2006). Some alleles of *TAC1* with different mutations can confer higher resistance to fluconazole and are termed hyperactive alleles (Coste et al., 2004, 2006, 2007). These hyperactive alleles contribute to resistance to fluconazole, but additional genomic changes are required to attain higher resistance. These include (i) homozygosis of hyperactive alleles by LOH, (ii) upregulation of *TAC1* by an increase in ploidy, and (iii) mutation of *ERG11* and increase in ploidy of that gene. Studies of the evolution of fluconazole resistance have been facilitated by the use of multiple sets of sequential isolates derived from parental Flu^S strains that progressively develop resistance upon fluconazole treatment in clinical settings.

Hyperactive *TAC1* alleles are codominant (Coste et al., 2004, 2006). Hyperactive/wild-type *TAC1* heterozygotes present a fluconazole sensitivity intermediate between those of the *TAC1* homozygotes. Codominance of alleles of genes involved in antifungal resistance is not unique to *TAC1*; it has also been reported for *ERG11* alleles for resistance to fluconazole (White, 1997; Sanglard et al., 1998) and for *FUR1* for resistance to flucytosine (Dodgson et al., 2004). A mechanism to increase resistance to fluconazole thus consists of gain-of-function mutations in *TAC1* and then homozygosis at *TAC1*. The acquisition of a hyperactive *TAC1* can be facultative, as a parental Flu^S isolate heterozygous hyperactive/wild type for *TAC1* has been reported (Coste et al., 2006). Homozygosis at *TAC1* can be generated by different mechanisms in different strains, and chromosome 5 loss and duplication, gene conversion in *TAC1*, and mitotic crossing over have each been reported for LOH at *TAC1* during acquisition of fluconazole resistance in a clinical setting (Coste et al., 2006, 2007; Selmecki et al., 2008). *TAC1* LOH is often associated with LOH at the *MTL* locus, which explains the initial association between *MTL* LOH and fluconazole resistance. Nevertheless, simultaneous LOH at both loci is not always due to a single recombination event; multiple gene conversions, which could be a consequence of increased recombination in response to fluconazole, have been noted in one case (Selmecki et al., 2008). The same event responsible for LOH at *TAC1* can also impact zygosity of *ERG11*, located approximately 250 kb from the *MTL* locus, toward the telomere (Coste et al., 2007). *ERG11* alleles can independently mutate to Flu^R alleles that can also become homozygous by the same LOH event as *TAC1* or independently (Coste et al., 2007).

Allelic mutations and LOH are sometimes not enough to attain the highest levels of fluconazole resistance. Increased gene dosage of *TAC1* and *ERG11* can play such a role. Ploidy levels of chromosome 5 or the left arm of chromosome 5 that are higher than diploid are frequently observed in Flu^R strains (Selmecki et al., 2006). Aneuploidy in Flu^R strains was seven times more frequent than in Flu^S strains (Selmecki et al., 2006). An overall increase in the number of whole-chromosome aneuploidies, as well as segmental aneuploidies, was observed over the entire genome of Flu^R strains, but chromosome 5 was most particularly affected. For chromosome 5, a total of 23 events were observed in 42 Flu^R strains compared to a single event in 28 Flu^S strains. Chromosome 5 aneuploidies were mostly due to trisomy of the entire chromosome, but a third of the cases involved segmental aneuploidy due to the presence of a chromosome 5 isochromosome. This isochromosome, i(5L), is composed of two left arms of chromosome 5, containing both *TAC1* and *ERG11*, around a chromosome 5 centromere that usually forms a new independent chromosome but can sometimes be fused at the telomere to a full-length chromosome 5 (Selmecki et al., 2006). While all strains with a i(5L) have an increased tolerance to fluconazole, a similar isochromosome formed of two right arms of chromosome 5 does not confer fluconazole resistance (Selmecki et al., 2006), suggesting a strong association between i(5L) and fluconazole resistance. In addition, i(5L) is unstable in cells grown in medium lacking fluconazole and this instability correlates with fluconazole resistance, since loss of i(5L) is associated with increased susceptibility to fluconazole (Selmecki et al., 2006; Selmecki et al., 2008). Depending upon whether a strain retained only one full-length chromosome 5 homologue or both, the presence of an isochromosome alters the ploidy of the left arm of chromosome 5 from diploidy to tri- or tetraploidy. This increase in ploidy results in increased expression of genes carried at the aneuploid region (Selmecki et al., 2006), including *TAC1* and *ERG11*. The increased copy number of both genes has been demonstrated to play an important role in fluconazole resistance, and the number of *TAC1* and/or *ERG11* gene copies positively correlates with the level of fluconazole resistance (Selmecki et al., 2008). The contribution of *TAC1* and *ERG11* to fluconazole resistance is additive. The acquisition of i(5L) has been documented in distinct series of isolates during the development of fluconazole resistance in clinical settings (Coste et al., 2007; Selmecki et al., 2008). While more frequent than strains with an i(5L), Flu^R strains with three copies of the entire chromosome 5 have not been extensively analyzed. The effect of entire chromosome 5 triploidy on fluconazole resistance should be very similar to that of strains with i(5L), since it also increases the copy numbers of *TAC1* and *ERG11*.

In conclusion, the development of resistance to fluconazole can involve mutations at *TAC1* and *ERG11*, as well as several genome plasticity events leading to LOH and aneuploidy that affect these two genes as well as additional genes on chromosome 5. Aneuploidies can be reversed in the absence of the selective pressures of fluconazole. This reversion could in part explain why resistance to fluconazole does not seem to be increasing among strains of *C. albicans*. The intensified and repeated use of fluconazole in the treatment of candidiasis and in prophylaxis against candidiasis has raised a major concern, namely, the possibility that fluconazole resistance may enrich in the global population of strains, rendering the entire species more resistant to fluconazole. While a few studies suggest that fluconazole resistance is slightly more frequent in the general *C. albicans* population (Bulik et al., 2011), a significant increase in fluconazole resistance has not been observed (Pfaller and Diekema, 2004; Ruan and Hsueh, 2009; Bulik et al., 2011). This is consistent with the hypothesis that acquisition of fluconazole resistance comes at a cost and that Flu^R strains are less competitive (i.e., are less fit) in the absence of fluconazole. The instability of i(5L) appears to be a way to reestablish higher fitness in the absence of fluconazole.

HETEROZYGOSITY AND LOSS OF HETEROZYGOSITY IN *C. ALBICANS*

The level of heterozygosity in strains of *C. albicans* is elevated. This has been demonstrated by analysis of the genome sequence of two strains (Jones et al., 2004; Butler et al., 2009) and by the observation of numerous heterozygosities in multiple strains fingerprinted by using codominant markers (reviewed by Pujol et al. [2005] and Bougnoux et al. [2007]). While analysis of heterozygosities in different *C. albicans* clades has indicated excesses of heterozygotes, demonstrating that heterozygosities are elevated and maintained in *C. albicans* strains (Bougnoux et al., 2008), LOH is relatively frequent in this species (Pujol et al., 2005; Bougnoux et al., 2007, 2008; Butler et al., 2009; Diogo et al., 2009). This represents a conundrum, as frequent LOH should lead to a clear deficit of heterozygotes, and suggests that despite frequent LOH, there is strong selective pressure to maintain heterozygosity in nature. Heterozygosity can be beneficial for several reasons, including (i) storage of genetic diversity, (ii) establishment of alleles with different functions, and (iii) heterosis or overdominance (i.e., higher fitness of a heterozygote than of either homozygote). There are no definitive data to demonstrate that any of these factors play a major role in the maintenance of heterozygosity, and there is very little work on heterozygosity in *C. albicans*. The analysis of the effect of a gene on phenotypes is commonly performed only after both alleles have been deleted and rarely on heterozygous mutant cells representing the two individual allelic deletions. There is, however, ample circumstantial evidence suggesting that heterozygosity is important. For example, it is now clear that LOH plays a major role in antifungal resistance.

Studies of the mechanisms of *MTL* homozygosis on chromosome 5 further suggest an important role for heterozygosity. *C. albicans* is diploid, and meiosis has not been observed. Hence, cells need to become homozygous at the *MTL* in order to mate. Initial studies suggested a frequency of 3 to 10% of *MTL* homozygotes in *C. albicans* populations (Lockhart et al., 2002; Legrand et al., 2004; Odds et al., 2007). A more recent study reported a frequency of 3% (Jacobsen et al., 2008a), and our unpublished analysis of 46 strains indicated a 2% frequency (C. Pujol, L. L. Hoyer, and D. R. Soll, unpublished observations). The estimates published by Legrand et al. (2004) and Odds et al. (2007) may not be as relevant, given that these authors used large collections of strains isolated over a time interval spanning 2 to 3 decades and strains appear to undergo *MTL* homozygosis during maintenance in the laboratory. In Table 1, evidence is presented strongly suggesting that increased frequencies of *MTL* homozygosis occur as strains age in a collection. The estimates by Lockhart et al. (2002), Jacobsen et al. (2008a), and our unpublished data were all obtained from strains recently isolated (isolated less than 2 years before analysis) and likely represent more accurate numbers. They indicate a frequency of 2 to 3% *MTL* homozygosis in natural populations. These numbers are very low considering that at least some strains can easily and spontaneously become homozygous in the laboratory during regular maintenance (Table 1) (Lockhart et al., 2002; Pujol et al., 2003; Wu et al., 2007). Because mating is rare in *C. albicans*, frequent loss of *MTL* heterozygosity should have led to an accumulation of *MTL*-homozygous strains in natural populations. Spontaneous loss of *MTL* heterozygosity in the laboratory is due mostly to loss of a chromosome 5 homologue followed by duplication of the retained homologue (alternatively, triploidy of chromosome 5 followed by loss of one chromosome cannot be ruled out) and is accompanied by a loss of virulence (Lockhart et al., 2005; Wu et al., 2005, 2007). This loss of virulence was initially thought to be due to an advantage conferred by *MTL* heterozygosity, a phenomenon that had previously been detected in *S. cerevisiae* (Birdsell and Wills, 1996). Further experiments suggested that this effect was also

TABLE 1 The proportion of *C. albicans MTL*-homozygous strains increases in older collections[a]

All isolates (1,293)	No. of isolates per decade isolated			
	2000s (738)	1990s (234)	1980s (95)	1970s (20)
*MTL***a**/α (1,182)	697	201	82	14
*MTL***a**/**a** (30)	11	9	5	0
*MTL*α/α (81)	30	24	8	6
MTL homozygotes (111)	41	33	13	6
% *MTL* homozygotes (8.6%)	5.5%	14.1%	13.7%	30.0%

[a]The data reported by Odds et al. (2007, Supplemental Table 1) were subdivided by decade and analyzed. *MTL* genotypes were available for 1,293 strains. Among these, the date of isolation was not available for 202 strains and 4 strains were isolated in the 1950s and 1960s. The proportion of *MTL*-homozygous strains was significantly lower among strains isolated since 2000 ($P < 10^{-2}$, Fisher's exact test) compared to strains isolated during any other decade (2000s versus 1990s, $P = 4.4 \times 10^{-5}$; 2000s versus 1980s, $P = 5 \times 10^{-3}$; 2000s versus 1970s, $P = 8.2 \times 10^{-4}$). The proportion of *MTL*-homozygous strains was highly significantly lower among strains isolated since 2000 than among strains isolated before 2000 ($P = 6 \times 10^{-7}$). The proportion of *MTL*-homozygous strains was significantly higher among strains isolated in the 1970s than among strains isolated since then ($P = 4.8 \times 10^{-3}$).

present in *C. albicans* but was not sufficient to explain the dramatic loss of virulence of spontaneous *MTL* homozygotes obtained through the loss of a chromosome 5 homologue (Wu et al., 2007). LOH affecting genes over the entire chromosome 5, including the *MTL* locus, resulted in a stronger defect; hence, LOH of genes other than *MTL* seems to play a major role. This was further supported by the analysis of a set of natural strains already *MTL* homozygous when isolated. These natural *MTL* homozygotes exhibited a level of virulence intermediate between that of natural *MTL***a**/α strains and that of spontaneous *MTL*-homozygous strains (Wu et al., 2007). Interestingly, none of the 10 natural *MTL* homozygotes had lost an entire chromosome 5 homologue and LOH at the *MTL* locus was associated with limited LOH around that locus, probably due to multiple mitotic recombinations or gene conversions (Wu et al., 2007). Spontaneous loss of an entire chromosome 5 in nature may be as frequent as that observed under laboratory conditions, but such strains may more rapidly become extinct. These results suggest that LOH over an entire chromosome 5 or large segments of that chromosome are selected against in nature. The selective pressure may act upon alleles with different relevant functions, deleterious alleles, heterosis, or overdominance or a combination of all or some of these.

The present evidence in *C. albicans* does not demonstrate that some loci may have evolved alleles with distinct functions, but, again, circumstantial evidence suggests that this may be the case at least for a few loci. We mention above the case of *ALS9* and the two very distinct alleles found at this locus in most strains (Zhao et al., 2003, 2007). One of the two alleles plays a role in adhesion to endothelial cells, while the second allele does not (Zhao et al., 2007). If the second allele has a different function, which seems likely, given that it is conserved in most strains, that function is unknown. Another candidate gene that may have evolved distinct alleles for different functions is *ALS3*, an additional member of the ALS gene family (Oh et al., 2005). ALS genes contain a region with different numbers of a 108-bp tandem repeat sequence within the central domain of the coding region (Hoyer, 2001). The number of tandem repeat sequences plays an important role in adhesion (Oh et al., 2005; Rauceo et al., 2006). In particular, alleles of *ALS3* containing 9 or 12 tandem repeats showed distinct adhesion properties (Oh et al., 2005). Characterization of the number of tandem repeats in alleles of a collection of 51 *C. albicans* isolates showed a bimodal distribution of the number of copies (Oh et al., 2005). This bimodal distribution observed over the global collection was also observed in each clade separately and was reflected in the genetic makeup of individual strains. Strains tended to be heterozygous for the number of tandem repeats and to carry a "long" allele besides a "short" one (Oh et al., 2005). "Long/short" *ALS3* heterozygotes were in significant excess, suggesting that "long" and "short" versions of *ALS3* may be conserved in parallel in most strains for distinct allelic functions. An analysis of *CDR2* zygosity has resulted in the same hypothesis (Holmes et al., 2006). Two types of alleles were identified, an A-type and a B-type. The B-type allele confers higher resistance to fluconazole than does the A-type. An analysis of a set of 69 strains indicated that the frequency of the two types of allele was similar but that A/B heterozygotes were in significant excess (81%), again suggesting that the two types of alleles have distinct primary functions (Holmes et al., 2006).

For other genes, while the function of the two alleles has not been reported to differ, regulation of each of the two alleles can diverge due to allelic differences in their promoter region. This has been reported for *CSH7* (Sanz et al., 2007) and *SAP2* (Staib et al., 2002). Allelism at *SAP2* is particularly interesting. Strain SC5314 has two alleles that differ in their promoter region. Both genes encode functional secreted proteinases, but the in vitro expression of *SAP2-1* is dependent on *SAP2-2* whereas that of *SAP2-2* does not depend on *SAP2-1* (Staib et al., 2002). In addition, in a mouse model of disseminated candidiasis, the *SAP2-2* allele was expressed first while the *SAP2-1* allele was activated only during the late stages of the infection (Staib et al., 2002). The differential regulation of these two alleles in vivo may be relevant to the virulence process.

Together, these observations support the idea that conservation of heterozygosity in *C. albicans* is advantageous and has a major impact on virulence. Population-based studies of haplotypes, however, suggest that LOH in *C. albicans* is relatively frequent (Bougnoux et al., 2008). In addition, LOH has been repeatedly detected between genetically related strains isolated from the same or related individuals, a phenomenon that is sometimes referred to as microevolution (Pujol et al., 2005; Bougnoux et al., 2007). These reports support the notion that LOH is relatively frequent in *C. albicans*. Recently, Diogo et al. (2009) characterized such LOH in five chromosomes from three sets of related isolates of commensal origin from the gastrointestinal tract of individuals with Crohn's disease. SNP analysis indicated that LOH occurred by the complete loss of one chromosome 6 homologue, mitotic crossover in three distinct chromosomes, and multiple short gene conversions in chromosome 1. High-resolution analysis of the boundary regions of recombination showed that recombination often occurred at or near LTR-retrotransposon sequences or close to tRNA genes (Diogo et al., 2009). One recombination occurred at an MRS locus. Due to the small sample size, this study does not definitely identify the preferred mechanism of recombination, but it does suggest that LOH over large DNA regions extending up to the telomere may be frequent and primarily due to mitotic crossing over. The sizes of LOH regions observed in this study are surprising. If they were the rule, it would suggest a progressive overall LOH in the long term, which does challenge the hypothesis that LOH over short DNA tracts is favored in order to maintain overall heterozygosity (Bougnoux et al., 2008). The strains analyzed in the Diogo et al. (2009) study were isolated from the digestive tract of individuals with Crohn's disease (Van Kruiningen et al., 2005; Bougnoux et al., 2006), a form of inflammatory bowel disease which involves chronic inflammation of the gastrointestinal tract. Thus, these strains can hardly be interpreted as being representative of the general commensal population, and a similar analysis performed on strains from healthy individuals with a larger sample size is warranted to clarify this question.

We propose the following hypothesis to reconcile frequent LOH and the general conservation of heterozygosity in *C. albicans*. LOH, and possibly other forms of chromosomal recombination, may represent a form of continuous experimentation. LOH is frequent and may be ongoing as a way of constantly generating new genetic combinations. Some of the descendants of any strain carry new LOHs. Most LOHs are deleterious as they affect gene combinations already adapted to the normal environment, and strains carrying those deleterious LOHs become extinct at a higher frequency than strains without LOHs. A few LOHs are neutral and are maintained in the population of offspring. These LOHs will likely be restrained to short DNA tracts and will have no effect. When conditions change, such as by the addition of an antifungal, the selective pressure can be altered and a LOH that would have been selected against under normal conditions would be favored.

GENOME PLASTICITY AND LABORATORY STRAINS

Genomic plasticity occurs in vivo and in vitro. It also occurs in laboratory strains, and aneuploidies have been reported during genetic manipulation as a consequence of DNA transformation or the use of 5-fluoroorotic acid (5-FOA), which is used to select for *ura3* cells (Chen et al., 2004; Selmecki et al., 2005; Wellington and Rustchenko, 2005). Due to diploidy, gene disruption in *C. albicans* involves two rounds of transformation and counterselection of the transformation marker. For more than a decade, the strategy of choice in *C. albicans* has been the "Ura-blaster" cassette (Fonzi and Irwin, 1993), which requires the use of 5-FOA for the counterselection step. In addition, spontaneous aneuploidy has been noted in strains maintained in the laboratory, such as trisomy in the *MTL*-homozygous strain WO-1, which affected *WOR1* function and the frequency of white-opaque switching (Ramírez-Zavala et al., 2008).

Genome plasticity in laboratory strains may be more consequential and less obvious than such gross chromosomal alterations. For example, the analysis of the number of repeats in *ALS3* genes (Oh et al., 2005) showed that laboratory type strains presented some atypical combinations. Three laboratory strains that have been commonly used for decades, 3153A, WO-1, and SC5314, were included in the analysis. SC5314 had one allele with 9 tandem repeats and one allele with 12 tandem repeats, and hence a 9/12 genotype. Two isolates of 3153A were found to be 9/12 and 10/13. Two isolates of WO-1 were found to be 9/12 and 9/9. Both alleles 9 and 12 were very rare in the general population. Only 11.5% and 7.3% of 191 recently isolated strains presented an allele 9 or 12, respectively, and none of these strains had both alleles simultaneously (Oh et al., 2005). Each of these alleles was significantly overrepresented in laboratory strains (Fisher's exact test; $P < 10^{-2}$). This, and the observation of different genotypes in two isolates each from 3153A and WO-1, suggests that the rare alleles 9 and 12 represent alterations of the original wild-type alleles under laboratory conditions. The number of tandem repeats is known to affect adherence (Oh et al., 2005; Rauceo et al., 2006). These two alleles are not favored in nature and are probably selected against in the host.

A last example of genomic alterations that has been noted to occur spontaneously in the laboratory is *MTL* LOH, which was discussed earlier in this chapter. All of these changes can affect gene function, and they likely do not represent the entire range of laboratory-acquired genomic plasticity. The use of laboratory strains is attractive because they represent extremely well characterized systems and in some cases have been genetically engineered for the generation of mutants, but how relevant these "benchmarks" are for understanding commensalism and the infectious process is in question. Laboratory strains should therefore be employed with extreme caution. The use of recently isolated strains may be more relevant, but even then, cells should be stored properly to avoid genomic changes. In this respect, the use of frozen stocks seems to be the best way to limit future genomic alterations.

CONCLUSIONS

C. albicans is capable of undergoing an array of genomic alterations, some of which can affect gene function. This genomic plasticity can often create deleterious outcomes, but it can also represent a crucial advantage under new selective pressures, such as adaptation to antifungals. Our understanding of the role and impact of genomic plasticity in commensal and infectious processes in the absence of antifungals is still limited. For example, we do not know if genomic plasticity increases during infection compared to commensalism. The new technologies developed for genomic analysis should greatly improve our future understanding of the complexity and role of genomic plasticity in *C. albicans*.

REFERENCES

Aanen, D. K., and R. F. Hoekstra. 2007. Why sex is good: on fungi and beyond, p. 527–534. *In* J. Heitman, J. W. Kronstad, J. W. Taylor, and L. A. Casselton (ed.), *Sex in Fungi: Molecular Determination and Evolutionary Implications.* ASM Press, Washington, DC.

Akins, R. A. 2005. An update on antifungal targets and mechanisms of resistance in *Candida albicans. Med. Mycol.* **43:**285–318.

Andaluz, E., J. Gómez-Raja, B. Hermosa, T. Ciudad, E. Rustchenko, R. Calderone, and G. Larriba. 2007. Loss and fragmentation of chromosome 5 are major events linked to the adaptation of *rad52*-ΔΔ strains of *Candida albicans* to sorbose. *Fungal Genet. Biol.* **44:**789–798.

Anderson, J. B., C. Wickens, M. Khan, L. E. Cowen, N. Federspiel, T. Jones, and L. M. Kohn. 2001. Infrequent genetic exchange and recombination in the mitochondrial genome of *Candida albicans. J. Bacteriol.* **183:**865–872.

Asakura, K., S. Iwaguchi, M. Homma, T. Sukai, K. Higashide, and K. Tanaka. 1991. Electrophoretic karyotypes of clinically isolated yeasts of *Candida albicans* and *C. glabrata. J. Gen. Microbiol.* **137:**2531–2538.

Barton, R. C., and S. Scherer. 1994. Induced chromosome rearrangements and morphologic variation in *Candida albicans. J. Bacteriol.* **176:**756–763.

Barton, R. C., A. van Belkum, and S. Scherer. 1995. Stability of karyotype in serial isolates of *Candida albicans* from neutropenic patients. *J. Clin. Microbiol.* **33:**794–796.

Bennett, R. J., and A. D. Johnson. 2003. Completion of a parasexual cycle in *Candida albicans* by induced chromosome loss in tetraploid strains. *EMBO J.* **22:**2505–2515.

Bennett, R. J., M. A. Uhl, M. G. Miller, and A. D. Johnson. 2003. Identification and characterization of a *Candida albicans* mating pheromone. *Mol. Cell. Biol.* **23;**8189–8201.

Birdsell, J., and C. Wills. 1996. Significant competitive advantage conferred by meiosis and syngamy in the yeast *Saccharomyces cerevisiae. Proc. Natl. Acad. Sci. USA* **93:**908–912.

Blignaut, E., C. Pujol, S. Lockhart, S. Joly, and D. R. Soll. 2002. Ca3 fingerprinting of *Candida albicans* isolates from human immunodeficiency virus-positive and healthy individuals reveals a new clade in South Africa. *J. Clin. Microbiol.* **40:**826–836.

Bougnoux, M.-E., C. Pujol, D. Diogo, C. Bouchier, D. R. Soll, and C. d'Enfert. 2008. Mating is rare within as well as between clades of the human pathogen *Candida albicans. Fungal Genet. Biol.* **45:**221–231.

Bougnoux, M.-E., D. Diogo, C. Pujol, D. R. Soll, and C. d'Enfert. 2007. Molecular epidemiology and population dynamics in *Candida albicans*, p. 51–70. *In* C. d'Enfert and B. Hube (ed.), *Candida: Comparative and Functional Genomics.* Caister Academic Press, Norwich, United Kingdom.

Bougnoux, M.-E., D. Diogo, N. François, B. Sendid, S. Veirmeire, J. F. Colombel, C. Bouchier, H. Van Kruiningen, C. d'Enfert, and D. Poulain. 2006. Multilocus sequence typing reveals intrafamilial transmission and microevolutions of *Candida albicans* isolates from the human digestive tract. *J. Clin. Microbiol.* **44:**1810–1820.

Bulik, C. C., J. D. Sobel, and M. D. Nailor. 2011. Susceptibility profile of vaginal isolates of *Candida albicans* prior to and following fluconazole introduction—impact of two decades. *Mycoses* **54:** 34–38.

Butler, G., M. D. Rasmussen, M. F. Lin, M. A. Santos, S. Sakthikumar, C. A. Munro, E. Rheinbay, M. Grabherr, A. Forche, J. L. Reedy, I. Agrafioti, M. B. Arnaud, S. Bates, A. J. Brown, S. Brunke, M. C. Costanzo, D. A. Fitzpatrick, P. W. de Groot, D. Harris, L. L. Hoyer, B. Hube, F. M. Klis, C. Kodira, N. Lennard, M. E. Logue, R. Martin, A. M. Neiman, E. Nikolaou, M. A. Quail, J. Quinn, M. C. Santos, F. F. Schmitzberger, G. Sherlock, P. Shah, K. A. Silverstein, M. S. Skrzypek, D. Soll, R. Staggs, I. Stansfield, M. P. Stumpf, P. E. Sudbery, T. Srikantha, Q. Zeng, J. Berman, M. Berriman, J. Heitman, N. A. Gow, M. C. Lorenz, B. W. Birren, M. Kellis, and C. A. Cuomo. 2009. Evolution of pathogenicity and sexual reproduction in eight *Candida* genomes. *Nature* **459:**657–662.

Chen, X., B. B. Magee, D. Dawson, P. T. Magee, and C. A. Kumamoto. 2004. Chromosome 1 trisomy compromises the virulence of *Candida albicans. Mol. Microbiol.* **51:**551–565.

Chibana, H., and P. T. Magee. 2009. The enigma of the major repeat sequence of *Candida albicans. Future Microbiol.* **4:**171–179.

Chibana, H., J. L. Beckerman, and P. T. Magee. 2000. Fine-resolution physical mapping of genomic diversity in *Candida albicans*. *Genome Res.* **10:**1865–1877.

Chindamporn, A., Y. Nakagawa, I. Mizuguchi, H. Chibana, M. Doi, and K. Tanaka. 1998. Repetitive sequences (RPS) in the chromosomes of *Candida albicans* are sandwiched between two novel stretches, HOK and RB2, common to each chromosome. *Microbiology* **144:**849–857.

Chu, W. S., B. B. Magee, P. T. Magee. 1993. Construction of an *Sfi*I macrorestriction map of the *Candida albicans* genome. *J. Bacteriol.* **175:**6637–6651.

Ciudad, T., E. Andaluz, O. Steinberg-Neifach, N. Lue, N. Gow, R. Calderone, and G. Larriba. 2004. Homologous recombination in *Candida albicans*: role of CaRad52p in DNA repair, integration of linear DNA fragments and telomere length. *Mol. Microbiol.* **53:**1177–1194.

Coste, A., A. Selmecki, A. Forche, D. Diogo, M.-E. Bougnoux, C. d'Enfert, J. Berman, and D. Sanglard. 2007. Genotypic evolution of azole resistance mechanisms in sequential *Candida albicans* isolates. *Eukaryot. Cell* **6:**1889–1904.

Coste, A. T., M. Karababa, F. Ischer, J. Bille, and D. Sanglard. 2004. *TAC1*, transcriptional activator of *CDR* genes, is a new transcription factor involved in the regulation of *Candida albicans* ABC transporters *CDR1* and *CDR2*. *Eukaryot. Cell* **3:**1639–1652.

Coste, A., V. Turner, F. Ischer, J. Morschhäuser, A. Forche, A. Selmecki, J. Berman, J. Bille, and D. Sanglard. 2006. A mutation in Tac1p, a transcription factor regulating CDR1 and CDR2, is coupled with loss of heterozygosity at Chromosome 5 to mediate antifungal resistance in *Candida albicans*. *Genetics* **172:**2139–2156.

Cowen, L. E., C. Sirjusingh, R. C. Summerbell, S. Walmsley, S. Richardson, L. M. Kohn, and J. B. Anderson. 1999. Multilocus genotypes and DNA fingerprints do not predict variation in azole resistance among clinical isolates of *Candida albicans*. *Antimicrob. Agents Chemother.* **43:**2930–2938.

Daniels, K. J., T. Srikantha, S. R. Lockhart, C. Pujol, and D. R. Soll. 2006. Opaque cells signal white cells to form biofilms in *Candida albicans*. *EMBO J.* **25:**2240–2252.

Dignard, D., A. L. El-Naggar, M. E. Logue, G. Butler, and M. Whiteway. 2007. Identification and characterization of *MFA1*, the gene encoding *Candida albicans* a-factor pheromone. *Eukaryot. Cell* **6:**487–494.

Diogo, D., C. Bouchier, C. d'Enfert, and M.-E. Bougnoux. 2009. Loss of heterozygosity in commensal isolates of the asexual diploid yeast *Candida albicans*. *Fungal Genet. Biol.* **46:**159–168.

Dodgson, A. R., K. J. Dodgson, C. Pujol, M. A. Pfaller, and D. R. Soll. 2004. Clade-specific flucytosine resistance is due to a single nucleotide change in the *FUR1* gene of *Candida albicans*. *Antimicrob. Agents Chemother.* **48:**2223–2227.

Doi, M., M. Homma, A. Chindamporn, and K. Tanaka. 1992. Estimation of chromosome number and size by pulsed-field gel electrophoresis (PFGE) in medically important *Candida* species. *J. Gen. Microbiol.* **138:**2241–2251.

Doi, M., M. Homma, S. I. Iwaguchi, K. Horibe, and K. Tanaka. 1994. Strain relatedness of *Candida albicans* strains isolated from children with leukemia and their bedside parent. *J. Clin. Microbiol.* **32:**2253–2259.

Dumitru, R., D. H. M. L. P. Navarathna, C. P. Semighini, C. G. Elowsky, R. V. Dumitru, D. Dignard, M. Whiteway, A. L. Atkin, and K. W. Nickerson. 2007. In vivo and in vitro anaerobic mating in *Candida albicans*. *Eukaryot. Cell* **6:**465–472.

Fischer, G., E. P. C. Rocha, F. Brunet, M. Vergassola, and B. Dujon. 2006. Highly variable rates of genome rearrangements between hemiascomycetous yeast lineages. *PLoS Genet.* **2:**e32.

Fonzi, W. A., and M. Y. Irwin. 1993. Isogenic strain construction and gene mapping in *Candida albicans*. *Genetics* **134:**717–728.

Forche, A., K. Alby, D. Schaefer, A. D. Johnson, J. Berman, and R. J. Bennett. 2008. The parasexual cycle in *Candida albicans* provides an alternative pathway to meiosis for the formation of recombinant strains. *PLoS Biol.* **6:**e110.

Forche, A., G. Schönian, Y. Gräser, R. Vilgalys, and T. G. Mitchell. 1999. Genetic structure of typical and atypical populations of *Candida albicans* from Africa. *Fungal Genet. Biol.* **28:**107–125.

Gee, S. G., S. Joly, D. R. Soll, J. F. G. M. Meis, P. E. Verweij, I. Polacheck, D. J. Sullivan, and D. C. Coleman. 2002. Identification of four distinct genotypes of *Candida dubliniensis* and detection of microevolution in vitro and in vivo. *J. Clin. Microbiol.* **40:**556–574.

Goddard, M. R. 2007. Why bother with sex? Answers from experiments with yeast and other organisms, p. 489–506. *In* J. Heitman, J. W. Kronstad, J. W. Taylor, and L. A. Casselton (ed.), *Sex in Fungi: Molecular Determination and Evolutionary Implications.* ASM Press, Washington, DC.

Goodwin, T. J. D., and R. T. M. Poulter. 2000. Multiple LTR-retrotransposon families in the asexual yeast *Candida albicans*. *Genome Res.* **10:**174–191.

Goodwin, T. J. D., J. E. Ormandy, and R. T. M. Poulter. 2001. L1-like non-LTR retrotransposons in the yeast *Candida albicans*. *Curr. Genet.* **39:**83–91.

Goodwin, T. J. D., J. N. Busby, and R. T. M. Poulter. 2007. A yeast model for target-primed (non-LTR) retrotransposition. *BMC Genomics* **8:**e263.

Gräser, Y., M. Volovsek, J. Arrington, G. Schönian, W. Presber, T. G. Mitchell, and R. Vilgalys. 1996. Molecular markers reveal that population structure of the human pathogen *Candida albicans* exhibits both clonality and recombination. *Proc. Natl. Acad. Sci. USA* **93:**12473–12477.

Hilton, C., D. Markie, B. Corner, E. Rikkerink, and R. Poulter. 1985. Heat shock induces chromosome loss in the yeast *Candida albicans. Mol. Gen. Genet.* **200:**162–168.

Holmes, A. R., S. Tsao, S.-W. Ong, E. Lamping, K. Niimi, B. C. Monk, M. Niimi, A. Kaneko, B. R. Holland, J. Schmid, and R. D. Cannon. 2006. Heterozygosity and functional allelic variation in the *Candida albicans* efflux pump genes *CDR1* and *CDR2. Mol. Microbiol.* **62:**170–186.

Hoyer, L. L. 2001. The ALS gene family of *Candida albicans. Trends Microbiol.* **9:**176–180.

Huang, G., H. Wang, S. Chou, X. Nie, J. Chen, and H. Liu. 2006. Bistable expression of *WOR1*, a master regulator of white–opaque switching in *Candida albicans. Proc. Natl. Acad. Sci. USA* **103:**12813–12818.

Huang, G., T. Srikantha, N. Sahni, S. Yi, and D. R. Soll. 2009. CO_2 regulates white-to-opaque switching in *Candida albicans. Curr. Biol.* **19:**330–334.

Hull, C. M., and A. D. Johnson. 1999. Identifcation of a mating type-like locus in the asexual pathogenic yeast *Candida albicans. Science* **285:**1271–1275.

Hull, C. M., R. M. Raisner, and A. D. Johnson. 2000. Evidence for mating of the "asexual" yeast *Candida albicans* in a mammalian host. *Science* **289:**307–310.

Ibrahim, A. S., B. B. Magee, D. C. Sheppard, M. Yang, S. Kauffman, J. Becker, J. E. Edwards, Jr., and P. T. Magee. 2005. Effects of ploidy and mating type on virulence of *Candida albicans. Infect. Immun.* **73:**7366–7374.

Iwaguchi, S.-I., M. Sato, B. B. Magee, P. T. Magee, K. Makimura, and T Suzuki. 2001. Extensive chromosome translocation in a clinical isolate showing the distinctive carbohydrate assimilation profile from a candidiasis patient. *Yeast* **18:**1035–1046.

Iwaguchi, S., M. Homma, and K. Tanaka. 1990. Variation in the electrophoretic karyotype analysed by the assignment of DNA probes in *Candida albicans. J. Gen. Microbiol.* **136:**2433–2442.

Iwaguchi, S., M. Homma, and K. Tanaka. 1992. Clonal variation of chromosome size derived from the rDNA cluster region in *Candida albicans. J. Gen. Microbiol.* **138:**1177–1184.

Iwaguchi, S., M. Suzuki, N. Sakai, Y. Nakagawa, P. T. Magee, and T. Suzuki. 2004. Chromosome translocation induced by the insertion of the URA blaster into the major repeat sequence (MRS) in *Candida albicans. Yeast* **21:**619–634.

Jacobsen, M. D., A. D Duncan, J. Bain, E. M. Johnson, J. R. Naglik, D. J. Shaw, N. A. R. Gow, and F. C. Odds. 2008a. Mixed *Candida albicans* strain populations in colonized and infected mucosal tissues. *FEMS Yeast Res.* **8:**1334–1338.

Jacobsen, M. D., A. M. J. Rattray, N. A. Gow, F. C. Odds, and D. J. Shaw. 2008b. Mitochondrial haplotypes and recombination in *Candida albicans. Med. Mycol.* **46:**647–654.

Janbon, G., F. Sherman, and E. Rustchenko. 1998. Monosomy of a specific chromosome determines L-sorbose utilization: a novel regulatory mechanism in *Candida albicans. Proc. Natl. Acad. Sci. USA* **95:**5150–5155.

Joly, S., C. Pujol, and D. R. Soll. 2002. Microevolutionary changes and chromosomal translocations are more frequent at RPS loci in *Candida dubliniensis* than in *Candida albicans. Infect. Genet. Evol.* **2:**19–37.

Joly, S., C. Pujol, M. Rysz, K. Vargas, and D. R. Soll. 1999. Development and characterization of complex DNA fingerprinting probes for the infectious yeast *Candida dubliniensis. J. Clin. Microbiol.* **37:**1035–1044.

Jones, T., N. A. Federspiel, H. Chibana, J. Dungan, S. Kalman, B. B. Magee, G. Newport, Y. R. Thorstenson, N. Agabian, P. T. Magee, R. W. Davis, and S. Scherer. 2004. The diploid genome sequence of *Candida albicans. Proc. Natl. Acad. Sci. USA* **101:**7329–7334.

Kanbe, T., T. Arishima, T Horii, and A. Kibuchi. 2003. Improvement of PCR-based identification targeting the DNA topoisomerase II gene to determine major species of the opportunistic fungi *Candida* and *Aspergillus fumigatus. Microbiol. Immunol.* **47:**631–638.

Kvaal, C. A., T. Srikantha, and D. R. Soll. 1997. Misexpression of the white-phase-specific gene *WH11* in the opaque phase of *Candida albicans* affects switching and virulence. *Infect. Immun.* **65:**4468–4475.

Kvaal, C., S. A. Lachke, T. Srikantha, K. Daniels, J. McCoy, and D. R. Soll. 1999. Misexpression of the opaque-phase-specific gene *PEP1* (*SAP1*) in the white phase of *Candida albicans* confers increased virulence in a mouse model of cutaneous infection. *Infect. Immun.* **67:**6652–6662.

Lasker, B. A., G. F. Carle, G. S. Kobayashi, and G. Medoff. 1989. Comparison of the separation of *Candida albicans* chromosome-sized DNA by pulsed-field gel electrophoresis techniques. *Nucleic Acids Res.* **17:**3783–3793.

Legrand, M., A. Forche, A. Selmecki, C. Chan, D. T. Kirkpatrick, and J. Berman. 2008. Haplotype mapping of a diploid non-meiotic organism using existing and induced aneuploidies. *PLoS Genet.* **4**:e1.

Legrand, M., P. Lephart, A. Forche, F.-M. C. Mueller, T. Walsh, P. T. Magee, and B. B. Magee. 2004. Homozygosity at the *MTL* locus in clinical strains of *Candida albicans*: karyotypic rearrangements and tetraploid formation. *Mol. Microbiol.* **52**:1451–1462.

Lephart, P. R., and P. T. Magee. 2006. Effect of the major repeat sequence on mitotic recombination in *Candida albicans. Genetics* **174**:1737–1744.

Lephart, P. R., H. Chibana, and P. T. Magee. 2005. Effect of the major repeat sequence on chromosome loss in *Candida albicans. Eukaryot. Cell* **4**:733–741.

Lockhart, S. R., B. Reed, and D. R. Soll. 1996. Most frequent scenario for recurrent *Candida* vaginitis is strain maintenance with "substrain shuffling": demonstration by sequential DNA fingerprinting with probes Ca3, C1, and CARE2. *J. Clin. Microbiol.* **34**:767–777.

Lockhart, S. R., C. Pujol, K. J. Daniels, M. G. Miller, A. D. Johnson, M. A. Pfaller, and D. R. Soll. 2002. In *Candida albicans*, white-opaque switchers are homozygous for mating type. *Genetics* **162**:737–745.

Lockhart, S. R., J. J. Fritch, A. S. Meier, K. Schröppel, T. Srikantha, R. Galask, and D. R. Soll. 1995. Colonizing populations of *Candida albicans* are clonal in origin but undergo microevolution through C1 fragment reorganization as demonstrated by DNA fingerprinting and C1 sequencing. *J. Clin. Microbiol.* **33**:1501–1509.

Lockhart, S. R., K. J. Daniels, R. Zhao, D. Wessels, and D. R. Soll. 2003a. Cell biology of mating in *Candida albicans. Eukaryot. Cell* **2**:49–61.

Lockhart, S. R., R. Zhao, K. J. Daniels, and D. R. Soll. 2003b. α-pheromone-induced "shmooing" and gene regulation require white-opaque switching during *Candida albicans* mating. *Eukaryot. Cell* **2**:847–855.

Lockhart, S. R., W. Wu, J. B. Radke, R. Zhao, and D. R. Soll. 2005. Increased virulence and competitive advantage of a/α over a/a or α/α offspring conserves the mating system of *Candida albicans. Genetics* **169**:1883–1890.

Lott, T. J., R. E. Fundyga, R. J. Kuykendall, and J. Arnold. 2005. The human commensal yeast, *Candida albicans*, has an ancient origin. *Fungal Genet. Biol.* **42**:444–451.

Magee, B. B., and P. T. Magee. 1987. Electrophoretic karyotypes and chromosome numbers in *Candida* species. *J. Gen. Microbiol.* **133**:425–430.

Magee, B. B., and P. T. Magee. 1997. WO-2, a stable aneuploid derivative of *Candida albicans* strain WO-1, can switch from white to opaque and form hyphae. *Microbiology* **143**:289–295.

Magee, B. B., M. D. Sanchez, D. Saunders, D. Harris, M. Berriman, and P. T. Magee. 2008. Extensive chromosome rearrangements distinguish the karyotype of the hypovirulent species *Candida dubliniensis* from the virulent *Candida albicans. Fungal Genet. Biol.* **45**:338–350.

McManus, B. A., D. C. Coleman, G. Moran, E. Pinjon, D. Diogo, M.-E. Bougnoux, S. Borecká-Melkusova, H. Bujdákova, P. Murphy, C. d'Enfert, and D. J. Sullivan. 2008. Multilocus sequence typing reveals that the population structure of *Candida dubliniensis* is significantly less divergent than that of *Candida albicans. J. Clin. Microbiol.* **46**:652–664.

Miller, M. G., and A. D. Johnson. 2002. White-opaque switching in *Candida albicans* is controlled by mating-type locus homeodomain proteins and allows efficient mating. *Cell* **110**:293–302.

Mishra, P. K., M. Baum, and J. Carbon. 2007. Centromere size and position in *Candida albicans* are evolutionarily conserved independent of DNA sequence heterogeneity. *Mol. Genet. Genomics* **278**:455–465.

Navarro-Garcia, F., R. M. Pérez-Diaz, B. B. Magee, J. Pla, C. Nombela, and P. Magee. 1995. Chromosome reorganization in *Candida albicans* 1001 strain. *J. Med. Vet. Mycol.* **33**:361–366.

Odds, F. C., M.-E. Bougnoux, D. J. Shaw, J. M. Bain, A. D. Davidson, D. Diogo, M. D. Jacobsen, M. Lecomte, S.-Y. Li, A. Tavanti, M. C. J. Maiden, N. A. R. Gow, and C. d'Enfert. 2007. Molecular phylogenetics of *Candida albicans. Eukaryot. Cell* **6**:1041–1052.

Oh, S.-H., G. Cheng, J. A. Nuessen, R. Jajko, K. M. Yeater, X. Zhao, C. Pujol, D. R. Soll, and L. L. Hoyer. 2005. Functional specificity of *Candida albicans* Als3p proteins and clade specificity of *ALS3* alleles discriminated by the number of copies of the tandem repeat sequence in the central domain. *Microbiology* **151**:673–681.

Olaiya, A. F., and S. J. Sogin. 1979. Ploidy determination of *Candida albicans. J. Bacteriol.* **140**:1043–1049.

Perea, S., J. L. López-Ribot, W. R. Kirkpatrick, R. K. McAtee, R. A. Santillán, M. Martínez, D. Calabrese, D. Sanglard, and T. F. Patterson. 2001. Prevalence of molecular mechanisms of resistance to azole antifungal agents in *Candida albicans* strains displaying high-level fluconazole resistance isolated from human immunodeficiency virus-infected patients. *Antimicrob. Agents Chemother.* **45**:2676–2684.

Perepnikhatka, V., F. J. Fischer, M. Niimi, R. A. Baker, R. D. Cannon, Y.-K. Wang, F. Sherman, and E. Rustchenko. 1999. Specific chromosome alterations in fluconazole-resistant mutants of *Candida albicans. J. Bacteriol.* **181**:4041–4049.

Pfaller, M. A., and D. J. Diekema. 2004. Twelve years of fluconazole in clinical practice: global trends in species distribution and fluconazole susceptibility of bloodstream isolates of *Candida*. *Clin. Microbiol. Infect.* **10**(Suppl. 1)**:**11–23.

Pujol, C., A. Dodgson, and D. R. Soll. 2005. Population genetics of ascomycetes pathogenic to humans and animals, p. 149–188. *In* J. Xu (ed.), *Evolutionary Genetics of Fungi*. Horizon Scientific Press, Norwich, United Kingdom.

Pujol, C., J. Reynes, F. Renaud, M. Raymond, M. Tibayrenc, F. J. Ayala, F. Janbon, M. Mallié, and J.-M. Bastide. 1993. The yeast *Candida albicans* has a clonal mode of reproduction in a population of infected human immunodeficiency virus-positive patients. *Proc. Natl. Acad. Sci. USA* **90:**9456–9459.

Pujol, C., M. Pfaller, and D. R. Soll. 2002. Ca3 fingerprinting of *Candida albicans* bloodstream isolates from the United States, Canada, South America, and Europe reveals a European clade. *J. Clin. Microbiol.* **40:**2729–2740.

Pujol, C., S. A. Messer, M. Pfaller, and D. R. Soll. 2003. Drug resistance is not directly affected by mating type locus zygosity in *Candida albicans*. *Antimicrob. Agents Chemother.* **47:**1207–1212.

Pujol, C., S. Joly, B. Nolan, T. Srikantha, and D. R. Soll. 1999. Microevolutionary changes in *Candida albicans* identified by the complex Ca3 fingerprinting probe involve insertions and deletions of the full-length repetitive sequence RPS at specific genomic sites. *Microbiology* **145:**2635–2646.

Pujol, C., S. Joly, S. R. Lockhart, S. Noel, M. Tibayrenc, and D. R. Soll. 1997. Parity among the randomly amplified polymorphic DNA method, multilocus enzyme electrophoresis, and Southern blot hybridization with the moderately repetitive DNA probe Ca3 for fingerprinting *Candida albicans*. *J. Clin. Microbiol.* **35:**2348–2358.

Ramírez-Zavala, B., O. Reuß, Y.-N. Park, K. Ohlsen, and J. Morschhäuser. 2008. Environmental induction of white-opaque switching in *Candida albicans*. *PLoS Pathog.* **4:**e1000089.

Ramsey, H., B. Morrow, and D. R. Soll. 1994. An increase in switching frequency correlates with an increase in recombination of the ribosomal chromosomes of *Candida albicans* strain 3153A. *Microbiology* **140:**1525–1531.

Rauceo, J. M., R. De Armond, H. Otoo, P. C. Kahn, S. A. Klotz, N. K. Gaur, and P. N. Lipke. 2006. Threonine-rich repeats increase fibronectin binding in the *Candida albicans* adhesin Als5p. *Eukaryot. Cell* **5:**1664–1673.

Reedy, J. L., A. M. Floyd, and J. Heitman. 2009. Mechanistic plasticity of sexual reproduction and meiosis in the *Candida* pathogenic species complex. *Curr. Biol.* **19:**891–899.

Robles, J. C., L. Koreen, S. Park, and D. S. Perlin. 2004. Multilocus sequence typing is a reliable alternative method to DNA fingerprinting for discriminating among strains of *Candida albicans*. *J. Clin. Microbiol.* **42:**2480–2488.

Ruan, S.-Y., and P.-R. Hsueh. 2009. Invasive candidiasis: an overview from Taiwan. *J. Formos. Med. Assoc.* **108:**443–451.

Rustad, T. R., D. A. Stevens, M. A. Pfaller and T. C. White. 2002. Homozygosity at the *Candida albicans MTL* locus associated with azole resistance. *Microbiology* **148:**1061–1072.

Rustchenko, E. P., D. H. Howard, and F. Sherman. 1994. Chromosomal alterations of *Candida albicans* are associated with the gain and loss of assimilating functions. *J. Bacteriol.* **176:**3231–3241.

Rustchenko, E. P., T. M. Curran, and F. Sherman. 1993. Variations in the number of ribosomal DNA units in morphological mutants and normal strains of *Candida albicans* and in normal strains of *Saccharomyces cerevisiae*. *J. Bacteriol.* **175:**7189–7199.

Rustchenko-Bulgac, E. P. 1991. Variations of *Candida albicans* electrophoretic karyotypes. *J. Bacteriol.* **173:**6586–6596.

Rustchenko-Bulgac, E. P., F. Sherman, and J. B. Hicks. 1990. Chromosomal rearrangements associated with morphological mutants provide a means for genetic variation in *Candida albicans*. *J. Bacteriol.* **172:**1276–1283.

Sadhu, C., M. J. McEachern, E. P. Rustchenko-Bulgac, J. Schmid, D. R. Soll, and J. B. Hicks. 1991. Telomeric and dispersed repeat sequences in *Candida* yeasts and their use in strain identification. *J. Bacteriol.* **173:**842–850.

Sahni, N., S. Yi, C. Pujol, and D. R. Sol. 2009. The white cell response to pheromone is a general characteristic of *Candida albicans* strains. *Eukaryot. Cell* **8:**251–256.

Sanglard, D., F. Ischer, L. Koymans, and J. Bille. 1998. Amino acid substitutions in the cytochrome P450 lanosterol 14α-demethylase (CYP51A1) from azole-resistant *Candida albicans* clinical isolates contributing to the resistance to azole antifungal agents. *Antimicrob. Agents Chemother.* **42:**241–253.

Sanz, M., R. Valle, and C. Roncero. 2007. Promoter heterozygosity at the *Candida albicans CHS7* gene is translated into differential expression between alleles. *FEMS Yeast Res.* **7:**993–1003.

Scherer, S., and D. A. Stevens. 1988. A *Candida albicans* dispersed, repeated gene family and its epidemiological applications. *Proc. Natl. Acad. Sci. USA* **85:**1452–1456.

Schmid, J., E. Voss, and D. R. Soll. 1990. Computer-assisted methods for assessing strain relatedness in *Candida albicans* by fingerprinting with the moderately repetitive sequence Ca3. *J. Clin. Microbiol.* **28:**1236–1243.

Selmecki, A., A. Forche, and J. Berman. 2006. Aneuploidy and isochromosome formation in drug-resistant *Candida albicans*. *Science* **313:**367–370.

Selmecki, A., M. Gerami-Nejad, C. Paulson, A. Forche, and J. Berman. 2008. An isochromosome confers drug resistance *in vivo* by amplification of two genes, *ERG11* and *TAC1*. *Mol. Microbiol.* **68:**624–641.

Selmecki, A., S. Bergmann, and J. Berman. 2005. Comparative genome hybridization reveals widespread aneuploidy in *Candida albicans* laboratory strains. *Mol. Microbiol.* **55:**1553–1565.

Snell, R. G., I. F. Hermans, R. J. Wilkins, and B. E. Cornerl. 1987. Chromosomal variations in *Candida albicans*. *Nucleic Acids Res.* **15:**3625.

Slutsky, B., J. Buffo, and D. R. Soll. 1985. High frequency switching of colony morphology in *Candida albicans*. *Science* **230:**666–669.

Slutsky, B., M. Staebell, J. Anderson, L. Risen, M. Pfaller, and D. R. Soll. 1987. "White-opaque transition": a second high-frequency switching system in *Candida albicans*. *J. Bacteriol.* **169:**189–197.

Soll, D. R. 1992. High-frequency switching in *Candida albicans*. *Clin. Microbiol. Rev.* **5:**183–203.

Soll, D. R. 2000. The ins and outs of DNA fingerprinting the infectious fungi. *Clin. Microbiol. Rev.* **13:**332–370.

Soll, D. R., and C. Pujol. 2003. *Candida albicans* clades. *FEMS Immunol. Med. Microbiol.* **39:**1–7.

Soll, D. R., C. J. Langtimm, J. McDowell, J. Hicks, and R. Galask. 1987. High-frequency switching in *Candida* strains isolated from vaginitis patients. *J. Clin. Microbiol.* **25:**1611–1622.

Soll, D. R., C. Pujol, and T. Srikantha. 2009. Sex: deviant mating in yeast. *Curr. Biol.* **19:**R509–R511.

Soll, D. R., R. Galask, J. Schmid, C. Hanna, K. Mac, and B. Morrow. 1991. Genetic dissimilarity of commensal strains carried in different anatomical locations of the same healthy women. *J. Clin. Microbiol.* **29:**1702–1710.

Srikantha, T., A. R. Borneman, K. J. Daniels, C. Pujol, W. Wu, M. R. Seringhaus, M. Gerstein, S. Yi, M. Snyder, and D. R. Soll. 2006. TOS9 regulates white-opaque switching in *Candida albicans*. *Eukaryot. Cell* **5:**1674–1687.

Staib, P., M. Kretschmar, T. Nichterlein, H. Hof, and J. Morschhäuser. 2002. Host versus *in vitro* signals and intrastrain allelic differences in the expression of a *Candida albicans* virulence gene. *Mol. Microbiol.* **44:**1351–1366.

Sudbery, P., N. Gow, and J. Berman. 2004. The distinct morphogenic states of *Candida albicans*. *Trends Microbiol.* **12:**317–324.

Sullivan, D. J., G. P. Moran, E. Pinjon, A. Al-Mosaid, C. Stokes, C. Vaughan, and D. C. Coleman. 2004. Comparison of the epidemiology, drug resistance mechanisms, and virulence of *Candida dubliniensis* and *Candida albicans*. *FEMS Yeast Res.* **4:**369–376.

Suzuki, T., S. Nishibayashi, T. Kuroiwa, T. Kanbe, and K. Tanaka. 1982. Variance of ploidy in *Candida albicans*. *J. Bacteriol.* **152:**893–896.

Tavanti, A., A. D. Davidson, M. J. Fordyce, N. A. Gow, M. C. Maiden, and F. C. Odds. 2005. Population structure and properties of *Candida albicans*, as determined by multilocus sequence typing. *J. Clin. Microbiol.* **43:**5601–5613.

Tavanti, A., N. A. R. Gow, M. C. J. Maiden, F. C. Odds, and D. J. Shaw. 2004. Genetic evidence for recombination in *Candida albicans* based on haplotype analysis. *Fungal Genet. Biol.* **41:**553–562.

Tsong, A. E., M. G. Miller, R. M. Raisner, and A. D. Johnson. 2003. Evolution of a combinatorial transcriptional circuit: a case study in yeasts. *Cell* **115:**389–399.

Tzung, K. W., R. M. Williams, S. Scherer, N. Federspiel, T. Jones, N. Hansen, V. Bivolarevic, L. Huizar, C. Komp, R. Surzycki, R. Tamse, R. W. Davis, and N. Agabian. 2001. Genomic evidence for a complete sexual cycle in *Candida albicans*. *Proc. Natl. Acad. Sci. USA* **98:**3249–3253.

Uhl, M. A., M. Biery, N. Craig, and A. D. Johnson. 2003. Haploinsufficiency-based large-scale forward genetic analysis of filamentous growth in the diploid human fungal pathogen *C. albicans*. *EMBO J.* **22:**2668–2678.

Van Kruiningen, H. J., M. Joossens, S. Vermeire, S. Joossens, S. Debeugny, C. Gower-Rousseau, A. Cortot, J. F. Colombel, P. Rutgeerts, and R. Vlietinck. 2005. Environmental factors in familial Crohn's disease in Belgium. *Inflamm. Bowel Dis.* **11:**360–365.

Welch, D. M., and M. Meselson. 2000. Evidence for the evolution of bdelloid rotifers without sexual reproduction or genetic exchange. *Science* **288:**1211–1215.

Wellington, M., and E. Rustchenko. 2005. 5-Fluoro-orotic acid induces chromosome alterations in *Candida albicans*. *Yeast* **22:**57–70.

Whelan, W. L., and D. R. Soll. 1982. Mitotic recombination in *Candida albicans*: recessive lethal alleles linked to a gene required for methionine biosynthesis. *Mol. Gen. Genet.* **187:**477–485.

White, T. C. 1997. The presence of an R467K amino acid substitution and loss of allelic variation correlate with an azole-resistant lanosterol 14-alpha-demethylase in *Candida albicans*. *Antimicrob. Agents Chemother.* **41:**1488–1494.

White, T. C., K. A. Marr, and R. A. Bowden. 1998. Clinical, cellular, and molecular factors that contribute to antifungal drug resistance. *Clin. Microbiol. Rev.* **11:**382–402.

Wickes, B., J. Staudinger, B. B. Magee, K.-J. Kwon-Chung, P. T. Magee, and S. Scherer. 1991.

Physical and genetic mapping of *Candida albicans*: several genes previously assigned to chromosome 1 map to chromosome R, the rDNA-containing linkage group. *Infect. Immun.* **59:**2480–2484.

Wilson, M. J., D. W. Williams, M. D. L. Forbes, I. G. Finlay, and M. A. O. Lewis. 2001. A molecular epidemiological study of sequential oral isolates of *Candida albicans* from terminally ill patients. *J. Oral Pathol. Med.* **30:**206–212.

Wu, W., C. Pujol, S. R. Lockhart, and D. R. Soll. 2005. Chromosome loss followed by duplication is the major mechanism of spontaneous mating-type locus homozygosis in *Candida albicans*. *Genetics* **169:**1311–1327.

Wu, W., S. R. Lockhart, C. Pujol, T. Srikantha, and D. R. Soll. 2007. Heterozygosity of genes on the sex chromosome regulates *Candida albicans* virulence. *Mol. Microbiol.* **64:**1587–1604.

Yi, S., N. Sahni, K. J. Daniels, C. Pujol, T. Srikantha, and D. R. Soll. 2008. The same receptor, G protein, and mitogen-activated protein kinase pathway activate different downstream regulators in the alternative white and opaque pheromone responses of *Candida albicans*. *Mol. Biol. Cell* **19:**957–970.

Yi, S., N. Sahni, C. Pujol, K. J. Daniels, T. Srikantha, N. Ma, and D. R. Soll. 2009. A *Candida albicans*-specific region of the α-pheromone receptor plays a selective role in the white cell pheromone response. *Mol. Microbiol.* **71:**925–947.

Zeyl, C. 2007. Ploidy and the sexual yeast genome in theory, nature, and experiment, p. 507–525. *In* J. Heitman, J. W. Kronstad, J. W. Taylor, and L. A. Casselton (ed.), *Sex in Fungi: Molecular Determination and Evolutionary Implications.* ASM Press, Washington, DC.

Zhao, X., C. Pujol, D. R. Soll, and L. L. Hoyer. 2003. Allelic variation in the contiguous loci encoding *Candida albicans ALS5, ALS1* and *ALS9*. *Microbiology* **149:**2947–2960.

Zhao, X., S.-H. Oh, and L. L. Hoyer. 2007. Unequal contribution of *ALS9* alleles to adhesion between *Candida albicans* and human vascular endothelial cells. *Microbiology* **153:**2342–2350.

Zordan, R. E., D. J. Galgoczy, and A. D. Johnson. 2006. Epigenetic properties of white–opaque switching in *Candida albicans* are based on a self-sustaining transcriptional feedback loop. *Proc. Natl. Acad. Sci. USA* **103:**12807–12812.

GENOME PLASTICITY OF *Aspergillus* SPECIES

Thorsten Heinekamp and Axel A. Brakhage

19

THE GENUS *ASPERGILLUS*

A member of the filamentous ascomycete fungi, the genus *Aspergillus* contains more than 200 species. Aspergilli occur worldwide in a wide variety of natural habitats and exhibit extraordinary diverse features. They have an important impact on humankind, both beneficial and detrimental. On the one hand, some *Aspergillus* species are used industrially for the production or refinement of beverages, enzymes, food additives, or pharmaceuticals (Baker and Bennett, 2008). The species *Aspergillus niger* and *Aspergillus oryzae* are the most prominent representatives of the beneficial aspergilli. On the other hand, 20 *Aspergillus* species are regarded as pathogenic or as having other adverse effects. The species *Aspergillus fumigatus* and *Aspergillus terreus* are important human pathogens. Another omnipresent representative of the harmful aspergilli is *Aspergillus flavus*, a well-known producer of the carcinogenic compound aflatoxin. *A. flavus* is also a human pathogen but is more often found as a contaminant in corn and peanut storage, causing economically relevant losses in agriculture.

A. fumigatus is exceptional because it is the main causative agent of invasive infections due to filamentous fungi in immunosuppressed patients (Brakhage, 2005; Hohl and Feldmesser, 2007). Generally, *A. fumigatus* is a ubiquitous soil inhabitant that feeds on organic matter. It is often found in compost or hay and is a key player in recycling carbon and nitrogen sources (Latge, 1999). Due to its thermotolerance and ability to use various nutrient resources, *A. fumigatus* occupies a wide variety of ecological niches (Rhodes, 2006). For efficient distribution, *A. fumigatus* produces asexual spores, conidia, with a characteristic gray-green color that are passively distributed via the air. Every conidium contains a single haploid nucleus enabling the isolation of clones (Brakhage and Langfelder, 2002). A typical *A. fumigatus* conidiophore, a specialized stalk from which the conidia are born, is shown in Fig. 1.

For many decades, only the asexual life cycle of *A. fumigatus* was known; i.e., sexual crossing was not observed. Therefore, the fungus was classified as one of the Deuteromycota, the imperfect fungi. However, the existence

Thorsten Heinekamp and Axel A. Brakhage, Department of Molecular and Applied Microbiology, Leibniz Institute for Natural Product Research and Infection Biology—Hans Knöll Institute, and Department of Microbiology and Molecular Biology, Friedrich Schiller University Jena, Beutenbergstraße 11a, 07745 Jena, Germany.

Genome Plasticity and Infectious Diseases,
Edited by J. Hacker, U. Dobrindt, and R. Kurth,

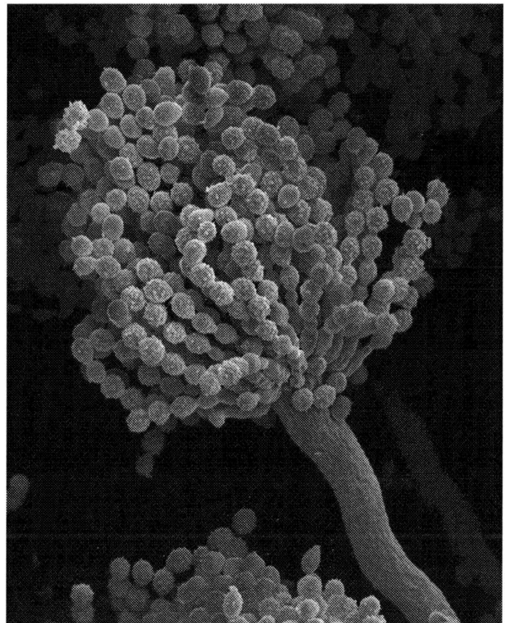

FIGURE 1 Electron micrograph of an *A. fumigatus* conidiophore. The conidiophore shows the typical columnar, uniseriate conidial head. Phialides are the conidiogenous cells which produce long chains of conidia in basipetal succession. Micrograph kindly provided by Jeannette Schmaler-Ripcke, Hans Knöll Institute and Center for Electron Microscopy, Friedrich Schiller University, Jena, Germany.

of two different mating types was observed and transcription of the mating-type-specific genes *MAT1-1* and *MAT1-2* as well as of genes encoding pheromone and pheromone receptors was verified, implying the possibility of sexuality (Paoletti et al., 2005, 2007). Finally, O'Gorman et al. (2009) discovered the sexual life cycle of *A. fumigatus* and identified the teleomorph *Neosartorya fumigata*. Admittedly, to induce sexual reproduction, special incubation conditions had to be applied. After a 6-month incubation on oatmeal agar plates at 30°C in the dark, two different mating types induced the formation of fruiting bodies. The so-called cleistothecia contained asci with ascopores of 4 to 5 µm. Germination of ascopores resulted in the formation of mycelium and asexual conidiation. The discovery of the sexual life cycle gives a reasonable explanation for the finding of intrapopulation genetic recombination in *A. fumigatus*. Prior to the discovery of the sexual cycle in *A. fumigatus*, it was assumed that transposable elements were the driving force behind the generation of genetic differences (Daboussi and Capy, 2003).

A. fumigatus produces small conidia that are distributed in the air and are continuously inhaled by breathing organisms. With a size of only 2 to 3 µm, they can easily reach the alveoli of the human lung. Every human inhales several hundred conidia during daily activities (Chazalet et al., 1998; Goodley et al., 1994; Hospenthal et al., 1998). Normally, conidia are cleared by the innate immune system. Symptoms of disease occur only if the host response is inadequate (Hohl and Feldmesser, 2007). In healthy individuals, *A. fumigatus* is confronted with two lines of defense. First, macrophages phagocytose and lyse spores. Second, hyphae are attacked by neutrophils. However, patients with a suppressed immune system are not able to clear inhaled spores and therefore are at high risk for an invasive infection with *A. fumigatus*. The incidence of invasive aspergillosis has increased over the last 2 decades, due to increasing numbers of patients with weakened immune system, e.g., as a result of solid-organ transplantation, cancer therapy, leukemia, or human immunodeficiency virus infection (Brakhage, 2005; Latge, 1999). Accordingly, *A. fumigatus* has become the most significant human-pathogenic filamentous fungus. It has developed specific features that enable it to survive in the human host. Although there are not many differences between *A. fumigatus* and other aspergilli and nonpathogenic filamentous fungi (Tekaia and Latge, 2005), *A. fumigatus* possesses several virulence determinants, e.g., adhesins, pigment biosynthesis, toxins, and iron acquisition mechanisms involved in invasive growth (Rhodes and Brakhage, 2006). During the infection process it is also essential that *A. fumigatus* adapt its physiology to the changing conditions in the host (Askew, 2008). Interestingly, *A. fumigatus* clinical isolates vary significantly in pathogenicity (Paisley et al., 2005). This is also reflected by the finding that in a murine infection model the total number of conidia necessary to induce similar mortality rates in the infected animals depends on the *A. fumigatus* isolate. For example, 3×10^4 conidia from clinical isolate CEA10 (CBS 144.89) are necessary to cause 80 to 90% mortality, whereas 6×10^4 conidia from strain ATCC 46645 and 2.5×10^5 conidia from isolate Af293 have to be applied (Liebmann et al., 2004; Bok et al., 2006; Kupfahl et al., 2006). The molecular mechanisms responsible for these differences in pathogenicity have still not been identified.

COMPARISON OF *ASPERGILLUS* GENOMES

Due to constant improvements in sequencing technologies and capacities in the recent past, several *Aspergillus* genomes have been sequenced and the sequences have been made publicly available. Starting in 2005 with the parallel publication of the *A. nidulans*, *A. fumigatus,* and *A. oryzae* genome sequences, the genomes of eight different *Aspergillus* species have been completely sequenced (Galagan et al., 2005; Machida et al., 2005; Nierman et al., 2005; Pel et al., 2007; Fedorova et al., 2008a). Furthermore, sequencing of several other *Aspergillus* strains and isolates is currently in progress, reflecting the importance of this genus. In detail, in addition to the *A. nidulans* (FGSCA4) genome, complete sequences of two different isolates of *A. fumigatus* (Af293 and A1163), its close relative *Neosartorya fischeri* (NRRL 181), and isolates of *A. oryzae* (RIB40), *A. niger* (CBS513.88 and ATCC 1015), *A. terreus* (NIH 2624), *A. flavus* (NRRL 3357), and *A. clavatus* (NRRL 1) are available. Detailed sequence features can be obtained from different internet based resources, e.g., via the Central *Aspergillus* Data Repository (CADRE; http://www.cadre.co.uk) or the *Aspergillus* Genome Database (AspGD) (Mabey et al., 2004; Arnaud et al., 2010). The main genome features of fully sequenced *Aspergillus* genomes are summarized in Table 1. In general, the genome size of aspergilli spans from 27.9 to 39.9 Mb and the number of predicted protein-encoding genes ranges from 9,121 (*A. clavatus* NRRL 1) to 14,086 (*A. niger* CBS513.88). The average number of exons per gene (2.8 to 3.5) is quite similar among the different *Aspergillus* species.

Previously, *A. fumigatus* isolates were described as having low genetic variation and no detectable population structure, unlike *N. fischeri* (Rydholm et al., 2006). The finding of several isolate-specific and polymorphic genes, however, contradict this hypothesis (Balajee et al., 2007; Levdansky et al., 2007; Nierman et al., 2005). Genomic and phenotypic comparison of the two *A. fumigatus* isolates Af293 and A1163 also revealed remarkable differences, e.g., in genome size and resistance to antifungal drugs. The genome size of isolate A1163 (29.1 Mb) is 1.1 % larger than that of isolate Af293. A total of 98% of the genomes can be aligned, and the nucleotide sequence identity is remarkably high (99.8% in the shared regions); 143 and 218 genes were assigned to be isolate specific for Af293 and A1163, respectively (Fedorova et al., 2008a). Although isolate-specific genes were located throughout the genome, these differences are concentrated in a region within 300 kb of the chromosome ends. Furthermore, the majority of species-specific genes are clustered in highly variable segments that contain numerous repeat elements and pseudogenes (Fedorova et al., 2008a). Species-specific genes may also attribute to phenotypic differences between isolates, e.g., with regard to resistance to antifungal agents. For example, *A. fumigatus* isolate A1163 is three times more resistant to hygromycin B than is isolate ATCC 45546.

Comparative genomics of the distantly related fungi *A. fumigatus*, *A. nidulans,* and *A. oryzae* showed an unexpected genetic variability of these species, reflected, among other differences (see below), by broad reorganization of the genome structure (Galagan et al., 2005). The average amino acid identity was less than 70% between each species pair. This suggests that these species are evolutionarily as distant from each other as are mammals and fish, which diverged 450 million years ago. The size of the genome and the number of predicted genes differ remarkably between the aspergilli. The genomes of *A. fumigatus* (28.8 Mb) and

TABLE 1 List of genome features of different aspergilli[a]

Species (strain or isolate)	Genome size (Mb)	No. of genes	Total no. of ITRs	No. of genes with ITRs	No. of genes in SM cluster	No. of genes			
						PKS	NRPS	Hybrid NRPS/PKS	DMAT
A. fumigatus (Af293)	28.8	9,630	222	207	30	15	18	1	7
A. fumigatus (A1163)	29.1	9,929	ND[b]	ND	28	14	18	1	7
N. fischeri (NRRL 181)	32.1	10,406	222	194	39	18	28	0	10
A. nidulans (FGSCA4)	30.1	10,546	215	200	46	28	23	1	6
A. oryzae (RIB 40)	37.2	12,074	204	182	56	27	32	2	8
A. niger (CBS513.88)	33.9	14,086	345	317	67	42	33	4	2
A. niger (ATCC 1015)	34.9	11,197	ND	ND	ND	ND	ND	ND	ND
A. clavatus (NRRL 1)	27.9	9,121	313	278	35	17	18	4	3
A. terreus (NIH 2624)	29.3	10,402	172	154	56	30	34	1	10
A. flavus (NRRL 3357)	39.9	13,487	235	210	55	28	32	2	8

[a]The genome data were collected from CADRE (http://www.cadre-genomes.org.uk), data for intragenic tandem repeats (ITRs) are from Gibbons and Rokas (2009). Data for secondary-metabolite gene clusters were obtained via the Web-based tool SMURF (http://jcvi.org/smurf).
[b]ND, not determined.

A. nidulans (30.1 Mb) are ~25 % smaller than those of *A. oryzae* (37.2 Mb) and *A. flavus* (39.9 Mb). It is speculated that these differences are most probably due to acquisition of sequences in *A. oryzae* and *A. flavus* rather than loss in the other aspergilli (Galagan et al., 2005).

In a comprehensive study, two isolates of *A. fumigatus,* Af293 and A1183, were compared in detail with their close relatives *N. fischeri* and *A. clavatus* (Fedorova et al., 2008a). Af293 contains eight chromosomes with a size of 1.8 to 4.9 Mb. The function of about one-third of the 9,630 predicted proteins is unknown. In comparison to *N. fischeri* and *A. clavatus,* more than 800 genes were found to be specific for *A. fumigatus*; i.e., no orthologs are present in the other genomes. These species-specific genes are located predominantly in subtelomeric regions. As evident by BLAST search analyses, several of the *A. fumigatus* species-specific genes have only bacterial or archaeal homologs (Fedorova et al., 2008a). They are mostly annotated as hypothetical proteins, hindering functional allocation. These genes probably contribute positively to the adaptation of the fungus to different environmental niches, such as compost heaps or the human lung.

Although *N. fischeri* is a very close relative of *A. fumigatus,* it is rarely found to be pathogenic. The genome of *N. fischeri* is more than 10% larger than that of *A. fumigatus*. However, the number of predicted gene transcripts is only 6 to 8% larger than that of Af293 or A1163. This discrepancy might be explained by the large number of transposable elements found in *N. fischeri*. Comparison to the Af293 and *A. clavatus* genomes revealed ca. 1,400 genes unique to *N. fischeri,* including several mycotoxin islands and paralogous gene families. The *A. clavatus* genome, with a size of only 27.9 Mb, is the smallest of the genomes of the sequenced aspergilli. Approximately 1,150 of the 9,379 genes were found to be specific for *A. clavatus* compared to *N. fischeri* and *A. fumigatus* (Fedorova et al., 2008a). In contrast to *A. fumigatus, A. clavatus* is rarely pathogenic, although it is a competent producer of mycotoxins and is implicated in respiratory disease in malt workers (Blyth et al., 1977).

As mentioned above, species-specific genes comprise 10 to 15% of the *Aspergillus* genomes. This is of especial interest with regard to the identification of virulence genes specific for *A. fumigatus*. However, none of these genes have been found to be involved in *A. fumigatus* virulence. By contrast, most genes that were identified as virulence determinants have orthologs in nonpathogenic filamentous ascomycetes or even more distantly related fungi such as the basidiomycete *Cryptococcus neoformans* (Fedorova et al., 2008b). The *A. fumigatus*-specific genes with an assigned function are associated with general processes of adaptation to environmental niches. Genes encoding proteins for secondary metabolite biosynthesis, detoxification processes, and carbohydrate metabolism and transport are often species specific. Another common feature of species-specific genes is their preferential localization in intrasyntenic plasticity zones. Since, in contrast to *Saccharomyces cerevisiae,* these plasticity zones are rather large, it has been suggested that this may be the genetic basis for the flexible adaptability of the aspergilli to different environments (Fedorova et al., 2008b).

Orthologous genes originate from a common ancestor and retain the same function during evolution. Therefore, they can be used to determine syntenic regions between genomes of different species. In the genomes of *A. fumigatus* Af293, *N. fischeri,* and *A. clavatus,* nearly 9,000 ortholog clusters were identified, of which around 7,500 were found in all three genomes (Fedorova et al., 2008a). The average amino acid identity of protein orthologs between Af293 and *N. fischeri* and *A. clavatus* is 94% and 80%, respectively, reflecting the phylogeny of these species as previously proposed by ribosomal DNA sequence analysis (Peterson, 2008).

The highest sequence identities are normally found for orthologous genes located in central regions of chromosomes. By contrast, orthologs located within a region of 300 kb from chromosome ends have a lower sequence identity, indicating an accelerated evolution process of these genes. Consistently, the chromosomal core genes encode proteins that often play important roles in essential functions of the organisms such as transcription and translation and organization of nuclear and chromatin structure. Also, genes for cell cycle-controlling processes are concentrated in the central chromosomal regions. The likelihood of finding genes belonging to these functional categories in the chromosomal center is six times higher than that of finding them within the subtelomeric regions. Furthermore, genes involved in other essential processes such as energy metabolism, signal transduction, and cytoskeleton assembly reveal a strong bias for location in the chromosomal core regions (Fedorova et al., 2008b).

Genes encoding central components of signal transduction cascades appear to be exceptionally highly conserved. An example is given by a comparison of members of the mitogen-activated protein kinase signaling pathways that are involved in regulating cell wall integrity in *A. fumigatus* and *S. cerevisiae*: the *A. fumigatus* mitogen-activated protein kinase MpkA reveals 68% identity to the *S. cerevisiae* Slt2/Mpk1 and the upstream kinases Mkk2 and Bck1 show 55% and 47% identity to the orthologous yeast genes (Rispail et al., 2009; Valiante et al., 2008, 2009). Furthermore, genes encoding cyclic AMP signaling components, such as adenylyl cyclase and protein kinase A catalytic subunit (Liebmann et al., 2003), as well as genes involved in calcium signaling via calcineurin (da Silva Ferreira et al., 2007; Steinbach et al., 2006), are also well conserved in fungi. Within all these genes the average identity between orthologs of *A. fumigatus* and yeast is ~50%, whereas the overall identity of orthologous genes is 39% (Fedorova et al., 2008b).

The subtelomeric diversity may be a potential driving force in the evolution of pathogenicity in *A. fumigatus*. This hypothesis is strengthened by the finding that transcription of one-third of the *A. fumigatus* species-specific and subtelomeric genes are induced during initiation of invasive aspergillosis (McDonagh et al., 2008).

SECONDARY METABOLITES IN *A. FUMIGATUS*

Fungi differ remarkably in their ability to produce secondary metabolites. These natural products comprise a broad range of effective drugs, e.g., antibiotics and immunosuppressive agents. However, several secondary metabolites also display strong toxic activities. Aflatoxin, produced by *A. flavus* and *A. parasiticus,* is an extremely carcinogenic and hepatotoxic substance. The function of most secondary metabolites in the producing organism is not known yet. As biologically active compounds they might protect the fungus against other soil inhabitants and may also contribute to weakening of the host immune system (Askew, 2008; Brakhage et al., 2008, 2009).

The numbers of nonribosomal peptid synthetase (NRPS), polyketide synthase (PKS), and dimethylallyl tryptophan synthase (DMAT) genes encoding central proteins for secondary-metabolite production differ remarkably in the *Aspergillus* genomes (Table 1). Genes involved in the production of secondary metabolites are often organized in a cluster. Besides core genes relevant for the production of metabolites such as NRPS, PKS, DMAT, or hybrid PKS-NRPS, these clusters often contain genes involved in transcriptional regulation and genes with a putative role in resistance such as those encoding efflux transporters. Putative secondary-metabolite gene clusters from several aspergilli were obtained from precomputed results by using the Web-based tool SMURF (Secondary Metabolite Unique Regions Finder; http://jcvi.org/smurf). The overall number of predicted secondary metabolite clusters as well as PKS, NRPS, and DMAT genes identified by this tool is in general larger than that found in previous studies. For example, SMURF identified 30 secondary metabolite clusters in *A. fumigatus* Af293, whereas prior to that only 22 or 23 were predicted (Fedorova et al., 2008b; Nierman et al., 2005). A common and striking result of these studies is that secondary metabolite clusters are not equally distributed all over the chromosomes; they are often located at the end of the chromosomes and are hardly ever found at the centers of the chromosomes. For example, in *A. fumigatus* 50% of secondary-metabolite clusters are located in subtelomeric regions of less than 300 kb close to the ends of chromosomes (Fig. 2).

Many (Brakhage et al., 2008, 2009) of the clusters for biosynthesis of secondary metabolites contain regulatory genes. The transcriptional regulators found in these clusters seem to be specific to their cluster due to missing similarities to other transcriptional regulators. In addition to the regulators directly connected to the cluster, so-called global regulators of secondary-metabolite synthesis are present in the genomes of aspergilli. Examples of such global regulators are the nuclear protein LaeA and the CCAAT-binding complex, which are found in all *Aspergillus* genomes. The *laeA* gene encodes a putative methyltransferase. In *A. fumigatus* 12 of the secondary metabolite gene clusters are at least partially regulated by LaeA (Perrin et al., 2007). The regulation of secondary metabolite gene clusters by LaeA is not correlated to the chromosomal localization of the cluster. LaeA is, e.g., responsible for transcription of genes for gliotoxin biosynthesis (1.5 Mb away from the telomere), dihydroxynaphthalene (DHN) melanin biosynthesis (200 kb away from the telomere), and fumitremorgin biosynthesis (100 kb away from the telomere). The *cis*-acting sequence CCAAT is located in a region 50 to 200 bp upstream from the transcriptional start point of approximately 30% of all eukaryotic genes (Bucher, 1990). An evolutionarily conserved heterotrimeric CCAAT-binding complex has been found in all eukaryotes analyzed so far. In *Aspergillus* species this complex is designated AnCF (Brakhage et al., 1999). In *A. nidulans* this factor regulates

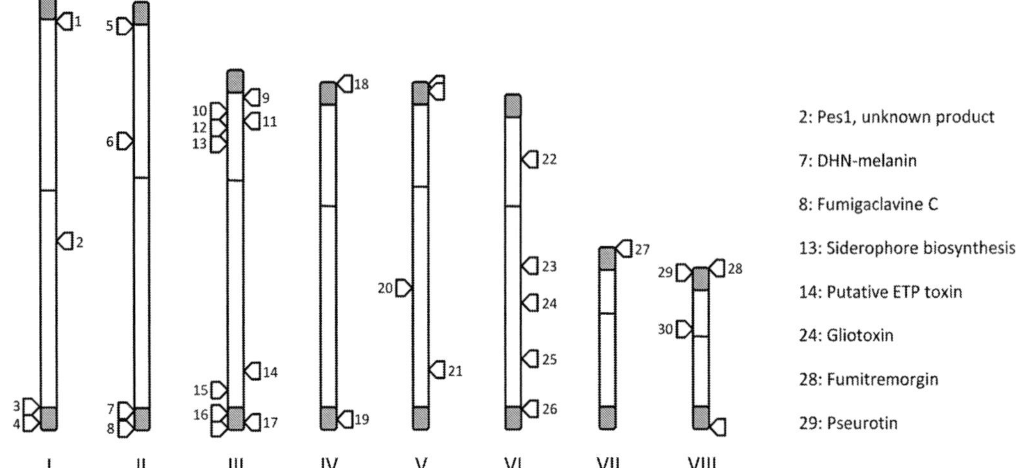

FIGURE 2 Chromosomal localization of secondary metabolite gene clusters in *A. fumigatus*. Putative secondary metabolite gene clusters from *A. fumigatus* were obtained from precomputed results of the Web-based tool SMURF. The positions of secondary metabolite clusters are depicted by arrowheads; the cluster number corresponds to the SMURF prediction. Arrowheads without a number show the positions of single NRPS or PKS genes. Telomeric regions are indicated in gray.

the expression of numerous genes, including *acvA, ipnA,* and *aatA,* responsible for penicillin biosynthesis (Litzka et al., 1996; Then Bergh and Brakhage, 1998).

The best known secondary metabolite produced by *A. fumigatus* is the compound gliotoxin, belonging to the class of epipolythiodioxopiperazine (ETP) toxins (Gardiner and Howlett, 2005). Putative ETP toxin biosynthesis clusters are widely distributed in ascomycete fungi (Patron et al., 2007). Gliotoxin production was reported for even distantly related fungi, i.e., *Trichoderma virens* and *Penicillium terlikowskii* (Anitha and Murugesan, 2005; Waring et al., 1987). Gliotoxin is produced during the infection process and exhibits immunosuppressive and cell-damaging activity. However, whether gliotoxin plays a central role in pathogenicity is still a matter of debate (Bok et al., 2006; Cramer et al., 2006; Kupfahl et al., 2006; Spikes et al., 2008; Sugui et al., 2007).

In several studies, different isolates of *A. fumigatus* were tested for their ability to produce gliotoxin (Lewis et al., 2005; Reeves et al., 2004; Kosalec and Pepeljnjak, 2005). Recently, Kupfahl and coworkers investigated 53 environmental and 47 clinical isolates and found that nearly all (98% and 96%, respectively) produced gliotoxin (Kupfahl et al., 2008). This study contradicts previous studies which claimed that clinical isolates were the predominant producers of gliotoxin. In contrast to *A. fumigatus,* the percentage of gliotoxin-producing isolates in other *Aspergillus* species is significantly lower. Only 56% of *A. niger*, 37% of *A. terreus,* and 13% of *A. flavus* strains produced gliotoxin under standardized laboratory conditions. The reason for being a nonproducing strain was not analyzed in detail, but some of the gliotoxin-negative strains lack the central NRPS. The ability to produce gliotoxin is of no obvious advantage or disadvantage for the fungus, leaving the biological function of this secondary metabolite unclear.

Another well-characterized secondary metabolite from *A. fumigatus* is the pigment DHN melanin, responsible for the characteristic gray-green color of the conidia. The polyketide synthase PksP is a key enzyme in the biosynthesis of this pigment. Mutants deficient for PksP produce white conidia and are strongly attenuated in virulence (Langfelder et al., 1998). Expression of the gene was found to occur predominantly in the conidia and phialides but was also detected in hyphae during the infection process (Langfelder et al., 2001). Products of biosynthesis genes have been shown to protect *A. fumigatus* against reactive oxygen intermediates, derived from host immune effector cells (Jahn et al., 2000; Langfelder et al., 2003), and are also involved in the inhibition of phagosome-lysosome fusion and thereby in the killing of *A. fumigatus* conidia.

In comparison to the 30 putative gene clusters for the biosynthesis of secondary metabolites that were identified in *A. fumigatus*, the genomes of *N. fischeri* and *A. clavatus* contain 28 and 35 putative secondary metabolite gene clusters, respectively. The repertoire of secondary metabolite gene clusters differs remarkably among these three species; i.e., many clusters were found that are unique to one *Aspergillus* species. *A. fumigatus* and *N. fischeri* share only 14 orthologous clusters, including the gliotoxin and putative pseurotin biosynthesis clusters. Only five clusters are similar between *A. fumigatus* and *A. clavatus*. Among these clusters only three were found to be orthologous among all three aspergilli. The common clusters are the ones containing genes for siderophore biosynthesis and pigment formation and the Pes-1-associated cluster (Fedorova et al., 2008a).

Besides the gliotoxin biosynthesis cluster, *A. fumigatus* and *N. fischeri* share a cluster putatively relevant for synthesis of another ETP toxin. Due to sequence similarities, it is likely that this cluster derived from segmental duplication of the gliotoxin cluster in a common ancestor of these aspergilli. Segmental duplication and accelerated divergence are, among others, important driving forces for the evolution of clusters. However, many secondary metabolite biosynthesis clusters unique to one *Aspergillus* species appear to be assembled de novo. They are often flanked by transposable elements and repeat sequences and neighboring nonsyntenic sequences (Fedorova et al., 2008a). Forces that may have contributed to de novo cluster assembly are the availability of spare elements and the enhanced occurrence of crossover events in genomic plasticity zones. Plasticity zones are dynamic chromosomal regions with typical high recombination rates and are found in many eukaryotic genomes. They facilitate frequent exchanges between nonhomologous chromosomes, and this may place appropriate genes in physical proximity for coregulated transcription. Secondary metabolite gene clusters are located predominantly in such zones; e.g., in *A. fumigatus* only the DHN melanin biosynthesis cluster and the Pes-1-associated cluster are not part of a plasticity zone (Fedorova et al., 2008a).

Although various secondary metabolites have been isolated from several aspergilli, their assignment to specific NRPS or PKS gene clusters is in its very early stages. Recently, several attempts were made to assign gene clusters to their corresponding produced metabolites (Brakhage et al., 2008; Chiang et al., 2009). Under normal laboratory cultivation conditions the vast majority of secondary metabolite gene clusters are silent; i.e., no transcripts are produced (Bergmann et al., 2007; Schroeckh et al., 2009). This is the reason why simple knockout strategies and subsequent metabolite analysis are usually not successful. Often, genes encoding transcription factors are part of the predicted gene cluster for the production of secondary metabolites. Therefore, a very promising approach is the inducible overproduction of the respective transcription factor and thereby the induced transcription of all genes of the cluster (Bergmann et al., 2007). The activity of many secondary metabolite gene clusters is subject to coregulation at the heterochromatin level. Therefore, another approach to activate silent-gene clusters is the global reorganization of euchromatin or heterochromatin regions (Bok and Keller, 2004; Lee et al., 2009).

As well as the PKS and NRPS genes which are obviously connected to a gene cluster for biosynthesis of secondary metabolites, the analysis of all sequenced *Aspergillus* genomes displayed the existence of a quite remarkable number of standalone PKS- and NRPS-like enzymes. The role of these enzymes, which are not part of an obvious gene cluster in secondary metabolite production, remains to be elucidated.

TRANSPOSABLE ELEMENTS IN ASPERGILLI

Transposable elements are ubiquitous mobile genetic elements and are present in all prokaryotic and eukaryotic genomes, including fungi. However, although the types of transposons are the same in all eukaryotes, the copy numbers of these elements are much lower in fungi.

Based on the genome sequence of *A. fumigatus, A. oryzae,* and *A. nidulans,* a large number of transposable elements were identified in these species (Clutterbuck et al., 2008). Remarkably, the localization of the transposable elements was found with a strong bias toward the telomeric and centromeric regions of the chromosomes. In these three aspergilli, only a small proportion of the genome was found to be made up of transposable elements. In *A. nidulans*, a total of 1,218 copies of transposable elements were identified, representing 2.5% of the genome. In *A. fumigatus,* 595 copies of transposable elements make up 2.9% of the genome. However, in the organism with the largest genome in this comparison, *A. oryzae* (37.2 Mb), only 857 copies of transposable elements were found, comprising only 1.2% of the genome. Regardless of the relative small proportion of transposable elements in the genome, the analyzed aspergilli include a wide spectrum of different types of transposable elements belonging to several transposable-element superfamilies, such as Copia, Mariner, and Gypsy. Members of the Gypsy-type retrotransposons are the most prominent transposable elements found in *A. nidulans* (73 copies) and *A. fumigatus* (190 copies), at 177 and 465 kb, respectively. In *A. oryzae*, Gypsy-type mobile elements account for 129 kb of the genome and represent the second most prominent family of transposons, outnumbered by Mariner-type transposons, which account for 214 kb in this *Aspergillus* species (Clutterbuck et al., 2008).

Although the *A. nidulans, A. fumigatus,* and *A. oryzae* genomes harbor several mobile elements from a wide variety of superfamilies, no identical elements are present in these species. Obviously, the panoply of transposable elements completely changed during the evolution of these species (Galagan et al., 2005). Although *A. nidulans* harbors the largest number of elements showing the widest overall diversity, a similar amount of the *A. fumigatus* genome consists of transposable elements, due to the presence of more intact large elements in the latter organism. In contrast, many of the transposable elements in *A. oryzae* are incomplete and highly degraded copies. Consequently, the proportion of the genome of *A. oryzae* composed of transposable elements is only half as much as that of *A. nidulans* and *A. fumigatus* (Clutterbuck et al., 2008).

Regardless of the rapid progress in collecting genome-sequencing information from different *Aspergillus* species, the literature about transposable elements in aspergilli is rather limited. Very few elements have been characterized in detail, such as the retrotransposon-like elements Afut1, Afut2, and Aft1 and the class II transposon Tafl (Hey et al., 2008; Neuveglise et al., 1996; Paris and Latge, 2001; Monroy and Sheppard, 2005) from *A. fumigatus*. In *A. niger* the elements ANiTa1 and Vader have been subject to more detailed analysis (Braumann et al., 2007, 2008).

Tafl is the only class II transposable element of *A. fumigatus* analyzed in detail so far (Monroy and Sheppard, 2005). In contrast to class I transposons, which transpose via a reverse-transcribed RNA intermediate, class II transposons transpose directly at the DNA level. Both class I and class II elements have been found in all *Aspergillus* species. However, active transposition is rather rare and was verified only for the class II elements Ant1, Tan1, and Vader (Glayzer et al., 1995; Amutan et al., 1996; Nyyssonen et al., 1996) of *A. niger*. The retrotransposons Afut1 and Afut from *A. fumigatus* have been shown to be inactive (Paris and Latge, 2001).

The class II transposon Tafl from *A. fumigatus*, belonging to the Mariner superfamily, is characterized by extremely long inverted repeats flanking the transposase gene. Strain Af293 contains multiple copies of Tafl, and transcription of this element was proven by reverse transcriptase PCR (Monroy and Sheppard, 2005). Examination of seven different clinical isolates by Southern blot analysis revealed a strain-specific signal pattern for Tafl fragments; i.e., Tafl is present in different locations and copy numbers within different isolates. Therefore, Taf1 insertions are polymorphic among *A. fumigatus* isolates, and it is proposed that Taf1 may be able to transpose actively. However, stimuli inducing active transposition of Taf1 have not been identified yet (Monroy and Sheppard, 2005).

Aft1 was identified and characterized as a further transposable element from the Mariner superfamily in *A. fumigatus* (Hey et al., 2008). The structure of Aft1 is typical for Mariner-type transposons, and the inverted repeats are 45 bp long. Aft1 has 65% identity to the active Tan1 element from *A. niger*. The Aft1 gene is 1.9 kb and is present in multiple and highly conserved copies in the *A. fumigatus* genome. Aft1 encodes an apparently functional transposase, and transcription of the transposase gene was verified in several *A. fumigatus* isolates. Aft1 is widely distributed among clinical isolates, but the genomic localization pattern differs considerably between the analyzed strains. BLAST analysis revealed the presence of Aft1-like elements in other aspergilli, e.g., the F2P08 hypothetical transposase of *A. nidulans* and the Tao2 element of *A. oryzae*. The latter has 70% identity on the amino acid level to the Aft1 transposase and was also found to be actively transcribed. In the *A. flavus* genome, multiple BLAST hits for Aft1 sequences were identified. In *A. clavatus*, only fragments but no intact copies of Aft1 elements could be identified (Hey et al., 2008). Sequence alignments of several transposons revealed that Aft1 is more closely related to *A. niger* Tan1 and *A. nidulans* F2P08 elements than to *A. fumigatus* Taf1, suggesting independent ancestry of Taf1.

INTRAGENIC TANDEM REPEATS

The human genome is composed of ca. 35% repetitive elements (Venter et al., 2001). Very often, these repeat elements are located in intergenic regions, but some are also present in protein-coding regions or pseudogenes. Therefore, this class of repetitive DNA elements is designated intragenic tandem repeats (ITRs). Characteristically, ITRs comprise three or more nucleotides repeated in tandem. ITRs can differ in the length of the repeat motif as well as in the total number of repeats. For example, ITRs are designated as microsatellites if they consist of simple sequence repeats, i.e., if a sequence of a few nucleotides is repeated 10 to 100 times (Ellegren, 2004; Li et al., 2004). Other ITRs (minisatellites) consist of longer repeat motifs containing tens to hundreds of nucleotides tandemly repeated. Generally, tandemly repeated DNA sequences are highly dynamic components of genomes (Verstrepen et al., 2005). ITR sequences are typically unstable and tend to expand or contract locally by processes of unequal recombination or slipped-strand mispairing (Levinson and Gutman, 1987; Schlotterer and Tautz, 1994; Bichara et al., 2006). This sequence instability leads to increased mutation rates of ITR-containing segments, combined with genotypic and phenotypic variations, relative to ITR-free genomic regions. This is especially true for sequences containing short ITRs (Dieringer and Schlotterer, 2003; Kashi and King, 2006; Moxon et al., 2006). The induced variations, at both the genotype and phenotype levels, have also been found in fungi (Balajee et al., 2007; Levdansky et al., 2007; Verstrepen et al., 2004, 2005; Fidalgo et al., 2006; Michael et al., 2007).

To further expand the analysis of ITRs for fungal genomes, the evolution and functional role of these repeat elements was examined in detail on the basis of the sequenced *Aspergillus* genomes (Gibbons and Rokas, 2009). Overall, around 2,000 ITRs were found among the eight different analyzed species. Both short (3 to 39 nucleotides) and long (40 to 500 nucleotides) ITRs in each of the screened *Aspergillus* genomes were identified. The total number of ITRs varied extensively between species, from 172 (*A. terreus*) to 345 (*A. niger* CBS513.88); the abundance of ITRs is not associated with genome size (Table 1). The number of ITR-containing genes in aspergilli ranged from 154 to 317. In many instances, individual genes harbored multiple ITRs. Generally, short ITRs were more abundant than ITRs with long repeat units. The regions containing ITRs are exceptionally variable, and the ITR-containing proteins are less conserved in comparison to the background proteome. Interestingly, several ITR-containing genes are known to play key roles in fungal lifestyle and pathogenicity (Gibbons and Rokas, 2009).

In eukaryotes ITRs are not equally distributed in protein-encoding genes but tend to be biased to the end of the protein. However, this does not apply for ITRs in most of the aspergilli. With the exception of *A. niger,* in which the ITRs do tend to be located at the end of the protein, the distribution of ITRs across protein lengths was random for all *Aspergillus* species.

Subdividing the entire proteome into genes encoding proteins harboring ITRs (the "ITR proteome") and ITR-free proteins (the "background proteome") (Gibbons and Rokas, 2009), it is intriguing that the background proteome is more conserved than the ITR proteome. This lack of conservation is especially true in a comparison of species that are closely related, such as *A. fumigatus* and *N. fischeri* or *A. flavus* and *A. oryzae*. In the latter, for 84% of all the background proteins an ortholog in the sister species is present, but in the ITR proteome only 75% shared an ortholog. Furthermore, only half of the ITR sequences within these orthologous proteins were conserved. Overall, only every fifth ITR was found to be present in a closely related species.

Gene products associated with the cell surface, e.g., proteins with GPI anchors and signal peptides, were overrepresented in the ITR proteome compared to the background proteome in all bioinformatically screened *Aspergillus* species. This is in accordance with previous studies suggesting that ITRs are associated with pathogenesis due to their potential to diversify the structure of cell surface proteins (Levdansky et al., 2007; Verstrepen et al., 2004, 2005).

The genomes of the four *Aspergillus* species *A. oryzae, A. terreus, A. fumigatus,* and *A. nidulans* were annotated according to FunCat (Ruepp et al., 2004). ITR-containing genes were significantly overrepresented in the following categories: transcription, cellular communication and signal transduction, and cell type differentiation. In the metabolism and energy categories, ITRs were underrepresented. However, no accumulation of microsatellites in genes belonging to the stress response category occurs in the aspergilli as was found for *Escherichia coli* and *S. cerevisiae* (Rocha et al., 2002; Bowen et al., 2005).

On the one hand, ITRs are frequently associated with genetic disease and pathogenesis (Sutherland and Richards, 1995; Verstrepen et al., 2005; Fondon and Garner, 2004; Pearson et al., 2005; Mirkin, 2007). On the other hand, they are also connected to environmental adaptation processes and phenotypic evolution (Oh et al., 2005; Verstrepen et al., 2004, 2005; Fidalgo et al., 2006; Michael et al., 2007). Therefore, it seems likely that since ITRs are present in such a wide range of functionally diverse proteins involved in transcriptional regulation and cell surface activities, they may play a major role in the amazing diversity of lifestyles found in the aspergilli.

REFERENCES

Amutan, M., E. Nyyssonen, J. Stubbs, M. R. Diaz-Torres, and N. Dunn-Coleman. 1996. Identification and cloning of a mobile transposon from *Aspergillus niger* var. *awamori*. *Curr. Genet.* **29:** 468–473.

Anitha, R., and K. Murugesan. 2005. Production of gliotoxin on natural substrates by *Trichoderma virens*. *J. Basic Microbiol.* **45:**12–19.

Arnaud, M. B., M. C. Chibucos, M. C. Costanzo, J. Crabtree, D. O. Inglis, A. Lotia, J. Orvis, P. Shah, M. S. Skrzypek, G. Binkley, S. R. Miyasato, J. R. Wortman, and G. Sherlock. 2010. The *Aspergillus* Genome Database, a curated comparative genomics resource for gene, protein and sequence information for the *Aspergillus* research community. *Nucleic Acids Res.* **38:**D420–D427.

Askew, D. S. 2008. *Aspergillus fumigatus*: virulence genes in a street-smart mold. *Curr. Opin. Microbiol.* **11:**331–337.

Baker, S. E., and J. W. Bennett. 2008. An overview of the genus *Aspergillus*, p. 3–13. *In* S. A. Osmani, and G. H. Goldman (ed.), *The Aspergilli: Genomics, Medical Aspects, Biotechnology, and Research Methods.* CRC Press. Boca Raton, FL.

Balajee, S. A., S. T. Tay, B. A. Lasker, S. F. Hurst, and A. P. Rooney. 2007. Characterization of a novel gene for strain typing reveals substructuring of *Aspergillus fumigatus* across North America. *Eukaryot. Cell* **6:**1392–1399.

Bergmann, S., J. Schumann, K. Scherlach, C. Lange, A. A. Brakhage, and C. Hertweck. 2007. Genomics-driven discovery of PKS-NRPS hybrid metabolites from *Aspergillus nidulans*. *Nat. Chem. Biol.* **3:**213–217.

Bichara, M., J. Wagner, and I. B. Lambert. 2006. Mechanisms of tandem repeat instability in bacteria. *Mutat. Res.* **598:**144–163.

Blyth, W., I. W. Grant, E. S. Blackadder, and M. Greenberg. 1977. Fungal antigens as a source of sensitization and respiratory disease in Scottish maltworkers. *Clin. Allergy* **7:**549–562.

Bok, J. W., D. Chung, S. A. Balajee, K. A. Marr, D. Andes, K. F. Nielsen, J. C. Frisvad, K. A. Kirby, and N. P. Keller. 2006. GliZ, a transcriptional regulator of gliotoxin biosynthesis, contributes to *Aspergillus fumigatus* virulence. *Infect. Immun.* **74:**6761–6768.

Bok, J. W., and N. P. Keller. 2004. LaeA, a regulator of secondary metabolism in *Aspergillus spp. Eukaryot. Cell* **3:**527–535.

Bowen, S., C. Roberts, and A. E. Wheals. 2005. Patterns of polymorphism and divergence in stress-related yeast proteins. *Yeast* **22:**659–668.

Brakhage, A. A. 2005. Systemic fungal infections caused by *Aspergillus* species: epidemiology, infection process and virulence determinants. *Curr. Drug Targets* **6:**875–886.

Brakhage, A. A., A. Andrianopoulos, M. Kato, S. Steidl, M. A. Davis, N. Tsukagoshi, and M. J. Hynes. 1999. HAP-Like CCAAT-binding complexes in filamentous fungi: implications for biotechnology. *Fungal Genet. Biol.* **27:**243–252.

Brakhage, A. A., and K. Langfelder. 2002. Menacing mold: the molecular biology of *Aspergillus fumigatus*. *Annu. Rev. Microbiol.* **56:**433–455.

Brakhage, A. A., J. Schuemann, S. Bergmann, K. Scherlach, V. Schroeckh, and C. Hertweck. 2008. Activation of fungal silent gene clusters: a new avenue to drug discovery. *Prog. Drug Res.* **66:** 3–12.

Brakhage, A. A., M. Thon, P. Sprote, D. H. Scharf, Q. Al-Abdallah, S. M. Wolke, and P. Hortschansky. 2009. Aspects on evolution of fungal beta-lactam biosynthesis gene clusters and recruitment of trans-acting factors. *Phytochemistry* **70:**1801–1811.

Braumann, I., M. van den Berg, and F. Kempken. 2007. Transposons in biotechnologically relevant strains of *Aspergillus niger* and *Penicillium chrysogenum*. *Fungal Genet. Biol.* **44:**1399–1414.

Braumann, I., M. A. van den Berg, and F. Kempken. 2008. Strain-specific retrotransposon-mediated recombination in commercially used *Aspergillus niger* strain. *Mol. Genet. Genomics* **280:** 319–325.

Bucher, P. 1990. Weight matrix descriptions of four eukaryotic RNA polymerase II promoter elements derived from 502 unrelated promoter sequences. *J. Mol. Biol.* **212:**563–578.

Chazalet, V., J. P. Debeaupuis, J. Sarfati, J. Lortholary, P. Ribaud, P. Shah, M. Cornet, H. Vu Thien, E. Gluckman, G. Brucker, and J. P. Latge. 1998. Molecular typing of environmental and patient isolates of *Aspergillus fumigatus* from various hospital settings. *J. Clin. Microbiol.* **36:** 1494–1500.

Chiang, Y. M., K. H. Lee, J. F. Sanchez, N. P. Keller, and C. C. Wang. 2009. Unlocking fungal cryptic natural products. *Nat. Product Commun.* **4:**1505–1510.

Clutterbuck, J. A., V. V. Kapitonov, and J. Jurka. 2008. Transposable elements and repeat induced point mutation in *Aspergillus nidulans*, *Aspergillus fumigatus*, and *Aspergillus oryzae*, p. 343–355. *In* S. A. Osmani and G. H. Goldman (ed.), *The Aspergilli: Genomics, Medical Aspects, Biotechnology, and Research Methods*. CRC Press, Boca Raton, FL.

Cramer, R. A., Jr., M. P. Gamcsik, R. M. Brooking, L. K. Najvar, W. R. Kirkpatrick, T. F. Patterson, C. J. Balibar, J. R. Graybill, J. R. Perfect, S. N. Abraham, and W. J. Steinbach. 2006. Disruption of a nonribosomal peptide synthetase in *Aspergillus fumigatus* eliminates gliotoxin production. *Eukaryot. Cell* **5:**972–980.

Daboussi, M. J., and P. Capy. 2003. Transposable elements in filamentous fungi. *Annu. Rev. Microbiol.* **57:**275–299.

da Silva Ferreira, M. E., T. Heinekamp, A. Hartl, A. A. Brakhage, C. P. Semighini, S. D. Harris, M. Savoldi, P. F. de Gouvea, M. H. de Souza Goldman, and G. H. Goldman. 2007. Functional characterization of the *Aspergillus fumigatus* calcineurin. *Fungal Genet. Biol.* **44:**219–230.

Dieringer, D., and C. Schlotterer. 2003. Two distinct modes of microsatellite mutation processes: evidence from the complete genomic sequences of nine species. *Genome Res.* **13:**2242–2251.

Ellegren, H. 2004. Microsatellites: simple sequences with complex evolution. *Nat. Rev. Genet.* **5:**435–445.

**Fedorova, N. D., N. Khaldi, V. S. Joardar, R. Maiti, P. Amedeo, M. J. Anderson, J. Crabtree, J. C. Silva, J. H. Badger, A. Albarraq, S. Angiuoli, H. Bussey, P. Bowyer, P. J. Cotty, P. S. Dyer, A. Egan, K. Galens, C. M. Fraser-Liggett, B. J. Haas, J. M. Inman, R. Kent, S. Lemieux, I. Malavazi, J. Orvis, T. Roemer, C. M. Ronning, J. P. Sundaram, G. Sutton, G. Turner, J. C. Venter, O. R. White, B. R. Whitty, P.

Youngman, K. H. Wolfe, G. H. Goldman, J. R. Wortman, B. Jiang, D. W. Denning, and W. C. Nierman. 2008a. Genomic islands in the pathogenic filamentous fungus *Aspergillus fumigatus*. *PLoS Genet.* **4:**e1000046.

Fedorova, N. D., W. C. Nierman, G. Turner, V. Joardar, R. Maiti, M. J. Anderson, D. W. Denning, and J. R. Wortman. 2008b. A comparative view of the genome of *Aspergillus fumigatus*, p. 25–42. *In* S. A. Osmani and G. H. Goldman (ed.), *The Aspergilli: Genomics, Medical Aspects, Biotechnology, and Research Methods.* CRC Press, Boca Raton, FL.

Fidalgo, M., R. R. Barrales, J. I. Ibeas, and J. Jimenez. 2006. Adaptive evolution by mutations in the FLO11 gene. *Proc. Natl. Acad. Sci. USA* **103:** 11228–11233.

Fondon, J. W., III, and H. R. Garner. 2004. Molecular origins of rapid and continuous morphological evolution. *Proc. Natl. Acad. Sci. USA* **101:**18058–18063.

Galagan, J. E., S. E. Calvo, C. Cuomo, L. J. Ma, J. R. Wortman, S. Batzoglou, S. I. Lee, M. Basturkmen, C. C. Spevak, J. Clutterbuck, V. Kapitonov, J. Jurka, C. Scazzocchio, M. Farman, J. Butler, S. Purcell, S. Harris, G. H. Braus, O. Draht, S. Busch, C. D'Enfert, C. Bouchier, G. H. Goldman, D. Bell-Pedersen, S. Griffiths-Jones, J. H. Doonan, J. Yu, K. Vienken, A. Pain, M. Freitag, E. U. Selker, D. B. Archer, M. A. Penalva, B. R. Oakley, M. Momany, T. Tanaka, T. Kumagai, K. Asai, M. Machida, W. C. Nierman, D. W. Denning, M. Caddick, M. Hynes, M. Paoletti, R. Fischer, B. Miller, P. Dyer, M. S. Sachs, S. A. Osmani, and B. W. Birren. 2005. Sequencing of *Aspergillus nidulans* and comparative analysis with *A. fumigatus* and *A. oryzae*. *Nature* **438:**1105–1115.

Gardiner, D. M., and B. J. Howlett. 2005. Bioinformatic and expression analysis of the putative gliotoxin biosynthetic gene cluster of *Aspergillus fumigatus*. *FEMS Microbiol. Lett.* **248:**241–248.

Gibbons, J. G., and A. Rokas. 2009. Comparative and functional characterization of intragenic tandem repeats in 10 *Aspergillus* genomes. *Mol. Biol. Evol.* **26:**591–602.

Glayzer, D. C., I. N. Roberts, D. B. Archer, and R. P. Oliver. 1995. The isolation of Ant1, a transposable element from *Aspergillus niger*. *Mol. Gen. Genet.* **249:**432–438.

Goodley, J. M., Y. M. Clayton, and R. J. Hay. 1994. Environmental sampling for aspergilli during building construction on a hospital site. *J. Hosp. Infect.* **26:**27–35.

Hey, P., G. Robson, M. Birch, and M. Bromley. 2008. Characterisation of Aft1 a Fot1/Pogo type transposon of *Aspergillus fumigatus*. *Fungal Genet. Biol.* **45:**117–126.

Hohl, T. M., and M. Feldmesser. 2007. *Aspergillus fumigatus*: principles of pathogenesis and host defense. *Eukaryot. Cell* **6:**1953–1963.

Hospenthal, D. R., K. J. Kwon-Chung, and J. E. Bennett. 1998. Concentrations of airborne *Aspergillus* compared to the incidence of invasive aspergillosis: lack of correlation. *Med. Mycol.* **36:** 165–168.

Jahn, B., F. Boukhallouk, J. Lotz, K. Langfelder, G. Wanner, and A. A. Brakhage. 2000. Interaction of human phagocytes with pigmentless *Aspergillus conidia*. *Infect. Immun.* **68:**3736–3739.

Kashi, Y., and D. G. King. 2006. Simple sequence repeats as advantageous mutators in evolution. *Trends Genet.* **22:**253–259.

Kosalec, I., and S. Pepeljnjak. 2005. Mycotoxigenicity of clinical and environmental *Aspergillus fumigatus* and *A. flavus* isolates. *Acta Pharm.* **55:**365–375.

Kupfahl, C., T. Heinekamp, G. Geginat, T. Ruppert, A. Hartl, H. Hof, and A. A. Brakhage. 2006. Deletion of the *gliP* gene of *Aspergillus fumigatus* results in loss of gliotoxin production but has no effect on virulence of the fungus in a low-dose mouse infection model. *Mol. Microbiol.* **62:**292–302.

Kupfahl, C., A. Michalka, C. Lass-Florl, G. Fischer, G. Haase, T. Ruppert, G. Geginat, and H. Hof. 2008. Gliotoxin production by clinical and environmental *Aspergillus fumigatus* strains. *Int. J. Med. Microbiol.* **298:**319–327.

Langfelder, K., B. Jahn, H. Gehringer, A. Schmidt, G. Wanner, and A. A. Brakhage. 1998. Identification of a polyketide synthase gene *(pksP)* of *Aspergillus fumigatus* involved in conidial pigment biosynthesis and virulence. *Med. Microbiol. Immunol.* **187:**79–89.

Langfelder, K., B. Philippe, B. Jahn, J. P. Latge, and A. A. Brakhage. 2001. Differential expression of the *Aspergillus fumigatus pksP* gene detected in vitro and in vivo with green fluorescent protein. *Infect. Immun.* **69:**6411–6418.

Langfelder, K., M. Streibel, B. Jahn, G. Haase, and A. A. Brakhage. 2003. Biosynthesis of fungal melanins and their importance for human pathogenic fungi. *Fungal Genet. Biol.* **38:**143–158.

Latge, J. P. 1999. *Aspergillus fumigatus* and aspergillosis. *Clin. Microbiol. Rev.* **12:**310–350.

Lee, I., J. H. Oh, E. K. Shwab, T. R. Dagenais, D. Andes, and N. P. Keller. 2009. HdaA, a class 2 histone deacetylase of *Aspergillus fumigatus*, affects germination and secondary metabolite production. *Fungal Genet. Biol.* **46:**782–790.

Levdansky, E., J. Romano, Y. Shadkchan, H. Sharon, K. J. Verstrepen, G. R. Fink, and N. Osherov. 2007. Coding tandem repeats generate diversity in *Aspergillus fumigatus* genes. *Eukaryot. Cell* **6:**1380–1391.

Levinson, G., and G. A. Gutman. 1987. Slipped-strand mispairing: a major mechanism for DNA sequence evolution. *Mol. Biol. Evol.* **4:**203–221.

Lewis, R. E., N. P. Wiederhold, M. S. Lionakis, R. A. Prince, and D. P. Kontoyiannis. 2005. Frequency and species distribution of gliotoxin-producing *Aspergillus* isolates recovered from patients at a tertiary-care cancer center. *J. Clin. Microbiol.* **43:**6120–6122.

Li, Y. C., A. B. Korol, T. Fahima, and E. Nevo. 2004. Microsatellites within genes: structure, function, and evolution. *Mol. Biol. Evol.* **21:**991–1007.

Liebmann, B., S. Gattung, B. Jahn, and A. A. Brakhage. 2003. cAMP signaling in *Aspergillus fumigatus* is involved in the regulation of the virulence gene *pksP* and in defense against killing by macrophages. *Mol. Genet. Genomics* **269:**420–435.

Liebmann, B., M. Muller, A. Braun, and A. A. Brakhage. 2004. The cyclic AMP-dependent protein kinase A network regulates development and virulence in *Aspergillus fumigatus. Infect. Immun.* **72:**5193–5203.

Litzka, O., K. Then Bergh, and A. A. Brakhage. 1996. The *Aspergillus nidulans* penicillin-biosynthesis gene aat *(penDE)* is controlled by a CCAAT-containing DNA element. *Eur. J. Biochem.* **238:**675–682.

Mabey, J. E., M. J. Anderson, P. F. Giles, C. J. Miller, T. K. Attwood, N. W. Paton, E. Bornberg-Bauer, G. D. Robson, S. G. Oliver, and D. W. Denning. 2004. CADRE: the Central *Aspergillus* Data REpository. *Nucleic Acids Res.* **32:**D401–D405.

Machida, M., K. Asai, M. Sano, T. Tanaka, T. Kumagai, G. Terai, K. Kusumoto, T. Arima, O. Akita, Y. Kashiwagi, K. Abe, K. Gomi, H. Horiuchi, K. Kitamoto, T. Kobayashi, M. Takeuchi, D. W. Denning, J. E. Galagan, W. C. Nierman, J. Yu, D. B. Archer, J. W. Bennett, D. Bhatnagar, T. E. Cleveland, N. D. Fedorova, O. Gotoh, H. Horikawa, A. Hosoyama, M. Ichinomiya, R. Igarashi, K. Iwashita, P. R. Juvvadi, M. Kato, Y. Kato, T. Kin, A. Kokubun, H. Maeda, N. Maeyama, J. Maruyama, H. Nagasaki, T. Nakajima, K. Oda, K. Okada, I. Paulsen, K. Sakamoto, T. Sawano, M. Takahashi, K. Takase, Y. Terabayashi, J. R. Wortman, O. Yamada, Y. Yamagata, H. Anazawa, Y. Hata, Y. Koide, T. Komori, Y. Koyama, T. Minetoki, S. Suharnan, A. Tanaka, K. Isono, S. Kuhara, N. Ogasawara, and H. Kikuchi. 2005. Genome sequencing and analysis of *Aspergillus oryzae. Nature* **438:**1157–1161.

McDonagh, A., N. D. Fedorova, J. Crabtree, Y. Yu, S. Kim, D. Chen, O. Loss, T. Cairns, G. Goldman, D. Armstrong-James, K. Haynes, H. Haas, M. Schrettl, G. May, W. C. Nierman, and E. Bignell. 2008. Sub-telomere directed gene expression during initiation of invasive aspergillosis. *PLoS Pathog.* **4:**e1000154.

Michael, T. P., S. Park, T. S. Kim, J. Booth, A. Byer, Q. Sun, J. Chory, and K. Lee. 2007. Simple sequence repeats provide a substrate for phenotypic variation in the *Neurospora crassa* circadian clock. *PloS One* **2:**e795.

Mirkin, S. M. 2007. Expandable DNA repeats and human disease. *Nature* **447:**932–940.

Monroy, F., and D. C. Sheppard. 2005. Tafl: a class II transposon of *Aspergillus fumigatus. Fungal Genet. Biol.* **42:**638–645.

Moxon, R., C. Bayliss, and D. Hood. 2006. Bacterial contingency loci: the role of simple sequence DNA repeats in bacterial adaptation. *Annu. Rev. Genet.* **40:**307–333.

Neuveglise, C., J. Sarfati, J. P. Latge, and S. Paris. 1996. Afut1, a retrotransposon-like element from *Aspergillus fumigatus. Nucleic Acids Res.* **24:**1428–1434.

Nierman, W. C., A. Pain, M. J. Anderson, J. R. Wortman, H. S. Kim, J. Arroyo, M. Berriman, K. Abe, D. B. Archer, C. Bermejo, J. Bennett, P. Bowyer, D. Chen, M. Collins, R. Coulsen, R. Davies, P. S. Dyer, M. Farman, N. Fedorova, N. Fedorova, T. V. Feldblyum, R. Fischer, N. Fosker, A. Fraser, J. L. Garcia, M. J. Garcia, A. Goble, G. H. Goldman, K. Gomi, S. Griffith-Jones, R. Gwilliam, B. Haas, H. Haas, D. Harris, H. Horiuchi, J. Huang, S. Humphray, J. Jimenez, N. Keller, H. Khouri, K. Kitamoto, T. Kobayashi, S. Konzack, R. Kulkarni, T. Kumagai, A. Lafon, J. P. Latge, W. Li, A. Lord, C. Lu, W. H. Majoros, G. S. May, B. L. Miller, Y. Mohamoud, M. Molina, M. Monod, I. Mouyna, S. Mulligan, L. Murphy, S. O'Neil, I. Paulsen, M. A. Penalva, M. Pertea, C. Price, B. L. Pritchard, M. A. Quail, E. Rabbinowitsch, N. Rawlins, M. A. Rajandream, U. Reichard, H. Renauld, G. D. Robson, S. Rodriguez de Cordoba, J. M. Rodriguez-Pena, C. M. Ronning, S. Rutter, S. L. Salzberg, M. Sanchez, J. C. Sanchez-Ferrero, D. Saunders, K. Seeger, R. Squares, S. Squares, M. Takeuchi, F. Tekaia, G. Turner, C. R. Vazquez de Aldana, J. Weidman, O. White, J. Woodward, J. H. Yu, C. Fraser, J. E. Galagan, K. Asai, M. Machida, N. Hall, B. Barrell, and D. W. Denning. 2005. Genomic sequence of the pathogenic and allergenic filamentous fungus *Aspergillus fumigatus. Nature* **438:**1151–1156.

Nyyssonen, E., M. Amutan, L. Enfield, J. Stubbs, and N. S. Dunn-Coleman. 1996. The transposable element Tan1 of *Aspergillus niger* var. *awamori*, a new member of the Fot1 family. *Mol. Gen. Genet.* **253:**50–56.

O'Gorman, C. M., H. T. Fuller, and P. S. Dyer. 2009. Discovery of a sexual cycle in the opportunistic fungal pathogen *Aspergillus fumigatus*. *Nature* **457:**471–474.

Oh, S. H., G. Cheng, J. A. Nuessen, R. Jajko, K. M. Yeater, X. Zhao, C. Pujol, D. R. Soll, and L. L. Hoyer. 2005. Functional specificity of *Candida albicans* Als3p proteins and clade specificity of ALS3 alleles discriminated by the number of copies of the tandem repeat sequence in the central domain. *Microbiology* **151:**673–681.

Paisley, D., G. D. Robson, and D. W. Denning. 2005. Correlation between in vitro growth rate and in vivo virulence in *Aspergillus fumigatus*. *Med. Mycol.* **43:**397–401.

Paoletti, M., C. Rydholm, E. U. Schwier, M. J. Anderson, G. Szakacs, F. Lutzoni, J. P. Debeaupuis, J. P. Latge, D. W. Denning, and P. S. Dyer. 2005. Evidence for sexuality in the opportunistic fungal pathogen *Aspergillus fumigatus*. *Curr. Biol.* **15:**1242–1248.

Paoletti, M., F. A. Seymour, M. J. Alcocer, N. Kaur, A. M. Calvo, D. B. Archer, and P. S. Dyer. 2007. Mating type and the genetic basis of self-fertility in the model fungus *Aspergillus nidulans*. *Curr. Biol.* **17:**1384–1389.

Paris, S., and J. P. Latge. 2001. Afut2, a new family of degenerate gypsy-like retrotransposon from *Aspergillus fumigatus*. *Med. Mycol.* **39:**195–198.

Patron, N. J., R. F. Waller, A. J. Cozijnsen, D. C. Straney, D. M. Gardiner, W. C. Nierman, and B. J. Howlett. 2007. Origin and distribution of epipolythiodioxopiperazine (ETP) gene clusters in filamentous ascomycetes. *BMC Evol. Biol.* **7:**174.

Pearson, C. E., K. Nichol Edamura, and J. D. Cleary. 2005. Repeat instability: mechanisms of dynamic mutations. *Nat. Rev.* **6:**729–742.

Pel, H. J., J. H. de Winde, D. B. Archer, P. S. Dyer, G. Hofmann, P. J. Schaap, G. Turner, R. P. de Vries, R. Albang, K. Albermann, M. R. Andersen, J. D. Bendtsen, J. A. Benen, M. van den Berg, S. Breestraat, M. X. Caddick, R. Contreras, M. Cornell, P. M. Coutinho, E. G. Danchin, A. J. Debets, P. Dekker, P. W. van Dijck, A. van Dijk, L. Dijkhuizen, A. J. Driessen, C. d'Enfert, S. Geysens, C. Goosen, G. S. Groot, P. W. de Groot, T. Guillemette, B. Henrissat, M. Herweijer, J. P. van den Hombergh, C. A. van den Hondel, R. T. van der Heijden, R. M. van der Kaaij, F. M. Klis, H. J. Kools, C. P. Kubicek, P. A. van Kuyk, J. Lauber, X. Lu, M. J. van der Maarel, R. Meulenberg, H. Menke, M. A. Mortimer, J. Nielsen, S. G. Oliver, M. Olsthoorn, K. Pal, N. N. van Peij, A. F. Ram, U. Rinas, J. A. Roubos, C. M. Sagt, M. Schmoll, J. Sun, D. Ussery, J. Varga, W. Vervecken, P. J. van de Vondervoort, H. Wedler, H. A. Wosten, A. P. Zeng, A. J. van Ooyen, J. Visser, and H. Stam. 2007. Genome sequencing and analysis of the versatile cell factory *Aspergillus niger* CBS 513.88. *Nat. Biotechnol.* **25:**221–231.

Perrin, R. M., N. D. Fedorova, J. W. Bok, R. A. Cramer, J. R. Wortman, H. S. Kim, W. C. Nierman, and N. P. Keller. 2007. Transcriptional regulation of chemical diversity in *Aspergillis fumigatus* by LaeA. *PLoS Pathog.* **3:**e50.

Peterson, S. W. 2008. Phylogenetic analysis of *Aspergillus* species using DNA sequences from four loci. *Mycologia* **100:**205–226.

Reeves, E. P., C. G. Messina, S. Doyle, and K. Kavanagh. 2004. Correlation between gliotoxin production and virulence of *Aspergillus fumigatus* in *Galleria mellonella*. *Mycopathologia* **158:**73–79.

Rhodes, J. C. 2006. *Aspergillus fumigatus*: growth and virulence. *Med. Mycol.* **44**(Suppl.):77–81.

Rhodes, J. C., and A. A. Brakhage. 2006. Molecular determinants of virulence in *Aspergillus fumigatus*, p. 333–345. *In* J. Heitman, S. G. Filler, J. E. Edwards, and A. P. Mitchell (ed.), *Molecular Principles of Fungal Pathogenesis*. ASM Press, Washington, DC.

Rispail, N., D. M. Soanes, C. Ant, R. Czajkowski, A. Grunler, R. Huguet, E. Perez-Nadales, A. Poli, E. Sartorel, V. Valiante, M. Yang, R. Beffa, A. A. Brakhage, N. A. Gow, R. Kahmann, M. H. Lebrun, H. Lenasi, J. Perez-Martin, N. J. Talbot, J. Wendland, and A. Di Pietro. 2009. Comparative genomics of MAP kinase and calcium-calcineurin signalling components in plant and human pathogenic fungi. *Fungal Genet. Biol.* **46:**287–298.

Rocha, E. P., I. Matic, and F. Taddei. 2002. Overrepresentation of repeats in stress response genes: a strategy to increase versatility under stressful conditions? *Nucleic Acids Res.* **30:**1886–1894.

Ruepp, A., A. Zollner, D. Maier, K. Albermann, J. Hani, M. Mokrejs, I. Tetko, U. Guldener, G. Mannhaupt, M. Munsterkotter, and H. W. Mewes. 2004. The FunCat, a functional annotation scheme for systematic classification of proteins from whole genomes. *Nucleic Acids Res.* **32:**5539–5545.

Rydholm, C., G. Szakacs, and F. Lutzoni. 2006. Low genetic variation and no detectable population structure in *Aspergillus fumigatus* compared to closely related *Neosartorya* species. *Eukaryot. Cell* **5:**650–657.

Schlotterer, C., and D. Tautz. 1994. Chromosomal homogeneity of Drosophila ribosomal DNA arrays suggests intrachromosomal exchanges drive concerted evolution. *Curr. Biol.* **4:**777–783.

Schroeckh, V., K. Scherlach, H. W. Nutzmann, E. Shelest, W. Schmidt-Heck, J. Schuemann, K. Martin, C. Hertweck, and A. A. Brakhage. 2009. Intimate bacterial-fungal interaction triggers biosynthesis of archetypal polyketides in *Aspergillus nidulans*. *Proc. Natl. Acad. Sci. USA* **106:**14558–14563.

Spikes, S., R. Xu, C. K. Nguyen, G. Chamilos, D. P. Kontoyiannis, R. H. Jacobson, D. E. Ejzykowicz, L. Y. Chiang, S. G. Filler, and G. S. May. 2008. Gliotoxin production in *Aspergillus fumigatus* contributes to host-specific differences in virulence. *J. Infect. Dis.* **197:**479–486.

Steinbach, W. J., R. A. Cramer, Jr., B. Z. Perfect, Y. G. Asfaw, T. C. Sauer, L. K. Najvar, W. R. Kirkpatrick, T. F. Patterson, D. K. Benjamin, Jr., J. Heitman, and J. R. Perfect. 2006. Calcineurin controls growth, morphology, and pathogenicity in *Aspergillus fumigatus*. *Eukaryot. Cell* **5:**1091–1103.

Sugui, J. A., J. Pardo, Y. C. Chang, K. A. Zarember, G. Nardone, E. M. Galvez, A. Mullbacher, J. I. Gallin, M. M. Simon, and K. J. Kwon-Chung. 2007. Gliotoxin is a virulence factor of *Aspergillus fumigatus*: *gliP* deletion attenuates virulence in mice immunosuppressed with hydrocortisone. *Eukaryot. Cell* **6:**1562–1569.

Sutherland, G. R., and R. I. Richards. 1995. Simple tandem DNA repeats and human genetic disease. *Proc. Natl. Acad. Sci. USA* **92:**3636–3641.

Tekaia, F., and J. P. Latge. 2005. *Aspergillus fumigatus*: saprophyte or pathogen? *Curr. Opin. Microbiol.* **8:**385–392.

Then Bergh, K., and A. A. Brakhage. 1998. Regulation of the *Aspergillus nidulans* penicillin biosynthesis gene *acvA (pcbAB)* by amino acids: implication for involvement of transcription factor PACC. *Appl. Environ. Microbiol.* **64:**843–849.

Valiante, V., T. Heinekamp, R. Jain, A. Hartl, and A. A. Brakhage. 2008. The mitogen-activated protein kinase MpkA of *Aspergillus fumigatus* regulates cell wall signaling and oxidative stress response. *Fungal Genet. Biol.* **45:**618–627.

Valiante, V., R. Jain, T. Heinekamp, and A. A. Brakhage. 2009. The MpkA MAP kinase module regulates cell wall integrity signaling and pyomelanin formation in *Aspergillus fumigatus*. *Fungal Genet. Biol.* **46:**909–918.

Venter, J. C., M. D. Adams, E. W. Myers, P. W. Li, R. J. Mural, G. G. Sutton, H. O. Smith, M. Yandell, C. A. Evans, R. A. Holt, J. D. Gocayne, P. Amanatides, R. M. Ballew, D. H. Huson, J. R. Wortman, Q. Zhang, C. D. Kodira, X. H. Zheng, L. Chen, M. Skupski, G. Subramanian, P. D. Thomas, J. Zhang, G. L. Gabor Miklos, C. Nelson, S. Broder, A. G. Clark, J. Nadeau, V. A. McKusick, N. Zinder, A. J. Levine, R. J. Roberts, M. Simon, C. Slayman, M. Hunkapiller, R. Bolanos, A. Delcher, I. Dew, D. Fasulo, M. Flanigan, L. Florea, A. Halpern, S. Hannenhalli, S. Kravitz, S. Levy, C. Mobarry, K. Reinert, K. Remington, J. Abu-Threideh, E. Beasley, K. Biddick, V. Bonazzi, R. Brandon, M. Cargill, I. Chandramouliswaran, R. Charlab, K. Chaturvedi, Z. Deng, V. Di Francesco, P. Dunn, K. Eilbeck, C. Evangelista, A. E. Gabrielian, W. Gan, W. Ge, F. Gong, Z. Gu, P. Guan, T. J. Heiman, M. E. Higgins, R. R. Ji, Z. Ke, K. A. Ketchum, Z. Lai, Y. Lei, Z. Li, J. Li, Y. Liang, X. Lin, F. Lu, G. V. Merkulov, N. Milshina, H. M. Moore, A. K. Naik, V. A. Narayan, B. Neelam, D. Nusskern, D. B. Rusch, S. Salzberg, W. Shao, B. Shue, J. Sun, Z. Wang, A. Wang, X. Wang, J. Wang, M. Wei, R. Wides, C. Xiao, C. Yan, et al. 2001. The sequence of the human genome. *Science* **291:**1304–1351.

Verstrepen, K. J., A. Jansen, F. Lewitter, and G. R. Fink. 2005. Intragenic tandem repeats generate functional variability. *Nat. Genet.* **37:**986–990.

Verstrepen, K. J., T. B. Reynolds, and G. R. Fink. 2004. Origins of variation in the fungal cell surface. *Nat. Rev. Microbiol.* **2:**533–540.

Waring, P., R. Eichner, U. Tiwari-Palni, and A. Mullbacher. 1987. Gliotoxin E: a new biologically active epipolythiodioxopiperazine from *Penicillium terlikowskii*. *Aust. J. Chem.* **40:**991–997.

HOST SUSCEPTIBILITY

IV

DNA POLYMORPHISMS AND THEIR RELEVANCE FOR INFECTIONS WITH HUMAN CYTOMEGALOVIRUS AND *Aspergillus fumigatus*

Markus Mezger, Hermann Einsele, and Juergen Loeffler

20

SINGLE-NUCLEOTIDE POLYMORPHISMS

A single-nucleotide polymorphism (SNP) is a genetic variation within a person's DNA sequence. Such an SNP variation occurs when a single nucleotide, for example, an A (adenine), is replaced by one of the other three nucleotides: C (cytosine), G (guanine), or T (thymine). Generally, these alterations of the DNA sequence have no functional impact, because most SNPs are found outside of coding or regulatory gene regions.

For researchers, SNPs located within a coding sequence are of especial interest because they can result in a nonsynonymous amino acid exchange and in consequence lead to modified proteins with reduced or, in certain cases, increased biological activity. Due to recent advances in genotyping technology, coupled with the increasing clinical importance of these genetic markers, tremendous efforts have been made to discover correlations between distinct SNPs and the course and outcome of various diseases. There are several well-studied SNPs where such a single-nucleotide exchange can have severe consequences. A very prominent example is sickle cell anemia, where GTG is replaced by GAG in the sixth codon of the β-globin gene, which results in the substitution of valine for glutamic acid and a wrong folding of the β-globin chain (Lee et al., 2005; Stuart and Nagel, 2004).

The fungal pathogen *Aspergillus fumigatus* and the human cytomegalovirus (HCMV) represent a great challenge for immunosuppressed patients (Einsele and Hebart, 2002; Marr et al., 2002). In this chapter, our current knowledge about the increasing number of genetic markers influencing the pathobiology of and susceptibility to *A. fumigatus* and HCMV is summarized.

CLINICAL RELEVANCE AND PATHOBIOLOGY OF *A. FUMIGATUS*

A. fumigatus is a mold with a worldwide distribution, which grows predominantly in soil and organic waste. The fungal conidiophores produce thousands of grey-green conidia that are easily distributed by the air (Latge, 1999). Every person is confronted with several hundred spores each day, which easily reach the respiratory system and the intestinal tract after inhalation or ingestion. In general, healthy

Markus Mezger, Kinderklinik, Hoppe-Seyler-Str. 1, 72076 Tübingen, Germany. *Hermann Einsele and Juergen Loeffler,* Medizinische Klinik and Poliklinik II, Josef-Schneider-Str. 2, 97070 Würzburg, Germany.

Genome Plasticity and Infectious Diseases,
Edited by J. Hacker, U. Dobrindt, and R. Kurth,

people do not develop clinical symptoms because the intact immune system is able to eliminate invading fungal cells. However, due to the immunosuppression of hematopoietic stem cell transplant recipients, *A. fumigatus* is not always eliminated but can be disseminated via the bloodstream to different organs (Latge, 2001). In spite of various safety precautions, after allogeneic stem cell transplantation (allo-SCT) between 10% and 30% of patients develop an invasive aspergillosis which is often lethal, with a mortality rate of up to 90% if patients are not treated in time with antifungal drugs.

As an opportunistic human pathogen in immunocompromised individuals, *A. fumigatus* is associated with allergic disorders, severe asthma, and sinusitis and can cause potentially lethal invasive infections. Once the spores have gained entry, conidia start to germinate, resulting in germ tubes and later in hyphae that can become invasive and are carried in the blood to various organs (Latge, 2001). Localized lung tissue damage and local thrombosis of the lungs are major complications after allo-SCT, occurring in up to 50% of transplant recipients and accounting for much of the transplant-related mortality (Paterson and Singh, 1999).

Further complications that arise after exposure to *A. fumigatus* include allergic bronchopulmonary aspergillosis (ABPA) with hypersensitivity reactions that often occur in immunocompetent hosts with asthma or cystic fibrosis (Gibson et al., 2006). Subacute forms of pulmonary aspergillosis often result in multiple expanding cavities in the lungs, appropriately named chronic cavitary pulmonary aspergillosis (CCPA). It is distinguished histologically from chronic necrotizing pulmonary aspergillosis (CNPA) by the lack of visible hyphal invasion of tissue (Vaid et al., 2007).

SNPs ASSOCIATED WITH *A. FUMIGATUS* INFECTIONS

Alveolar macrophages, monocytes, and polymorphonuclear neutrophils have been shown to be essential for capable clearance of fungal cells. It is undisputed that efficient killing of fungi requires recognition by different immune receptors. In the last decade, several families of immune receptors have been discovered which are involved in the recognition of fungi. These receptors include the family of the Toll-like receptors (TLRs). TLR2 and TLR4 have been implicated as important components of the initial host immune response to fungal pathogens (Romani, 2004; Pamer, 2008).

The relevance of genetic markers in TLR genes is controversial. Kesh et al. (2005) showed an association of IA after allo-SCT with defined SNPs in *TLR1* and *TLR6*, whereas no involvement of markers (896 A/G and 1196 C/T) in *TLR4* was observable. This observation is in agreement with our own results; no association with IA after allo-SCT was detectable for the following five SNPs in *TLR4*: rs1927911 (7764 G/A), rs4986790 (896 A/G), rs2737191 (1256 A/G), rs5030728 (12823 A/G), and rs1554973 (19353 C/T) (Mezger et al., 2008a). In contrast, Bochud et al. (2008) analyzed two similar patient cohorts and found an association of a haplotype in the third exon of *TLR4* consisting of rs4986790 (1063 A/G) and rs4986791 (1363 C/T). However, these findings were subsequently questioned by several authors; Levitz and coworkers hypothesized that application of amphotericin B may activate phagocytotic cells by stimulation of TLR4, which in turn contributes to its antifungal activity (Levitz et al., 2009; Sau et al., 2003). In addition, Cervera et al. (2009) suggested that HCMV infection could be an intermediate variable in the association with TLR4 polymorphisms with aspergillosis and Asakura and Komatsu (2009) raised the question of the frequency of these markers in TLR4, as the relevant SNPs rs4986790 and rs4986791 are missing in the Asian population, where IA is also a common life-threatening complication after allo-SCT. The findings of Asakura and Komatsu (2009) confirmed data obtained by Carvalho et al. (2008) that revealed an association of the nucleotide substitution rs4986790 with CCPA. The same group (Carvalho et al., 2009) recently presented a significant association between the presence of the cosegregating Asp-299Gly/Thr399Ile polymorphisms (in *TLR4*) and fungal colonization ($P = 0.003$; odds ratio

[OR] = 10.6). In parallel, susceptibility to fungal infections, predominantly fungal pneumonia, was significantly decreased in the presence of the same polymorphisms ($P = 0.03$; OR = 0.23).

After internalization of fungi and upon direct contact, various cytokine and chemokine genes are differentially expressed, including *IL-1, IL-6, IL-10, IL-12,* and *TNF-α* (Roilides et al., 1998). There are a limited number of reports that SNPs in cytokine and cytokine receptor genes are involved in the efficiency of an immune response to *A. fumigatus*. Sainz et al. (2007b, 2008a) identified rs1143627 in *IL-1β* and a variable number of tandem repeats (at position −322) in the promoter region of *TNFR2* as a possible risk factor for IA in hematology patients, whereas SNPs in the TNFR2 ligands *TNF-α* (positions −308 and +489) and *LT-α* (position +252) (encoding lymphotoxin α) were not associated with IA. In addition, the genetic variants at positions −174 (C/G) and −634 (G/C) in the promoter of *IL-6* were not associated with susceptibility to IA in hematological patients (Sainz et al., 2008b).

Furthermore, genetic markers involved in the pathogenesis of IA were discovered in the promoter region of the *IL-10* gene. Interleukin-10 (IL-10) is an anti-inflammatory cytokine, which down-regulates the expression of Th1 cytokines, major histocompatibility complex class II antigens, and costimulatory molecules. The promoter of *IL-10* contains several polymorphisms from which SNPs at positions −1082, −819, and −592 have been intensively investigated (Turner et al., 1997). Haplotype analysis identified a protective role of the ACC haplotype in the development of IA after allo-SCT (Seo et al., 2005). Confirming these findings, our own group was able to find a statistical association between rs1800896 (−1082, G/A) and rs1878672 (2068, G/C) and the occurrence of IA (Mezger et al., 2008a). The polymorphism at position −1082 has been previously reported to produce higher levels of IL-10 if the G allele is present and lower levels if the A allele is present (Turner et al., 1997; Tagore et al., 1999).

In a large screening of 18 genes encoding cytokines and cytokine receptors (*CCL2, CCR1, CCR5, CCR6, CCR7, CLEC7A, CXCL10, ICAM-1, IFNG, IL-4, IL-6, IL-10, IL-12B, IL-18, SCYA20, TLR2, TLR4,* and *TNF-α*), 84 polymorphisms were analyzed for a possible association with the occurrence of IA in patients after allo-SCT (Mezger et al., 2008a). Three markers (rs1554013, rs3921, and rs4257674) in *CXCL10* (IFN-γ -inducible 10-kDa protein) and one marker (rs2069705) in *IFN-γ* were associated with a risk of contracting IA ($P <$ 0.010). CXCL10 is an inflammatory mediator, induced by IFN-γ, which stimulates the directional migration of Th1 cells as well as increasing T-cell adhesion to the endothelium (Loetscher et al., 1996). Haplotype analysis for rs1554013 (C/T), rs3921 (C/G), rs4859588 (A/G), and rs4257674 (A/G) in *CXCL10* confirmed the single-marker analysis and clearly identified "CGAG" as the high-risk haplotype. Furthermore, functional analysis revealed that immature dendritic cells exposed to *A. fumigatus* germlings showed higher *CXCL10* expression if carrying the wild-type genotype compared to the "CGAG" high-risk haplotype. In addition, in a small preliminary study, serum from patients with proven or probable IA showed increased levels of CXCL10 compared to serum from matched immunocompromised patients without evidence of IA.

Furthermore, the serum protein mannose-binding lectin (MBL) is a key molecule during fungal infection, enhancing innate immune mechanisms by binding to cell wall components of *A. fumigatus* (Vaid et al., 2007). Attachment to fungal cells is a strong signal for phagocytosis by immune effector cells and for activation of the lectin complement pathway, as well as for release of proinflammatory cytokines (Takahashi et al., 2008).

One defined genetic marker (rs36203921, 1011 A/G) in the *MBL* gene was found to contribute to allergic ABPA by influencing the level of MBL in plasma and the protein activity (Kaur et al., 2006, 2007). The group demonstrated that patients homozygous for the 1011 A allele showed significantly higher plasma MBL levels and activity in comparison to patients homozygous for the G allele. As this

TABLE 1 Association between defined genetic polymorphisms and an increased risk to suffer from diseases with *A. fumigatus*

Gene	dbSNP no.	SNP position[a]	No. Asp positive	No. Asp negative	*P* value[a]	Population	Disease[b]	Reference
CXCL10 (4q21)	rs1554013	11101 **C**/T* (downstream)	51	49	0.007	Caucasian	IA after HSCT (EORTC/IFICG)	Mezger et al. (2008a)
	rs3921	1642 C/**G*** (3′ UTR)	39	46	0.003			
	rs4257674	-1101 A/**G*** (promoter)	52	44	0.001			
IFN-γ (12q14)	rs2069705	-1616 C/**T*** (promoter)	69	56	0.010			
IL-10 (1q31-q32)	rs1800896	-1082 A/**G** (promoter)	58	55	0.046			
	rs1878672	2068 C/**G*** (intron)	67	57	0.025			
	rs1800896	-1082 A/**G** (promoter)	119 *Af* col. 27 ABPA	232	0.020	Caucasian	Colonization with *A. fumigatus* or ABPA after CF	Brouard et al. (2005)
	rs1800896	-1082 A/**G**	9	96	0.012	Korean	IPA after HSCT (EORTC/MSG)	Seo et al. (2005)
	rs1800871 rs1800872 (haplotype)	-819 C/**T** -592 **A**/C (promoter)						
	rs1800896	-1082 A/**G** (promoter)	59	61	0.052	Caucasian	IPA in hematologic patients (EORTC/IFICG)	Sainz et al. (2007a*)
IL-1β (2q14)	rs1143627	-511 C/**T** (promoter)	59	51	0.095	Caucasian	IPA in hematologic patients (EORTC/IFICG)	Sainz et al. (2008a)
IL-4Rα (16p12.1-p11.2)	rs1805010	4679 A/C/G/T (75 I/L/F/V)	40	56	0.008	Caucasian	ABPA	Knutsen et al. (2006)
MBL (10q11.2-q21)	rs5030737	868 C/**T** (52 C/R)	15	82	0.020	Caucasian	CCPA	Vaid et al. (2007)
	rs36203921	1011 **A**/G (intron)	11	84	<0.003	Indian	ABPA	Kaur et al. (2006)
	rs5030737	868 C/**T** (52 C/R)	10	82	0.015	Caucasian	CNPA	Crosdale et al. (2001)

Plg (6q26)	rs4252125	28904 **A**/G* (472 N/D)	83	147	<0.001	Caucasian	IA after HSCT (EORTC/IFICG)	Zaas et al. (2008)
SFTPA2 (10q22.3)	rs17886221	1660 A/**G** (94 R/R)	10	11	0.058	Indian	ABPA	Saxena et al. (2003)
	rs17886395	1649 C/**G** (91 A/P)			0.031			Madan et al. (2005)
	rs17880349	1492 C/**T** (intron)	7	46	0.090	Caucasian	ABPA	Vaid et al. (2007)
TLR1 (4p14)	rs5743611	239 C/**G** (80 R/T)	22	105	<0.001	Caucasian	IA after HSCT (EORTC/IFICG)	Kesh et al. (2005)
	rs4833095	743 **A**/G (248 S/N)						
TLR4 (9q32-q33)	rs4986790	1063 A/**G** (299 D/G)	103	263	0.020	Caucasian	IA after HSCT (EORTC)	Bochud et al. (2008)
	rs4986791 (haplotype)	1363 C/**T** (399 I/T)						
	rs4986790	1063 A/**G** (299 D/G)	40	80	0.003	Caucasian	CCPA	Carvalho et al. (2008)
TLR6 (4p14)	rs5743810	745 **C**/T (249 S/P)	22	105	See *TLR1*	Caucasian	IA after HSCT (EORTC/IFICG)	Kesh et al. (2005)
TLR9 (3p21.3)	rs5743836	-1237 **C**/T (promoter)	22	80	0.043	Caucasian	ABPA	Carvalho et al. (2008)
TNFR2 (1p36.3-p36.2)	VNTR	-322 (promoter)	54	48	0.029	Caucasian	IPA in hematologic patients (EORTC/IFICG)	Sainz et al. (2007b)

[a]Significant *P* values ($p < 0.050$) as obtained by statistical tests are indicated, respectively. In all markers, risk alleles are labeled in bold type. *, positions of the SNPs have been determined at http://snpper.chip.org/. Please note that localization of SNPs might differ from localizations indicated in other databases.

[b]VNTR, variable number of tandem repeats; IPA, invasive pulmonary aspergillosis; CF, cystic fibrosis; EORTC European Organization for Research and Treatment of Cancer; IFICG, Invasive Fungal Infections Cooperative Group; MSG, Mycoses Study Group (Ascioglu et al., 2002).

polymorphism is situated in an intron, further SNPs in exons or the promoter region of the *MBL* gene might be in linkage disequilibrium and account for the elevated MBL levels.

Additional data supporting the relevance of MBL have been published by Vaid et al. (2007) and Crosdale et al., (2001); both groups observed an association of the rs5030737 marker (868 C/T) with CCPA or CNPA in the Caucasian population, respectively. The nonsynonymous amino acid exchange from arginine to cysteine (at position 52) results in lower levels of functional MBL in serum.

Besides *MBL*, further C-type lectin genes were analyzed, leading to the identification of an association between ABPA and the variants rs17886395 (1649 C/G) and rs17886221 (1660 A/G) of the surfactant protein A2 *(SFPTPA2)* gene (Madan et al., 2005; Saxena et al., 2003). Pulmonary surfactant consists of a complex mixture of lipids and proteins, for example, the surfactant proteins SP-A and SP-D, which can bind to *A. fumigatus* conidia in alveolar fluid (Allen et al., 1999). In consequence, allergic responses are inhibited by reducing cellular lung infiltration in murine models (Kishore et al., 2006). However, in this study, only a small cohort of Indian patients (10 with ABPA and 11 without ABPA) was investigated and analyses of the National Center for Biotechnology Information (NCBI) databases revealed that this marker is very rare in the European population.

In contrast, there are data supporting the notion that the SNP rs17880349 (1492 C/T) in *SFPTPA2* might be a risk factor for ABPA, as revealed by Vaid et al. (2007): despite a small cohort of patients with ABPA (n = 7), they found an association in the Caucasian population. Further work with a larger number of patients might confirm these results.

Other studies of the role of surfactant proteins in the context of allergic airway responses have been published recently. Brandt et al. (2008) proposed that a polymorphism (Met11Thr) in the surfactant protein D gene (*SFTPD*) is associated with atopy in the black population and potentially with lower asthma susceptibility in white subjects.

Among many other factors, blood coagulation is regulated by plasminogen. Recently, it was demonstrated that plasminogen binds directly to *A. fumigatus* in a dose-dependent manner, influencing the pathogenesis of invasive fungal infections (Zaas et al., 2008). The same group was also able to demonstrate a correlation between an SNP in the plasminogen gene and the risk of contracting IA (Asp472Asn) (Zaas et al., 2008). Their association study was performed with a cohort of 236 allo-SCT recipients. It can be hypothesized that binding of plasminogen to the fungal cell wall leads to activation of this enzyme, which in turn mediates local destruction of the lung tissue, thereby promoting pathogen invasion and pulmonary hemorrhage (Sun et al., 2004).

In Table 1, our current knowledge about genetic markers that have an impact on *Aspergillus*-mediated diseases is summarized.

CLINICAL RELEVANCE AND PATHOBIOLOGY OF HCMV

Besides *A. fumigatus*, immunosuppressed patients have an increased risk for infections with the betaherpesvirus HCMV. After primary infection, the virus is not completely eliminated by the host immune system and remains hidden in different cell types until reactivation occurs when the immune system is not able to prevent the progress of HCMV infection.

HCMV is one of the most demanding complications after allo-SCT. Roughly half of the patients with HCMV infection not receiving antiviral chemotherapy experience HCMV reactivation and disease (Hebart and Einsele, 2004). Various clinical parameters have been identified as being associated with an increased risk for HCMV reactivation and disease (Anasetti, 2008). The enrichment of $CD34^+$ cells prior to transplantation leads to a delayed immune reconstitution because of a parallel depletion of B and T cells in the transplant. Furthermore, severe acute and chronic graft-versus-host disease, as well as treatment with corticosteroids, is significantly related to HCMV disease. The highest risk for patients after transplantation exists when stem cells from an HCMV-negative donor are transferred into an HCMV-positive recipient, because the new developing immune system has never been confronted with HCMV before.

Throughout acute and latent infection, HCMV interacts with various target cells. The ability of HCMV to recognize and enter a wide range of cells, including dendritic cells, monocytes, macrophages, endothelial cells, epithelial cells, muscle cells, and fibroblasts, suggests that it uses different receptors. During the complex entry path, HCMV initially binds to heparan sulfate proteoglycans on the host cell surface (Compton, 2004). A stronger connection is mediated by binding of glycoprotein B (gB), a major compound of the viral capsid, to one of the cellular receptors. Virus entry receptors include epidermal growth factor receptor (Wang et al., 2003), integrins (Feire et al., 2004), and the dendritic cell-specific ICAM3-grabbing nonintegrin (DC-SIGN) (Halary et al., 2002).

In response to infection, both innate and adaptive immune mechanisms are activated, including interferon (IFN) production and $CD8^+$ T-lymphocyte-mediated clearance of infected cells. For early detection of HCMV, TLR2 has been described as an important innate immune receptor for induction of the proinflammatory cytokine response after recognition of gB (Compton et al., 2003).

SNPs INFLUENCING SUSCEPTIBILITY TO HCMV

For exploration of HCMV risk markers, 90 SNPs of 17 immune-related gene loci *(IL-4, IL-6, IL-10, IL-12p40, IL-18, IFN-γ, TNF-α, CCL2, MCP1, CXCL10, CCR1, CCR5, CCR6, CCR7, ICAM1, TLR2,* and *TLR4)* have been genotyped by our group to investigate an association between defined SNPs and HCMV reactivation (DNAemia) and HCMV disease. We found no significant association between 71 of 80 markers and the occurrence of HCMV reactivation or disease in patients after allo-SCT. However, the other nine SNPs showed a significant association with HCMV reactivation and/or disease. These markers are located in *CCR5, MCP-1,* and *IL-10* (Loeffler et al., 2006).

The SNP rs1800896 (-1082 A/G) in *IL-10* was identified as a genetic risk factor, which contributes to a higher risk for HCMV disease after allo-SCT. This observation is supported by Alakulppi et al. (2006), who observed an association of rs1800896 with HCMV infection after kidney transplantation. Interestingly, the same SNP has already been reported to be associated with an increased risk for invasive aspergillosis (see above). In addition, the haplotype ATA at positions −1082, −819, and −592 protects against early Epstein-Barr virus infection by influencing IL-10 levels (Helminen et al., 2001). On the basis of these data, the influence of promoter polymorphisms in *IL-10* seems to be undisputed and might be one valuable target for realizing the concept of screening for high-risk patients and personalized medicine. Additionally, interesting in vitro experiments using transfected HeLa cell clones have identified two common variants (rs3135932 [A/G → Ser159Gly] and rs2229113 [A/G → Gly351Arg]) in the IL-10 receptor 1, which reduce signaling activity of these receptor types after binding of IL-10 (Gruber et al., 2008).

Protein tyrosine phosphatase nonreceptor type 22 (PTPN22) is an important negative regulator of T-cell activation. A C/T transition in *PTPN22* at position 1858 (rs2476601) results in an amino acid substitution from arginine to tryptophan (Arg620Trp) and has been shown to be associated with several autoimmune diseases (Vang et al., 2008). However, a recent study revealed no association with HCMV and fungal infections in 192 bone marrow transplant recipients (Azarian et al., 2008). Also, in a normal Chinese Han population, the marker rs16375 (now merged into rs1704) with a 14-bp insertion/deletion in the *human leukocyte antigen-G (HLA-G)* gene was found to be a susceptible polymorphism for active HCMV infection (Zheng et al., 2009).

HCMV reactivation is common in immunocompromised patients, for example in human immunodeficiency virus-infected individuals with fewer than 100 $CD4^+$ cells/μl (Moenkemeyer et al., 2009). There are several studies describing a correlation between defined genetic variations and a higher risk for severe HCMV reactivation in human immunodeficiency virus-infected patients: Moenkemeyer et al. (2009) reported an association between an additional nucleotide insertion in exon 5 of the major histocompatibility complex class I chain-related A (MICA) gene. Additionally, polymorphogenic sites spanning the region near the *TNF* locus are associated with retinitis in AIDS patients (Deghaide et al., 2009).

A very large cohort of HCMV-positive tested individuals (n = 188) has been analyzed by Hoffmann et al. (2008) for the marker rs3212227 in the *IL-12p40* gene. The authors could demonstrate that HCMV infection more often occurred after kidney transplantation, when the high-risk allele (C→A) was present (Hoffmann et al., 2009). This SNP is located in the 3′ untranslated region (UTR) of *IL-12p40* and has been shown to influence the stability of mRNA and protein production (Stanilova and Miteva, 2005). In a further study, in 469 kidney graft recipients a SNP (rs11568821) within intron 4 of a gene called *programmed death 1* (*PD-1*) was found to contribute to HCMV infections, even in combination with the IL-12p40 3′ UTR SNP rs3212227 (Hoffmann et al., 2009). PD-1 is an inhibitor of IFN-γ production, and, interestingly, another group could demonstrate that patients after allo-SCT with a defined microsatellite polymorphism in the first intron of *IFN-γ* (13-CA-repeat) had more frequent HCMV reactivation and a higher viral load (Jaskula et al., 2009).

The analysis of association between defined SNPs (n = 14) in TLR genes *(TLR3, TLR8,* and *TLR9),* as well as important entry receptor genes (i.e., *EGFR, ITGB3,* and *DC-SIGN*) and asymptomatic HCMV reactivation and disease in patients after allo-SCT revealed interesting data. Two SNPs (rs735240, G→A; rs2287886, C→T) in the promoter region of *DC-SIGN* showed significant association with an increased risk for the development of HCMV reactivation and disease. Furthermore, these genetic markers influenced the expression levels of *DC-SIGN* on immature dendritic cells, and decreased expression reduced HCMV infection efficiency (Mezger et al., 2008b).

In addition, a recent report by Carvalho et al. (2009) suggested that the presence of one marker (rs5743836) at position −1237 (C/T) in the *TLR9* gene influenced susceptibility to viral pneumonia in patients after allo-SCT. The same marker was found a year earlier by the same group to be associated with ABPA (Carvalho et al., 2008).

Furthermore, a specific SNP (rs5743708) in *TLR2* results in an amino acid substitution from arginine to glutamine and a functional defect in stimulation with the TLR2 ligand lipopeptide (von Aulock et al., 2004). Kijpittayarit et al. (2007) found a statistical association between this mutation and HCMV replication and disease after liver transplantation in patients with underlying chronic hepatitis C infection. The association was attributable to impaired TLR2-mediated immune signaling in response to HCMV gB (Brown et al., 2009). On the other hand, from the point of view of the virus, new data show that different gB genotypes (gB1 through gB4) had no effect on virological or clinical HCMV recurrence after solid-organ transplantation, as well as on specific clinical presentation or organ involvement in infants (Manuel et al., 2009; Mewara et al., 2009). The authors concluded that no specific gB genotype confers a virulence advantage, although mixed gB infections contributed to higher viral loads and delayed viral clearance (Manuel et al., 2009).

Concerning SNPs in *TLR4*, the two well-characterized markers rs4986790 (Asp299Gly) and rs4986791 (Thr399Ile) showed a trend of the mutant group toward a greater incidence of HCMV disease in renal transplant recipients (Cervera et al., 2007). Supporting data were reported by Ducloux et al. (2005), who observed an association of these markers with HCMV infection in a similar patient cohort. However, a limitation of both studies is the small number of *TLR4* polymorphism carriers suffering from HCMV disease; it therefore seems reasonable to increase the sample size for confirmation of previous observations.

In Table 2, our current knowledge about genetic markers that have an impact on HCMV-mediated diseases is summarized.

TABLE 2 Association between defined genetic polymorphisms and an increased risk to suffer from diseases with HCMV

Gene	dbSNP no.	SNP position[a]	No. HCMV positive	No. HCMV negative	*P* value[a]	Population	Disease	Reference
CCR5 (3p21)	rs2734648	-2554 **G**/T* (intron)	67	69	0.014	Caucasian	HCMV disease after HSCT[b]	Loeffler et al. (2006)
	rs1800023	-2086 **A**/G* (5′ UTR)	64	68	0.011			
DC-SIGN (19p13)	rs2287886	-139 **C**/T* (promoter)	76	39	0.003		HCMV disease after HSCT	Mezger et al. (2008b)
	rs735240	-939 A/**G*** (promoter)	73	36	0.010		HCMV reactivation after HSCT	
HLA-G (6p21.3)	rs1704	2961 C/T (3′ UTR)	54	165	0.002	Chinese Han	HCMV infection	Zheng et al. (2009)
IL-10 (1q31-q32)	rs1800896	-1082 A/**G** (promoter)	61	61	0.001		HCMV disease after HSCT	Loeffler et al. (2006)
	rs1878672	2068 C/**G*** (intron)	63	70	0.003		HCMV disease after HSCT	
	rs1800896	-1082 A/**G** (promoter)	62	71	0.031		HCMV infection after kidney transplantation	Alakulppi et al. (2006)
IL-12p40 (5q31.1-q33.1)	rs3212227	16974 A/**C** (3′ UTR)	188	281	0.031		HCMV infection after kidney transplantation	Hoffmann et al. (2008)
MCP-1 (17q11.2-q21.1)	rs1024611	-2581 **C**/T* (promoter)	106	91	0.029		HCMV reactivation after HSCT	Loeffler et al. (2006)
	rs13900	1543 C/**T*** (3′ UTR)	99	90	0.014		HCMV disease after HSCT	
PD-1 (2q37.3)	rs11568821	7079 A/G (Intron 4)	188	281	0.006		HCMV infection after kidney transplantation	Hoffmann et al. (2008)
TLR2 (4q32)	rs5743708	2258 A/G* (753 R/Q)	25	67	0.080		HCMV infection after liver transplantation	Kijpittayarit et al. (2007)
TLR4 (9q32-q33)	rs4986790	1063 A/**G** (299 D/G)	61	177	0.080		HCMV disease after kidney transplantation	Ducloux et al. (2005)
	rs4986791 (haplotype)	1063 A/**G** (299 D/G)						
TLR9 (3p21.3)	rs5743836	-1237 **C**/T (promoter)	87	134	0.040		HCMV disease after HSCT	Carvalho et al. (2009)

[a]Significant *P* values ($P < 0.050$) as obtained by statistical tests are indicated, respectively. In all markers, risk alleles are labeled in bold type. *, positions of the SNPs were determined at http://snpper.chip.org/. Please note that localization of SNPs might differ from localizations indicated in other databases.
[b]HSCT, hematopoietic stem cell transplantation.

CONCLUSIONS

Future work has to be done to clarify whether the genetic markers identified so far show significant associations in other patient cohorts as well. We propose that, beyond discovering studies, functional analysis has to follow for every SNP (not yet done) to underline its relevance in the context of fungal infections.

Another interesting point is the importance of ethnicity in susceptibility to fungal and viral infections. Although *A. fumigatus* and HCMV have a worldwide distribution, it seems obvious that vulnerability is usually controlled from variants in several immunorelevant genes, which mostly show altered frequency and biological significance in different populations. Moreover, it might be interesting to determine cross talks and antagonistic and/or synergistic effects of the so far identified SNPs on the risk for fungal and/or viral infections. Finally, the hope for early identification of patients at risk for *A. fumigatus* and/or HCMV infection is legitimate and might have an impact on individualization of antifungal and antiviral prophylaxis and treatment in the near future.

REFERENCES

Alakulppi, N. S., L. E. Kyllonen, H. M. Salo, J. Partanen, K. T. Salmela, and J. T. Laine. 2006. The impact of donor cytokine gene polymorphisms on the incidence of cytomegalovirus infection after kidney transplantation. *Transpl. Immunol.* **16:**258–262.

Allen, M. J., R. Harbeck, B. Smith, D. R. Voelker, and R. J. Mason. 1999. Binding of rat and human surfactant proteins A and D to *Aspergillus fumigatus* conidia. *Infect. Immun.* **67:**4563–4569.

Anasetti, C. 2008. What are the most important donor and recipient factors affecting the outcome of related and unrelated allogeneic transplantation? *Best Pract. Res. Clin. Haematol.* **21:**691–697.

Asakura, Y., and T. Komatsu. 2009. Toll-like receptor 4 polymorphisms and aspergillosis. *N. Engl. J. Med.* **360:**635; author reply 635–636.

Ascioglu, S., J. H. Rex, B. de Pauw, J. E. Bennett, J. Bille, F. Crokaert, D. W. Denning, J. P. Donnelly, J. E. Edwards, Z. Erjavec, D. Fiere, O. Lortholary, J. Maertens, J. F. Meis, T. F. Patterson, J. Ritter, D. Selleslag, P. M. Shah, D. A. Stevens, and T. J. Walsh. 2002. Defining opportunistic invasive fungal infections in immunocompromised patients with cancer and hematopoietic stem cell transplants: an international consensus. *Clin. Infect. Dis.* **34:**7–14.

Azarian, M., M. Busson, V. Rocha, P. Ribaud, R. Peffault de Latour, H. Bleux, V. Lepage, D. Charron, A. Toubert, G. Socié, and P. Loiseau. 2008. The PTPN22 R620W polymorphism is associated with severe bacterial infections after human leukocyte antigen geno-identical haematopoietic stem-cell transplantations. *Transplantation* **85:**1859–1862.

Bochud, P. Y., J. W. Chien, K. A. Marr, W. M. Leisenring, A. Upton, M. Janer, S. D. Rodrigues, S. Li, J. A. Hansen, L. P. Zhao, A. Aderem, and M. Boeckh. 2008. Toll-like receptor 4 polymorphisms and aspergillosis in stem-cell transplantation. *N. Engl. J. Med.* **359:**1766–1777.

Brandt, E. B., M. K. Mingler, M. D. Stevenson, N. Wang, G. K. Khurana Hershey, J. A. Whitsett, and M. E. Rothenberg. 2008. Surfactant protein D alters allergic lung responses in mice and human subjects. *J. Allergy Clin. Immunol.* **121:**1140–1147.

Brouard, J., N. Knauer, P. Y. Boelle, H. Corvol, A. Henrion-Caude, C. Flamant, F. Bremont, B. Delaisi, J. F. Duhamel, C. Marguet, M. Roussey, M. C. Miesch, K. Chadelat, M. Boule, B. Fauroux, F. Ratjen, H. Grasemann, and A. Clement. 2005. Influence of interleukin-10 on *Aspergillus fumigatus* infection in patients with cystic fibrosis. *J. Infect. Dis.* **191:**1988–1991.

Brown, R. A., J. H. Gralewski, and R. R. Razonable. 2009. The R753Q polymorphism abrogates toll-like receptor 2 signaling in response to human cytomegalovirus. *Clin. Infect. Dis.* **49:**96–99.

Carvalho, A., C. Cunha, A. Carotti, T. Aloisi, O. Guarrera, M. Di Ianni, F. Falzetti, F. Bistoni, F. Aversa, L. Pitzurra, F. Rodrigues, and L. Romani. 2009. Polymorphisms in Toll-like receptor genes and susceptibility to infections in allogeneic stem cell transplantation. *Exp. Hematol.* **37:**1022–1029.

Carvalho, A., A. C. Pasqualotto, L. Pitzurra, L. Romani, D. W. Denning, and F. Rodrigues. 2008. Polymorphisms in toll-like receptor genes and susceptibility to pulmonary aspergillosis. *J. Infect. Dis.* **197:**618–621.

Cervera, C., F. Lozano, N. Saval, I. Gimferrer, A. Ibanez, B. Suarez, L. Linares, F. Cofan, M. J. Ricart, N. Esforzado, M. A. Marcos, T. Pumarola, F. Oppenheimer, J. M. Campistol, and A. Moreno. 2007. The influence of innate immunity gene receptors polymorphisms in renal transplant infections. *Transplantation* **83:**1493–1500.

Cervera, C., A. Moreno, and F. Lozano. 2009. Toll-like receptor 4 polymorphisms and aspergillosis. *N. Engl. J. Med.* **360:**634–635; author reply 635–636.

Compton, T. 2004. Receptors and immune sensors: the complex entry path of human cytomegalovirus. *Trends Cell Biol.* **14:**5–8.

Compton, T., E. A. Kurt-Jones, K. W. Boehme, J. Belko, E. Latz, D. T. Golenbock, and R. W. Finberg. 2003. Human cytomegalovirus activates inflammatory cytokine responses via CD14 and Toll-like receptor 2. *J. Virol.* **77:**4588–4596.

Crosdale, D. J., K. V. Poulton, W. E. Ollier, W. Thomson, and D. W. Denning. 2001. Mannose-binding lectin gene polymorphisms as a susceptibility factor for chronic necrotizing pulmonary aspergillosis. *J. Infect. Dis.* **184:**653–656.

Deghaide, N. H., M. D. L. Rodrigues, E. C. Castelli, C. T. Mendes-Junior, J. F. Figueiredo, and E. A. Donadi. 2009. Tumor necrosis factor region polymorphisms are associated with AIDS and with cytomegalovirus retinitis. *AIDS* **23:**1641–1647.

Ducloux, D., M. Deschamps, M. Yannaraki, C. Ferrand, J. Bamoulid, P. Saas, A. Kazory, J. M. Chalopin, and P. Tiberghien. 2005. Relevance of Toll-like receptor-4 polymorphisms in renal transplantation. *Kidney Int.* **67:**2454–2461.

Einsele, H., and H. Hebart. 2002. Cellular immunity to viral and fungal antigens after stem cell transplantation. *Curr. Opin. Hematol.* **9:**485–489.

Feire, A. L., H. Koss, and T. Compton. 2004. Cellular integrins function as entry receptors for human cytomegalovirus via a highly conserved disintegrin-like domain. *Proc. Natl. Acad. Sci. USA* **101:**15470–15475.

Gibson, P. G. 2006. Allergic bronchopulmonary aspergillosis. *Semin. Respir. Crit. Care Med.* **27:**185–191.

Gruber, S. G., M. Gloria Luciani, P. Grundtner, A. Zdanov, and C. Gasche. 2008. Differential signaling of cmvIL-10 through common variants of the IL-10 receptor 1. *Eur. J. Immunol.* **38:**3365–3375.

Halary, F., A. Amara, H. Lortat-Jacob, M. Messerle, T. Delaunay, C. Houles, F. Fieschi, F. Arenzana-Seisdedos, J. F. Moreau, and J. Dechanet-Merville. 2002. Human cytomegalovirus binding to DC-SIGN is required for dendritic cell infection and target cell trans-infection. *Immunity* **17:**653–664.

Hebart, H., and H. Einsele. 2004. Clinical aspects of CMV infection after stem cell transplantation. *Hum. Immunol.* **65:**432–436.

Helminen, M. E., S. Kilpinen, M. Virta, and M. Hurme. 2001. Susceptibility to primary Epstein-Barr virus infection is associated with interleukin-10 gene promoter polymorphism. *J. Infect. Dis.* **184:**777–780.

Hoffmann, T. W., J. M. Halimi, M. Buchler, F. Velge-Roussel, A. Al-Najjar, J. F. Marliere, Y. Lebranchu, and C. Baron. 2009. Impact of a polymorphism in the IL-12p40 gene on the outcome of kidney transplantation. *Transplant. Proc.* **41:**654–656.

Hoffmann, T. W., J. M. Halimi, M. Buchler, F. Velge-Roussel, A. Goudeau, A. Al-Najjar, J. F. Marliere, Y. Lebranchu, and C. Baron. 2010. Association between a polymorphism in the human programmed death-1 (PD-1) gene and CMV infection after kidney transplantation. *J. Med. Genet.* **47:**54–58.

Hoffmann, T. W., J. M. Halimi, M. Buchler, F. Velge-Roussel, A. Goudeau, A. Al Najjar, M. D. Boulanger, T. S. Houssaini, J. F. Marliere, Y. Lebranchu, and C. Baron. 2008. Association between a polymorphism in the IL-12p40 gene and cytomegalovirus reactivation after kidney transplantation. *Transplantation* **85:**1406–1411.

Jaskula, E., D. Dlubek, D. Duda, K. Bogunia-Kubik, A. Mlynarczewska, and A. Lange. 2009. Interferon gamma 13-CA-repeat homozygous genotype and a low proportion of CD4(+) lymphocytes are independent risk factors for cytomegalovirus reactivation with a high number of copies in hematopoietic stem cell transplantation recipients. *Biol. Blood Marrow Transplant.* **15:**1296–1305.

Kaur, S., V. K. Gupta, A. Shah, S. Thiel, P. U. Sarma, and T. Madan. 2006. Elevated levels of mannan-binding lectin [corrected] (MBL) and eosinophilia in patients of bronchial asthma with allergic rhinitis and allergic bronchopulmonary aspergillosis associate with a novel intronic polymorphism in MBL. *Clin. Exp. Immunol.* **143:**414–419.

Kaur, S., V. K. Gupta, S. Thiel, P. U. Sarma, and T. Madan. 2007. Protective role of mannan-binding lectin in a murine model of invasive pulmonary aspergillosis. *Clin. Exp. Immunol.* **148:**382–389.

Kesh, S., N. Y. Mensah, P. Peterlongo, D. Jaffe, K. Hsu, M. van den Brink, R. O'Reilly, E. Pamer, J. Satagopan, and G. A. Papanicolaou. 2005. TLR1 and TLR6 polymorphisms are associated with susceptibility to invasive aspergillosis after allogeneic stem cell transplantation. *Ann. NY Acad. Sci.* **1062:**95–103.

Kijpittayarit, S., A. J. Eid, R. A. Brown, C. V. Paya, and R. R. Razonable. 2007. Relationship between Toll-like receptor 2 polymorphism and cytomegalovirus disease after liver transplantation. *Clin. Infect. Dis.* **44:**1315–1320.

Kishore, U., T. J. Greenhough, P. Waters, A. K. Shrive, R. Ghai, M. F. Kamran, A. L. Bernal, K. B. Reid, T. Madan, and T. Chakraborty. 2006. Surfactant proteins SP-A and SP-D: structure, function and receptors. *Mol. Immunol.* **43:**1293–1315.

Knutsen, A. P., B. Kariuki, J. D. Consolino, and M. R. Warrier. 2006. IL-4 alpha chain receptor (IL-4Ralpha) polymorphisms in allergic bronchopulmonary aspergillosis. *Clin. Mol. Allergy* **4:**3.

Latge, J. P. 1999. *Aspergillus fumigatus* and aspergillosis. *Clin. Microbiol. Rev.* **12:**310–350.

Latge, J. P. 2001. The pathobiology of *Aspergillus fumigatus. Trends. Microbiol.* **9:**382–389.

Lee, J. E., J. H. Choi, J. H. Lee, and M. G. Lee. 2005. Gene SNPs and mutations in clinical genetic testing: haplotype-based testing and analysis. *Mutat. Res.* **573:**195–204.

Levitz, S. M., S. Shoham, and J. D. Cleary. 2009. Toll-like receptor 4 polymorphisms and aspergillosis. *N. Engl. J. Med.* **360:**634; author reply, **360:**635–636.

Loeffler, J., M. Steffens, E. M. Arlt, M. R. Toliat, M. Mezger, A. Suk, T. F. Wienker, H. Hebart, P. Nurnberg, M. Boeckh, P. Ljungman, R. Trenschel, and H. Einsele. 2006. Polymorphisms in the genes encoding chemokine receptor 5, interleukin-10, and monocyte chemoattractant protein 1 contribute to cytomegalovirus reactivation and disease after allogeneic stem cell transplantation. *J. Clin. Microbiol.* **44:**1847–1850.

Loetscher, M., B. Gerber, P. Loetscher, S. A. Jones, L. Piali, I. Clark-Lewis, M. Baggiolini, and B. Moser. 1996. Chemokine receptor specific for IP10 and mig: structure, function, and expression in activated T-lymphocytes. *J. Exp. Med.* **184:**963–969.

Madan, T., S. Kaur, S. Saxena, M. Singh, U. Kishore, S. Thiel, K. B. Reid, and P. U. Sarma. 2005. Role of collectins in innate immunity against aspergillosis. *Med. Mycol.* **43:**155–163.

Manuel, O., A. Asberg, X. Pang, H. Rollag, V. C. Emery, J. K. Preiksaitis, D. Kumar, M. D. Pescovitz, A. A. Bignamini, A. Hartmann, A. G. Jardine, and A. Humar. 2009. Impact of genetic polymorphisms in cytomegalovirus glycoprotein B on outcomes in solid-organ transplant recipients with cytomegalovirus disease. *Clin. Infect. Dis.* **49:**1160–1166.

Marr, K. A., R. A. Carter, M. Boeckh, P. Martin, and L. Corey. 2002. Invasive aspergillosis in allogeneic stem cell transplant recipients: changes in epidemiology and risk factors. *Blood* **100:**4358–4366.

Mewara, A., B. Mishra, R. K. Ratho, and P. Kumar. 2009. Cytomegalovirus glycoprotein B gene polymorphism and its association with clinical presentations in infants. *Southeast Asian J. Trop. Med. Public Health* **40:**759–764.

Mezger, M., M. Steffens, M. Beyer, C. Manger, J. Eberle, M. R. Toliat, T. F. Wienker, P. Ljungman, H. Hebart, H. J. Dornbusch, H. Einsele, and J. Loeffler. 2008a. Polymorphisms in the chemokine (C-X-C motif) ligand 10 are associated with invasive aspergillosis after allogeneic stem-cell transplantation and influence CXCL10 expression in monocyte-derived dendritic cells. *Blood* **111:**534–536.

Mezger, M., M. Steffens, C. Semmler, E. M. Arlt, M. Zimmer, G. I. Kristjanson, T. F. Wienker, M. R. Toliat, T. Kessler, H. Einsele, and J. Loeffler. 2008b. Investigation of promoter variations in dendritic cell-specific ICAM3-grabbing non-integrin (DC-SIGN) (CD209) and their relevance for human cytomegalovirus reactivation and disease after allogeneic stem-cell transplantation. *Clin. Microbiol. Infect.* **14:**228–234.

Moenkemeyer, M., H. Heiken, R. E. Schmidt, and T. Witte. 2009. Higher risk of cytomegalovirus reactivation in human immunodeficiency virus-1-infected patients homozygous for MICA5.1. *Hum. Immunol.* **70:**175–178.

Pamer, E. G. 2008. TLR polymorphisms and the risk of invasive fungal infections. *N. Engl. J. Med.* **359:**1836–1838.

Paterson, D. L., and N. Singh. 1999. Invasive aspergillosis in transplant recipients. *Medicine* (Baltimore) **78:**123–138.

Roilides, E., A. Dimitriadou-Georgiadou, T. Sein, I. Kadiltsoglou, and T. J. Walsh. 1998. Tumor necrosis factor alpha enhances antifungal activities of polymorphonuclear and mononuclear phagocytes against *Aspergillus fumigatus. Infect. Immun.* **66:**5999–6003.

Romani, L. 2004. Immunity to fungal infections. *Nat. Rev. Immunol.* **4:**1–23.

Sainz, J., L. Hassan, E. Perez, A. Romero, A. Moratalla, E. Lopez-Fernandez, S. Oyonarte, and M. Jurado. 2007a. Interleukin-10 promoter polymorphism as risk factor to develop invasive pulmonary aspergillosis. *Immunol. Lett.* **109:**76–82.

Sainz, J., E. Perez, S. Gomez-Lopera, and M. Jurado. 2008a. IL1 gene cluster polymorphisms and its haplotypes may predict the risk to develop invasive pulmonary aspergillosis and modulate C-reactive protein level. *J. Clin. Immunol.* **28:**473–485.

Sainz, J., E. Perez, S. Gomez-Lopera, E. Lopez-Fernandez, L. Moratalla, S. Oyonarte, and M. Jurado. 2008b. Genetic variants of IL6 gene promoter influence on C-reactive protein levels but are not associated with susceptibility to invasive pulmonary aspergillosis in haematological patients. *Cytokine* **41:**268–278.

Sainz, J., E. Perez, L. Hassan, A. Moratalla, A. Romero, M. D. Collado, and M. Jurado. 2007b. Variable number of tandem repeats of TNF receptor type 2 promoter as genetic biomarker of susceptibility to develop invasive pulmonary aspergillosis. *Hum. Immunol.* **68:**41–50.

Sau, K., S. S. Mambula, E. Latz, P. Henneke, D. T. Golenbock, and S. M. Levitz. 2003. The antifungal drug amphotericin B promotes inflammatory cytokine release by a Toll-like receptor- and

CD14-dependent mechanism. *J. Biol. Chem.* **278:** 37561–37568.

Saxena, S., T. Madan, A. Shah, K. Muralidhar, and P. U. Sarma. 2003. Association of polymorphisms in the collagen region of SP-A2 with increased levels of total IgE antibodies and eosinophilia in patients with allergic bronchopulmonary aspergillosis. *J. Allergy Clin. Immunol.* **111:**1001–1007.

Seo, K. W., D. H. Kim, S. K. Sohn, N. Y. Lee, H. H. Chang, S. W. Kim, S. B. Jeon, J. H. Baek, J. G. Kim, J. S. Suh, and K. B. Lee. 2005. Protective role of interleukin-10 promoter gene polymorphism in the pathogenesis of invasive pulmonary aspergillosis after allogeneic stem cell transplantation. *Bone Marrow Transplant.* **36:**1089–1095.

Stanilova, S., and L. Miteva. 2005. Taq-I polymorphism in 3′UTR of the IL-12B and association with IL-12p40 production from human PBMC. *Genes Immun.* **6:**364–366.

Stuart, M. J., and R. L. Nagel. 2004. Sickle-cell disease. *Lancet* **364:**1343–1360.

Sun, H., U. Ringdahl, J. W. Homeister, W. P. Fay, N. C. Engleberg, A. Y. Yang, L. S. Rozek, X. Wang, U. Sjöbring, and D. Ginsburg. 2004. Plasminogen is a critical host pathogenicity factor for group A streptococcal infection. *Science* **305:**1283–1286.

Tagore, A., W. M. Gonsalkorale, V. Pravica, A. H. Hajeer, R. McMahon, P. J. Whorwell, P. J. Sinnott, and I. V. Hutchinson. 1999. Interleukin-10 (IL-10) genotypes in inflammatory bowel disease. *Tissue Antigens* **54:**386–390.

Takahashi, M., D. Iwaki, K. Kanno, Y. Ishida, J. Xiong, M. Matsushita, Y. Endo, S. Miura, N. Ishii, K. Sugamura, and T. Fujita. 2008. Mannose-binding lectin (MBL)-associated serine protease (MASP)-1 contributes to activation of the lectin complement pathway. *J. Immunol.* **180:**6132–6138.

Turner, D. M., D. M. Williams, D. Sankaran, M. Lazarus, P. J. Sinnott, and I. V. Hutchinson. 1997. An investigation of polymorphism in the interleukin-10 gene promoter. *Eur. J. Immunogenet.* **24:**1–8.

Vaid, M., S. Kaur, H. Sambatakou, T. Madan, D. W. Denning, and P. U. Sarma. 2007. Distinct alleles of mannose-binding lectin (MBL) and surfactant proteins A (SP-A) in patients with chronic cavitary pulmonary aspergillosis and allergic bronchopulmonary aspergillosis. *Clin. Chem. Lab. Med.* **45:**183–186.

Vang, T., A. V. Miletic, Y. Arimura, L. Tautz, R. C. Rickert, and T. Mustelin. 2008. Protein tyrosine phosphatases in autoimmunity. *Annu. Rev. Immunol.* **26:**29–55.

von Aulock, S., N. W. J. Schröder, S. Traub, K. Gueinzius, E. Lorenz, T. Hartung, R. R. Schumann, and C. Hermann. 2004. Heterozygous Toll-like receptor 2 polymorphism does not affect lipoteichoic acid-induced chemokine and inflammatory responses. *Infect. Immun.* **72:**1828–1831.

Wang, X., S.-M. Huong, M. L. Chiu, N. Raab-Traub, and E.-S. Huang. 2003. Epidermal growth factor receptor is a cellular receptor for human cytomegalovirus. *Nature* **424:**456–461.

Zaas, A. K., G. Liao, J. W. Chien, C. Weinberg, D. Shore, S. S. Giles, K. A. Marr, J. Usuka, L. H. Burch, L. Perera, J. R. Perfect, G. Peltz, and D. A. Schwartz. 2008. Plasminogen alleles influence susceptibility to invasive aspergillosis. *PLoS Genet.* **4:**e1000101.

Zheng, X. Q., F. Zhu, W. W. Shi, A. Lin, and W. H. Yan. 2009. The HLA-G 14 bp insertion/deletion polymorphism is a putative susceptible factor for active human cytomegalovirus infection in children. *Tissue Antigens* **74:**317–321.

HOST GENETIC VARIATION, INNATE IMMUNITY, AND SUSCEPTIBILITY TO URINARY TRACT INFECTION

Bryndís Ragnarsdóttir and Catharina Svanborg

21

The clinical manifestations and consequences of infectious disease differ markedly among individuals. While such differences often reflect socioeconomic factors and access to health care worldwide, the frequency, severity, and sequels of infectious diseases are also determined by exquisitely regulated molecular interactions between host and microbe. Microbial determinants of acute-disease severity and tissue damage have been extensively studied, but less is known about genetic variation influencing host susceptibility, especially susceptibility to the most common infections.

Defects in specific immunity are known to have profound effects on host susceptibility to infectious disease (Casanova and Abel, 2007). Inherited or acquired T-cell deficiencies increase susceptibility to a variety of infections by viruses, intracellular bacteria, and fungi. The inherited defects manifest themselves in the neonatal period or later during the first year of life, after loss of maternal antibodies. The acquired T-cell defects, resulting from human immunodeficiency virus (HIV) infection, malignancy, or immunosuppressive therapy, increase susceptibility to infections by *Pneumocystis jirovecii*, *Toxoplasma gondii*, neurotropic viruses, and bacteria, to name a few. B-cell defects dysregulate immunoglobulin production, for example in patients with hypogammaglobulinemias, immunoglobulin G (IgG) subclass deficiencies, or hyper-IgM syndrome. B-cell deficiencies increase the susceptibility to encapsulated bacteria, mainly in the respiratory tract, as well as the risk of sepsis and meningitis caused by such pathogens. Defects in specific immunity do not explain the variation in susceptibility to many other common infections, however.

It is becoming increasingly clear that defects in innate immunity may create strong, disease-prone phenotypes, exemplified by meningococcal meningitis in complement-deficient individuals (Fijen et al., 1989; Morgan and Orren, 1998; Sjoholm et al., 2006). Blood group-dependent variation influences susceptibility to malaria, and protection is associated with α-thalassemia and the hemoglobin A/E mutation,

Bryndís Ragnarsdóttir, Department of Microbiology, Immunology and Glycobiology, Institute of Laboratory Medicine, Lund University, Sölvegatan 23, S-223 62 Lund, Sweden. *Catharina Svanborg*, Department of Microbiology, Immunology and Glycobiology, Institute of Laboratory Medicine, Lund University, Sölvegatan 23, S-223 62 Lund, Sweden, and Singapore Immunology Network (SIgN), Biomedical Sciences Institutes, Agency for Science, Technology, and Research (A*STAR), 8A Biomedical Grove, Immunos, Biopolis, Singapore 138648.

Genome Plasticity and Infectious Diseases,
Edited by J. Hacker, U. Dobrindt, and R. Kurth,

while non-O blood groups are emerging as significant risk factors for life-threatening malaria (Chotivanich et al., 2002; Rowe et al., 2009). We identified blood group-dependent variation as the first human urinary tract infection (UTI) susceptibility determinant (Lomberg et al., 1981, 1983; Stapleton et al., 1992); individuals of blood group P1 express glycolipid receptors for P-fimbriated *Escherichia coli* and run a much higher risk of infection with such bacteria than do individuals of other blood groups (Lomberg et al., 1983). More recently, we identified polymorphisms in the chemokine receptor gene *CXCR1* and reduced receptor expression as risk factors in pyelonephritis-prone individuals (Frendeus et al., 2000; Lundstedt et al., 2007b). Since then, other primary deficiencies in innate immunity have been shown to predispose children to infection. Mutations in IκB kinase (IKKγ or NEMO) result in X-linked recessive anhidrotic ectodermal dysplasia with immunodeficiency (Doffinger et al., 2001). Autosomal-recessive interleukin-1 (IL-1) receptor-associated kinase 4 (IRAK-4) and MyD88 deficiencies affect the Toll-like receptor (TLR) pathway (Picard et al., 2003; von Bernuth et al., 2008). IRAK-4 deficiency results in 40% mortality during childhood, mostly due to invasive infections by gram-positive bacteria (*Streptococcus pneumoniae* and *Staphylococcus aureus*). Surprisingly, gram-negative bacterial, viral, or fungal infections are rare in MyD88- and IRAK-4-deficient patients. Most of the mutations that cause monogenic diseases occur within the coding regions and drastically impair their function, resulting in a high disease penetrance. The contribution and inheritance patterns of other types of genetic variants may be more difficult to discern.

HUMAN GENETICS AND UTI SUSCEPTIBILITY

UTIs provide a relevant and suitable model to identify determinants of host susceptibility and genetic variants affecting disease severity. UTIs are common in all societies and age groups, and susceptibility varies among individuals. The clinical manifestations of disease differ markedly. Asymptomatic bacteriuria (ABU) is the most common form of UTI, occurring at higher frequencies in the elderly (20%) and pregnant women (2 to 11%), in 1% of girls, and at lower frequencies in boys and men. ABU is considered protective without pathologic effects. A small group of highly susceptible individuals develop life-threatening, septic infections (acute pyelonephritis [APN]), and their dysregulated innate immune response combined with recurrent infections may cause renal scarring and loss of kidney function. These two extremes of the disease spectrum have proven very useful in identifying positive and negative regulators of UTI susceptibility. The long-term aim is to compensate for the defects and prevent severe, recurrent disease by designing appropriate therapies.

To identify genes involved in human disease, we have used a combination of cellular models and mutant mice, with defects in candidate innate immune response genes. In this chapter, we discuss two candidate genes with strong effects on the innate immune response and the antibacterial defense in the urinary tract and with major but opposite effects on UTI susceptibility. We propose that defects in TLR4 expression are protective and associated with ABU while defects in CXCR1 expression promote APN and renal scarring.

Experimental Approach to Identifying Specific Genetic Defects

Early studies showed that T-cell-deficient *(nu/nu)* and X-linked-immunodeficient *(xid)* mice are resistant to UTI (Hagberg et al., 1985; Svanborg Eden et al., 1985), suggesting that innate rather than adaptive immunity is essential to maintain the sterility of the urinary tract. These findings were later confirmed in studies with TCRαβ and γδ knockout and RAG-1 mice with defects in T-lymphocyte, immunoglobulin, or total-lymphocyte function (Frendeus et al., 2001b; Svanborg Eden et al., 1985). C3H/HeJ mice, then known as lipopolysaccharide (LPS)-nonresponder mice, had an increased susceptibility to UTI, as shown by delayed bacterial clearance, and had an impaired innate immune response, suggesting that defects in innate immunity are of great importance for the antibacterial defense of the urinary tract (Hagberg et al., 1985). In addition, C3H/HeJ mice remained chronically infected but without evidence of tissue damage, linking innate immunity to the inflammatory response and potentially to tissue damage (Frendeus et al., 2001b; Hagberg et al., 1985; Hedlund et al., 2001; Hopkins et al., 1998; Schilling et al., 2003; Shahin et al., 1987). The Lps gene defect in C3H/HeJ mice was subsequently identified as a point mutation in the intracellular Toll/interleukin-1 receptor (TIR) domain, which is required for signaling (Poltorak et al., 1998), and the importance of Tlr4 in UTI was confirmed in studies of *Tlr4*$^{-/-}$ mice (Fischer et al. 2007). Other studies have suggested that TLR5 contributes to the antibacterial defence against flagellated bacteria (Hawn et al., 2003), and Tlr11 has also been identified as an important host response regulator in murine UTI (Zhang et al., 2004). The TLR11 sequences are present in the human genome, but a stop codon in the putative TLR11 open reading frame indicates that TLR11 may not be expressed.

TLR4 AND ADAPTOR PROTEIN SIGNALING

The studies of the murine model showed that the antibacterial defense of the urinary tract mucosa relies on innate immunity and that Tlr4 plays a central role in the early host defense against infection. TLR4 is a transmembrane glycoprotein composed of three major domains: a leucine-rich repeat (LRR) ectodomain, a transmembrane domain, and an intracellular domain known as the TIR domain. The LRR domain is essential for microbial ligand recognition (Kawai and Akira, 2009; Matsushima et al., 2007), and crystallization studies have revealed that the LRR domain of TLR4 contains a β-strand and an α-helix linked by loops, forming a horseshoe-like structure (Kim et al., 2007). The TLRs have a short region of about 22 uncharged amino acids that is predicted to form a membrane-spanning α-helix (Gay and Gangloff, 2008), and the cytoplasmic side linking the transmembrane domain to the first secondary-structure element of the TIR domain varies from 20 amino acids in TLR4 to 30 amino acids in TLR5 (Gay and Gangloff, 2008).

The TIR domain is shared between the TLRs and their five adaptors as well as the IL-1 receptor family and is highly conserved in plants, mammals, and insects (Anderson et al., 1985). Recently, TIR domain-containing proteins have also been identified in bacteria and viruses (Bowie et al., 2000; Cirl et al., 2008). The five intracellular adaptors are the TIR domain-containing adaptor protein inducing beta interferon (TRIF), TRIF-related adaptor molecule (TRAM), myeloid differentiation factor 88 (MyD88), TIR domain-containing adaptor protein (TIRAP), and sterile alpha- and armadillo-motif-containing protein (SARM) (Dunne et al., 2003; Sheedy and O'Neill, 2007). The TIR domains are characterized by three main conserved sequences, designated boxes 1, 2, and 3. Box 1 is the signature sequence of all TLRs and the most highly conserved. The praline-to-histidine mutation that renders C3H/HeJ mice hyporesponsive to gram-negative bacterial stimuli is in box 2 (Poltorak et al., 1998). The death domain loop mutation in TLR2 has been shown to abrogate signal transduction in response to yeasts and gram-positive bacteria (Lien et al., 1999; Underhill et al., 1999). The crystal structures and models of other TIR domains from TLRs and cognate adaptor proteins reveal substantial differences in the surface charge distribution, which may influence the specificity for adaptor proteins and downstream signaling (Dunne et al., 2003).

MYD88-DEPENDENT SIGNALING

MyD88 is common to all the TLRs as well as IL-1R and consists of a C-terminal TIR and an N-terminal death domain, linked by an intermediate domain (Burns et al., 1998; Kawai et al., 1999). After binding of LPS to the TLR4 complex (Fig. 1), TIRAP plays an important role in recruiting MyD88 to the cytoplasmic portion of TLR4 (Fitzgerald et al., 2001; Horng et al., 2001). This is due to a phosphatidylinositol 4,5-bisphosphate (PIP2)-binding domain in its N terminus, which recruits TIRAP to PIP2-rich areas in the plasma membrane, thereby

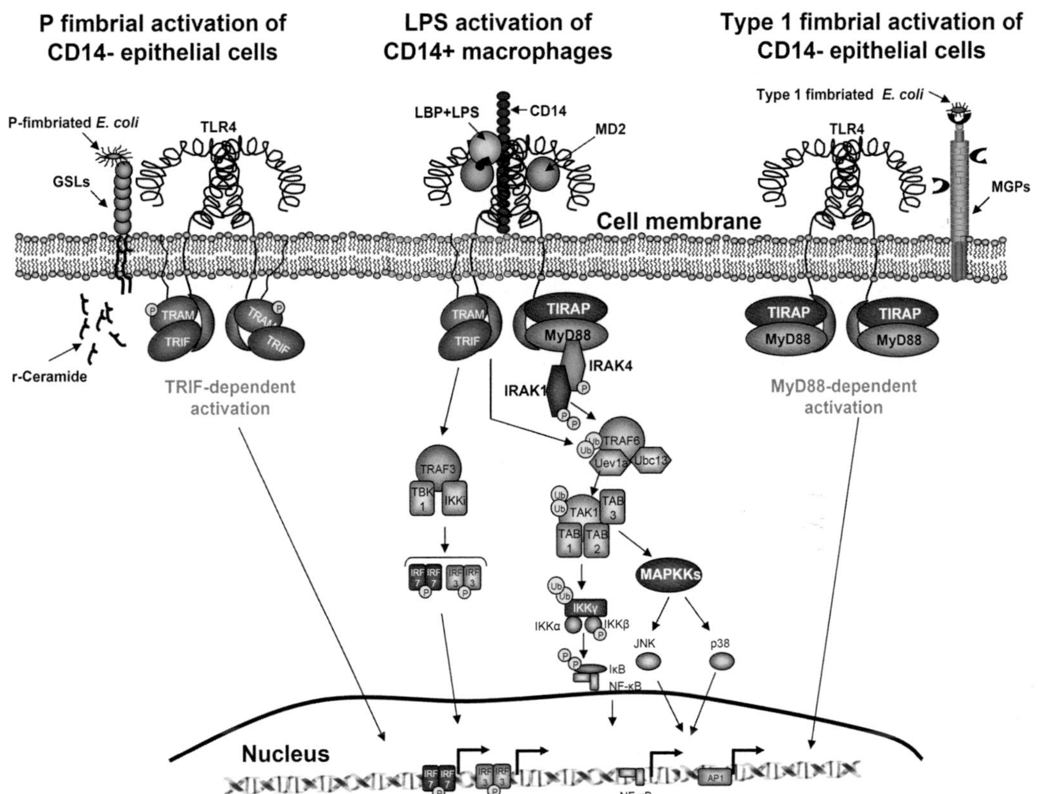

FIGURE 1 TLR4 is crucial for recognition of gram-negative bacteria and is best known as the LPS receptor. CD14 is a coreceptor for TLR4 and is essential for LPS recognition. Epithelial cells are, unlike macrophages and polymorphonuclear neutrophils, CD14 negative and as a result do not respond to LPS or commensal-like bacteria. However, epithelial cells respond in a pathogen-specific way and are activated by both P- and type 1-fimbriated *E. coli* but in different ways. P fimbriae bind to the Galα1-4Galβ receptor epitope in the globoseries of glycosphingolipids (GSLs), resulting in ceramide release and activation of epithelial cells through a TLR4 and the TRIF/TRAM-dependent pathway. Type 1 fimbriae bind α-mannosylated glycoproteins (MGPs) and activate epithelial cells through TLR4 but through MyD88-dependent mechanisms.

enabling the delivery of MyD88 to an activated TLR4 (Kagan and Medzhitov, 2006). Upon TLR4 stimulation, TIRAP is phosphorylated by Bruton's tyrosine kinase (Btk), and this is crucial for LPS-induced NF-κB activation (Gray et al., 2006). Signaling is initiated by the TLR4/MyD88 interaction through TIR-TIR association, resulting in the recruitment of IRAK-4 to MyD88 through death domain association. The intermediate domain is also crucial since an alternative splice variant of MyD88 lacking this region, MyD88s, fails to recruit IRAK-4 and therefore acts as a negative regulator of TLR signaling (Janssens et al., 2003). IRAK-4 interacts with IRAK-1, resulting in phosphorylation and activation of IRAK-4. The phosphorylation of IRAK-4 induces autophosphorylation of IRAK-1, which disassociates from the complex and binds TRAF6 to the complex through a TRAF6-binding motif in its TIR domain. TRAF6 (Cao et al., 1996) is the link between the TLR4 adaptor complex and the subsequent kinase signaling (Kawai et al., 2004) and is activated after interaction with two ubiquitin-conjugating enzymes (Uev1A and Ubc13), resulting in polyubiquitinilation of TRAF6 (Deng et al., 2000) and its association with the downstream proteins, TAK1 and the

TAK1-binding proteins, TAB1, TAB2, and TAB3 (Wang et al., 2001). TAK1 is then ubiquitinated and phosphorylates the inhibitor of the NF-κB (IκB) kinase (IKK) complex, which is polyubiquinated by Uev1A/Ubc13/TRAF6. Inactive IKK sequesters NF-κB in the cytoplasm, but the activated IKKs phosphorylate the IκB protein(s), which release NF-κB to translocate to the nucleus and induce inflammatory-gene expression. The most common dimer of NF-κB consists of two proteins, p50 and p65 (also known as RelA); p65 is important for transactivation of gene expression, while p50 is responsible for interaction with IκBα. In MyD88-dependent signaling, IκBα becomes phosphorylated, polyubiquitinated, and then degraded (Brikos and O'Neill, 2008; Karin and Ben-Neriah, 2000).

TRIF-DEPENDENT SIGNALING

TRIF has a TIR domain as well as several TRAF6-binding regions on the N terminus and a C-terminal RIP homotypic interaction motif (RHIM) (Fitzgerald et al., 2003; Sato et al., 2003; Yamamoto et al., 2003). The TRIF-dependent pathway is dependent on TRAM (Fig. 1) (Fitzgerald et al., 2003; Yamamoto et al., 2003), which has a myristoylated N terminus that associates with the plasma membrane. PKCε (protein kinase Cε) phosphorylation of serine residues 6 and 16 is essential for the activation of TRAM (McGettrick et al., 2006; Rowe et al., 2006). TRAM differs from the other adaptors by being TLR4 specific, acting as a bridge between TLR4 and TRIF. Although not as well documented as the MyD88-dependent pathway, the TRIF pathway can activate both NF-κB and IRF3/7 (Fitzgerald et al., 2003). Following TRAM-dependent activation of TLR4, TRIF forms a complex with TRAF3, IRAK-1, an IKK-like kinase named the TRAF family member-associated NF-κB activator (TANK)-binding kinase 1 (TBK1), and the IKK homolog IKKε, leading to the phosphorylation of IRF3 at its C terminus (Fitzgerald et al., 2003; Oganesyan et al., 2006). Consequently, IRF3 binds to the interferon-stimulated response element (ISRE) on target genes and induces the production of alpha/beta interferon (IFN-α/β) (Sato et al., 2003). Similar to IRF3, IRF7 becomes activated via its phosphorylation by TBK1 and IKKε, and induces the expression of genes, by binding to their ISREs (Kawai et al., 2004).

TLR4 RECEPTOR LIGANDS

The TLRs bind to conserved microbial patterns (pathogen-associated molecular patterns [PAMPs]) and in some cases endogenous ligands or damage-associated molecular patterns (DAMPs) (Bianchi, 2007; Mogensen, 2009). In addition, activation of the TLRs depends on the presence of coreceptors, which first bind microbial ligands and then serve as a signaling intermediate to activate TLRs (Table 1). LPS is the classical TLR4 agonist where the LPS-LPS-binding protein complex binds CD14 and MD2 (Fig. 1) (Pugin et al., 1993; Shimazu et al., 1999). After dimerization (Ozinsky et al., 2000), TLR4 recruits IRAK-4 via the adaptors MyD88 and TIRAP. In addition, MyD88-independent TLR4 activation through TRIF/TRAM regulates other aspects of the innate response (Fitzgerald et al., 2003; Hoebe et al., 2003; Yamamoto et al., 2002, 2003). Mucosal epithelial cells lack cell surface-bound CD14, however, and therefore the response to LPS is impaired (Hedlund et al., 1999; Samuelsson et al., 2004). The cells can still respond to LPS but only if sCD14 is added as a cofactor (Backhed et al., 2002). We think the lack of CD14 and LPS recognition by epithelial cells protects the mucosal TLR4 from pattern recognition and the urinary tract from responding to LPS-bearing, asymptomatic carrier strains.

MECHANISM OF EPITHELIAL TLR4 ACTIVATION BY P-FIMBRIATED, UROPATHOGENIC *E. COLI*: GSL RECEPTORS AND CERAMIDE RELEASE

P fimbriae are critical virulence factors of uropathogenic *E. coli* and activate a TLR4-dependent mucosal response (Svanborg et al., 2006). In the human inoculation model, P fimbriae have been shown to act as independent virulence factors and to fulfill the molecular Koch postulates (Bergsten et al., 2004, 2005).

TABLE 1 Some of the known TLR ligands (PAMPs)

TLR	Bacteria	Viruses[a]	Fungi	Endogenous ligands
TLR1/2	Triacyl lipopeptides			
TLR2	Lipopeptides, lipoproteins Peptidoglycan Lipoarabinomannan Lipoteichoic acid Porin (PorB)	Envelope proteins	Phosopholipomannan	
TLR3		Double-stranded RNA Poly I:C		
TLR4	LPS Flavolipin Hsp60	Fusion protein (RSV) Envelope proteins (MMTV)	Glucuronoxylomannan	Hsp60, Hsp70 Hyaluronic acid Heparan sulfate Fibrinogen Fibronectin
TLR5	Flagellin			
TLR2/6	Diacyl lipopeptides		Zymosan	
TLR7		Single-stranded RNA		Imidazoquinolines (hTLR7)
TLR8		Single-stranded RNA		Imidazoquinolines (hTLR8)
TLR9	Unmethylated CpG DNA	Unmethylated CpG DNA	Unmethylated CpG DNA	Chromatin-IgG complexes
TLR10				
TLR11	UPEC (mTLR11)		Profilin (mTLR11)	
TLR12	Unknown ligands			
TLR13	Unknown ligands			

[a]RSV, respiratory syncytial virus; MMTV, mouse mammary tumor virus.

PapG-mediated adherence enables the host to sense the attacking pathogen and to activate TLR4 signaling and the innate mucosal response in the human urinary tract.

TLR4 activation by P-fimbriated *E. coli* requires a ligand-binding receptor and TLR4 as coreceptors to activate transmembrane signaling (Fig. 1). The glycosphingolipids (GSLs) are ceramide-anchored and extracellular oligosaccharides that provide recognition epitopes for the PapG adhesin. In response to P-fimbriated *E. coli*, the intracellular levels of free ceramide increase, and ceramide has been shown to act as a signaling intermediate between the glycolipid receptors and TLR4 (Fig. 1) (Hedlund et al., 1996, 1998). Using isolated ceramide and stably transfected HEK cells, we have shown that exogenous ceramide activates a TLR4-dependent response, and similar results were obtained by releasing endogenous ceramide with sphingomyelinases (Fischer et al., 2007). Consistent with these studies, ceramide was shown to act as a lipid second messenger when released from plasma membrane sphingolipids by acid sphingomyelinase (Schenck et al., 2007). TLR4 signaling can thus be activated by P-fimbriated uropathogenic *E. coli* and by other agonists that modify membrane glycolipids (Fischer et al., 2007).

P-fimbrial binding to GSL receptors provides a pathogen-specific mechanism to circumvent the LPS unresponsiveness of the mucosa (Hedlund et al., 1998; Samuelsson et al., 2004).

Membrane-bound CD14 is not expressed by human uroepithelial cells, and unless soluble CD14 is added, LPS is a poor activator of the mucosal TLR4 response. P fimbriae do not activate TLR4 through LPS, however, as shown in experiments using *E. coli* strains expressing detoxified lipid A (Bergsten et al., 2004; Hedlund et al., 1999). Thus, the fimbrial ligands change the quality of TLR4 signaling in a pathogen-specific rather than PAMP-dependent manner.

Genetic Variation Affecting *TLR4*

TLR structure and function are tightly regulated at the genetic level, as expected from the role of these receptors as sentinels of the innate immune response. Numerous studies have attempted to find genetic variants and correlations to disease, but so far these studies have given unclear results.

STRUCTURAL GENE POLYMORPHISMS

Very few structural *TLR* mutations have been documented, but a stop codon polymorphism in the ligand-binding domain of *TLR5* (*TLR5*^{392STOP}) has been shown to abrogate flagellin-induced signaling and to increase the susceptibility to experimental *Legionella pneumophila* pneumonia (Hawn et al., 2003). Many groups have tried to link *TLR4* polymorphisms to disease, and two cosegregating polymorphisms of the human *TLR4* gene, Asp299Gly and Thr399Ile, were shown to be more common among individuals who are hyporesponsive to inhaled LPS than in controls (Arbour et al., 2000). Two subsequent studies failed to find a link between these single-nucleotide polymorphisms (SNPs) and meningococcal susceptibility, however (Allen et al., 2003; Read et al., 2001).

A large number of in vitro studies have suggested that this Asp299Gly polymorphism in *TLR4* may influence the efficiency of LPS recognition. Crystallization studies have identified two highly conserved LPS/MD-2-binding regions (Kim et al., 2007), and while Asp299Gly is not in the MD-2-binding domain, it has been proposed to increase the rotational freedom of the peptide bond and to change the negatively charged area at position 299, thus affecting LPS binding (Rallabhandi et al., 2006). Karoly et al. (2007) showed that patients with UTI had a higher prevalence of Asp299Gly than did controls ($P = 0.041$). The SNP tended to occur more frequently in patients with recurrent UTI without vesicoureteral reflux than in patients with vesicoureteral abnormalities ($P = 0.067$). Hawn et al. (2009a) suggested that Asp299Gly was associated with protection from rUTI, but not pyelonephritis. Furthermore, they showed that a *TLR5*_(C1174T) polymorphism was associated with an increased risk of recurrent UTI but not pyelonephritis while a polymorphism in *TLR1*_(G1805T) was associated with protection from pyelonephritis. Furthermore, a recent study by the same group reported that a *TLR2*_(G2258A) polymorphism, which has been associated with decreased lipopeptide-induced signaling, was associated with an increased risk of ABU. Other associations include respiratory syncytial virus infection (Tal et al., 2004), severe malaria (Mockenhaupt et al., 2006), and myocardial infarction (Edfeldt et al., 2004). Despite this, in vivo studies have shown little effect of the Asp299Gly/Thr399Ile SNPs (Calvano et al., 2006; Marsik et al., 2005), and one study that examined cytokine production by individuals carrying the Asp-299Gly mutation showed a stronger rather than weaker cytokine response (Ferwerda et al., 2007), suggesting that other mechanisms of TLR4 regulation might be relevant.

LOW TLR4 EXPRESSION IN PATIENTS WITH ABU

TLR4 controls the innate immune response to *E. coli* UTI, and *Tlr4*$^{-/-}$ mice develop ABU rather than severe infection, suggesting that reduced mucosal TLR4 function may protect the host against symptomatic infection. To examine whether ABU might be associated with variant TLR4 expression, we examined children with a consistent UTI pattern. Children with primary ABU (no previous symptomatic UTI) had lower TLR4 expression than did controls and children with secondary ABU following a previous symptomatic UTI episode (Ragnarsdottir et al., 2007). The ABU group also had increased TRIF protein levels, but TRAM and MyD88 expression was not changed (Ragnarsdottir et al., 2007). The results suggested TLR4 low responders may enjoy the benefits of asymptomatic carriage while avoiding the destructive effects of the innate host defense.

In transgenic mice, differences in Tlr4 expression levels influence the early stages of *Salmonella* infection (Bihl et al., 2003; Kalis et al., 2003; Roy et al., 2006). Mice carrying one, two, or three copies of Tlr4 had incremental protective responses against acute gram-negative bacterial sepsis, but higher levels of Tlr4 expression gave no benefits (Roy et al., 2006). Mice with low Tlr4 copy numbers survived high levels of LPS, and the sensitivity increased with the Tlr4 copy number (Kalis et al., 2003). A linear relationship between the response and the logarithm of TLR4-MD-2 levels and the LPS-induced cytokine (IL-6) response in macrophages has been proposed (Kalis et al., 2003).

TLR4 PROMOTER VARIATION AND TLR4 EXPRESSION

To explain the low TLR4 expression at the genetic level, we sequenced *TLR4* in patients with UTI. *TLR4* is ca. 19 kb and is located on chromosome 9q33.1; the protein comprises 839 amino acids. Polymorphic sites other than the known Asp299Gly were not observed, and this site was polymorphic in one control only. The low expression levels were thus not explained by structural-gene variation.

We have subsequently identified a new mechanism for human TLR variation, based on *TLR4* promoter polymorphisms that influence expression dynamics in vitro and innate immune response dynamics in patients with ABU. The results suggest that reduced TLR4 expression attenuates the innate mucosal response, thus promoting an asymptomatic carrier state rather than severe disease. The results also suggest that genetic variation of the *TLR4* promoter is an essential, largely overlooked mechanism to influence TLR4 expression and UTI susceptibility. The results have not been published, however, and thus more detailed data cannot be revealed at this time.

The human *TLR4* promoter is 4.3 kb and lacks a TATA box, typical Sp1 sites, and CCAAT box sequences (Rehli et al., 2000). Instead it contains multiple binding sites for PU.1, a member of the Ets family of transcription factors, as well as octamer-binding factors and composite interferon response factor/Ets motifs. Two proximal PU.1-binding sites were needed for *TLR4* promoter activity, and transient transfection revealed that the region, 75 bp upstream of the major transcription initiation site, is sufficient to induce maximal luciferase activity in THP-1 cells while a negative regulatory region was predicted to reside between nucleotides −3228 and −743. Rehli and coworkers did not, however, explain how TLR4 expression was activated in nonmyeloid cells, such as epithelial cells and fibroblasts. Furthermore, they suggested that the proximal promoter (−75 bp upstream) showed a high degree of conservation between human and mouse *TLR4* genes (Lichtinger et al., 2007; Roger et al., 2001, 2005). Lichtinger et al. (2007) described an additional distal promoter in the murine *Tlr4* model, exclusively used by nonmyeloid cells, while human epithelial cells use both the "myeloid" proximal promoter and, to a lesser extent, the distal promoter. This distal promoter comprises a conserved E-box element where upstream stimulatory factors or microphthalmia TFE factors are thought to be the dominant binding factors.

REGULATORS OF TLR4 SIGNALING

Inflammation is crucial to control the growth of pathogenic organisms, but excessive inflammation and cytokine production is always harmful to the host and can in some cases be fatal. It is therefore essential to have tight regulation of the inflammatory response. There are several known negative regulators of TLR signaling, including SIGIRR, MyD88s, IRAK-M, SOCS1, Triad3A, and SARM. SIGIRR, MyD88s, and IRAK-M are all involved in blocking MyD88-dependent activation, while Triad3A and SARM block the TRIF-dependent pathway. Recently, a splice variant of TRAM was identified as a new negative regulator (Palsson-McDermott et al., 2009).

SIGIRR has an extracellular domain consisting of a single immunoglogbulin domain, and the TIR domain resembles MyD88 but lacks two important amino acids needed for signaling (Thomassen et al., 1999; Wald et al., 2003). The cytosolic domain of SIGIRR blocks TLR4 signaling through TIR-TIR interactions between SIGIRR and TLR4, thus preventing the recruitment of IRAK and TRAF6 to MyD88 and the resulting inflammatory process (Wald et al., 2003). MyD88s is a splice variant of MyD88 that affects, like SIGIRR, MyD88-dependent activation of TLR4. MyD88s is lacking the intermediate domain (ID), that is found in MyD88, allowing it to bind IRAK but unable to induce IRAK phosphorylation and NF-κB activation, thereby hindering host activation (Burns et al., 2003). IRAK-M prevents dissociation of IRAK and IRAK-4 from MyD88 and formation of IRAK-TRAF6 complexes (Kobayashi et al., 2002). Triad3A is an E3 ubiquitin-protein ligase that has been shown to interact with TIR domains of TLRs as well as TRIF, TIRAP, and RIP1 (Fearns et al., 2006), and SARM blocks gene induction downstream of TRIF (Carty et al., 2006). There are thus many additional targets where polymorphisms might contribute to susceptibility to human disease. In addition, bacteria modify TLR4 signaling to their advantage. Recently, we identified molecules that actively inhibit the TLR-dependent innate host defense (Cirl et al., 2008). TcpC, the TIR-homologous protein in uropathogenic *E. coli*, inhibits innate immunity by binding to MyD88 as well as TRIF, thereby influencing both the NF-κB- and the IRF3-dependent signaling pathways (Yadav et al., 2010).

CHEMOKINE RECEPTOR POLYMORPHISMS AND UTI SUSCEPTIBILITY

Epithelial cells are the first to encounter mucosal pathogens and respond to microbial challenge by producing a variety of proinflammatory mediators. The chemokine gradient and neutrophil activation result in high-affinity binding to intercellular adhesion molecules on the surface of activated endothelial cells, and the neutrophils penetrate through the endothelial layer and migrate to mucosal sites of infection (Agace et al., 1993a, 1993b; Ko et al., 1993). The mechanisms of neutrophil recruitment in the urinary tract have been extensively studied (Godaly et al., 2000; Haraoka et al., 1999), and CXCL8 has been shown to support neutrophil migration across infected uroepithelial cell layers (Godaly et al., 1997), as well as the phagocytosis of bacteria. CXCL8 responses in patients are correlated to urine neutrophil numbers (Agace et al., 1993b).

Chemokines function as chemotactic cytokines and are divided into four subfamilies—CXC, CC, C, and CX3C—according to the number and position of conserved cysteine residues (Olson and Ley, 2002). Chemokine receptors are defined by the class of chemokines that they bind (CXCR, CCR, CR, and CX3CR1) (Baggiolini et al., 1998). CXCL8 (also known as IL-8) is essential for the innate response to UTI and is produced by a variety of cells. Its biological effects are mediated through the binding of CXCL8 to the cell surface G protein-coupled receptors CXCR1 and CXCR2 (Holmes et al., 1991; Murphy and Tiffany, 1991; Baggiolini, 1998). Signals are transmitted across the membrane through ligand-induced conformational changes, exposing epitopes on the intracellular loops and carboxy-terminal tail of the receptor that promote coupling to functional heterotrimeric G proteins. CXCR1 is activated only by IL-8 and granulocyte chemotactic protein 2 (GCP-2), while CXCR2 is activated by multiple CXC chemokines. CXCR1 activation leads to cell migration, granule release, and an oxidative burst, depending on the IL-8 concentration; low levels stimulate cell migration, while higher CXCL8 levels are needed for granule release (Smith et al., 1992) and even higher concentrations stimulate internalization of cell surface CXCR1 (Chuntharapai and Kim, 1995).

CXCR1 plays a crucial role in bacterial clearance from the urinary tract (Frendeus et al, 2000; Godaly et al., 2001; Hang et al., 2000; Svensson et al., 2005). The murine IL-8 receptor homologue (mIL-8rh, also known as mCXCR2) is an ortholog of the human CXCR2 gene but functionally resembles CXCR1 (Fu et al., 2005; Moepps et al., 2006). In the murine UTI model, mCXCR2 is an essential determinant of severe UTI (APN). The m*CXCR2*$^{-/-}$ mice developed acute, septic pyelonephritis with about 50% mortality, and surviving mice showed chronic tissue damage resembling renal scarring. In m*CXCR2*$^{-/-}$ mice, neutrophil recruitment into the kidneys was slow and there was a delay in neutrophil exit across the mucosal lining into the urine (Frendeus et al., 2000), resulting in neutrophil entrapment underneath the mucosa, leading to tissue damage and renal scarring (Hang et al., 2000; Svensson et al., 2005). The dramatic phenotype in m*CXCR2*$^{-/-}$ mice suggested that a single gene defect is sufficient to increase susceptibility to acute pyelonephritis and chronic morbidity and thus to control the resistance to acute kidney infection and renal scarring in mice.

Genetic Variation Affecting *CXCR1* and UTI Susceptibility

In a first pilot study of UTI-prone patients, we examined the neutrophil CXCR1 and CXCR2 surface expression and mRNA levels and found reduced levels of CXCR1 (Frendeus et al., 2000). In a subsequent study, we included APN-prone children and adults as well as age-matched controls without known UTI (Lundstedt et al., 2007b). We found that the protein expression was reduced and additionally the level of CXCR1 transcript and protein expression was lower in this new subset of pediatric patients. Direct sequencing of the *CXCR1* gene revealed five *CXCR1* gene variants in the APN group: variant 1 was located in the intronic region, variant 2 was located in the coding region (CDS) of exon 2, and variants 3 to 5 were located in the 3′ untranslated region with a cumulative frequency of 38%. In contrast to the APN-prone children, only variants 1 and 2 were found in the controls, with a cumulative freqency of 4% ($P < 0.005$), indicating that these changes were selective to the APN patients. Furthermore, the frequency of *CXCR1* variants 1 and 2 was confirmed in the adult APN-prone individuals (25% and 28%, respectively) compared to the adult controls (8%; $P < 0.0056$ for SNP1 and $P < 0.0018$ for SNP2), clearly showing that these *CXCR1* variants are associated with APN susceptibility (Lundstedt et al., 2007b). The *CXCR1* promoter has previously been described as containing a TATA box equivalent, GC-rich areas that may serve as SP-1 and AP.2 sites, and finally a binding site for PU.1 that is adjacent to the transcription start site (TSS). Most of the promoter activity is determined to be close to the TSS, −56 to +50, with positive regulatory elements at −126 to +50 and negative regulatory elements upstream (−640 to −126) (Sprenger et al., 1994; Wilkinson and Navarro, 1999). We found no disease-associated promoter polymorphisms, however (Lundstedt et al., 2007b).

The identified SNPs were examined to define evolutionarily conserved regions and potential transcription factor-binding sites (Lundstedt et al., 2007b). All SNPs except for the exonic variant were located in sequences potentially controlling transcription and mRNA stability or processing. The predicted reduction in RUNX1 binding due to variant 1 was confirmed by electrophoretic mobility shift assay, and the specificity was confirmed by competition with cold RUNX1-binding-site probe (wt-probe). The bound protein was identified as RUNX1 by using specific antibody. Furthermore, the loss of the RUNX1-binding site was shown to reduce transcription in a luciferase reporter assay. CXCR1 has two alternative poly(A) sites, resulting in a long or short transcript of CXCR1 (Ahuja and Murphy, 1996). Reverse transcriptase PCR (RT-PCR) analysis has been used to examine the predicted effect of variant 5 on the two alternative poly(A) sites. Variant 5 results in a G-to-A transition at position +3665, between the first poly(A) signal and the poly(A) sites. If variant 5 had the predicted effect, the levels of the long CXCR1 transcripts would be reduced. The long and total CXCR1 transcripts were quantified by RT-PCR and showed that mRNAs from a patient carrying variant 5 and the mother with the same mutation contained reduced levels of the CXCR1 large transcript compared to the control, thus confirming the predicted effect of variant 5 (Lundstedt et al., 2007b). Furthermore, we have investigated the susceptibility to APN in three-generation pedigrees of APN-prone families and controls not prone to UTI (Lundstedt et al., 2007a) (Fig. 2). Our results demonstrated clearly that family members of APN-prone children have lower CXCR1 expression and increased frequency of APN compared to control families (Fig. 2). In a case-control study, Hawn et al. (2009b) looked for polymorphisms in *CXCR1* and *CXCR2* to associate with ABU susceptibility but did not find any associations. However, several *CXCR1* polymorphisms were associated with ABU caused by gram-positive pathogens.

CXCR1 and *CXCR2* are clustered on chromosome 2q35, the same area that has been mapped as a susceptibility locus for several human disorders including rheumatoid arthritis, systemic lupus erythematosus, and insulin-dependent diabetes mellitus (Copeman et al., 1995; Cornelis et al., 1998; Gaffney et al., 1998). The *CXCR1* gene comprises two exons that are interrupted by a 1.7-kb intron, but the entire coding region is located in exon 2. Most of the genetic studies of *CXCR1* have investigated the frequency of two SNPs in the coding region of *CXCR1*, a serine-to-threonine amino acid change at location 276 (827G/C) and an arginine-to-cysteine change at position 335 (1003C/T). However, these SNPs and two other rare mutations were not observed at increased frequencies in Japanese patients with rheumatoid arthritis (Kato et al., 2000). Furthermore, no difference was seen in 827G/C patients with persistent hepatitis B virus infection (Cheong et al., 2007) or Kawasaki disease (Breunis et al., 2007). A positive association has been made, however, between a *CXCR1* haplotype carrying two nonsynonymous SNPs (92T/G and 1003C/T) and protection against rapid disease progression in HIV-1^+ patients (Vasilescu et al., 2007). Smithson and colleagues (2005) reported CXCR1 expression levels in premenopausal women with recurrent UTI but found no SNPs in the *CXCR1* promoter; the SNPs found in the coding regions (92T/G and 1003C/T) did not differ between the patients and controls. Vasilescu et al. (2007) found three promoter SNPs in their HIV-1^+ patients and controls, but their frequency did not vary between groups. In view of the critical role of chemokines and their receptors, it can be speculated that polymorphisms might contribute to immunological/inflammatory diseases.

Does Specific Immunity Play a Role in UTI?

For many years, the specific immune response to UTI was a target of investigation by many groups. The aim was to develop a vaccine with effects on mucosal as well as systemic aspects of disease. The work was motivated by clinical studies showing that APN patients developed a rapid systemic immune response to bacterial antigens, including O antigens defined by their LPS structure and K antigens defined by the capsular polysaccharides (Kaijser et al., 1978). There was no immediate association between the systemic antibody response and disease progression, however. In experimental rat and rabbit studies, several bacterial surface O and K antigens were shown to trigger a protective immune response (Hanson et al., 1977, Kaijser, 1977, 1983; Silverblatt and Cohen, 1979), and in later studies antibodies against fimbriae were also shown to prevent or reduce the severity of infection (Pecha et al., 1989; Silverblatt and Cohen, 1979). Detailed studies of patients with recurrent UTI by Uehling and coworkers assessed the efficiency of vaginal mucosal immunization with a multivalent bacterial vaccine (Hopkins et al., 1999; Uehling et al., 1994, 1997, 2001, 2003). Although not always significant compared to placebo treatment, a degree of beneficial effect of the vaccine was documented. A significant improvement was detected in women who received vaccine with boosters, were sexually active, were less than 52 years old, and had not undergone hysterectomy. This group had *E. coli* UTIs at a much lower rate than women given placebo only, indicating that the vaccine may provide the greatest benefit to sexually active women in the 20- to 50-year-old

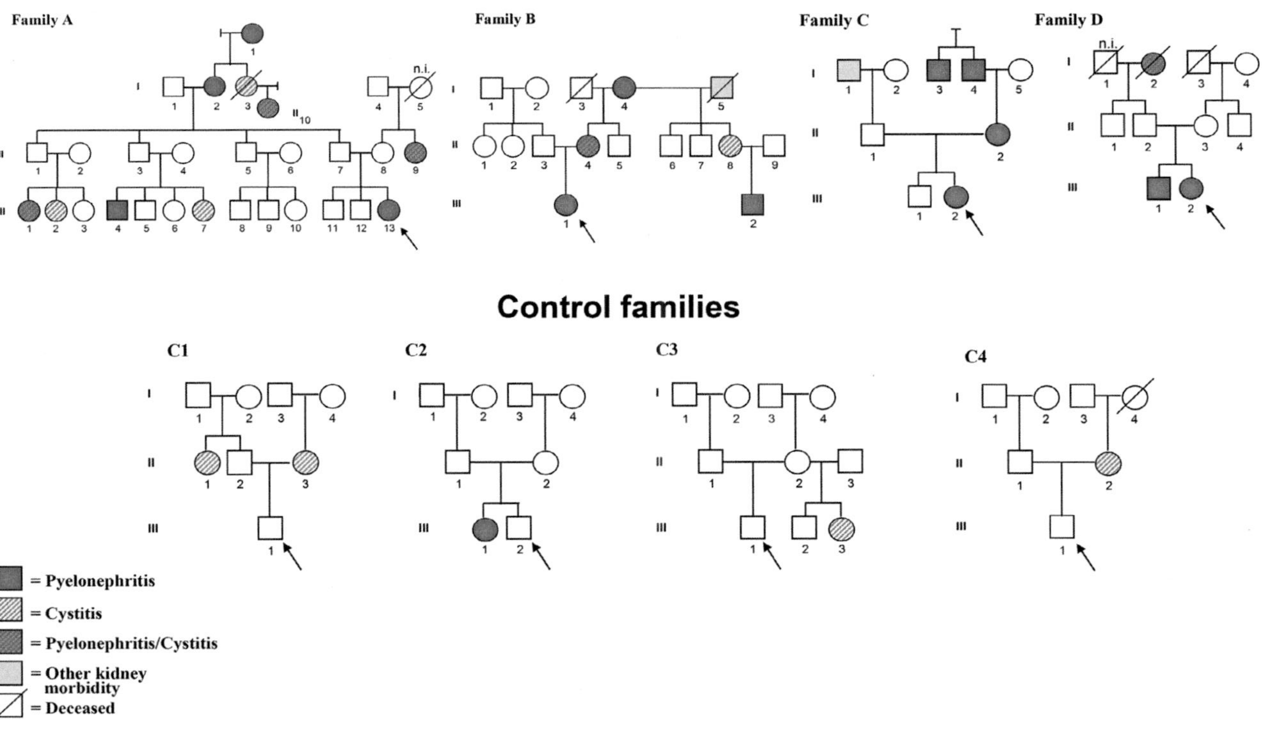

FIGURE 2 Three-generation pedigrees reveal a genetic predisposition to UTI. An accumulation of pyelonephritis was found in the relatives of the APN-prone patients (shown in red), while most of the UTI incidents in the control families were single episodes of cystitis (shown in gray), often associated with pregnancy. The arrows indicate the index APN-prone children. Partially reprinted from the *Journal of Infectious Diseases* (Lundstedt et al., 2007a) with permission of the publisher.

age group (Hopkins et al., 2007). Other studies have implicated adaptive immunity involvement in UTI, where recruitment of activated T cells and development of specific IgG antibody in the serum and urine were observed after reinfection with the same *E. coli* strain (Thumbikat et al., 2006). Furthermore, immunization against the FimH adhesion of type 1-fimbriated *E. coli* gave protective immunity in the murine model and nonhuman primates (Langermann et al., 1997, 2000). The human trial data have not been published, as far as we know. It still remains possible and interesting that patients with the innate immune defects defined by us and others might benefit from vaccination to prevent infection or reduce its destructive effects in this targeted patient group.

SUMMARY AND CONCLUSIONS

The contribution of bacterial pathogens to disease and the resulting damage to the host depend on their virulence factor repertoire. Classical virulence factors include adhesins, toxins, capsular polysaccharides, and iron-sequestering systems (Hacker and Kaper, 2000; Wiles et al., 2008), while bacterial genome analysis has identified novel factors, including molecules that actively inhibit the TLR-dependent innate host defense (Cirl et al., 2008). Less is known about the determinants of host susceptibility to common infections and about genetic variation influencing host defense. In this chapter, we have summarized available information on the innate immune response to UTI as a model of mucosal disease pathogenesis. We have shown that TLR4 variation may be protective and that promoter polymorphisms can cause reduced expression levels and promote asymptomatic bacterial carriage. Dysregulated innate immunity leading to aggravated acute infection and tissue damage may, on the other hand, be caused by chemokine receptor variants that disturb neutrophil migration and bacterial clearance.

There is a great clinical need to identify genetic variants that improve resistance or increase susceptibility to infectious pathogens. We hope that the types of molecular markers presented here and additional markers discovered in the future may help to identify patients who are susceptible to common infections, both symptomatic and asymptomatic. Further clinical studies are needed to define whether detection of polymorphisms in *TLR4* and *CXCR1* or protein expression variation can be used to distinguish susceptible from resistant individuals.

REFERENCES

Agace, W., S. Hedges, U. Andersson, J. Andersson, M. Ceska, and C. Svanborg. 1993a. Selective cytokine production by epithelial cells following exposure to *Escherichia coli*. *Infect. Immun.* **61:**602–609.

Agace, W., S. Hedges, M. Ceska, and C. Svanborg. 1993b. IL-8 and the neutrophil response to mucosal Gram negative infection. *J. Clin. Investig.* **92:**780–785.

Ahuja, S. K., and P. M. Murphy. 1996. The CXC chemokines growth-regulated oncogene (GRO) alpha, GRObeta, GROgamma, neutrophil-activating peptide-2, and epithelial cell-derived neutrophil-activating peptide-78 are potent agonists for the type B, but not the type A, human interleukin-8 receptor. *J. Biol. Chem.* **271:**20545–20550.

Allen, A., S. Obaro, K. Bojang, A. A. Awomoyi, B. M. Greenwood, H. Whittle, G. Sirugo, and M. J. Newport. 2003. Variation in Toll-like receptor 4 and susceptibility to group A meningococcal meningitis in Gambian children. *Pediatr. Infect. Dis. J.* **22:**1018–1019.

Anderson, K. V., G. Jurgens, and C. Nusslein-Volhard. 1985. Establishment of dorsal-ventral polarity in the Drosophila embryo: genetic studies on the role of the Toll gene product. *Cell* **42:**779–789.

Arbour, N. C., E. Lorenz, B. C. Schutte, J. Zabner, J. N. Kline, M. Jones, K. Frees, J. L. Watt, and D. A. Schwartz. 2000. TLR4 mutations are associated with endotoxin hyporesponsiveness in humans. *Nat. Genet.* **25:**187–191.

Backhed, F., L. Meijer, S. Normark, and A. Richter-Dahlfors. 2002. TLR4-dependent recognition of lipopolysaccharide by epithelial cells requires sCD14. *Cell. Microbiol.* **4:**493-501.

Baggiolini, M. 1998. Chemokines and leukocyte traffic. *Nature* **392:**565–568.

Bergsten, G., M. Samuelsson, B. Wullt, I. Leijonhufvud, H. Fischer, and C. Svanborg. 2004. PapG-dependent adherence breaks mucosal inertia and triggers the innate host response. *J. Infect. Dis.* **189:**1734–1742.

Bergsten, G., B. Wullt, and C. Svanborg. 2005. Escherichia coli, fimbriae, bacterial persistence and host response induction in the human urinary tract. *Int. J. Med. Microbiol.* **295:**487–502.

Bianchi, M. E. 2007. DAMPs, PAMPs and alarmins: all we need to know about danger. *J. Leukoc. Biol.* **81:**1–5.

Bihl, F., L. Salez, M. Beaubier, D. Torres, L. Lariviere, L. Laroche, A. Benedetto, D. Martel, J. M. Lapointe, B. Ryffel, and D. Malo. 2003. Overexpression of Toll-like receptor 4 amplifies the host response to lipopolysaccharide and provides a survival advantage in transgenic mice. *J. Immunol.* **170:**6141–6150.

Bowie, A., E. Kiss-Toth, J. A. Symons, G. L. Smith, S. K. Dower, and L. A. O'Neill. 2000. A46R and A52R from vaccinia virus are antagonists of host IL-1 and toll-like receptor signaling. *Proc. Natl. Acad. Sci. USA* **97:**10162–10167.

Breunis, W. B., M. H. Biezeveld, J. Geissler, I. M. Kuipers, J. Lam, J. Ottenkamp, A. Hutchinson, R. Welch, S. J. Chanock, and T. W. Kuijpers. 2007. Polymorphisms in chemokine receptor genes and susceptibility to Kawasaki disease. *Clin. Exp. Immunol.* **150:**83–90.

Brikos, C., and L. A. O'Neill. 2008. Signalling of toll-like receptors. *Handb. Exp. Pharmacol.* **2008**(183):21–50.

Burns, K., S. Janssens, B. Brissoni, N. Olivos, R. Beyaert and J. Tschopp. 2003. Inhibition of interleukin 1 receptor/Toll-like receptor signaling through the alternatively spliced, short form of MyD88 is due to its failure to recruit IRAK-4. *J. Exp. Med.* **197:**263–268.

Burns, K., F. Martinon, C. Esslinger, H. Pahl, P. Schneider, J. L. Bodmer, F. Di Marco, L. French, and J. Tschopp. 1998. MyD88, an adapter protein involved in interleukin-1 signaling. *J. Biol. Chem.* **273:**12203–12209.

Calvano, J. E., D. J. Bowers, S. M. Coyle, M. Macor, M. T. Reddell, A. Kumar, S. E. Calvano, and S. F. Lowry. 2006. Response to systemic endotoxemia among humans bearing polymorphisms of the Toll-like receptor 4 (hTLR4). *Clin. Immunol.* **121:**186–190.

Cao, Z., J. Xiong, M. Takeuchi, T. Kurama, and D. V. Goeddel. 1996. TRAF6 is a signal transducer for interleukin-1. *Nature* **383:**443–446.

Carty, M., R. Goodbody, M. Schroder, J. Stack, P. N. Moynagh, and A. G. Bowie. 2006. The human adaptor SARM negatively regulates adaptor protein TRIF-dependent Toll-like receptor signaling. *Nat. Immunol.* **7:**1074–1081.

Casanova, J. L., and L. Abel. 2007. Primary immunodeficiencies: a field in its infancy. *Science* **317:**617–619.

Cheong, J. Y., S. W. Cho, J. Y. Choi, J. A. Lee, M. H. Kim, J. E. Lee, K. B. Hahm, and J. H. Kim. 2007. RANTES, MCP-1, CCR2, CCR5, CXCR1 and CXCR4 gene polymorphisms are not associated with the outcome of hepatitis B virus infection: results from a large scale single ethnic population. *J. Korean Med. Sci.* **22:**529–535.

Chotivanich, K., R. Udomsangpetch, K. Pattanapanyasat, W. Chierakul, J. Simpson, S. Looareesuwan, and N. White. 2002. Hemoglobin E: a balanced polymorphism protective against high parasitemias and thus severe P falciparum malaria. *Blood* **100:**1172–1176.

Chuntharapai, A., and K. J. Kim. 1995. Regulation of the expression of IL-8 receptor A/B by IL-8: possible functions of each receptor. *J. Immunol.* **155:**2587–2594.

Cirl, C., A. Wieser, M. Yadav, S. Duerr, S. Schubert, H. Fischer, D. Stappert, N., Wantia, N. Rodriguez, H. Wagner, C. Svanborg, and T. Miethke. 2008. Subversion of Toll-like receptor signaling by a unique family of bacterial Toll/interleukin-1 receptor domain-containing proteins. *Nat. Med.* **14:**399–406.

Copeman, J. B., F. Cucca, C. M. Hearne, R. J. Cornall, P. W. Reed, K. S. Ronningen, D. E. Undlien, L. Nistico, R. Buzzetti, R. Tosi, et al. 1995. Linkage disequilibrium mapping of a type 1 diabetes susceptibility gene (IDDM7) to chromosome 2q31-q33. *Nat. Genet.* **9:**80–85.

Cornelis, F., S. Faure, M. Martinez, J. F. Prud'homme, P. Fritz, C. Dib, H. Alves, P. Barrera, N. de Vries, A. Balsa, D. Pascual-Salcedo, K. Maenaut, R. Westhovens, P. Migliorini, T. H. Tran, A. Delaye, N. Prince, C. Lefevre, G. Thomas, M. Poirier, S. Soubigou, O. Alibert, S. Lasbleiz, S. Fouix, C. Bouchier, F. Liote, M. N. Loste, V. Lepage, D. Charron, G. Gyapay, A. Lopes-Vaz, D. Kuntz, T. Bardin, and J. Weissenbach. 1998. New susceptibility locus for rheumatoid arthritis suggested by a genome-wide linkage study. *Proc. Natl. Acad. Sci. USA* **95:**10746–10750.

Deng, L., C. Wang, E. Spencer, L. Yang, A. Braun, J. You, C. Slaughter, C. Pickart, and Z. J. Chen. 2000. Activation of the IkappaB kinase complex by TRAF6 requires a dimeric ubiquitin-conjugating enzyme complex and a unique polyubiquitin chain. *Cell* **103:**351–361.

Doffinger, R., A. Smahi, C. Bessia, F. Geissmann, J. Feinberg, A. Durandy, C. Bodemer, S. Kenwrick, S. Dupuis-Girod, S. Blanche, P. Wood, S. H. Rabia, D. J. Headon, P. A. Overbeek, F. Le Deist, S. M. Holland, K. Belani, D. S. Kumararatne, A. Fischer, R. Shapiro, M. E. Conley, E. Reimund, H. Kalhoff, M. Abinun,

A. Munnich, A. Israel, G. Courtois, and J. L. Casanova. 2001. X-linked anhidrotic ectodermal dysplasia with immunodeficiency is caused by impaired NF-kappaB signaling. *Nat. Genet.* **27:**277–285.

Dunne, A., M. Ejdeback, P. L. Ludidi, L. A. O'Neill, and N. J. Gay. 2003. Structural complementarity of Toll/interleukin-1 receptor domains in Toll-like receptors and the adaptors Mal and MyD88. *J. Biol. Chem.* **278:**41443–41451.

Edfeldt, K., A. M. Bennet, P. Eriksson, J. Frostegard, B. Wiman, A. Hamsten, G. K. Hansson, U. de Faire, and Z. Q. Yan. 2004. Association of hypo-responsive toll-like receptor 4 variants with risk of myocardial infarction. *Eur. Heart J.* **25:**1447–1453.

Fearns, C., Q. Pan, J. C. Mathison, and T. H. Chuang. 2006. Triad3A regulates ubiquitination and proteasomal degradation of RIP1 following disruption of Hsp90 binding. *J. Biol. Chem.* **281:**34592–34600.

Ferwerda, B., M. B. McCall, S. Alonso, E. J. Giamarellos-Bourboulis, M. Mouktaroudi, N. Izagirre, D. Syafruddin, G. Kibiki, T. Cristea, A. Hijmans, L. Hamann, S. Israel, G. ElGhazali, M. Troye-Blomberg, O. Kumpf, B. Maiga, A. Dolo, O. Doumbo, C. C. Hermsen, A. F. Stalenhoef, R. van Crevel, H. G. Brunner, D. Y. Oh, R. R. Schumann, C. de la Rua, R. Sauerwein, B. J. Kullberg, A. J. van der Ven, J. W. van der Meer, and M. G. Netea. 2007. TLR4 polymorphisms, infectious diseases, and evolutionary pressure during migration of modern humans. *Proc. Natl. Acad. Sci. USA* **104:**16645–16650.

Fijen, C. A., E. J. Kuijper, A. J. Hannema, A. G. Sjoholm, and J. P. van Putten. 1989. Complement deficiencies in patients over ten years old with meningococcal disease due to uncommon serogroups. *Lancet* **ii:**585–588.

Fischer, H., P. Ellstrom, K. Ekstrom, L. Gustafsson, M. Gustafsson, and C. Svanborg. 2007. Ceramide as a TLR4 agonist; a putative signalling intermediate between sphingolipid receptors for microbial ligands and TLR4. *Cell. Microbiol.* **9:**1239–1251.

Fitzgerald, K. A., E. M. Palsson-McDermott, A. G. Bowie, C. A. Jefferies, A. S. Mansell, G. Brady, E. Brint, A. Dunne, P. Gray, M. T. Harte, D. McMurray, D. E. Smith, J. E. Sims, T. A. Bird, and L. A. O'Neill. 2001. Mal (MyD88-adapter-like) is required for Toll-like receptor-4 signal transduction. *Nature* **413:**78–83.

Fitzgerald, K. A., D. C. Rowe, B. J. Barnes, D. R. Caffrey, A. Visintin, E. Latz, B. Monks, P. M. Pitha, and D. T. Golenbock. 2003. LPS-TLR4 signaling to IRF-3/7 and NF-kappaB involves the toll adapters TRAM and TRIF. *J. Exp. Med.* **198:**1043–1055.

Frendeus, B., G. Godaly, L. Hang, D. Karpman, A. C. Lundstedt, and C. Svanborg. 2000. Interleukin 8 receptor deficiency confers susceptibility to acute experimental pyelonephritis and may have a human counterpart. *J. Exp. Med.* **192:**881–890.

Frendeus, B., G. Godaly, L. Hang, D. Karpman, and C. Svanborg. 2001a. Interleukin-8 receptor deficiency confers susceptibility to acute pyelonephritis. *J. Infect. Dis.* **183**(Suppl. 1):S56–S60.

Frendeus, B., C. Wachtler, M. Hedlund, H. Fischer, P. Samuelsson, M. Svensson, and C. Svanborg. 2001b. Escherichia coli P fimbriae utilize the Toll-like receptor 4 pathway for cell activation. *Mol. Microbiol.* **40:**37–51.

Fu, W., Y. Zhang, J. Zhang, and W. F. Chen. 2005. Cloning and characterization of mouse homolog of the CXC chemokine receptor CXCR1. *Cytokine* **31:**9–17.

Gaffney, P. M., G. M. Kearns, K. B. Shark, W. A. Ortmann, S. A. Selby, M. L. Malmgren, K. E. Rohlf, T. C. Ockenden, R. P. Messner, R. A. King, S. S. Rich, and T. W. Behrens. 1998. A genome-wide search for susceptibility genes in human systemic lupus erythematosus sib-pair families. *Proc. Natl. Acad. Sci. USA* **95:**14875–14879.

Gay, N. J., and M. Gangloff. 2008. Structure of toll-like receptors. *Handb. Exp. Pharmacol.* **2008** (183):181–200.

Godaly, G., G. Bergsten, L. Hang, H. Fischer, B. Frendeus, A. C. Lundstedt, M. Samuelsson, P. Samuelsson, and C. Svanborg. 2001. Neutrophil recruitment, chemokine receptors, and resistance to mucosal infection. *J. Leukoc. Biol.* **69:**899–906.

Godaly, G., L. Hang, B. Frendeus, and C. Svanborg. 2000. Transepithelial neutrophil migration is CXCR1 dependent in vitro and is defective in IL-8 receptor knockout mice. *J. Immunol.* **165:** 5287–5294.

Godaly, G., A. E. Proudfoot, R. E. Offord, C. Svanborg, and W. W. Agace. 1997. Role of epithelial interleukin-8 (IL-8) and neutrophil IL-8 receptor A in *Escherichia coli*-induced transuroepithelial neutrophil migration. *Infect. Immun.* **65:**3451–3456.

Gray, P., A. Dunne, C. Brikos, C. A. Jefferies, S. L. Doyle, and L. A. O'Neill. 2006. MyD88 adapter-like (Mal) is phosphorylated by Bruton's tyrosine kinase during TLR2 and TLR4 signal transduction. *J. Biol. Chem.* **281:**10489–10495.

Hacker, J., and J. B. Kaper. 2000. Pathogenicity islands and the evolution of microbes. *Annu. Rev. Microbiol.* **54:**641–679.

Hagberg, L., D. Briles, and C. Svanborg-Edén. 1985. Evidence for separate genetic defects in

C3H/HeJ and C3HeB/FeJ mice that affect the susceptibility to Gram-negative infections. *J. Immunol.* **134:**4118–4122.

Hang, L., B. Frendeus, G. Godaly, and C. Svanborg. 2000. Interleukin-8 receptor knockout mice have subepithelial neutrophil entrapment and renal scarring following acute pyelonephritis. *J. Infect. Dis.* **182:**1738–1748.

Hanson, L. A., S. Ahlstedt, A. Fasth, U. Jodal, B. Kaijser, P. Larsson, U. Lindberg, S. Olling, A. Sohl-Akerlund, and C. Svanborg-Eden. 1977. Antigens of Escherichia coli, human immune response, and the pathogenesis of urinary tract infections. *J. Infect. Dis.* **136**(Suppl.)**:**S144–S149.

Haraoka, M., L. Hang, B. Frendeus, G. Godaly, M. Burdick, R. Strieter, and C. Svanborg. 1999. Neutrophil recruitment and resistance to urinary tract infection. *J. Infect. Dis.* **180:**1220–1229.

Hawn, T. R., D. Scholes, S. S. Li, H. Wang, Y. Yang, P. L. Roberts, A. E. Stapleton, M. Janer, A. Aderem, W. E. Stamm, L. P. Zhao, and T. M. Hooton. 2009a. Toll-like receptor polymorphisms and susceptibility to urinary tract infections in adult women. *PLoS One* **4:**e5990.

Hawn, T. R., D. Scholes, H. Wang, S. S. Li, A. E. Stapleton, M. Janer, A. Aderem, W. E. Stamm, L. P. Zhao, and T. M. Hooton. 2009b. Genetic variation of the human urinary tract innate immune response and asymptomatic bacteriuria in women. *PLoS One* **4:**e8300.

Hawn, T. R., A. Verbon, K. D. Lettinga, L. P. Zhao, S. S. Li, R. J. Laws, S. J. Skerrett, B. Beutler, L. Schroeder, A. Nachman, A. Ozinsky, K. D. Smith, and A. Aderem. 2003. A common dominant TLR5 stop codon polymorphism abolishes flagellin signaling and is associated with susceptibility to legionnaires' disease. *J. Exp. Med.* **198:**1563–1572.

Hedlund, M., B. Frendeus, C. Wachtler, L. Hang, H. Fischer, and C. Svanborg. 2001. Type 1 fimbriae deliver an LPS- and TLR4-dependent activation signal to CD14-negative cells. *Mol. Microbiol.* **39:**542–552.

Hedlund, M., Å. Nilsson, R. D. Duan, and C. Svanborg. 1998. Sphingomyelin, glycosphingolipids and ceramide signalling in cells exposed to P fimbriated *Escherichia coli*. *Mol. Microbiol.* **29:**1297–1306.

Hedlund, M., M. Svensson, A. Nilsson, R. D. Duan, and C. Svanborg. 1996. Role of the ceramide-signaling pathway in cytokine responses to P-fimbriated Escherichia coli. *J. Exp. Med.* **183:** 1037–1044.

Hedlund, M., C. Wachtler, E. Johansson, L. Hang, J. E. Somerville, R. P. Darveau, and C. Svanborg. 1999. P fimbriae-dependent, lipopolysaccharide-independent activation of epithelial cytokine responses. *Mol. Microbiol.* **33:**693–703.

Hoebe, K., X. Du, P. Georgel, E. Janssen, K. Tabeta, S. O. Kim, J. Goode, P. Lin, N. Mann, S. Mudd, K. Crozat, S. Sovath, J. Han, and B. Beutler. 2003. Identification of Lps2 as a key transducer of MyD88-independent TIR signalling. *Nature* **424:**743–748.

Holmes, W. E., J. Lee, W. J. Kuang, G. C. Rice, and W. I. Wood. 1991. Structure and functional expression of a human interleukin-8 receptor. *Science* **253:**1278–1280.

Hopkins, W. J., J. Elkahwaji, L. M. Beierle, G. E. Leverson, and D. T. Uehling. 2007. Vaginal mucosal vaccine for recurrent urinary tract infections in women: results of a phase 2 clinical trial. *J. Urol.* **177:**1349–1353; quiz 1591.

Hopkins, W. J., A. Gendron-Fitzpatrick, E. Balish, and D. T. Uehling. 1998. Time course and host responses to *Escherichia coli* urinary tract infection in genetically distinct mouse strains. *Infect. Immun.* **66:**2798–2802.

Hopkins, W. J., D. T. Uehling, and D. S. Wargowski. 1999. Evaluation of a familial predisposition to recurrent urinary tract infections in women. *Am. J. Med. Genet.* **83:**422–424.

Horng, T., G. M. Barton, and R. Medzhitov. 2001. TIRAP: an adapter molecule in the Toll signaling pathway. *Nat. Immunol.* **2:**835–841.

Janssens, S., K. Burns, E. Vercammen, J. Tschopp, and R. Beyaert. 2003. MyD88S, a splice variant of MyD88, differentially modulates NF-κB- and AP-1-dependent gene expression. *FEBS Lett.* **548:**103–107.

Kagan, J. C., and R. Medzhitov. 2006. Phosphoinositide-mediated adaptor recruitment controls Toll-like receptor signaling. *Cell* **125:**943–955.

Kaijser, B., S. Ahlstedt, U. Jodal, and S. Mårild. 1978. Possible clinical significance of O and K antibodies against infecting Escherichia coli in antimicrobial treatment of acute childhood pyelonephritis. *Infection* **6:**S125–S128.

Kaijser, B., L. A. Hanson, U. Jodal, G. Lidin-Janson, and J. B. Robbins. 1977. Frequency of E. coli K antigens in urinary-tract infections in children. *Lancet* **i:**663–666.

Kaijser, B., P. Larsson, S. Olling, and R. Schneerson. 1983. Protection against acute, ascending pyelonephritis caused by *Escherichia coli* in rats, using isolated capsular antigen conjugated to bovine serum albumin. *Infect. Immun.* **39:**142–146.

Kalis, C., B. Kanzler, A. Lembo, A. Poltorak, C. Galanos, and M. A. Freudenberg. 2003. Toll-like receptor 4 expression levels determine the degree of LPS-susceptibility in mice. *Eur. J. Immunol.* **33:**798–805.

Karin, M., and Y. Ben-Neriah. 2000. Phosphorylation meets ubiquitination: the control of NF-κB activity. *Annu. Rev. Immunol.* **18:**621–663.

Karoly, E., A. Fekete, N. F. Banki, B. Szebeni, A. Vannay, A. J. Szabo, T. Tulassay, and G. S. Reusz. 2007. Heat shock protein 72 (HSPA1B) gene polymorphism and Toll-like receptor (TLR) 4 mutation are associated with increased risk of urinary tract infection in children. *Pediatr. Res.* **61:**371–374.

Kato, H., N. Tsuchiya, and K. Tokunaga. 2000. Single nucleotide polymorphisms in the coding regions of human CXC-chemokine receptors CXCR1, CXCR2 and CXCR3. *Genes Immun.* **1:**330–337.

Kawai, T., O. Adachi, T. Ogawa, K. Takeda, and S. Akira. 1999. Unresponsiveness of MyD88-deficient mice to endotoxin. *Immunity* **11:**115–122.

Kawai, T., and S. Akira. 2009. The roles of TLRs, RLRs and NLRs in pathogen recognition. *Int. Immunol.* **21:**317–337.

Kawai, T., S. Sato, K. J. Ishii, C. Coban, H. Hemmi, M. Yamamoto, K. Terai, M. Matsuda, J. Inoue, S. Uematsu, O. Takeuchi, and S. Akira. 2004. Interferon-alpha induction through Toll-like receptors involves a direct interaction of IRF7 with MyD88 and TRAF6. *Nat. Immunol.* **5:**1061–1068.

Kim, H. M., B. S. Park, J. I. Kim, S. E. Kim, J. Lee, S. C. Oh, P. Enkhbayar, N. Matsushima, H. Lee, O. J. Yoo, and J. O. Lee. 2007. Crystal structure of the TLR4-MD-2 complex with bound endotoxin antagonist Eritoran. *Cell* **130:**906–917.

Ko, Y. C., N. Mukaida, S. Ishiyama, A. Tokue, T. Kawai, K. Matsushima, and T. Kasahara. 1993. Elevated interleukin-8 levels in the urine of patients with urinary tract infections. *Infect. Immun.* **61:**1307–1314.

Kobayashi, K., L. D. Hernandez, J. E. Galan, C. A. Janeway, Jr., R. Medzhitov, and R. A. Flavell. 2002. IRAK-M is a negative regulator of Toll-like receptor signaling. *Cell* **110:**191–202.

Langermann, S., R. Mollby, J. E. Burlein, S. R. Palaszynski, C. G. Auguste, A. DeFusco, R. Strouse, M. A. Schenerman, S. J. Hultgren, J. S. Pinkner, J. Winberg, L. Guldevall, M. Soderhall, K. Ishikawa, S. Normark, and S. Koenig. 2000. Vaccination with FimH adhesin protects cynomolgus monkeys from colonization and infection by uropathogenic Escherichia coli. *J. Infect. Dis.* **181:**774–778.

Langermann, S., S. Palaszynski, M. Barnhart, G. Auguste, J. S. Pinkner, J. Burlein, P. Barren, S. Koenig, S. Leath, C. H. Jones, and S. J. Hultgren. 1997. Prevention of mucosal *Escherichia coli* infection by FimH-adhesin-based systemic vaccination. *Science* **276:**607–611.

Lichtinger, M., R. Ingram, M. Hornef, C. Bonifer, and M. Rehli. 2007. Transcription factor PU.1 controls transcription start site positioning and alternative TLR4 promoter usage. *J. Biol. Chem.* **282:**26874–26883.

Lien, E., T. J. Sellati, A. Yoshimura, T. H. Flo, G. Rawadi, R. W. Finberg, J. D. Carroll, T. Espevik, R. R. Ingalls, J. D. Radolf, and D. T. Golenbock. 1999. Toll-like receptor 2 functions as a pattern recognition receptor for diverse bacterial products. *J. Biol. Chem.* **274:**33419–33425.

Lomberg, H., L. A. Hanson, B. Jacobsson, U. Jodal, H. Leffler, and C. S. Eden. 1983. Correlation of P blood group, vesicoureteral reflux, and bacterial attachment in patients with recurrent pyelonephritis. *N. Engl. J. Med.* **308:**1189–1192.

Lomberg, H., U. Jodal, C. Svanborg-Edén, H. Leffler, and B. Samuelsson. 1981. P1 blood group and urinary tract infection. *Lancet* **i:**551–552.

Lundstedt, A. C., I. Leijonhufvud, B. Ragnarsdottir, D. Karpman, B. Andersson, and C. Svanborg. 2007a. Inherited susceptibility to acute pyelonephritis: a family study of urinary tract infection. *J. Infect. Dis.* **195:**1227–1234.

Lundstedt, A. C., S. McCarthy, M. C. Gustafsson, G. Godaly, U. Jodal, D. Karpman, I. Leijonhufvud, C. Linden, J. Martinell, B. Ragnarsdottir, M. Samuelsson, L. Truedsson, B. Andersson, and C. Svanborg. 2007b. A genetic basis of susceptibility to acute pyelonephritis. *PLoS One* **2:**e825.

Marsik, C., B. Jilma, C. Joukhadar, C. Mannhalter, O. Wagner, and G. Endler. 2005. The Toll-like receptor 4 Asp299Gly and Thr399Ile polymorphisms influence the late inflammatory response in human endotoxemia. *Clin. Chem.* **51:**2178–2180.

Matsushima, N., T. Tanaka, P. Enkhbayar, T. Mikami, M. Taga, K. Yamada, and Y. Kuroki. 2007. Comparative sequence analysis of leucine-rich repeats (LRRs) within vertebrate toll-like receptors. *BMC Genomics* **8:**124.

McGettrick, A. F., E. K. Brint, E. M. Palsson-McDermott, D. C. Rowe, D. T. Golenbock, N. J. Gay, K. A. Fitzgerald, and L. A. O'Neill. 2006. Trif-related adapter molecule is phosphorylated by PKCε during Toll-like receptor 4 signaling. *Proc. Natl. Acad. Sci. USA* **103:**9196–9201.

Mockenhaupt, F. P., J. P. Cramer, L. Hamann, M. S. Stegemann, J. Eckert, N. R. Oh, R. N. Otchwemah, E. Dietz, S. Ehrhardt, N. W. Schroder, U. Bienzle, and R. R. Schumann. 2006. Toll-like receptor (TLR) polymorphisms in African children: common TLR-4 variants predispose to severe malaria. *Proc. Natl. Acad. Sci. USA* **103:**177–182.

Moepps, B., E. Nuesseler, M. Braun, and P. Gierschik. 2006. A homolog of the human chemokine receptor CXCR1 is expressed in the mouse. *Mol. Immunol.* **43:**897–914.

Mogensen, T. H. 2009. Pathogen recognition and inflammatory signaling in innate immune defenses. *Clin. Microbiol. Rev.* **22:**240–273.

Morgan, B. P., and A. Orren. 1998. Vaccination against meningococcus in complement-deficient individuals. *Clin. Exp. Immunol.* **114:**327–329.

Murphy, P. M., and H. L. Tiffany. 1991. Cloning of complementary DNA encoding a functional human interleukin-8 receptor. *Science* **253:**1280–1283.

Oganesyan, G., S. K. Saha, B. Guo, J. Q. He, A. Shahangian, B. Zarnegar, A. Perry, and G. Cheng. 2006. Critical role of TRAF3 in the Toll-like receptor-dependent and -independent antiviral response. *Nature* **439:**208–211.

Olson, T. S., and K. Ley. 2002. Chemokines and chemokine receptors in leukocyte trafficking. *Am. J. Physiol. Regul. Integr. Comp. Physiol.* **283:**R7–R28.

Ozinsky, A., K. D. Smith, D. Hume, and D. M. Underhill. 2000. Co-operative induction of pro-inflammatory signaling by Toll-like receptors. *J. Endotoxin Res.* **6:**393–396.

Palsson-McDermott, E. M., S. L. Doyle, A. F. McGettrick, M. Hardy, H. Husebye, K. Banahan, M. Gong, D. Golenbock, T. Espevik, and L. A. O'Neill. 2009. TAG, a splice variant of the adaptor TRAM, negatively regulates the adaptor MyD88-independent TLR4 pathway. *Nat. Immunol.* **10:**579–586.

Pecha, B., D. Low, and P. O'Hanley. 1989. Gal-Gal pili vaccines prevent pyelonephritis by piliated Escherichia coli in a murine model. Single-component Gal-Gal pili vaccines prevent pyelonephritis by homologous and heterologous piliated E. coli strains. *J. Clin. Investig.* **83:**2102–2108.

Picard, C., A. Puel, M. Bonnet, C. L. Ku, J. Bustamante, K. Yang, C. Soudais, S. Dupuis, J. Feinberg, C. Fieschi, C. Elbim, R. Hitchcock, D. Lammas, G. Davies, A. Al-Ghonaium, H. Al-Rayes, S. Al-Jumaah, S. Al-Hajjar, I. Z. Al-Mohsen, H. H. Frayha, R. Rucker, T. R. Hawn, A. Aderem, H. Tufenkeji, S. Haraguchi, N. K. Day, R. A. Good, M. A. Gougerot-Pocidalo, A. Ozinsky, and J. L. Casanova. 2003. Pyogenic bacterial infections in humans with IRAK-4 deficiency. *Science* **299:**2076–2079.

Poltorak, A., X. He, I. Smirnova, M. Y. Liu, C. Van Huffel, X. Du, D. Birdwell, E. Alejos, M. Silva, C. Galanos, M. Freudenberg, P. Ricciardi-Castagnoli, B. Layton, and B. Beutler. 1998. Defective LPS signaling in C3H/HeJ and C57BL/10ScCr mice: mutations in Tlr4 gene. *Science* **282:**2085–2088.

Pugin, J., M. Schürer, D. Leturcq, A. Moriarty, R. J. Ulevitch, and P. S. Tobias. 1993. Lipopolysaccharide activation of human endothelial and epithelial cells is mediated by lipopolysaccharide-binding protein and soluble CD14. *Proc. Natl. Acad. Sci. USA* **90:**2744–2748.

Ragnarsdottir, B., M. Samuelsson, M. C. Gustafsson, I. Leijonhufvud, D. Karpman, and C. Svanborg. 2007. Reduced toll-like receptor 4 expression in children with asymptomatic bacteriuria. *J. Infect. Dis.* **196:**475–484.

Rallabhandi, P., J. Bell, M. S. Boukhvalova, A. Medvedev, E. Lorenz, M. Arditi, V. G. Hemming, J. C. Blanco, D. M. Segal, and S. N. Vogel. 2006. Analysis of TLR4 polymorphic variants: new insights into TLR4/MD-2/CD14 stoichiometry, structure, and signaling. *J. Immunol.* **177:**322–332.

Read, R. C., J. Pullin, S. Gregory, R. Borrow, E. B. Kaczmarski, F. S. di Giovine, S. K. Dower, C. Cannings, and A. G. Wilson. 2001. A functional polymorphism of toll-like receptor 4 is not associated with likelihood or severity of meningococcal disease. *J. Infect. Dis.* **184:**640–642.

Rehli, M., A. Poltorak, L. Schwarzfischer, S. W. Krause, R. Andreesen, and B. Beutler. 2000. PU.1 and interferon consensus sequence-binding protein regulate the myeloid expression of the human Toll-like receptor 4 gene. *J. Biol. Chem.* **275:**9773–9781.

Roger, T., J. David, M. P. Glauser, and T. Calandra. 2001. MIF regulates innate immune responses through modulation of Toll-like receptor 4. *Nature* **414:**920–924.

Roger, T., I. Miconnet, A. L. Schiesser, H. Kai, K. Miyake, and T. Calandra. 2005. Critical role for Ets, AP-1 and GATA-like transcription factors in regulating mouse Toll-like receptor 4 (Tlr4) gene expression. *Biochem. J.* **387:**355–365.

Rowe, D. C., A. F. McGettrick, E. Latz, B. G. Monks, N. J. Gay, M. Yamamoto, S. Akira, L. A. O'Neill, K. A. Fitzgerald, and D. T. Golenbock. 2006. The myristoylation of TRIF-related adaptor molecule is essential for Toll-like receptor 4 signal transduction. *Proc. Natl. Acad. Sci. USA* **103:**6299–6304.

Rowe, J. A., D. H. Opi, and T. N. Williams. 2009. Blood groups and malaria: fresh insights into pathogenesis and identification of targets for intervention. *Curr. Opin. Hematol.* **16:**480–487.

Roy, M. F., L. Lariviere, R. Wilkinson, M. Tam, M. M. Stevenson, and D. Malo. 2006. Incremental expression of Tlr4 correlates with mouse resistance to Salmonella infection and fine regulation of relevant immune genes. *Genes Immun.* **7:**372–383.

Samuelsson, P., L. Hang, B. Wullt, H. Irjala, and C. Svanborg. 2004. Toll-like receptor 4 expression and cytokine responses in the human urinary tract mucosa. *Infect. Immun.* **72:**3179–3186.

Sato, S., M. Sugiyama, M. Yamamoto, Y. Watanabe, T. Kawai, K. Takeda, and S. Akira. 2003. Toll/IL-1 receptor domain-containing adaptor inducing IFN-beta (TRIF) associates with TNF receptor-associated factor 6 and TANK-binding kinase 1, and activates two distinct transcription factors, NF-kappa B and IFN-regulatory factor-3, in the Toll-like receptor signaling. *J. Immunol.* **171:**4304–4310.

Schenck, M., A. Carpinteiro, H. Grassme, F. Lang, and E. Gulbins. 2007. Ceramide: physiological and pathophysiological aspects. *Arch. Biochem. Biophys.* **462:**171–175.

Schilling, J. D., S. M. Martin, C. S. Hung, R. G. Lorenz, and S. J. Hultgren. 2003. Toll-like receptor 4 on stromal and hematopoietic cells mediates innate resistance to uropathogenic *Escherichia coli. Proc. Natl. Acad. Sci. USA* **100:**4203–4208.

Shahin, R., I. Engberg, L. Hagberg, and C. Svanborg-Edén. 1987. Neutrophil recruitment and bacterial clearance correlated with LPS responsiveness in local gram-negative infection. *J. Immunol.* **10:**3475–3480.

Sheedy, F. J., and L. A. O'Neill. 2007. The Troll in Toll: Mal and Tram as bridges for TLR2 and TLR4 signaling. *J. Leukoc. Biol.* **82:**196–203.

Shimazu, R., S. Akashi, H. Ogata, Y. Nagai, K. Fukudome, K. Miyake, and M. Kimoto. 1999. MD-2, a molecule that confers lipopolysaccharide responsiveness on Toll-like receptor 4. *J. Exp. Med.* **189:**1777–1782.

Silverblatt, F., and L. Cohen. 1979. Anti pili antibody affords protection against experimental ascending pyelonephritis. *J. Clin. Investig.* **64:** 333–336.

Sjoholm, A. G., G. Jonsson, J. H. Braconier, G. Sturfelt, and L. Truedsson. 2006. Complement deficiency and disease: an update. *Mol. Immunol.* **43:**78–85.

Smith, R. J., L. M. Sam, K. L. Leach, and J. M. Justen. 1992. Postreceptor events associated with human neutrophil activation by interleukin-8. *J. Leukoc. Biol.* **52:**17–26.

Smithson, A., M. R. Sarrias, J. Barcelo, B. Suarez, J. P. Horcajada, S. M. Soto, A. Soriano, J. Vila, J. A. Martinez, J. Vives, J. Mensa, and F. Lozano. 2005. Expression of interleukin-8 receptors (CXCR1 and CXCR2) in premenopausal women with recurrent urinary tract infections. *Clin. Diagn. Lab. Immunol.* **12:**1358–1363.

Sprenger, H., A. R. Lloyd, R. G. Meyer, J. A. Johnston, and D. J. Kelvin. 1994. Genomic structure, characterization, and identification of the promoter of the human IL-8 receptor A gene. *J. Immunol.* **153:**2524–2532.

Stapleton, A., E. Nudelman, H. Clausen, S. Hakomori, and W. E. Stamm. 1992. Binding of uropathogenic *Escherichia coli* R45 to glycolipids extracted from vaginal epithelial cells is dependent on histo-blood group secretor status. *J. Clin. Investig.* **90:**965–972.

Svanborg, C., G. Bergsten, H. Fischer, G. Godaly, M. Gustafsson, D. Karpman, A. C. Lundstedt, B. Ragnarsdottir, M. Svensson, and B. Wullt. 2006. Uropathogenic Escherichia coli as a model of host-parasite interaction. *Curr. Opin. Microbiol.* **9:**33–39.

Svanborg Eden, C., D. Briles, L. Hagberg, J. McGhee, and S. Michalec. 1985. Genetic factors in host resistance to urinary tract infection. *Infection* **13**(Suppl. 2)**:**S171–S176.

Svensson, M., H. Irjala, P. Alm, B. Holmqvist, A.-C. Lundstedt, and C. Svanborg. 2005. Natural history of renal scarring in susceptible mIL-8Rh−/− mice. *Kidney Int.* **67:**103–110.

Tal, G., A. Mandelberg, I. Dalal, K. Cesar, E. Somekh, A. Tal, A. Oron, S. Itskovich, A. Ballin, S. Houri, A. Beigelman, O. Lider, G. Rechavi, and N. Amariglio. 2004. Association between common Toll-like receptor 4 mutations and severe respiratory syncytial virus disease. *J. Infect. Dis.* **189:**2057–2063.

Thomassen, E., B. R. Renshaw, and J. E. Sims. 1999. Identification and characterization of SIGIRR, a molecule representing a novel subtype of the IL-1R superfamily. *Cytokine* **11:**389–399.

Thumbikat, P., C. Waltenbaugh, A. J. Schaeffer, and D. J. Klumpp. 2006. Antigen-specific responses accelerate bacterial clearance in the bladder. *J. Immunol.* **176:**3080–3086.

Uehling, D. T., W. J. Hopkins, E. Balish, Y. Xing, and D. M. Heisey. 1997. Vaginal mucosal immunization for recurrent urinary tract infection: phase II clinical trial. *J. Urol.* **157:**2049–2052.

Uehling, D. T., W. J. Hopkins, L. M. Beierle, J. V. Kryger, and D. M. Heisey. 2001. Vaginal mucosal immunization for recurrent urinary tract infection: extended phase II clinical trial. *J. Infect. Dis.* **183**(Suppl. 1)**:**S81–S83.

Uehling, D. T., W. J. Hopkins, L. A. Dahmer, and E. Balish. 1994. Phase I clinical trial of vaginal mucosal immunization for recurrent urinary tract infection. *J. Urol.* **152:**2308–2311.

Uehling, D. T., W. J. Hopkins, J. E. Elkahwaji, D. M. Schmidt, and G. E. Leverson. 2003. Phase 2 clinical trial of a vaginal mucosal vaccine for urinary tract infections. *J. Urol.* **170:**867–869.

Underhill, D. M., A. Ozinsky, A. M. Hajjar, A. Stevens, C. B. Wilson, M. Bassetti, and A. Aderem. 1999. The Toll-like receptor 2 is recruited to macrophage phagosomes and discriminates between pathogens. *Nature* **401:**811–815.

Vasilescu, A., Y. Terashima, M. Enomoto, S. Heath, V. Poonpiriya, H. Gatanaga, H. Do, G. Diop,

T. Hirtzig, P. Auewarakul, D. Lauhakirti, T. Sura, P. Charneau, S. Marullo, A. Therwath, S. Oka, S. Kanegasaki, M. Lathrop, K. Matsushima, J. F. Zagury, and F. Matsuda.** 2007. A haplotype of the human CXCR1 gene protective against rapid disease progression in HIV-1 patients. *Proc. Natl. Acad. Sci. USA* **104:**3354–3359.

von Bernuth, H., C. Picard, Z. Jin, R. Pankla, H. Xiao, C. L. Ku, M. Chrabieh, I. B. Mustapha, P. Ghandil, Y. Camcioglu, J. Vasconcelos, N. Sirvent, M. Guedes, A. B. Vitor, M. J. Herrero-Mata, J. I. Arostegui, C. Rodrigo, L. Alsina, E. Ruiz-Ortiz, M. Juan, C. Fortuny, J. Yague, J. Anton, M. Pascal, H. H. Chang, L. Janniere, Y. Rose, B. Z. Garty, H. Chapel, A. Issekutz, L. Marodi, C. Rodriguez-Gallego, J. Banchereau, L. Abel, X. Li, D. Chaussabel, A. Puel, and J. L. Casanova. 2008. Pyogenic bacterial infections in humans with MyD88 deficiency. *Science* **321:**691–696.

Wald, D., J. Qin, Z. Zhao, Y. Qian, M. Naramura, L. Tian, J. Towne, J. E. Sims, G. R. Stark, and X. Li. 2003. SIGIRR, a negative regulator of Toll-like receptor-interleukin 1 receptor signaling. *Nat. Immunol.* **4:**920–927.

Wang, C., L. Deng, M. Hong, G. R. Akkaraju, J. Inoue, and Z. J. Chen. 2001. TAK1 is a ubiquitin-dependent kinase of MKK and IKK. *Nature* **412:**346–351.

Wiles, T. J., R. R. Kulesus, and M. A. Mulvey. 2008. Origins and virulence mechanisms of uropathogenic Escherichia coli. *Exp. Mol. Pathol.* **85:**11–19.

Wilkinson, N. C., and J. Navarro. 1999. PU.1 regulates the CXCR1 promoter. *J. Biol. Chem.* **274:**438–443.

Yadav, M., J. Zhang, H. Fischer, W. Huang, N. Lutay, C. Cirl, J. Lum, T. Miethke, and C. Svanborg. 2010. Inhibition of TIR domain signaling by TcpC: MyD88-dependent and independent effects on *Escherichia coli* virulence. *PLoS Pathog.* **6:**e1001120.

Yamamoto, M., S. Sato, H. Hemmi, K. Hoshino, T. Kaisho, H. Sanjo, O. Takeuchi, M. Sugiyama, M. Okabe, K. Takeda, and S. Akira. 2003. Role of adaptor TRIF in the MyD88-independent toll-like receptor signaling pathway. *Science* **301:**640–643.

Yamamoto, M., S. Sato, H. Hemmi, S. Uematsu, K. Hoshino, T. Kaisho, O. Takeuchi, K. Takeda, and S. Akira. 2003. TRAM is specifically involved in the Toll-like receptor 4-mediated MyD88-independent signaling pathway. *Nat. Immunol.* **4:**1144–1150.

Yamamoto, M., S. Sato, K. Mori, K. Hoshino, O. Takeuchi, K. Takeda, and S. Akira. 2002. Cutting edge: a novel Toll/IL-1 receptor domain-containing adapter that preferentially activates the IFN-beta promoter in the Toll-like receptor signaling. *J. Immunol.* **169:**6668–6672.

Zhang, D., G. Zhang, M. S. Hayden, M. B. Greenblatt, C. Bussey, R. A. Flavell, and S. Ghosh. 2004. A toll-like receptor that prevents infection by uropathogenic bacteria. *Science* **303:**1522–1526.

INDEX